Recent Progress in Veterinary Medicine

Recent Progress in Veterinary Medicine

Edited by Ryan Jaxon

hayle medical
New York

Hayle Medical,
750 Third Avenue, 9th Floor,
New York, NY 10017, USA

Visit us on the World Wide Web at:
www.haylemedical.com

ISBN: 978-1-63241-819-7

The publisher's policy is to use permanent paper from mills that operate a sustainable forestry policy. Furthermore, the publisher ensures that the text paper and cover boards used have met acceptable environmental accreditation standards.

Printed in China.

Cataloging-in-Publication Data

Recent progress in veterinary medicine / edited by Ryan Jaxon.
p. cm.
Includes bibliographical references and index.
ISBN 978-1-63241-819-7
1. Veterinary medicine. 2. Animals--Diseases. 3. Animal health. I. Jaxon, Ryan.
SF745 .R43 2019
636.089--dc23

Table of Contents

Preface IX

Chapter 1 **Phenotypic classification of variability of non-syndromic congenital cleft lip and jaw in Vorderwald × Montbéliarde cattle** 1
Sina Reinartz, Maren Hellige, Karsten Feige, Peter Wenning and Ottmar Distl

Chapter 2 **The reproductive pattern and potential of free ranging female wild boars (*Sus scrofa*)** 7
Anna Malmsten, Gunnar Jansson, Nils Lundeheim and Anne-Marie Dalin

Chapter 3 **Farm characteristics and management routines related to neonatal porcine diarrhoea: a survey among Swedish piglet producers** 14
Jenny Larsson, Nils Fall, Maria Lindberg and Magdalena Jacobson

Chapter 4 **Kinematic and spatiotemporal assessment of habituation to treadmill walking in Labrador retrievers** 24
Pia Gustås, Kjerstin Pettersson, Sofia Honkavaara, Anne-Sofie Lagerstedt and Anna Byström

Chapter 5 **Identification and characterization of cancer stem cells in canine mammary tumors** 32
Agata Rybicka and Magdalena Król

Chapter 6 **Correlations between cresty neck scores and post-mortem nape fat measurements in horses, obtained after photographic image analysis** 39
Severiano R. Silva, Rita Payan-Carreira, Cristina M. Guedes, Simão Coelho and Ana Sofia Santos

Chapter 7 **Computed tomography of the thorax in rabbits: a prospective study in ten clinically healthy New Zealand White rabbits** 45
Désirée Müllhaupt, Sandra Wenger, Patrick Kircher, Nadja Pfammatter, Jean-Michel Hatt and Stefanie Ohlerth

Chapter 8 **A survey of straw use and tail biting in Swedish pig farms rearing undocked pigs** 54
Torun Wallgren, Rebecka Westin and Stefan Gunnarsson

Chapter 9 **In vitro investigations on extracellular proteins secreted by *Aphanomyces invadans*, the causative agent of epizootic ulcerative syndrome** 65
Muhammad Majeed, Gokhlesh Kumar, Sarah Schlosser, Mansour El-Matbouli and Mona Saleh

Chapter 10 **Blood pressure and heart rate during ovariohysterectomy in pyometra and control dogs: a preliminary investigation** 73
Odd Viking Höglund, Johanna Lövebrant, Ulf Olsson and Katja Höglund

Chapter 11 **Ability of vaccine strain induced antibodies to neutralize field isolates of caliciviruses from Swedish cats** 80
Jonas Johansson Wensman, Ayman Samman, Anna Lindhe, Jean-Christophe Thibault, Louise Treiberg Berndtsson and Margaret J. Hosie

Chapter 12 ***Toxoplasma gondii* seroprevalence in breeding pigs**....84
Azzurra Santoro, Maarja Tagel, Kärt Must, Miia Laine, Brian Lassen and Pikka Jokelainen

Chapter 13 **Preventive measures aimed at minimizing the risk of African swine fever virus spread in pig farming systems**....91
Silvia Bellini, Domenico Rutili and Vittorio Guberti

Chapter 14 **Glycaemic and insulinemic response to dietary carbohydrates in horses** 100
Christine Brøkner, Dag Austbø, Jon A. Næsset, Dominique Blache, Knud Erik B. Knudsen, Hanne H. Hansen and Anne-Helene Tauson

Chapter 15 **Prevalence of subclinical mastitis in Finnish dairy cows: changes during recent decades and impact of cow and herd factors**....105
Heidi Hiitiö, Johanna Vakkamäki, Heli Simojoki, Tiina Autio, Jouni Junnila, Sinikka Pelkonen and Satu Pyörälä

Chapter 16 **The response of mute swans (*Cygnus olor*, Gm. 1789) to vaccination against avian influenza with an inactivated H5N2 vaccine**....119
Beata Dolka, Artur Żbikowski, Izabella Dolka and Piotr Szeleszczuk

Chapter 17 **Cross-sectional survey on the use and impact of the Danish national antibiotic use guidelines for companion animal practice**....128
Lisbeth Rem Jessen, Tina Møller Sørensen, Zenia Littau Lilja, Maja Kristensen, Tine Hald and Peter Damborg

Chapter 18 **Cross-sectional study on risk factors for Porcine Reproductive and Respiratory Syndrome virus sow herd instability in German breeding herds** 137
Christina Nathues, Eltje Janssen, Andrea Duengelhoef, Heiko Nathues and Elisabeth grosse Beilage

Chapter 19 **α-Tocopherol and β-carotene concentrations in feed, colostrum, cow and calf serum in Swedish dairy herds with high or low calf mortality** 145
Maria Torsein, Ann Lindberg, Catarina Svensson, Sören Krogh Jensen, Charlotte Berg and Karin Persson Waller

Chapter 20 **Clinical evaluation of constant rate infusion of alfaxalone–medetomidine combined with sevoflurane anesthesia in Thoroughbred racehorses undergoing arthroscopic surgery**....159
Hirotaka Tokushige, Asuka Kushiro, Atsushi Okano, Tatsuya Maeda, Hideki Ito, Ai Wakuno, Shun-ichi Nagata and Minoru Ohta

Chapter 21 **Development of the Finnish neurological function testing battery for dogs and its intra-and inter-rater reliability**....166
Anna Fredrika Boström, Heli Katariina Hyytiäinen, Petteri Koho, Sigitas Cizinauskas and Anna Katrina Hielm-Björkman

Chapter 22 **A veterinary perspective on One Health in the Arctic 174**
Christian Sonne, Robert James Letcher, Bjørn Munro Jenssen, Jean-Pierre Desforges, Igor Eulaers, Emilie Andersen-Ranberg, Kim Gustavson, Bjarne Styrishave and Rune Dietz

Chapter 23 **Protective role of the vulture facial skin and gut microbiomes aid adaptation to scavenging 185**
Marie Lisandra Zepeda Mendoza, Michael Roggenbuck, Karla Manzano Vargas, Lars Hestbjerg Hansen, Søren Brunak, M. Thomas P. Gilbert and Thomas Sicheritz-Pontén

Chapter 24 **Determination of the expression of three fimbrial subunit proteins in cultured *Trueperella pyogenes* 204**
Mengcheng Liu, Bing Wang, Hongmin Liang, Bo Ma, Junwei Wang and Wenlong Zhang

Chapter 25 ***Salmonella enterica* subspecies *enterica* serovar Choleraesuis in a German wild boar population: occurrence and characterisation 213**
Ulrich Methner, Sabine Merbach and Martin Peters

Chapter 26 **Descriptive study for culling and mortality in five high-producing Spanish dairy cattle farms (2006–2016) 220**
Ramon Armengol and Lorenzo Fraile

Chapter 27 **Canine angiostrongylosis in Sweden: a nationwide seroepidemiological survey by enzyme-linked immunosorbent assays and a summary of five-year diagnostic activity (2011-2015) 231**
Giulio Grandi, Eva Osterman Lind, Roland Schaper, Erik Ågren and Manuela Schnyder

Permissions

List of Contributors

Index

Preface

The subspecialty of medicine concerned with animal diseases is known as veterinary medicine. It focuses on the prevention, diagnosis and treatment of injuries, diseases and disorders in animals. The management of zoonotic diseases also falls under this domain. Professionals in this field are veterinary physicians, veterinary technicians and nurses. They deal with various kinds of animals, including livestock, zoo animals, companion animals, etc. Some common procedures performed by veterinary physicians include declawing of cats, cropping of ears, debarking and docking of tails. This book aims to shed light on some of the unexplored aspects of veterinary medicine and the recent researches in this field. It studies, analyzes and upholds the pillars of veterinary medicine and its utmost significance in modern times. This book will prove to be immensely beneficial to students and researchers in this field.

Various studies have approached the subject by analyzing it with a single perspective, but the present book provides diverse methodologies and techniques to address this field. This book contains theories and applications needed for understanding the subject from different perspectives. The aim is to keep the readers informed about the progresses in the field; therefore, the contributions were carefully examined to compile novel researches by specialists from across the globe.

Indeed, the job of the editor is the most crucial and challenging in compiling all chapters into a single book. In the end, I would extend my sincere thanks to the chapter authors for their profound work. I am also thankful for the support provided by my family and colleagues during the compilation of this book.

Editor

Phenotypic classification of variability of non-syndromic congenital cleft lip and jaw in Vorderwald × Montbéliarde cattle

Sina Reinartz[1], Maren Hellige[2], Karsten Feige[2], Peter Wenning[3] and Ottmar Distl[1*]

Abstract

Background: Non-syndromic congenital cleft lip and jaw (CLJ) is a condition reported in several cattle breeds, but a detailed classification system does not exist for cattle. The objective of the present study was to describe the phenotypic variability of this orofacial malformation in Vorderwald × Montbéliarde cattle. For this purpose, a classification system of CLJ was developed on examination of five orofacial structures: (1) lips, (2) the *processus* (*proc.*) *nasalis* of the *os incisivum*, (3) the dental plate with adjacent segments of the hard palate, (4) the facial bones (*os incisivum*, *os maxillare*, *os nasale* and *os palatinum*) and (5) the mandibles. Each structure was given a score reflecting the degree of the lesion from absent (score 0) to severe.

Results: Nine cases were included in the study and they shared absence of the abaxial rostral part of the *processus* (*proc.*) *nasalis* of the *os incisivum*, partial loss of the *rugae palatinae* and the dental plate. A sigmoid curvature of the rostral lower jaw as well as a lateral deviation of the face and rostral lower jaw was highly variable in their expression. These deformations were present in eight of nine cases. In addition to the complete CLJ, three animals had an incomplete CLJ on the contralateral site with variable defects of the rostral part of the *proc. nasalis* of the *os incisivum*.

Conclusions: A complete CLJ is obviously accompanied by a loss of parts of the *proc. nasalis* of the *os incisivum*. Extent and localization of the missing parts of the *proc. nasalis* were similar in all cases. A precise classification of the various CLJ forms is necessary.

Keywords: Vorderwald cattle, Cleft lip and jaw, Phenotypic variability, Orofacial malformation

Background

Non-syndromic congenital cleft lip and jaw (CLJ) is rarely reported in cattle. Cases of CLJ have been reported in Austrian Simmental, Charolais, Czech Red Pied, German Holstein, Gir, Hereford, Japanese Brown, Shorthorn and Vorderwald × Montbéliarde cattle [1–14]. According to the location and morphology, CLJ can be classified into three main groups, i.e. unilateral CLJ on the right or left side, median CLJ and bilateral CLJ with a cleft palate. In addition, syndromic forms show bilateral CLJ with malformations in other organs [11, 13].

CLJ is generally diagnosed easily by the externally obvious lesions in the lip and upper jaw, but presence and grade of lesions vary among cases when examined in detail. Koch et al. [15] described orofacial malformations in humans and developed a system to record morphological details thus allowing accurate phenotyping. Accurate phenotyping is essential for understanding the epidemiology and etiology of congenital malformations, particularly, if phenotypic expression varies [16] and precise recording is necessary to be able to distinguish among closely related phenotypes [17]. In human medicine, different systems with descriptors and symbolic representations for orofacial malformations exist [15, 18–24].

Three cases of unilateral CLJ have been ascertained in Vorderwald × Montbéliarde cattle in 2009–2010 [13] and further six cases were reported by farmers in

*Correspondence: ottmar.distl@tiho-hannover.de
[1] University of Veterinary Medicine Hannover, Foundation, Institute for Animal Breeding and Genetics, Bünteweg 17p, 30559 Hannover, Germany
Full list of author information is available at the end of the article

the following years. CLJ was not known in this breed before and the frequency of this condition was seemingly increasing. The objective of the present study was to develop a classification system for CLJ in Vorderwald × Montbéliarde cattle for fast characterization of the anomaly as well as ensuring a consistent recording of the underlying defects.

Methods

Nine Vorderwald × Montbéliarde cattle (cases 1–9) showing congenital CLJ had been sampled from 2009 to 2013, including three cases reported by Lupp et al. [13].

The sex ratio was 4 males and 5 females (0.8:1), the calves were born on different farms and were the first cases of CLJ in the respective herds according to the owners. All cases with exception of case 2 underwent a detailed examination based on either computed tomography (CT) scanning (cases 3–9) or digital radiography (case 1). Age at CT scanning was 3–6 months and 12 months at radiology. The CT scanning image acquisition was performed under general anaesthesia with the animal positioned in sternal recumbency on the CT table. CT scans were acquired with a multislice helical CT scanner (Brilliance-™-CT BigBore, Oncology, Philips Healthcare, Best, The Netherlands) using conventional settings (90 kV, 100 mAs) and 2 mm slice thickness.

The study was conducted according to national and international guidelines for animal welfare. The study was approved by the Institutional Animal Care and Use Committee of Lower Saxony, the State Veterinary Office Niedersächsisches Landesamt für Verbraucherschutz und Lebensmittelsicherheit, Oldenburg, Germany (Registration Number 33.9-42502-04-12/1036).

The classification system of CLJ was based on examination of five orofacial structures: (1) lips, (2) the *processus* (*proc.*) *nasalis* of the *os incisivum*, (3) the dental plate with adjacent segments of the hard palate, (4) the facial bones (*os incisivum*, *os maxillare*, *os nasale* and *os palatinum*) and (5) the mandibles. Each structure was given a score reflecting the degree of the lesion from absent (score 0) to severe. We distinguished the site of the cleft lip (SITE), the depth of cleft lip (DEPTH), the width of cleft lip (WIDTH), changes at the dental plate and hard palate (DEN-HAP), the deviation of the face from the midline (DEVIATION), the lateral curvature of the mandibles (CURVATURE), the slope of the anterior part of the lower jaw (SLOPE) and the extend of loss of the *proc. nasalis* of the *os incisivum* (INCISIVUM). A detailed description of the scoring system is provided in Additional file 1.

Results

All cases had complete unilateral or bilateral CLJ (Table 1), while median CLJ was not found. In two cases with a left-sided complete CLJ, and in one case with a right-sided complete CLJ, an incomplete cleft lip on the contralateral side was seen (Figs. 1, 2, 3, 4). An overview of the classification of the cases is given in Table 2.

Absence of about 1/3 of the dental plate on the ipsilateral side of the CLJ was observed in all cases. Minor and major forms of cleft lips were not accompanied by a partial loss of the dental plate. On the hard palate adjacent to the complete CLJ, missing *rugae palatinae* were noticed in all cases (Fig. 5). The lateral deviation of the face and mandibles concomitantly occurred consistently but in varying degrees in all cases.

A sigmoid flexure of the rostral part of the mandibles was identified in all cases except case 8 (Fig. 4). This curvature had the steepest slope in case 6 with a complete bilateral CLJ and in the right-sided complete CLJ cases 1, 2, 3 and 5. The largest angular deviation of the occlusal plane was also found in the right-sided CLJ cases and the bilateral CLJ case.

In all cases, the same segment of the *proc. nasalis* was missing on the ipsilateral side as the complete CLJ. This segment includes the rostral abaxial part of the *os incisivum*. Further changes of the *proc. nasalis* in the presence of incomplete cleft lips were located in the middle of the rostral abaxial part of the *proc. nasalis*. In case 9, a small notch ventrally at the *proc. nasalis* corresponded to the minor form of a cleft lip (Additional file 2). A large notch of 2.5 × 0.8 cm in size was present ventrally at the *proc. nasalis* underlying the major form of a cleft lip in case 4 (Additional file 3). Case 7 revealed a ring-like bone loss in the *proc. nasalis* with only a thin bone bridge remaining (Additional file 4).

Discussion

In Vorderwald × Montbéliarde cattle phenotypic expression of CLJ includes unilateral (right- or left-sided) and bilateral cases. In cases with a unilateral complete CLJ, the abaxial rostral part of the *proc. nasalis*, approximately 1/3 of the dental plate and the *rugae palatinae* of the adjacent hard palate were missing. All cases examined using X-rays or CT scanning (n = 8) had similar changes of the *os incisivum*, the dental plate and the hard palate in the ipsilateral to the complete CLJ. The deficit of the middle segment of the *proc. nasalis* was consistently observed in these cases ipsilateral to the complete CLJ. Rieke [6] also described the absence of this segment of the *proc. nasalis* in German Holstein calves but also a progression of this defect through the middle of the corpus of the premaxilla. The macerated heads of CLJ cases reported by Moritomo et al. [11] also showed a partial loss of the *proc. nasalis*. A female Japanese Brown calf with a left-sided CLJ missed this segment. Furthermore, the outward curvature of the *os incisivum* was also

Table 1 Description of the cleft lip and jaw (CLJ) cases in nine Vorderwald × Montbéliarde cattle

Case no.	Orofacial cleft				Sex	
	Complete CLJ		Incomplete CLJ		Male	Female
	Right	Left	Right	Left		
1	+				+	
2	+					+
3	+					+
4		+	+		+	
5	+					+
6	+	+			+	
7	+			+		+
8		+				+
9		+	+		+	

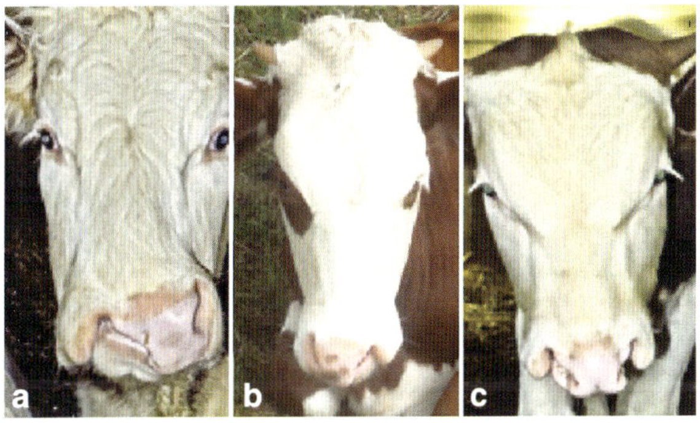

Fig. 1 Vorderwald × Montbéliarde cattle showing complete cleft lip and jaw (CLJ). **a** Case 3 shows a complete *right*-sided CLJ with a lateral curvature of the mandibles to the *left* side. **b** Case 8 shows a complete *left*-sided CLJ without lateral curvature of the mandibles. **c** Case 6 shows a complete bilateral CLJ with a slight lateral curvature of the mandibles to the *left* side

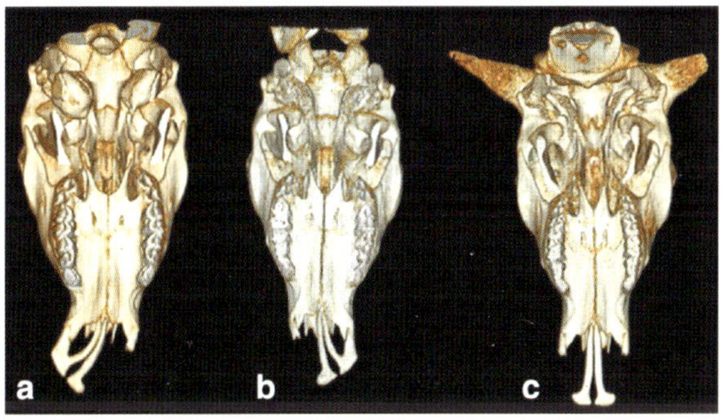

Fig. 3 Computed tomography scanning images of the head for Vorderwald × Montbéliarde cattle showing the ventral view of the skull excluding the mandibles. **a** Case 3 shows a complete *right*-sided CLJ. **b** Case 8 shows a complete *left*-sided CLJ. **c** Case 6 shows a complete bilateral CLJ

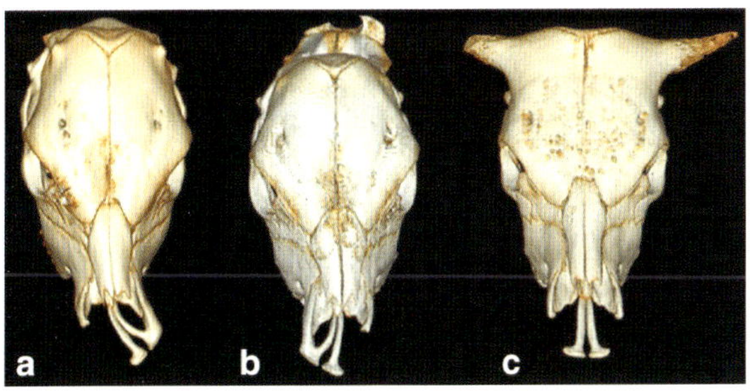

Fig. 2 Computed tomography scanning images of the head for Vorderwald × Montbéliarde cattle. **a** Case 3 with a complete *right*-sided cleft lip and jaw, **b** case 8 with a complete *left*-sided CLJ and **c** case 6 with a complete bilateral CLJ. Dorsal view of the skull excluding the mandibles

associated with unilateral CLJ on the contralateral side of the muzzle in the cases presented by Moritomo et al. [11].

In agreement with Rieke [25], unilateral CLJ was most frequent. Unilateral CLJ is also most common in humans and laboratory rodents [26, 27]. In six CLJ affected Japanese Brown cattle, three had unilateral CLJ, one had bilateral CLJ and two had median CLJ [11]. Right-sided CLJ were more frequent than left-sided in the present study. Rieke [25] observed 33.3 % right-sided CLJ and 21.7 % left-sided CLJ which is in contrast to humans and laboratory animals having a majority of left sided CLJ [26, 27].

The term "cleft lip" includes complete and incomplete clefts of the upper lip independent of whether the maxillary alveolus is affected [28]. In human medicine,

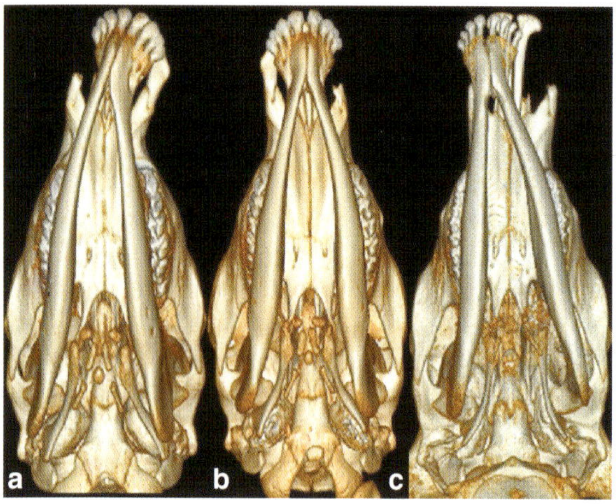

Fig. 4 Computed tomography scanning images of the head for Vorderwald × Montbéliarde cattle affected by cleft lip and jaw (CLJ) showing the lateral curvature of the mandibles. **a** Case 3 shows a complete *right*-sided CLJ with a lateral curvature of the mandibles to the *left* side. **b** Case 8 shows a complete *left*-sided CLJ without lateral curvature of the mandibles. **c** Case 6 shows a complete bilateral CLJ with a slight lateral curvature of the mandibles to the *left* side

notches <3 mm were defined as microforms [29]. In microform clefts the functional tissue layer such as the muscle for the lip, cartilage of the nose and the septum or bone of the maxillary alveolus are not affected [15]. Minor forms in humans include defects extending 3 mm or more but <1/2 of the vertical dimension of the lip and the nostril floor [29]. A complete cleft is defined as a cleft which includes the upper lip and nostril floor in total [30], while an incomplete cleft is defined as involving only a part of the upper lip. Incomplete cleft lips on the contralateral side were present in 3/9 of the affected Vorderwald × Montbéliarde cattle. This could have particular importance for ascertainment of possible cases with incomplete cleft lip. Mayr et al. [5] described a three-years-old Fleckvieh bull with an incomplete cleft lip. This Austrian bull sired 55 descendants of which 32 had a complete CLJ. Therefore, in cattle each cleft lips should be registered as a mild form of a CLJ. Phenotypic variants like lip pits, prints or microforms of cleft lips should be considered as an anomaly and may have consequences for selective breeding, particularly, if relatives with CLJ are observed.

On the side with the complete CLJ, the size of the missing parts of the dental plate and of the hard palate was very similar in all cases. Swartz et al. [7] studied two Angus calves with unilateral left-sided CLJ with variable defects of the dental plate and hard palate. The dental plate was completely missing on the left side and a segment on the right side lacked in one case. Furthermore,

Table 2 Scores according to the classification system for cleft lip and jaw in nine Vorderwald × Montbéliarde cattle

Case	SITE	DEPTH	WIDTH	DEN-HAP	DEVIATION		CURVATURE		SLOPE		INCISIVUM
					To left	To right	To left	To right	Left-to-right	Right-to-left	
Score range	0–4	0–5	0–6	0–9	0–3	0–3	0–3	0–3	0–3	0–3	0–9
1	1	5	3	2	3			x	3		5
2	1	5	3	2	3			x	3		5
3	1	5	4	2	3			3	2		5
5	1	5	3	2	3			2	3		5
7	1	5	5	2	2			1		0	5
		3	4								1
8	2	5	2	2		1		0		1	5
4	2	5	2	2		2	3			1	5
		3	4								3
9	2	5	4	2		2	2			2	5
		2	6								2
6	4	5	1	2	1		3		2		5
		5	1								5

The nine CLJ-affected Vorderwald × Montbéliarde cattle were scored for the site of cleft lip (SITE), depth of cleft lip (DEPTH), width of cleft lip (WIDTH), changes of the dental plate and hard palate (DEN-HAP), deviation of the face from the midline (DEVIATION), degree of the lateral curvature of the mandibles (CURVATURE), slope of the anterior part of the lower jaw (SLOPE) and bone loss at the *proc. nasalis* of the *os incisivum* (INCISIVUM). Score 0 represents no lesions, while increasing scores reflect increasing severity. See Additional file 1 for details on the scoring system. A right-sided minor form and a right-sided major-form of a cleft lip with a vertical dimension <1/2 accompanied cases 4 and 9 with a complete left CLJ. Case 7 with a complete right-sided CLJ had an incomplete cleft lip with a vertical dimension <1/2 on the left side. Animals with a complete right-sided CLJ (cases 1, 2, 3, 5) exhibited the highest degree of deviation of the face including the mandibles. Cases with a complete unilateral CLJ and a minor or major form of cleft lip on either side (cases 4, 7, 9) had a moderate lateral deviation of the face and mandibles. Complete left-sided (case 8) and complete bilateral CLJ (case 6) were associated with the mildest degree of deviation of the face

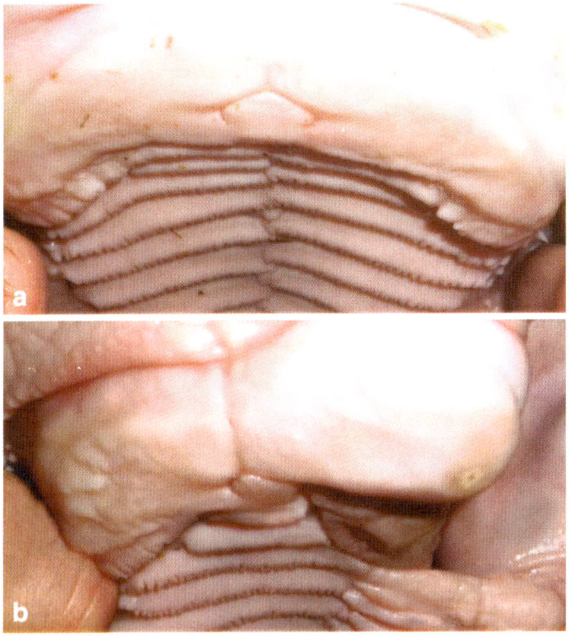

Fig. 5 Roofs of the oral cavity of a control and a cleft lip and jaw (CLJ) affected Vorderwald × Montbéliarde cattle. **a** Normally formed roof of an oral cavity of a control without a CLJ. In the foreground, the *papilla incisiva* is visible on the dental plate. Behind the dental plate, the connection to the hard palate and the *rugae palatinae* on both sides are visible. **b** The oral cavity of Vorderwald × Montbéliarde cattle (case 8) with a *left*-sided CLJ is shown. Approximately 1/3 of the dental plate is missing on the *left*. On the adjacent hard palate, *rugae palatinae* are missing

a V-shaped wedge of the hard palate lacked in this case. The second case was lacking approximately the same proportion of the dental plate as observed in Vorderwald × Montbéliarde cattle.

The curvature of the lower jaw may be a secondary deformation that develops due to the absence of the pressing surface between the mandibles and the missing segment of the *os incisivum* contralateral to the CLJ [10]. However, among the nine cases, the bull with a complete bilateral CLJ (case 6) showed the most pronounced rostral curvature of the mandibles. This latter case is apparently in contrast to the assumption of an induced malformation through the missing pressure of the upper jaw on this part of the mandibles.

Lateral deviation of the face was obviously associated with CLJ as reported previously [7, 10, 25] and in all the present cases. A severe deviation of the face may cause respiratory distress due to reduced size of the nostril and air-conducting ways. Thielscher [10] reported unilateral nasal obstruction and dyspnea in a Red and White Spotted calf with right-sided CLJ. One case with a left sided CLJ mentioned by Swartz et al. [7] showed extreme right curvature of the rostral end of the nose and muzzle. In this case, the dorsal alar cartilage on the left nostril dropped ventrally and reduced further the opening to the nares. The consequences of the lateral deviation of the face in the affected cattle were limited to dental anomalies in form of wiggling teeth with sporadic tooth loss, probably due to pathological friction. This was particularly noticed in the bull with a complete left-sided CLJ and a right-sided minor form (case 9) at an age of one year and in the two right-sided CLJ cows (cases 3 and 5) when they reached an age of 3 and 4 years, respectively.

Conclusions

Complete CLJ was accompanied by loss of parts of the *proc. nasalis* of the *os incisivum.* The extent and localization of the missing parts of the *proc. nasalis* were similar in all cases. The accompanying orofacial defects like lateral deviation of the face and rostral lower jaw as well as the sigmoid curvature of the rostral lower jaw showed a high degree of variability. A precise documentation of the changes, e.g. based on CT scanning, facilitates precise identification of different forms of CLJ and correct classification of animals with morphologically identical orofacial malformations for further analyses.

Additional files

Additional file 1. Explanation of the scoring system for cleft lips and accompanying malformations in the face. The system distinguishes the site of the cleft lip (SITE), the depth of cleft lip (DEPTH), the width of cleft lip (WIDTH), changes at the dental plate and hard palate (DEN-HAP), the deviation of the face from the midline (DEVIATION), the lateral curvature of the mandibles (CURVATURE), the slope of the anterior part of the lower jaw (SLOPE) and the extend of loss of the *proc. nasalis* of the *os incisivum* (INCISIVUM).

Additional file 2. a) The picture shows the muzzle of case 9 with a complete left-sided cleft lip and a minor form on the right side of the lip. b) Computed tomography scanning image of the head showing the lateral view of the skull. The arrow marks the deficit of bony substance (25 %) ventral to the bone shaft corresponded to the minor form of a cleft lip.

Additional file 3. a) The picture shows the muzzle of case 4 with a complete left-sided cleft lip and a macroform on the right side of the lip. b) Computed tomography scanning image of the head showing the lateral view of the skull. The arrow marks the deficit of bony substance (50 %) ventral to the bone shaft corresponded to the macroform of a cleft lip.

Additional file 4. a) The picture shows the muzzle of case 7 with a complete right-sided cleft lip and a macroform on the left side of the lip. b) Computed tomography scanning image of the head showing the lateral view of the skull. The arrow marks the deficit of bony substance in form of a ring-like bone loss corresponded to the macroform of a cleft lip.

Abbreviations

CLJ: cleft lip and jaw; CT: computer tomography; CURVATURE: lateral curvature of the mandibles; DEN-HAP: dental plate and hard palate; DEPTH: depth of cleft lip; INCISIVUM: *proc. nasalis* of the os incisivum; Proc: *processus*; DEVIATION: deviation of the face from the midline; SLOPE: slope of the anterior part of the lower jaw; WIDTH: width of cleft lip.

Authors' contributions

SR, PW and OD did the clinical investigation. MH and KF performed the CT scannings. SR, OD, PW and MH prepared the manuscript. All authors read and approved the final manuscript.

Author details

[1] University of Veterinary Medicine Hannover, Foundation, Institute for Animal Breeding and Genetics, Bünteweg 17p, 30559 Hannover, Germany. [2] University of Veterinary Medicine Hannover, Foundation, Clinic for Horses, Bünteweg 9, 30559 Hannover, Germany. [3] University of Veterinary Medicine Hannover, Foundation, Clinic for Cattle, Bischofsholer Damm 15, 30173 Hannover, Germany.

Acknowledgements

The authors are gratefully to Michaela Reinhardt and Franz Maus, Landratsamt Schwarzwald-Baar-Kreis, Sachgebiet Tierzucht, for their support in ascertainment of the cases and the farmers for providing the animals.

Competing interests

The authors declare that they have no competing interests.

References

1. Wheat JD. Harelip in Shorthorn cattle. J Hered. 1960;51:99–101.
2. Hidiroglou M. Note sur deux cas de bec de lièvre constatés parmi des veaux Shorthorn. Can J Comp Med Vet Sci. 1962;26:180.
3. Shupe JL, James LF, Balls L, Binns W, Keeler RF. A probable hereditary skeletal deformity in Hereford cattle. J Hered. 1967;58:311–3.
4. Labik K. Hereditarily conditioned anomalies of the facial part of the animal head. Acta Vet (Brno). 1972;41:167–76.
5. Mayr B, Hofecker G, Zach E, Pilz E, Themessl H, Wöckl F, Leitner K, Stur I, Schleger W. Dominanter Erbgang von Lippenkieferspalten beim Rind. Züchtungskunde. 1979;51:192.
6. Rieke H. Erbliche Lippenkieferspalten kombiniert mit Kryptorchismus beim schwarzbunten Rind. Dtsch Tierärztl Wschr. 1979;86:108–13.
7. Swartz H, Vogt D, Kintner L. Chromosome evaluation of Angus calves with unilateral congenital cleft lip and jaw (cheilognathoschisis). Am J Vet Res. 1982;43:729–31.
8. Hámori D. Labio-palatoschisis. Constitutional disorders and hereditary diseases in domestic animals. New York: Elsevier; 1983. p. 430–4.
9. Loeffler K. Lippenkieferspalte beim Kalb. Anmerkungen zu dem Artikel "Cornea-Dermoide und Doppelmißbildung der Nasenlöcher bei einem Rind" von C. Neophytou. Berl Münch Tierärztl Wschr. 1990;103:297–8.
10. Thielscher HH. Bildbericht. Cheilognathoschisis superior lat. beim Kalb. Tierärztl Umsch. 1991;46:103.
11. Moritomo Y, Tsuda T, Miyamoto H. Craniofacial skeletal abnormalities in anomalous calves with clefts of the face. J Vet Med Sci. 1999;61:1147–52.
12. Huston K, Saperstein G, Steffen D, Millar P, Lauvergne J. Clinical, pathological and other visible traits loci except coat colour (category 2). In: Lauvergne JJ, Dolling CHS, Millar P, editors. Mendelian inheritance in cattle 2000—EAAP 101, vol. 101. Wageningen: Wageningen Press; 2000. p. 216–8, p. 24–30.
13. Lupp B, Kuiper H, Abfalter K, Reinhardt M, Maus F, Distl O. Einseitig laterale Oberlippenkieferspalte und Gesichtsskoliose in einer ingezüchteten Familie von Vorderwälder Rindern. Prakt Tierarzt. 2011;7:1086–92.
14. Lupp B, Reinhardt M, Maus F, Hellige M, Feige K, Distl O. Right-sided cleft lip and jaw in a family of Vorderwald × Montbéliarde cattle. Vet J. 2012;192:520–2.
15. Koch H, Grzonka M, Koch J. Cleft malformation of lip, alveolus, hard and soft palate, and nose (LAHSN)—a critical view of the terminology, the diagnosis and gradation as a basis for documentation and therapy. Br J Oral Maxillofac Surg. 1995;33:51–8.
16. Dixon MJ, Marazita ML, Beaty TH, Murray JC. Cleft lip and palate: understanding genetic and environmental influences. Nat Rev Genet. 2011;12:167–78.
17. Cox TC, Luquetti DV, Cunningham ML. Perspectives and challenges in advancing research into craniofacial anomalies. Am J Med Genet C Semin Med Genet. 2013;163:213–7.
18. Kernahan DA, Stark RB. A new classification for cleft lip and cleft palate. Plast Reconstr Surg. 1958;22:435–41.
19. Kernahan DA. The striped Ya symbolic classification for cleft lip and palate. Plast Reconstr Surg. 1971;47:469–70.
20. Friedman HI, Sayetta RB, Coston GN, Hussey JR. Symbolic representation of cleft lip and palate. Cleft Palate Craniofac J. 1991;28:252–60.
21. Schwartz S, Kapala JT, Rajchgot H, Roberts GL. Accurate and systematic numerical recording system for the identification of various types of lip and maxillary clefts (RPL system). Cleft Palate Craniofac J. 1993;30:330–2.
22. Ortiz-Posadas M, Vega-Alvarado L, Maya-Behar J. A new approach to classify cleft lip and palate. Cleft Palate Craniofac J. 2001;38:545–50.
23. Anastassov Y, Chipkov C. Analysis of nasal and labial deformities in cleft lip, alveolus and palate patients by a new rating scale: preliminary report. J Craniomaxillofac Surg. 2003;31:299–303.
24. Koul R. Describing cleft lip and palate using a new expression system. Cleft Palate Craniofac J. 2007;44:585–9.
25. Rieke H. Die Gesichtsspalten (Cheilognathoschisis und Palatoschisis) in der hessischen Rinderpopulation. Morphologie, Aetiologie, Statistik. Dissertation, Justus-Liebig-Universität Gießen, 1982.
26. Murray JC, Daack-Hirsch S, Buetow KH, Munger R, Espina L, Paglinawan N, Birgfeld CB, Fitzsimons DA, Cox TC. Clinical and epidemiologic studies of cleft lip and palate in the Philippines. Cleft Palate Craniofac J. 1997;34:7–10.
27. Brydon CA, Conway J, Kling R, Mehta L, Jabs EW, Taub PJ. Cleft lip and/or palate: one organization's experience with more than a quarter million surgeries during the past decade. J Craniofac Surg. 2014;25:1601–9.
28. Wang KH, Heike CL, Clarkson MD, Mejino JL, Brinkley JF, Tse RW, Villanueva E, Rary J, Magee K, Magee W. Evaluation and integration of disparate classification systems for clefts of the lip. Front Physiol. 2014;5:163.
29. Yuzuriha S, Mulliken JB. Minor-form, microform, and mini-microform cleft lip: anatomical features, operative techniques, and revisions. Plast Reconstr Surg. 2008;122:1485–93.
30. Elsahy NI. The modified striped Y—a systematic classification for cleft lip and palate. Cleft Palate J. 1973;10:247–50.

2

The reproductive pattern and potential of free ranging female wild boars (*Sus scrofa*) in Sweden

Anna Malmsten[1*], Gunnar Jansson[2], Nils Lundeheim[3] and Anne-Marie Dalin[1]

Abstract

Background: The number and spatial distribution of wild boars (*Sus scrofa*) has increased remarkably in Sweden as well as in other European countries. To understand the population dynamics of the wild boar, knowledge of its reproductive period, oestrus cycle and reproductive success is essential. The aim of this study was therefore to describe the seasonal reproductive pattern and reproductive potential of a wild boar population in Sweden. The study was based on findings from macroscopic examinations of the reproductive organs from 575 hunter-harvested female wild boars (>30 kg body weight). Samples were collected between December 2011 and December 2015 in the southern and middle parts of Sweden. The age of the sampled animals was determined and dressed weight was noted. The stage of the reproductive cycle was defined according to ovarian structures and in relation to the appearance of/and findings in the uterus. The crown-rump length (CRL) of the embryos/foetuses was used to calculate the oestrus/mating month and month for the expected farrowing.

Results: The macroscopic examination revealed a seasonal variation of reproductive stages, although cyclic and pregnant females were found in all seasons. Moreover, the estimated oestrus/mating and farrowing months based on the CRL showed that mating and farrowing may occur 'off-season'. The average litter size (no. of embryos or foetuses) per pregnant female was 5.4. Sow weight and age had significant effect on both the reproductive potential (ovulation rate and litter size) and pregnancy rate, respectively.

Conclusions: The reproductive potential in the studied wild boar population was high compared to studies from other countries and farrowing may occur 'off-season'. This suggests that the environmental conditions in Sweden, including supplemental feeding, are favourable for wild boar reproduction.

Keywords: Litter size, Ovulation rate, Pregnancy rate, Seasonality, Supplemental feeding

Background

The number and spatial distribution of wild boars has increased remarkably in Sweden as well as in other European countries during the last decades [1–5]. Besides the generalist behaviour of wild boars such as wide feed and habitat selection, the main reasons for this rapid increase are thought to be the high reproductive potential of the wild boar [6] in combination with extensive supplemental feeding and relatively low harvest rates.

*Correspondence: anna.malmsten@slu.se
[1] Division of Reproduction, Department of Clinical Sciences, Swedish University of Agricultural Sciences, Box 7054, 750 07 Uppsala, Sweden
Full list of author information is available at the end of the article

To understand the population dynamics of a game species such as the wild boar, knowledge of its reproductive period, oestrus cycle and reproductive success is essential [7, 8]. Wild boar biology has been studied in several countries with a long history of wild boar populations. Based on European studies, pure breeds of wild boars without a history of hybridization with domestic pigs (that are poly-oestral throughout the year) have a reproduction that is clearly seasonal [9]. The wild boars are so-called short-day breeders. During the summer months, the majority of the female wild boars are anoestral [9–11]. In continental Europe, the summer anoestrus coincides with high ambient temperatures, long days and restricted access to feed [12]. In the autumn, as a result of shortened day length, the oestrus period begins [9]. However, the first oestrus of the breeding season may take place at different time in different years depending on natural feed availability and other environmental and climatic factors [9, 11, 13]. For example, it appears that earliness or delay in the onset of the breeding season is related to the level of available feed in that a high access to feed can cause a shortened anoestrus period [10]. In a natural environment, without any human impact, there is normally only one oestrus peak in the autumn/winter [12]. However, a bimodal pattern of oestrus and consequently farrowing can also occur [2, 14]. In addition, some studies show that farrowing may occur throughout the year when feed is available all year round [15, 16].

The current wild boar population in Sweden originates from an unknown number of individuals that escaped enclosures in the 1970s and 1980s. Since, the population has steadily and rapidly increased. During the last 20 years, the annual number of harvested wild boars in Sweden has increased from 5000 to 100,000 animals [5]. The knowledge about Swedish wild boar and its management is limited, and only a few studies have been published. These studies have mainly described wild boar movement patterns, behaviour, and habitat selection [17–20], but few include data on reproduction [7, 21], i.e. reproductive performance and reproductive potential of the species in Sweden.

The aim of this study was to describe the reproductive pattern and potential of free ranging female wild boars in Sweden.

Methods

Study area

Samples were collected between December 2011 and December 2015 at seven hunting estates in four different regions (Skåne, Blekinge, Södermanland, and Uppland) in southern and central Sweden (Additional file 1).

The size of the estates varied from 10 to 87 km^2 and the population density of wild boars estimated by the wildlife manager at each estate ranged from 5 to 40 animals per km^2 among the estates. Similar management strategies for the wild boars were applied at all estates, including supplemental feeding throughout the year. The types of feed used were corn, grain, mixes of cereal and sugar beets, and silage (anaerobic fermentation with wheat and oats grains, peas, and clover). Meteorological data (monthly mean precipitation and temperature) were obtained from local meteorological services [22]. During the study period, the weather conditions in the sampling regions were similar with mean temperatures in January and July of −1 and 18 °C respectively, and mean precipitation in January and July was 49 and 58 mm, respectively (Additional file 2).

Hunting methods and Swedish wild boar hunting legislation

Sampling occurred during ordinary hunting. The hunting methods used were beat/drive hunts and stalking. Beat/drive hunts were the most common method in the study areas during the main hunting season (October until February) and resulted in considerable hunting bags (30–100 animals per day). Stalking was used during spring and summer and animals were most often shot while feeding at open field/grazing-ground, i.e. hunting was used mainly as a crop preventive action.

For practical reasons, the sampling effort was biased towards the main hunting season (October–February). In Sweden, the hunting season of adult wild boars range between 16th of April and 15th of February. The wild boar hunting is allowed 24 h, i.e. day and night, and hunting with dogs is allowed between 1st of August and 31st of January. Hunting of yearlings is allowed throughout the year, whereas females with dependent piglets are protected [23].

Data collection

Body weight (BW) and field dressed weight (FDW, weight of the eviscerated animal with skin) were recorded. Sampling included all females with BW ≥30 kg. For animals where only BW was noted, FDW were estimated using the equation FDW = −1.855 + 0.810*BW, based on the known relationship between BW and FDW of 296 animals [Lundeheim, unpublished data]. Altogether, FDW was noted for 540 animals. Age was determined for 442 of the animals based on tooth eruption and replacement pattern [24] and the animals were subdivided into juveniles (<1 year), yearlings (1–2 years) and adults (>2 years).

Macroscopic examinations of reproductive organs

The collected reproductive organs were frozen at −20 °C until the macroscopic laboratory examination [7]. The size and weight of the uterus and ovaries were recorded as were the ovarian structures (follicles and *corpora lutea*, CL). Ovulation rate (OR) was defined as the total number of active CL from both ovaries. The uteri were cut open and the contents examined. The reproductive stage was determined based on the data from the macroscopic examination [7]. Animals in prooestrus, oestrus, metoestrus and dioestrus were classified as cyclic. In pregnant females, from about 18 days of pregnancy (when embryos in the foetal membranes could be clearly observed), the number of embryos or foetuses were counted. Litter size was defined as the total number of embryos or foetuses. The OR and litter size were considered as two measurements of reproductive potential. The crown-rump length

(CRL), weight, gender and development of the embryos/foetus were noted. The estimated oestrus/mating months and expected farrowing months were calculated based on the CRL of the embryos/foetuses [25].

Statistical analyses

The statistical analyses were carried out in SAS (SAS Institute Inc. Cary, N. C). In the analyses, year was divided into four seasons as: spring (March–May), summer (June–August), autumn (September–November) and winter (December–February). Analysis of variance [both PROC GLM (general linear model) and PROC GLIMMIX (generalized linear mixed model)] were used for the statistical analyses.

Primary statistics showed that there was a high variation and poor overlapping in number of observations among seasons and age classes (Table 1). To overcome the statistical problems this raises in the analyses, monofactorial analyses were performed.

Sub-analysis 1

Analyses of the effect of season and age class on the continuous variables weight (dressed), OR and litter size. The statistical model included either the fixed effect of season (4 classes) or age class (3 classes). These analyses was performed using PROC GLM, and were based on 421, 139 and 71 observations, respectively.

Sub-analysis 2

For the analyses of the three binary variables, indicating the reproductive stage (anoestrus, cyclic or pregnant), fixed effects of season and age class were included in the model, one at a time. In these analyses prepubertal animals and animals with disrupted cycles were excluded. These analyses were performed using PROC GLIMMIX, and were based on 357 (for season) and 261 (for age class) observations. Using this approach, the effect of age class on the pregnancy rate of female wild boars was also analysed (442 observations). The pregnancy rate was defined as the proportion of pregnant females per age class of the sampled population. P-values less than 0.05 were considered as significant.

Results

In total, 617 female wild boars were collected and 575 individuals met the requirements to be included in this study, i.e. a complete set of reproductive organs available for examination. The number of animals sampled in each season and in relation to age and sampling region is presented in Table 1. The number of animals in the different reproductive stages were: 207 prepubertal (36.0%), 131 anoestral (22.8%), cyclic 104 (18.1%), 123 pregnant (21.2%), and 11 had a disrupted ovarian cyclic pattern (1.9%). The levels of significance for the effects included in the statistical analyses are presented in Table 2. The proportion of animals in different reproductive stages (prepubertal animals and animals with disrupted oestrus cycle excluded) was significantly affected by season ($P < 0.0001$, Fig. 1).

Pregnancy was detected in 122 animals. After excluding 11 pregnant females with embryo mortality and 10 animals in an early pregnancy state (<2.5 weeks), the mean number of CL was 6.4 (range 2–11; n = 101) and the mean number of embryos/foetuses was 5.4 (range 1–9). The estimated oestrus/mating- and farrowing months based on the CRL of embryos/foetuses

Table 2 The levels of significance for the effects of season and age class on weight, reproductive potential, reproductive stage and pregnancy rate of the sampled female wild boars

Variable	Season	Age class
Weight	***	***
Reproductive potential		
OR	Ns	***
Litter size	Ns	***
Reproductive stage		
Anoestrus	***	**
Cyclic	***	Ns
Pregnant	***	Ns
Pregnancy rate	–	***

Levels of significance: *ns* not significant

P < 0.05; ** P ≤ 0.01; *** P ≤ 0.001

Table 1 The number of sampled female wild boars in total, per season, per age class, and per sampling region

Season	Total	Age class				Region			
		Juvenile	Yearling	Adult	Unknown	Skåne	Blekinge	Södermanland	Uppland
Spring	76	11	16	8	41	0	5	59	12
Summer	48	7	17	8	16	0	2	44	2
Autumn	345	109	100	101	35	38	149	78	80
Winter	106	23	15	27	41	45	2	31	28
Total	575	150	148	144	133	83	158	212	122

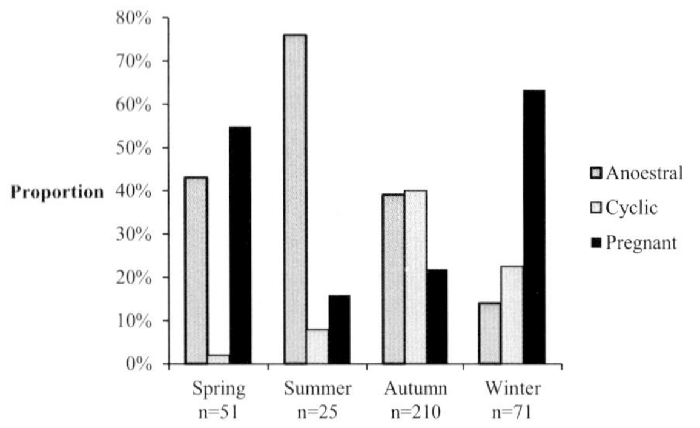

Fig. 1 The proportion of female wild boar in different reproductive stages in relation to culling season (prepubertal animals and animals with disrupted ovarian cyclic pattern excluded)

from 105 pregnant female wild boars sampled between November 2012 and December 2014, are illustrated in Fig. 2.

Age class and weight was highly associated (Table 2). The reproductive potential (OR and litter size) in relation to weight class for 99 of the pregnant animals, for which the FDW was noted and the pregnancy had proceeded over 18 days, is illustrated in Fig. 3. The reproductive potential increased significantly with age class. Age was determined in 442 animals of which 78 were pregnant, and the pregnancy rate in relation to age class is presented in Table 3. The pregnancy rate increased significantly per age class ($P < 0.001$).

Discussion

To identify the population dynamics of a game species in order to conduct a proper management, understanding of its reproductive period, oestrus cycle and the mean reproductive outcome is essential. In the present study, the reproductive pattern and potential among free ranging female wild boars in Sweden is described.

The reproductive potential indicated by ovulation rates and litter size of the studied wild boars was high (6.4 and 5.4, respectively), compared to litter sizes reported from other countries, e.g. Portugal 4.2 [15], Iberian Peninsula 3.6 [26], Switzerland 4.8 [27], and Italy 5.0 [1], but not as high as in a recent German study; 6.6 [8]. The reproductive potential of wild boars can be affected by many factors such as feed availability, climate [6, 26, 28, 29], the genetic background including influence of domestic pigs [14, 30, 31], and the weight and age of gilts and sows [9, 29]. High natural feed availability may increase the litter size [32] as well as the availability of supplementary feed [26, 29]. In Sweden, although controversial, supplemental feeding is to a varying extent applied throughout the wild boar range. This makes studies of the direct effects of supplemental feeding on free ranging wild boars, including controls (in areas without supplementary feeding), more or less impossible to conduct in Sweden. Moreover, the availability of natural feed in Sweden is high for wild boars, both in forests and agricultural habitats, and especially in the southern and central parts of Sweden. During winter, the scarcity of natural feed is compensated by supplemental feeding. Compared to southern and central

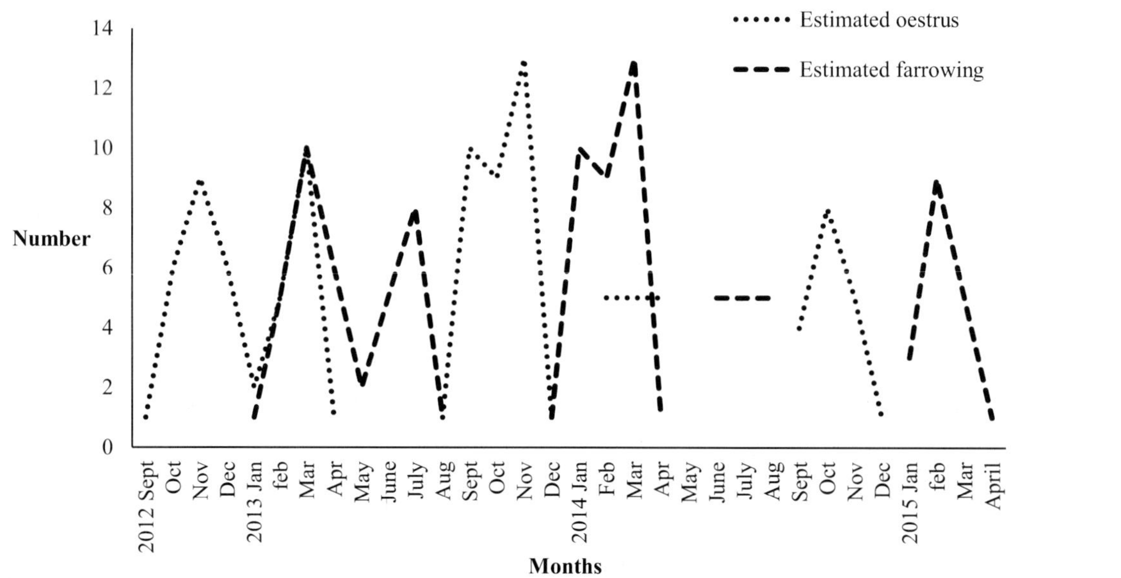

Fig. 2 The estimated oestrus/mating—and farrowing months based on the crown-rump-length (CRL) of embryos/fetuses from 105 pregnant wild boars

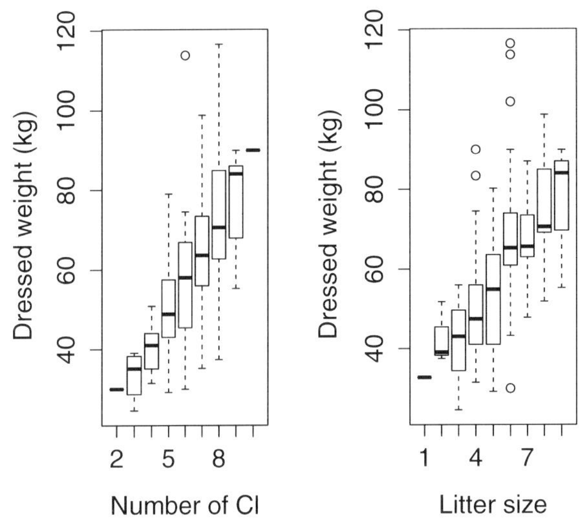

Fig. 3 The number of *corpora lutea* (ovulation rate) and litter size in relation to maternal field dressed weight in kg. Box and whisker plots show median (*point within box*), 25% (interquartile range 1) and 75% (interquartile range 3) percentiles (box) and the range (whiskers). *Circles* indicate statistical outliers

Table 3 Pregnancy rate of the examined female wild boars in relation to age class

Age class	Number examined	Number (%) pregnant
Juvenile	150	10 (6.7)
Yearling	148	30 (20.3)
Adult	144	38 (26.4)
Total	442	78 (17.7)

Europe [12], Swedish summers are (due to mild climate) not likely to constitute a regulating season for wild boar populations. Instead, the summer conditions in the south and central Sweden normally result in a long vegetation period without long periods of high ambient temperatures or drought [22]. Such conditions are favorable for wild boars [8, 28] and possibly contribute to the large litter sizes.

The genetic background and possible influence of domestic pigs in the wild boar population is known to affect the litter size and growth rate [30]. Bergman et al. [33] found genetic signs in Swedish wild boars that possibly could indicate interbreeding between wild boars and domestic pigs. Still, further studies to identify the occurrence of genetic introgression from domestic pig into the Swedish wild boar populations are required for wider conclusions.

The age/weight of the sows in the wild boar population can also affect the observed litter size. Younger and lighter individuals have smaller litters than older/heavier individuals [12, 26]. In agreement with previous studies [1, 8, 15, 26, 34], we also found that pregnancy rate and reproductive potential increased with age and weight. The proportion of old/heavy sows, included in the studied material, is highly linked to management in Sweden. The Swedish hunting regulations [35] prohibit culling of females with piglets, and large females (also without piglets) are often voluntarily banned from culling by hunters. Therefore, it is possible that the age and weight composition of the sampled animals was not representative for the actual age and weight composition of the wild boar population in the sampled areas. Instead, it is likely that the proportion of large, adult females was higher in the population than in the studied material, and the average reproductive potential presented here might be underestimated.

Although the majority of the studied female wild boars showed a seasonal pattern in accordance to previous studies [2, 9], cyclic and pregnant females were found in all seasons. This pattern was further confirmed by the estimated oestrus/mating and farrowing months based on the CRL of embryos/fetuses (Fig. 2). These observations show that farrowing may occur 'off-season' in Sweden, as also suggested by studies describing the corresponding pattern when feed is accessible throughout the year [15, 36]. Despite the lack of material from a few months, a tendency of at least two peak periods for oestrus/mating (one in November and one in March) is seen in the material from 2013 and evident, but not as pronounced in 2014 (Fig. 2). This would give (if the animals had stayed alive), peaks of farrowing in March and July. Breeding in March is not considered to be normal for "short-day breeders", such as wild boars. However, this bimodal distribution of birth has been described in other studies [2, 14]. Other authors explain this second peak as a result of (1) some factors that make an early spring litter die and the sow then goes into oestrus again and become pregnant, (2) involvement of young females in reproduction during spring, (juveniles that did not reach the necessary weight at the time of the mating season), and (3) genetic influences of domestic pigs in the wild boar population that also can affect the seasonality of reproduction [14], a factor that still is to be investigated in the Swedish wild boar population. In the first explanation, harsh weather conditions, scarcity of feed, or diseases are factors that may affect the litter survival. In our case, the female boars involved in the second birth peak (June–July) had a mean live weight of 54.3 kg ($n = 13$, range 34–70.6 kg), which may contribute to the second theory. Moreover, scarcity of feed would not be an explanation to the second peak because the studied population was supplementary fed throughout the study period. However, during January and February 2013, game managers at the different estates, observed a lot of piglets that later on disappeared. The results of the macroscopical examination of the reproductive tract of female wild boars from this period confirm these observations. We found that a large proportion (17%, n = 84 in 2013) and (26%, n = 27 in 2014) of the females that were shot between January and May (both included), recently had been pregnant. In practice this means that these individuals either (1) had lost their piglets shortly after birth due to piglet death (because of disease, predation, starvation, or frostbite) or the sows had left their piglets of unknown cause; (2) had aborted, i.e. lost their litter before birth due to poor body condition or disease; or (3) were shot although their piglets were alive (unlikely when hunters neither seen piglets or quoted drawn teats of sows). Harsh weather conditions and infectious diseases may contribute to the annual loss of wild boar litters. Still, the appearance and possible effect of infectious diseases on wild boar reproduction, i.e. porcine parvovirus and porcine circovirus type 2 is still to be investigated.

Litters produced all year round complicate wild boar hunting and may thus infer difficulties to meet management goals. Adult sows which, if targeted by hunting, would be the animal category most effective to harvest if a population decrease is aimed for, are protected from culling if accompanied by piglets. Further, piglets present during hunting season, may be injured and/or killed by hunting dogs, which is an important issue of ethical and animal welfare to acknowledge.

Conclusions

This descriptive study of wild boar reproduction showed that the reproductive potential in the studied population was high and that farrowing may occur 'off-season'. We suggest that the general high feed availability and environmental conditions in Sweden is favorable for wild boars. The possible effect of introgression of domestic pigs should not be neglected as a possible contributing factor to the high reproductive potential presented in this study.

Additional files

Additional file 1. Map of Sweden highlighting the regions where female wild boars were sampled. a) Skåne, b) Blekinge c) Södermanland, d) Uppland.

Additional file 2. Mean temperature and percipitation in four Swedish counties, measured in January and July in the years of 2013–2015.

Authors' contributions

AM, AMD, and GJ were involved in the design and coordination of the study, AM and AMD collected the data and performed the organ examination. NL performed the statistical analyses. All authors contributed in drafting the manuscript. All authors read and approved the final manuscript.

Author details

[1] Division of Reproduction, Department of Clinical Sciences, Swedish University of Agricultural Sciences, Box 7054, 750 07 Uppsala, Sweden. [2] Grimsö Wildlife Research Station, Department of Ecology, Swedish University of Agricultural Sciences, 730 91 Riddarhyttan, Sweden. [3] Department of Animal Breeding and Genetics, Swedish University of Agricultural Sciences, Box 7054, 750 07 Uppsala, Sweden.

Acknowledgements

We thank all of the estate owners for permitting collection and the wildlife managers and hunters for their engagement and contribution in this project. The authors wish to thank Andreas Karlsson and Bertil Malmsten who assisted in the sample collection.

Competing interests

The authors declare that they have no competing interests.

Funding

This work was supported by the Swedish Environmental Protection Agency, and the Swedish Association for Hunting and Wildlife Management.

References

1. Boitani L, Trapanese P, Mattei L. Demographic patterns of a wild boar (*Sus scrofa* L.) population in Tuscany, Italy. IBEX J Mount Ecol. 1995;3:197–201.
2. Ježek M, Štípek K, Kušta T, Červený J, Vícha J. Reproductive and morphometric characteristics of wild boar (*Sus scrofa*) in the Czech Republic. J For Sci. 2011;57:285–92.
3. Keuling O, Baubet E, Duscher A, Ebert C, Fisher C, Monaco A, et al. Mortality rates of wild boar *Sus scrofa* L. in central Europe. Eur J Wildl Res. 2013;59:805–14.
4. Massei G, Kindberg J, Licoppe A, Cačić D, Šprem N, Kamler J, Baubet E, et al. Wild boar populations up, numbers of hunters down? A review of trends and implications for Europe. Pest Manag Sci. 2015;71:492–500.
5. Svenska Jägareförbundet [The Swedish Hunting Association]. 2014. http://svenskjakt.se/Start/Nyheter/2014/08/hur-mycket-vilt-har-vi-egentligen/. Accessed 19 July 2016.
6. Servanty S, Gaillard JM, Allaine D, Brandt D, Baubet E. Litter size and fetal sex ratio adjustment in a highly polytocous species: the wild boar. Behav Ecol. 2007;18:427–32.
7. Malmsten A, Jansson G, Dalin AM. Postmortem examination of the reproductive organs of female wild boars (*Sus scrofa*) in Sweden. Reprod Dom Anim. 2017. doi:10.1111/rda.12947.
8. Frauendorf M, Gethöffer F, Siebert U, Keuling O. The influence of environmental and physiological factors on the litter size of wild boar (*Sus scrofa*) in an agriculture dominated area in Germany. Sci Total Environ. 2016;541:877–82.
9. Mauget R. Seasonality of reproduction in the wild boar. In: Cole DJA, Foxcroft GR, editors. Control of pig reproduction. London: Butterworth Scientific; 1982. p. 509–26.
10. Pépin D, Spitz F, Janeau G, Valet G. Dynamics of reproduction and development of weight in the wild boar (*Sus scrofa*) in South-West France. Z Säugetierk. 1987;52:21–30.
11. Delcroix I, Mauget R, Signoret JP. Existence of synchronization of reproduction at the level of the social group of the European wild boar (*Sus scrofa*). J Reprod Fert. 1990;89:613–7.

12. Mauget R. Seasonal reproductive activity of the European wild boar. Comparison with the domestic sow. In: Assenmacher I, Farner DS, editors. Environmental endocrinology. Berlin: Springer; 1978. p. 79–80.
13. Macchi E, Starvaggi Cucuzza A, Badino P, Odore R, Re F, Bevilacqua L, Malfatti A. Seasonality of reproduction in wild boar (*Sus scrofa*) were assessed by fecal and plasmatic steroids. Theriogenology. 2010;73:1230–7.
14. Mauget R. Observations sur la reproduction du sanglier (*Sus scrofa* L.) a l'état sauvage. Ann Biol Anim Biochem Biophys. 1972;12:195–202.
15. Fonseca C, Santos P, Monzón A, Bento P, Alves da Silva A, Alves J, et al. Reproduction in the wild boar (*Sus scrofa* Linnaeus, 1758) populations of Portugal. Galemys. 2004;16:53–65.
16. Orlowska L, Rembacz W, Florek C. Carcass weight, condition and reproduction of wild boar harvested in north-western Poland. Pest Manage Sci. 2012. doi:10.1002/ps.3355.
17. Lemel J, Truvé J, Söderberg B. Variation in ranging and activity behavior of European wild boar *Sus scrofa* in Sweden. Wildl Biol. 2003;9:29–36.
18. Truvé J, Lemel J. Timing and distance of natal dispersal for wild boar *Sus scrofa* in Sweden. Wildl Biol. 2003;9:51–7.
19. Thurfjell H, Ball JP, Åhlén PA, Kornacher P, Dettki H, Sjöberg K. Habitat use and spatial patterns of wild boar *Sus scrofa*: agricultural fields and edges. Eur J Wildl Res. 2009;55:517–23.
20. Welander J. Spatial and temporal dynamics of wild boar (*Sus scrofa*) rooting in a mosaic landscape. J Zool. 2000;252:263–71.
21. Malmsten A, Dalin AM. Puberty in female wild boar (*Sus scrofa*) in Sweden. Acta Vet Scand. 2016;58:55. doi:10.1186/s13028-016-0236-1.
22. SMHI.se. 2016. Vegetationperiod. http://www.smhi.se/kunskapsbanken/klimat/vegetationsperiod-1.6270. Accessed 30 June 2016.
23. Naturvårdsverket. 2016. http://www.naturvardsverket.se/Var-natur/Jakt/Jakt-pa-klovvilt/Jakt-pa-vildsvin/. Accessed 13 Sept 2016.
24. Matschke GH. Ageing European wild hogs by dentition. J Wildl Manag. 1967;31:109–13.
25. Henry VG. Fetal development in European wild hogs. J Wildl Manag. 1968;32:966–70.
26. Fernández-Llario P, Mateos-Quesada P. Body size and reproductive parameters in the wild boar *Sus scrofa*. Acta Theriol. 1998;43:439–44.
27. Moretti M. Birth distribution, structure and dynamics of a hunted mountain population of wild boars (*Sus scrofa* L.), Ticino, Switzerland. IBEX J Mount Ecol. 1995;3:192–6.
28. Geisser H, Reyer HU. The influence of food and temperature on population density of wild boar *Sus scrofa* in the Thurgau (Switzerland). J Zool. 2005;267:89–96.
29. Fernández-Llario P, Carranza J. Reproductive performance of the wild boar in a Mediterranean ecosystem under drought conditions. Ethol Ecol Evol. 2000;12:335–43.
30. Booth WD. Wild boar farming in the United Kingdom. IBEX J Mount Ecol. 1995;3:245–8.
31. Gongora J, Peltoniemi OAT, Tammen I, Raadsma H, Moran C. Analyses of possible domestic pig contribution in two populations of finnish farmed wild boar. Acta Agric Scand. 2003;53:161–5.
32. Massei G, Genov PV, Staines BW. Diet, food availability and reproduction of wild boar in a Mediterranean coastal area. Acta Theriol. 1996;41:307–20.
33. Bergman IM, Sandholm K, Nilsson Ekdahl K, Okumura N, Uenishi H, Guldbrandtsen B, et al. MBL1 genotypes in wild boar populations from Sweden, Austria, the Czech Republic, and Japan. Int J Immunogenet. 2012. doi:10.1111/j.1744-313X.2012.0113240:131.
34. Santos P, Fernández-Llario P, Fonseca C, Monzón A, Bento P, Soares AMVM, et al. Habitat and reproductive phenology of wild boar (*Sus scrofa*) in the western Iberian Peninsula. Eur J Wildl Res. 2006;52:207–12.
35. Jaktförordning. 1987:905. https://www.notisum.se/rnp/sls/lag/19870905.htm#B1. Accessed 2 Feb 2017.
36. Bieber C, Ruf T. Population dynamics in wild boar *Sus scrofa*: ecology, elasticity of growth rate and implications for management of pulsed resource consumers. J Appl Ecol. 2005;42:1203–13.

Farm characteristics and management routines related to neonatal porcine diarrhoea: a survey among Swedish piglet producers

Jenny Larsson[1*], Nils Fall[1], Maria Lindberg[2] and Magdalena Jacobson[1]

Abstract

Background: In recent years reports from a number of countries, including Sweden, describe problems with diarrhoea in newborn piglets despite the use of previously effective preventive measures. This seemingly altered disease pattern of neonatal porcine diarrhoea (NPD) warrants investigations on the magnitude and manifestation of the problem. The aim of the present study was to investigate the herd-level prevalence of NPD in Sweden and to describe disease characteristics and intervention strategies used in affected herds. To obtain this information a questionnaire was developed and sent out to 170 randomly selected herds. The presence of NPD in the herds was specified as "Yes", "No" or "Occasional cases" during the preceding year.

Results: A response rate of 58% (98/170) was achieved. The total prevalence of farmer experienced NPD, including occasional cases was 79.6% (95% CI 70.6–86.4%). Most herds (85%; 83/98) employed maternal vaccination against enterotoxigenic *Escherichia coli* (ETEC). The most common treatment regimens used in affected herds included antimicrobials only (43%; 18/42) or antimicrobials in combination with supplementary fluids (33%; 14/42). Trimethoprim in combination with a sulphonamide was the drug of choice in 57% (24/42) of the affected herds whereas the remaining herds used a broad range of other antimicrobials (neomycin, amoxicillin, fluoroquinolones, penicillin, and tylosin). Furthermore, the risk of experiencing NPD was found to be higher in herds with >200 sows (OR = 4.0) compared to herds with <200 sows and in herds where more ambitious efforts (such as providing supplemental colostrum or practicing split-suckling) were made to save weak-born piglets (OR = 4.4).

Conclusions: The results of the present study indicate that Swedish farmers commonly experience NPD in their herds, often despite vaccination against ETEC. Considering the extent of this problem and its contribution to antimicrobial usage, improving alternative control strategies for NPD needs to be prioritized.

Keywords: New neonatal porcine diarrhoea, Neonatal porcine diarrhoea, Prevalence, Risk factors, Pigs, Swine, Treatment, Prevention

Background

Neonatal porcine diarrhoea (NPD) is a common and serious problem causing significant production losses in pig farming worldwide [1–3]. A number of infectious agents have been associated with NPD, however the occurrence of diarrhoea in newborn piglets should be viewed as the result of a multitude of interacting factors [4]. Major determinants for the manifestation of NPD are for instance the infection pressure exerted by specific pathogens present in the herd, the environmental temperature, and the passive immunity transferred by colostrum [4–8]. Many management practices and herd characteristics may hence be associated with either an increased or decreased risk of disease [9–14].

In Sweden, well-known causes of NPD include enterotoxigenic *Escherichia coli* (ETEC) and *Clostridium perfringens* type C, two agents that can be prevented by maternal vaccination combined with a high level of

*Correspondence: jenny.larsson@slu.se
[1] Department of Clinical Sciences, Swedish University of Agricultural Sciences, Box 7054, SE-75007 Uppsala, Sweden
Full list of author information is available at the end of the article

hygiene in the farrowing units [1, 15, 16]. In recent years however, reports from a number of countries, including Sweden, describe problems with NPD despite the use of previously effective preventive measures [17–20]. The underlying causes for this problem, by some referred to as new neonatal porcine diarrhoea syndrome (NNPDS), is currently unknown and hitherto well-known porcine enteropathogens seem to be of minor importance [17, 19, 20].

This seemingly altered disease pattern of NPD warrants further investigations on the magnitude and manifestation of the problem. The aim of the present study was hence to investigate the prevalence of NPD in Sweden and to describe disease characteristics and intervention strategies used in affected herds. Furthermore, we aimed to identify herd characteristics and herd management practices that differentiate herds experiencing a problem with neonatal porcine diarrhoea from herds not experiencing NPD.

Methods

Study design and data collection

A questionnaire was developed to obtain information on farm characteristics, management routines, and, in affected herds, disease manifestation and intervention strategies. The questionnaire was designed to be filled in by the farmers assisted by their veterinarian, and was pilot-tested in six piglet-producing herds to improve the comprehensiveness of the questions. These responses were not included in subsequent analysis.

The study population was piglet-producing herds supervised by the Swedish Animal Health Service (presently known as Farm and Animal Health) or by Lunden's Animal Health Service. In 2011, 740 piglet-producing herds (all production types including sows) were supervised by the Swedish Animal Health Service, and 59 by Lunden's Animal Health Service (personal communication, S.O. Dimander, Swedish Animal Health Service, and E. Lindahl, Lunden's Animal Health Service). This corresponded to approximately 86% of the total number of herds keeping sows in Sweden during 2011 [21]. We hypothesised that a higher response rate would be achieved if the questionnaires were distributed by the veterinarians at their routine herd visits, compared to distributing the questionnaires per mail.

In agreement with the 17 veterinarians participating in the study, an average of ten questionnaires was assigned per veterinarian. The sample size of 170 was hence indirectly decided by the study design. The random selection of herds (from the 799 in total) was however not stratified and resulted in four to 16 herds per veterinarian. Herds that had less than ten sows or had ceased their piglet production were replaced.

The final questionnaire included 59 questions divided into two sections—"production and management routines", and "disease characteristics and treatment of neonatal diarrhoea". The section on production and management covered type of production, age of farrowing stables, number of sows in production, number of employees, recording of production data and production results, employment of all in-all out in the farrowing unit, washing and disinfection of the farrowing unit, vaccination routines against NPD, employment of nurse sows, entry of sows to the farrowing unit, treatment of post–partum dysgalactia syndrome (PPDS), monitoring of farrowing, and management of newborn piglets and their environment. The section on disease characteristics and treatment of NPD in affected herds included proportion of piglets affected, changes in prevalence of NPD, prevalence in litters from first parity sows, time point for the occurrence of diarrhoea, treatment of diarrhoea, efforts made to investigate the cause, and employment of prophylactic measures.

The questionnaire design included multiple choice or dichotomous questions as well as a smaller number of open-ended or semi-open questions. Respondents were requested to base their answers on an average farrowing batch during the preceding year. The full questionnaire (in Swedish) is available upon request from the corresponding author.

Questionnaires and a stamped, addressed return envelope, as well as a short missive with instructions to the veterinarians, were distributed by mail during February 2012 to the 16 veterinarians employed by the Swedish Animal Health Service. A reminder to the veterinarians was sent out in May. In November, a second reminder was sent out to individual veterinarians by e-mail together with a list of herds from which responses were missing. Three veterinarians withdrew from the study. Following an initial telephone contact, these questionnaires were instead distributed to the corresponding herds by mail. A similar procedure was employed for herds supervised by Lunden's Animal Health Service ($n = 11$).

Data editing

In total, the 59 questions in the questionnaire corresponded to 63 different variables (including the outcome) as some questions included information on more than one parameter. Due to poor question design or low response rates (>25% missingness), 14 questions were discarded (10 and 4, respectively). See Fig. 1 for an overview.

All answers were treated as categorical variables. To facilitate the analyses, some answers were amalgamated into fewer categories. Answers on interval scale was categorised in quartiles ("sow batch size"). Other semi-open questions with numerical answers were often given in intervals, e.g. 2–3, and were categorised accordingly ("entry of sows to the farrowing unit" and "desired temperature in the farrowing unit"). The outcome "presence of neonatal diarrhoea", was specified in the questionnaire as diarrhoea in piglets younger than seven days with the possible responses "Yes", "No", and "Occasional cases". In the analyses, the outcome was treated as a binomial variable where "No" and "Occasional cases" were merged.

Most variables (Tables 1, 2, 3) are self-explanatory but some clarifications may be needed. "Efforts made to save weak-born piglets" were categorized as "none/some efforts" and "moderate/ambitious efforts" Criteria for categorising the answers as "some" were: one or two simple measures such as placing the piglet under the heat lamp or by the udder. Criteria for categorising the answers as "moderate/ambitious" were: two or more simple measures as stated above or providing

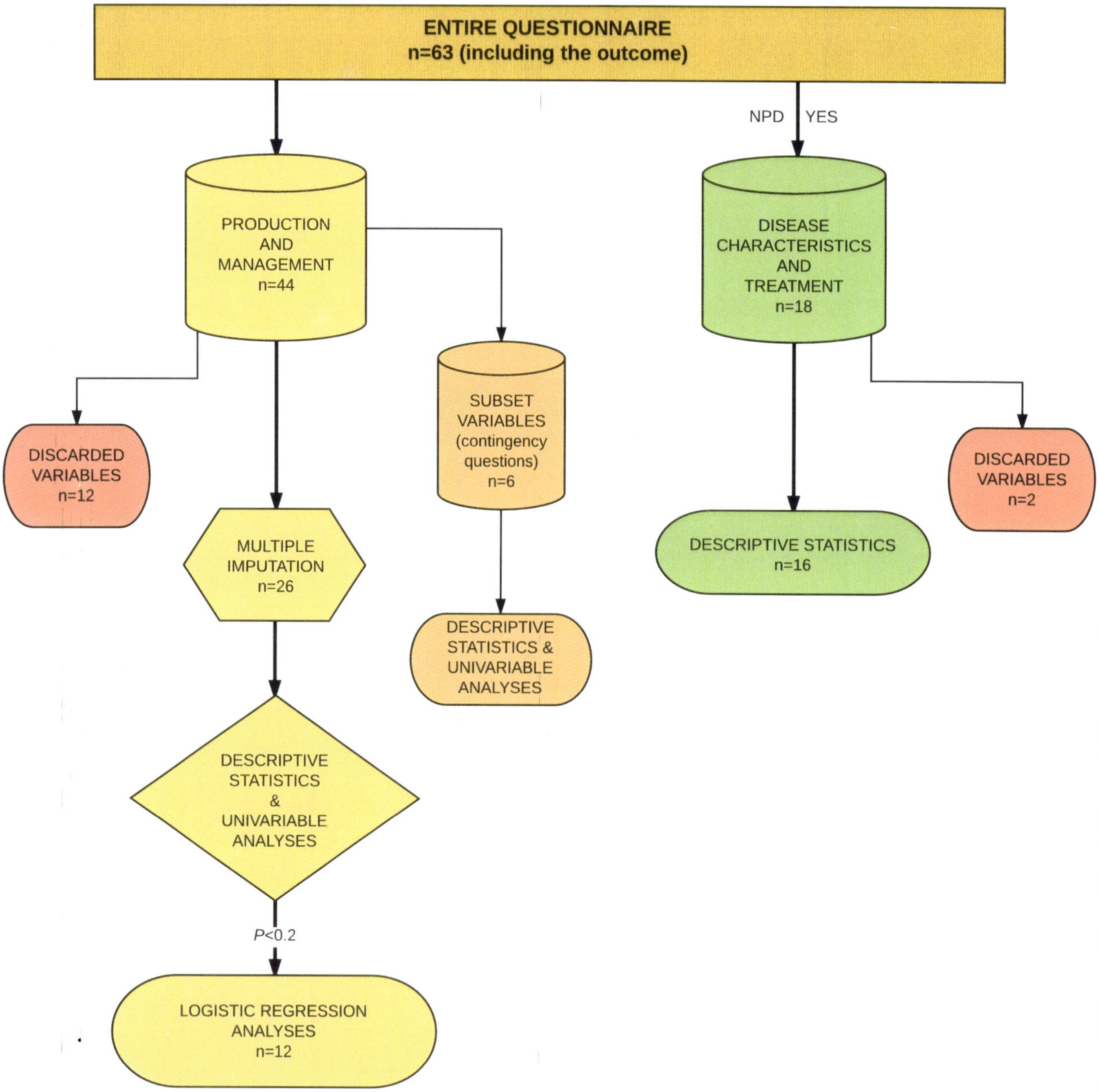

Fig. 1 Overview of data processing and analyses. The questionnaire included a total of 59 questions corresponding to 63 variables (including the outcome), as some questions included information on more than one parameter. In the illustration above "n" denotes the number of variables in the different sections of the questionnaire and in the following data processing and statistical analyses

Table 1 Distribution and univariable analysis of herd characteristics in 42 herds experiencing neonatal porcine diarrhoea (NPD herds) and 56 herds with no or occasional cases (non-NPD herds)

Variable[a]	NPD herds n (%)	Non-NPD herds n (%)	*P* value[b]
Building or renovation of stables used as farrowing units			0.05[d]
Earlier than 1990	3 (7)	11 (20)	
1990–2000	7 (17)	18 (32)	
Varies between units	12 (29)	10 (18)	
Later than 2000	20 (48)	17 (30)	
Number of sows in production			<0.01[c]
<200	20 (48)	44 (79)	
>200	22 (52)	12 (21)	
Batch size			<0.01[c]
<20	6 (14)	23 (41)	
20–34	9 (21)	16 (29)	
>34–46	12 (29)	11 (20)	
>46	15 (36)	6 (11)	
Recording of production results			0.02[d]
Yes	40 (95)	44 (79)	
No	2 (5)	12 (21)	
Level of gilt recruitment			0.18[c]
<30%	9 (21)	18 (32)	
30–40%	10 (24)	19 (34)	
>40%	16 (39)	11 (20)	
Unknown	7 (17)	8 (14)	

[a] Respondents were requested to base their answers on an average farrowing batch during the last 12 months

[b] P value of the entire variable

[c] χ^2-test

[d] Fisher's exact test

Table 2 Distribution and univariable analysis of management routines in 42 herds experiencing neonatal porcine diarrhoea (NPD herds) and 56 herds with no or occasional cases (Non-NPD herds)

Variable[a]	NPD herds n (%)	Non-NPD herds n (%)	*P* value[b]
Manual cleaning of the farrowing unit (times/day)[c]			0.12[d]
0–1	27 (64)	26 (46)	
2–3	15 (36)	30 (58)	
Washing of the farrowing unit between batches			<0.01[e]
Always	35 (83)	32 (57)	
During summer	5 (12)	9 (16)	
No	2 (5)	15 (27)	
Disinfection of the farrowing unit between batches			0.07[d]
Yes	28 (67)	26 (46)	
No	14 (33)	30 (54)	
Maternal vaccination against NPD			0.02[e]
Yes	40 (95)	43 (83)	
No	2 (5)	13 (25)	
Employment of nurse sows			0.01[d]
Yes	24 (57)	17 (30)	
No	18 (43)	39 (70)	
Monitoring of farrowings			0.17[e]
Only if indicated	3 (7)	11 (20)	
During daytime	35 (83)	38 (68)	
During day and night	4 (10)	7 (13)	
Efforts made to save weak-born piglets			<0.01[d]
None/some	18 (43)	43 (77)	
Moderate/ambitious	24 (57)	13 (23)	
Type of supplemental heating in the creep area			0.19[e]
Heat lamp	11 (26)	24 (43)	
Floor heating	4 (10)	6 (10)	
Lamp and floor heating	27 (64)	25 (45)	
Other	0 (0)	1 (2)	

[a] Respondents were requested to base their answers on an average farrowing batch during the last 12 months

[b] P value of the entire variable

[c] First week after farrowing

[d] χ^2-test

[e] Fisher's exact test

supplemental colostrum, providing active heating of piglets such as placement in warm water, or practicing split-suckling. Vaccination routines were categorised based on compliance with the current recommendations. For questions related to production, only data from respondents systematically recording data using PigWin Sugg [22] were included. From these production parameters, "number of live born piglets/sow" and "number of weaned piglets/sow" were selected and the answers compared with the national averages (includes data from 58 657 sows from 149 Swedish herds) of 13.2 and 10.8, respectively [23]. The answers were categorized as "good": both parameters above average, or one parameter above and one on average, "intermediate": one parameter above average and one below, or "low": both parameters below average, or one on average and one below.

Statistics

Prior to statistical analyses, missing values for explanatory variables in the section "production and management routines" were managed by multiple imputation (MI) using a nonparametric method in the CRAN package MissForest [24, 25]. In MI, missing values are

Table 3 Disease characteristics and management of neonatal porcine diarrhoea (NPD) in 42 herds experiencing more than occasional NPD-cases

Variable	Responses n (%)
Age of affected piglets	
First 24 h	2 (5)
1–3 days	26 (62)
3–7 days	9 (21)
Varied	3 (7)
Missing	2 (5)
Higher prevalence of NPD in litters from first parity sows	
Yes	34 (81)
No	7 (17)
Not known	1 (2)
Treatment of NPD	
Antimicrobials	18 (43)
Antimicrobials and fluids	14 (33)
Antimicrobials and fluids, and NSAID	2 (5)
"Injection"	3 (7)
Prophylactic treatment with antimicrobials	1 (2)
Missing	4 (10)
First choice of antimicrobial to treat NPD	
Amoxicillin	5 (12)
Penicillin	2 (5)
Fluoroquinolones	3 (7)
Neomycin	6 (14)
Trimethoprim/sulphonamide (sulfadiazine or sulfadoxine)	24 (57)
Tylosin	1 (2)
Missing	1 (2)
Prophylactic measures used against NPD	
Changed vaccination routines	5 (12)
Hygienic measures	6 (14)
Vaccination	2 (5)
Vaccination and hygienic measures	2 (5)
Faecal feedback	6 (14)
No specific measures	20 (48)
Missing	1 (2)

predicted based on the observed values for other variables in the dataset. The imputed dataset hence maintains the overall variability in the population while preserving relationships with other variables. The dataset for imputation only contained variables applicable for all respondents and hence, answers to contingency questions corresponding to six variables were removed before imputation. The dataset therefore totalled 26 explanatory variables for which the maximum missingness of any individual variable was 10% (Fig. 1).

The associations between the explanatory variables and NPD were initially analysed univariably (χ^2 –test or Fisher's exact tests in case of cell frequencies <5). The results were compared with equivalent analyses on the original non-imputed data with no considerable differences (see Additional file 1: Table S1). Variables with an association to NPD of $P < 0.2$ in the univariable analyses were subsequently examined by logistic regression models. The variable "number of sows per farrowing batch" was, however, excluded as sows in production (SIP) was considered a better measure of herd size. Hence, a total of 12 explanatory variables were included (Tables 1, 2). To check the selected explanatory variables for multicollinearity, variance inflation factors (VIF) were calculated using the CRAN package car [26], interpreting a VIF >5 as indicative for multicollinearity. No variable was removed due to multicollinearity. As herd size may be assumed to be associated with differences in production and management routines, the relationship between these variables and SIP was evaluated. Out of the 11 variables, all but "disinfection between farrowing batches" and "monitoring of farrowings" were significantly associated with SIP in univariable tests (see Additional file 2: Table S2 for descriptive data and univariable analyses). Due to these inter variable relationships the effect of SIP was estimated in a univariable logistic regression model whereas the other variables were analysed in a multivariable logistic regression model. Multivariable model building was done by backward stepwise elimination with re-entering based on Wald-tests of main effects until all remaining effects were significant at $P < 0.05$. Potential confounding was considered in each step by comparing the estimates of the variables with and without the possible confounder. A change of >30% in the estimates was interpreted as confounding, in which case the variable was retained in the model.

Apart from variables included in the imputed dataset, descriptive statistics and univariable analysis of associations with NPD are presented for subset variables from the sections "production and management". Variables from the section "disease characteristics and treatment of NPD in affected herds" are presented descriptively. All statistical analyses were performed in R version 3.2.2 [27].

Results

Of the 101 questionnaires returned by April 2013 one was blank. Further, information on the presence of NPD in the herd was missing from two respondents. The number of usable questionnaires therefore totalled 98 (response rate of 58%). Forty-two herds reported experience of more than occasional cases of NPD during the previous year, 36 reported occasional cases and 20 reported no occurrence. Hence, the total prevalence of farmer experienced NPD, including occasional cases was 79.6% (95% CI 70.6–86.4%) whereas the prevalence of herds experiencing a recurrent problem with NPD was 43% (95% CI 33.5–52.7%).

Herd characteristics and management routines

Of the 98 herds included in the study, 43 had integrated or partially integrated production, 34 were specialised piglet producers, 18 were satellite herds in sow pool-systems, and three were specialised gilt-producing or nucleus herds. The majority of herds (n = 64) had less than 200 sows in production. Of the 63 herds that recorded production results with PigWin Sugg, 23 had production results that were classified as "good", 10 had "intermediate" results, and 21 had production results that was lower than average (information was lacking from 9 herds). There was no statistical difference between NPD and non-NPD herds ($P = 0.68$).

All in-all out was practiced in the farrowing unit in 86 of the 98 herds and 67 washed the farrowing units between each batch. Maternal vaccination against agents associated with NPD was routinely performed in 83 of the herds. All vaccinating herds used vaccines against ETEC, seven in combination with *C. perfringens* type C and three in combination with *C. perfringens* type A and C (information was lacking from six herds). Eleven herds had changed vaccine during the last year. Most herds vaccinated sows and gilts at least three weeks prior to farrowing (68 and 52 out of the 83, respectively). However, in ten herds (four NPD and six non-NPD herds), gilts were only vaccinated once. Supplemental heating of the creep area was provided in all herds. However, in herds using heat lamps as the only heat source (n = 34), lamps with a low wattage (≤150 W) were more common in herds with NPD ($P = 0.02$).

Herd characteristics and management routines with associations to NPD of $P < 0.2$ in univariable tests are presented in Tables 1 and 2, respectively. Data on additional variables applicable for all 98 herds are available in Additional file 1: Table S1.

Analysis of potential risk factors for neonatal porcine diarrhoea on herd level

The univariable logistic regression analysis on the effect of herd size (number of sows in production, SIP) on the presence of NPD showed that herds with >200 SIP had a higher risk of having NPD compared with herds <200 SIP ($P < 0.01$). The estimated odds ratio for herds with >200 SIP was 4.0 (95% CI 1.7–10).

The multivariable logistic regression analysis of management factors rendered a final model which only included the variable "efforts made to save weak-born piglets" ($P < 0.01$). Herds where moderate to ambitious efforts were made to take care of weak piglets had a higher risk of having NPD compared with herds where none or only some efforts were made. The estimated odds ratio for herds where moderate to ambitious efforts were made was 4.4 (95% CI 1.9–11).

Disease characteristics and treatment of NPD

Among the 42 herds with more than occasional cases of NPD, the majority (33 out of 42) estimated that less than 25% of the piglets were affected by diarrhoea in an average farrowing batch. Diarrhoea was most common 1–3 days after birth (26 out of 42) and did often affect more than 50% of piglets in diarrhoeic litters (29 out of 42). The mortality due to NPD was estimated to be <10% in most herds (30 out of 42). In 29 of the 42 herds, the occurrence of diarrhoea in the herd was described as constant (18) or intermittent (11), whereas ten stated that the diarrhoea had decreased, and three that it had increased during the last year. Seasonal variations were only described in four herds (more during winter and spring). Diarrhoeic piglets were most commonly treated with antimicrobials only, or antimicrobials in combination with supplemental fluids (18 out of 42 and 14 out of 42, respectively). The drug of choice was trimethoprim/sulphonamide (24 out of 42) and 34 stated that treatment was successful in more than 75% of the cases. In case of poor response to initial treatment, 19 stated that they used fluoroquinolones as a second drug of choice. Efforts to investigate the cause of NPD had been undertaken in 13 out of 42 herds during the preceding year and three stated that the cause of diarrhoea had been established.

The prophylactic measures used to prevent NPD were grouped as "changed vaccination routines" (5), "hygienic measures" (6), "vaccination" (2), "vaccination and hygienic measures" (2), "faecal feedback" (6), and "no specific measures" (20). Hygienic measures were often not specified, and although most herds with diarrhoea vaccinated against NPD, only two respondents mentioned vaccination alone as a specific prophylactic measure. Among the 21 respondents reporting that specific prophylactic measures were employed, the effect was appreciated to be poor by two, moderate by 12, and successful by five (three missing answers). Measures with successful effect were hygienic measures and/or vaccination. Faecal back feeding was estimated to have poor (2) or moderate effect (4). An overview of disease characteristics and treatment of NPD in affected herds are presented in Table 3.

Discussion

The total herd-level prevalence of farmer experienced NPD (79.6%; 95% CI 70.6–86.4%) indicates that diarrhoea in neonatal piglets is common among Swedish piglet-producing herds. Interestingly, many herds experienced more than occasional NPD cases, despite maternal vaccination against ETEC or ETEC and *C. perfringens* (93% of the 42 herds with more than occasional cases of NPD). Moreover, a broad range of different antimicrobials were used for treatment (trimethoprim/sulphonamide, neomycin, amoxicillin, fluoroquinolones, penicillin, and tylosin). Taken together, these results suggest that NPD is a substantial problem and that prophylaxis and treatment regimens recommended against ETEC are not always efficient. Further, the results indicated that larger herd size (>200 SIP) and making more efforts to save weak-born piglets could be potential risk factors for experiencing NPD on herd-level.

The estimated prevalence of diarrhoea on herd level

Previous studies on the herd-level prevalence of NPD are lacking and epidemiological studies on pre-weaning diarrhoea have hitherto focused on incidence rates on litter level [10, 11, 28, 29]. In the present study, presence of NPD in a herd was subjectively estimated by the individual farmer as "Yes", "No", or "Occasional cases" during the preceding year. Thus, the prevalence reported in this study estimates how Swedish farmers experienced the problem with NPD in their herds rather than being an objective measure of the occurrence of diarrhoea. Moreover, the reported "farmer experienced" herd-level prevalence of 79.6% (including occasional cases) may be influenced by selection bias since farmers from herds with NPD might have been more motivated to complete the questionnaire. However, even if all of the 72 non-responders were herds without NPD, the prevalence would still be considerable (45.9%, 95% CI 38.6–53.4%).

Association of NPD with herd characteristics and management routines

To investigate whether presence of NPD on herd level could be associated with certain herd characteristics or management routines we wanted to compare herds experiencing a more recurrent problem with NPD from herds with less prominent or no problems. Thus, for these analyses the categories "occasional cases" and "no" were merged.

Before statistical analyses, missing data was handled by MI as MI analyses generally produce less biased and more precise (smaller standard errors) results than complete case analyses [30].

In the present study, larger herds (>200 SIP) were found to be significantly associated with experiencing NPD (OR = 4.0). The categorisation of herds size as <200 or >200 SIP was based on the average Swedish herd size of 186 sows [31]. Associations between herd size and risk for disease have previously been described for a number of infectious porcine diseases including pre-weaning diarrhoea [9, 11, 32]. The relationship has been discussed to not only depend on differences in the number of animals but also on environmental factors and management routines that may differ between smaller and larger herds [32]. This is supported by the present results where herd size was significantly associated with most of the herd characteristics and management routines that had a univariable association with NPD of $P < 0.2$ (see Additional file 2: Table S2). Assuming that these differences may partially explain the association between herd size and NPD, such factors could be considered as intervening variables. Statistical analysis of such interrelated variables is problematic. It is therefore recommended not to include intervening variables when investigating the association between explanatory variables (predictors) of interest and the outcome by multivariate modelling [33]. The association between herd size and NPD was hence analysed separately.

By multivariate analysis of other herd characteristics and management routines (n = 11), efforts made to save week-born piglets were shown to have a significant effect on the likelihood of experiencing NPD ($P < 0.01$). Interestingly, making more ambitious efforts to save weak piglets was associated with a higher risk of experiencing diarrhoea (OR = 4.4). One explanation for this may be that an increased handling of piglets could lead to an increased spread of pathogens between litters. However, it could also be that more ambitious animal caretakers were more likely to report NPD, or that newborn piglets were given extra attention because the herd had a NPD-problem. Lastly, it cannot be excluded that promoting survival of weak piglets indirectly could lead to an increased number of NPD-cases as these pigs may be more prone to develop diarrhoea.

Other factors significantly associated with NPD in the univariable tests were maternal vaccination against NPD, age of the farrowing building(s), recording of production results, washing of the farrowing unit, and employment of nurse sows (see Tables 1, 2). Maternal vaccination against ETEC was more common in herds with recurrent NPD as compared to herds with no or occasional cases ($P = 0.02$, see Table 2). As the presence of NPD is the incentive to vaccinate this is not surprising. However, the presence of more than occasional cases in vaccinating herds is notable (39 herds in total). Furthermore, 21% of the 39 vaccinating herds with NPD estimated that the average proportion of piglets affected per batch was >25%, thus indicating a substantial problem. The use of faecal back-feeding as a preventive measure against NPD in six of these herds further underlines that the effect of commercial vaccines was considered unsatisfactory. Possible explanations include inadequate vaccination routines, inadequate colostrum intake, or that piglets contracted diarrhoea despite a satisfactory passive immune status against ETEC and *C. perfringens* type C. Further, both the use of nurse sows and more rigorous washing routines (washing between each farrowing batch) were more common in herds experiencing more than occasional cases of NPD. These results hence follow the same trend as "efforts made to save weak-born piglets" suggesting that an increased use of zootechnical interventions could be associated with NPD. Again, it is however not possible to make any causal inferences from the present investigation. Nonetheless, a high level of intervention measures has previously been suggested as a contributing factor to recurrent NPD problems in high-performance herds [18, 34]. Thus, further investigations are needed.

Taken together, these results underline that the presence of NPD may be influenced by several aspects with complex interrelationships. It should however be stressed that the outcome in the present study reflects "farmer-experienced" NPD. Whereas this gives interesting descriptive information on how the presence of NPD is perceived, the subjective estimates of NPD-presence as "Yes", "No", or "Occasional cases" may not be consistent between herds. An objective classification of the presence of NPD should therefore be employed in future investigations of the potential risk factors suggested by the present study.

Disease manifestation and intervention strategies

In accordance with previous studies, most farmers stated that diarrhoea was more common in first-parity sow litters [29, 35, 36]. This is probably a reflection of first-parity sows having a poorly developed immunity against pathogens present in the farrowing unit [37]. However, since the question was phrased in a way which may be considered leading (Is diarrhoea more common in litters from first parity sows?), the answers might have been skewed.

Treatment of NPD commonly included antimicrobials only (43%; 18/42) or combined with supplementary fluids (33%; 14/42). A smaller proportion (7%; 3/42) had only stated "by injection" which likely could be interpreted as injection with antimicrobials. Notably, microbiological investigations of NPD had only been undertaken in 31% (13/42) of the affected herds during the preceding year. In addition, one respondent stated that all piglets were treated with antimicrobials after birth to prevent NPD. This frequent use of antimicrobials against NPD makes the development of alternative control strategies a necessity. Highlighting this need, a study of antimicrobial usage in Swedish pig herds recently showed that the highest treatment incidence occurs in suckling piglets [38]. Targeted health improvements in this age group may therefore be the most efficient way to further decrease the use of antibiotics.

The drug of choice in the present investigation was trimethoprim in combination with sulfadiazine/sulfadoxine (57%; 24/42), which is the recommended treatment against ETEC. Interestingly, however, 40% (17/42) of the herds used other antimicrobials (one missing answer). This could suggest an unsatisfactory effect by trimethoprim/sulphonamide treatment due to resistant ETEC, or that the treatment targeted bacteria other than *E. coli* (e.g. the use of penicillin or tylosin). Since many herds also reported more than occasional cases of NPD despite ETEC vaccination, the results suggest that prophylaxis and treatment regimens recommended against ETEC not always are efficient. This corresponds to recent pathological and microbiological studies, demonstrating occurrence of NPD unrelated to the presence of previously well-known enteropathogens in Sweden and Denmark [17, 19]. Prevalence studies on enteropathogens associated with NPD would hence be of great interest.

Considerations on the study design

The distribution of the questionnaire via the herd veterinarians was chosen as we hypothesised that this would yield a higher response rate as compared to distribution by mail. However, some veterinarians (4 out of 17) were not able to complete the study and thus, the corresponding questionnaires were instead distributed directly to the herds by mail. Due to the small number of questionnaires per veterinarian, differences between veterinarians and distribution method were however not included in the analysis and hence, these potential confounders should be kept in mind when interpreting the results. Furthermore, we do not know if responder and non-responder herds differed in terms of size, production results etc. since no data from non-responders were available. A nationwide, up-to-date register of pig herds in Sweden including information on herd size would greatly facilitate this type of studies. However, in the 63 herds using PigWin Sugg, production data was comparable to the average results reported by Swedish PigWin users during 2012.

Some information was not obtained due to inadequately designed questions (n = 10). Unfortunately, this included treatment frequencies of post-partum dysgalactia syndrome (PPDS) that is a known risk factor for NPD [10, 11, 28, 39]. The major reasons for the exclusion of questions were misinterpretation, or that the respondent had marked more than one response option making it impossible to create mutually exclusive categories. These problems could probably have been avoided by a more extensive pilot testing of the questionnaire. Moreover, one question excluded due to a low response rate (>25% missingness) was temperature in the creep area which possibly reflects that the temperature was not known by the respondents. This is noteworthy considering that the ambient temperature is known to be of great importance for the survival of the newborn pig [40–42].

Conclusions

The results of the present study indicate that Swedish farmers commonly experience NPD in their herds, often despite vaccination against ETEC. Considering that antimicrobials are frequently used as treatment, preventive measures against NPD need to be improved. To find rational means for intervention, identification of factors potentially related to the disease is important. In the present study, larger herd size and making more ambitious efforts to save weak-born piglets were suggested as potential risk factors and further studies of the underlying biological reasons for these relationships are warranted.

Additional files

Additional file 1: Table S1. Comparison of original and imputed data. Descriptive data and univariable associations between 26 variables and neonatal porcine diarrhoea in 98 herds (42 herds experiencing NPD and 56 experiencing no or only occasional cases) before and after multiple imputation of missing values for explanatory variables.

Additional file 2: Table S2. Associations with herd size. Descriptive data and univariable associations between herd size (<200 and >200 sows in production) and explanatory variables selected for regression analyses.

Authors' contributions

JL, ML, and MJ planned the study and the questionnaire. JL organised the data collection and carried out the statistical analyses together with NF. JL wrote the first draft of the manuscript while NF, ML, and MJ contributed to finalizing the manuscript. All authors read and approved the final manuscript.

Author details

[1] Department of Clinical Sciences, Swedish University of Agricultural Sciences, Box 7054, SE-75007 Uppsala, Sweden. [2] Farm and Animal Health, Kungsängens Gård hus 6 B, SE-753 23 Uppsala, Sweden.

Acknowledgements

The authors would like to acknowledge all participating farmers as well as veterinarians from the Farm and Animal Health organisation and Lunden's Animal Health Ltd.

Competing interests

The authors declare that they have no competing interests.

Funding

This research received no specific grant from any funding agency, commercial or not-for-profit sectors.

References

1. Thomson JR, Friendship RM. Digestive system. In: Zimmerman JJ, Karriker LA, Ramirez A, Schwartz KJ, Stevenson GW, editors. Diseases of Swine. 10th ed. Chichester: Wiley-Blackwell; 2012. p. 216–8.
2. Sjölund M, Zoric M, Wallgren P. Financial impact of disease on pig production. Part III. Gastrointestinal disorders. In: proceedings of the 6th European symposium of Porcine Health Management. Italy: Sorrento; 2014.
3. Carvajal A, Argüello H, Martínez-Lobo FJ, Costillas S, Miranda R, de Nova PJ, et al. Porcine epidemic diarrhoea: new insights into an old disease. Porcine Health Manag. 2015;1:1–8.
4. Martineau GP, Vaillancourt JP, Broes A. Principal Neonatal Diseases. In: Varley MA, editor. The Neonatal Pig-Development and Survival. Wallingford: CAB International; 1995. p. 239–64.
5. Drew M, Owen B. The provision of passive immunity to colostrum-deprived piglets by bovine or porcine serum immunoglobulins. Can J Anim Sci. 1988;68:1277–84.
6. Sarmiento JI. Environmental temperature: a predisposing factor in the enterotoxigenic Escherichia coli-induced diarrhea of the newborn pig. Diss. Guelph: University of Guelph; 1983.
7. Blecha F, Kelley KW. Cold stress reduces the acquisition of colostral immunoglobulin in piglets. J Anim Sci. 1981;52:594–600.
8. Kelley KW, Blecha F, Regnier JA. Cold exposure and absorption of colostral immunoglobulins by neonatal pigs. J Anim Sci. 1982;55:363–8.
9. Dewey CE, Wittum TE, Hurd HS, Dargatz D, Hill GW. Herd-and litter-level factors associated with the incidence of diarrhea morbidity and mortality in piglets 4–14 days of age. Swine Health Prod. 1995;3:105–12.
10. Wittum TE, Dewey CE, Hurd HS, Dargatz DA, Hill GW. Herd-and litter-level factors associated with the incidence of diarrhea morbidity and mortality in piglets 1–3 days of age. Swine Health Prod. 1995;3:99–104.
11. Svensmark B, Jorsal S, Nielsen K, Willeberg P. Epidemiological studies of piglet diarrhoea in intensively managed Danish sow herds. I. Pre-weaning diarrhoea. Acta Vet Scand. 1988;30:43–53.
12. Malmkvist J, Pedersen LJ, Damgaard BM, Thodberg K, Jørgensen E, Labouriau R. Does floor heating around parturition affect the vitality of piglets born to loose housed sows? Appl Anim Behav Sci. 2006;99:88–105.
13. Westin R, Holmgren N, Hultgren J, Ortman K, Linder A, Algers B. Post-mortem findings and piglet mortality in relation to strategic use of straw at farrowing. Prev Vet Med. 2015;119:141–52.
14. Devillers N, Le Dividich J, Prunier A. Influence of colostrum intake on piglets survival and immunity. Animal. 2011;5:1605–12.
15. Söderlind O, Thafvelin B, Möllby R. Virulence factors in *Escherichia coli* strains isolated from Swedish piglets with diarrhea. J Clin Microbiol. 1988;26:879–84.
16. Swedish board of Agriculture. Annual report on notifiable diseases of animals 2012. Sweden: Swedish board of Agriculture 2012. http://webbutiken.jordbruksverket.se/sv/artiklar/ovr310v12.html. Acessed 12 July 2016.
17. Kongsted H, Jonach B, Haugegaard S, Angen Ø, Jorsal SE, Kokotovic B, et al. Microbiological, pathological and histological findings in four Danish pig herds affected by a new neonatal diarrhoea syndrome. BMC Vet Res. 2013;9:206.
18. Gin T, Le Guennec J, Morvan H, Martineau G-P. Clinical and laboratory investigations in 10 French pig herds dealing with enzootic neonatal diarrhoea. In: proceedings of the 21st International Pig Veterinary Society Congress. Vancouver; 2010.
19. Larsson J, Aspán A, Lindberg R, Grandon R, Båverud V, Fall N, et al. Pathological and bacteriological characterization of neonatal porcine diarrhoea of uncertain aetiology. J Med Microbiol. 2015;64:916–26.
20. Jonach B, Boye M, Stockmarr A, Jensen TK. Fluorescence in situ hybridization investigation of potentially pathogenic bacteria involved in neonatal porcine diarrhea. BMC Vet Res. 2014;10:68.
21. Statistics Sweden. Yearbook of agricultural statistics 2012 including food statistics. Sweden: official statistics of Sweden 2012. https://www.jordbruksverket.se/omjordbruksverket/statistik/jordbruksstatistisksammanstallning. Accessed 12 July 2016.
22. WinPig startsida. http://www.gardochdjurhalsan.se/sv/winpig/. Accessed 4 April 2016.
23. Farm and animal health. Medeltal suggor 2012. Sweden: Farm and animal health 2012. http://www.gardochdjurhalsan.se/sv/winpig/medeltal-och-topplistor/medeltal-suggor/. Accessed 12 July 2016.

24. Stekhoven DJ. MissForest: nonparametric missing value imputation using random forest. Astrophys Sour Code Libr. 2015;1:05011.
25. Stekhoven DJ, Bühlmann P. MissForest—non-parametric missing value imputation for mixed-type data. Bioinformatics. 2012;28:112–8.
26. Fox J, Weisberg S. An R companion to applied regression. 2nd ed. Thousand Oaks: Sage; 2011.
27. R Core Team. R: a language and environment for statistical computing. Vienna: R Foundation for Statistical Computing; 2015.
28. Halgaard C. Epidemiologic factors in piglet diarrhea. Nord Vet Med. 1980;33:403–12.
29. Urcelay S, Hird D, Huffman E, Parker K, Farver T. Patterns of preweaning diarrhea in piglets on a central California ranch. Can J Comp Med. 1984;48:394.
30. Dohoo IR, Nielsen CR, Emanuelson U. Multiple imputation in veterinary epidemiological studies: a case study and simulation. Prev Vet Med. 2016;129:35–47.
31. Statistics Sweden. Yearbook of agricultural statistics 2013 including food statistics. Sweden: Official statistics of Sweden 2013. https://www.jordbruksverket.se/omjordbruksverket/statistik/jordbruksstatistisksammanstallning. Acessed 12 July 2016.
32. Gardner IA, Willeberg P, Mousing J. Empirical and theoretical evidence for herd size as a risk factor for swine diseases. Anim Health Res Rev. 2002;3:43–55.
33. Martin W. Making valid causal inferences from observational data. Prev Vet Med. 2014;113:281–97.
34. Goillandeau R, Vila T, Martineau GP. Neonatal diarrheas: a paradigmatic change. In: proceedings of the 19st International Pig Veterinary Society Congress. Copenhagen; 2006.
35. Kongsted H, Toft N, Nielsen JP. Risk factors and epidemiological characteristics of new neonatal porcine diarrhoea syndrome in four Danish herds. BMC Vet Res. 2014;10:151.
36. Wallgren P, Merza M. New neonatal porcine diarrhoea. I. clinical outcome in an affected herd. In: proceedings of the 22nd International pig veterinary society congress. Jeju; 2012.
37. Kruse PE. The importance of colostral immunoglobulins and their absorption from the intestine of the newborn animals. Ann Rech Vet. 1983;14:349–53.
38. Sjölund M, Backhans A, Greko C, Emanuelson U, Lindberg A. Antimicrobial usage in 60 Swedish farrow-to-finish pig herds. Prev Vet Med. 2015;121:257–64.
39. Svendsen J, Bille N, Nielsen N, Larsen J, Riising H. Preweaning mortality in pigs 4. Diseases of the gastrointestinal tract in pigs. Nord Vet Med. 1975;27:85–101.
40. Le Dividich J, Noblet J. Thermoregulation and energy metabolism in the neonatal pig. Ann Rech Vet. 1983;14:375–81.
41. Trayhurn P, Temple NJ, Van Aerde J. Evidence from immunoblotting studies on uncoupling protein that brown adipose tissue is not present in the domestic pig. Can J Physiol Pharmacol. 1989;67:1480–5.
42. Herpin P, Le Dividich J, Berthon D, Hulin JC. Assessment of thermoregulatory and postprandial thermogenesis over the first 24 hours after birth in pigs. Exp Physiol. 1994;79:1011–9.

Kinematic and spatiotemporal assessment of habituation to treadmill walking in Labrador retrievers

Pia Gustås[1*], Kjerstin Pettersson[2], Sofia Honkavaara[1,4], Anne-Sofie Lagerstedt[1] and Anna Byström[3]

Abstract

Background: This study investigated differences in kinematic and spatiotemporal variables in Labrador retrievers during introduction to treadmill walking, with the aim to determine the time required for them to become habituated. Twenty-five healthy, treadmill-naive Labrador retrievers participated in the study. The total angular displacement of the carpus, elbow, tarsus and stifle, as well as stride time and stance duration were calculated from the 3-D tracking of skin mounted reflective markers recorded with 6 infrared light emitting video cameras at 240 Hz. The measurements were done at two walking speeds, 0.78 and 0.96 m/s, in six sessions on the treadmill during two consecutive days.

Results: With a 1–2 min acclimatization period following each treadmill speed change, mean values of the study variables were significantly different from the last training session mainly in the first session on the first day. However, between-stride variability was significantly larger for at least one variable even in the fourth session for the slower walking speed, and in the fifth session for the higher walking speed.

Conclusions: The results show the importance of proper pre-training of dogs in locomotion studies at walk using a treadmill, and the need to consider not only variable mean values but also between-stride variability, in order to ensure that dogs are sufficiently accustomed to allow collection of reliable data.

Keywords: Canine, Kinematics, Locomotion, Orthopaedics, Rehabilitation

Background

A gait is formed through complex interactions between the musculoskeletal and the central and peripheral nervous system, where ambulation requires constant adaptation to both intrinsic and extrinsic factors. Orthopedic and other conditions that affect the function of either the nervous or the musculoskeletal system typically disrupt these interactions and thus lead to gait disturbances. To describe any such changes in a dog's locomotor function, a systematic approach with good repeatability of the selected gait variables is required. Because of movement variability, i.e. the inherent variation between strides present even within a stable gait pattern, it is necessary to record data from several strides to obtain a representative mean value [1–5]. Further, the influence of extrinsic factors, which may increase this variability, should be minimized during data collection, to obtain reproducible results from a minimum number of strides [6–10].

In order to record several strides from a stable gait, a treadmill has been found to be a useful tool, in human [11] and equine [12] as well as in canine [13] locomotion research. The advantage of a treadmill is that it provides a well-controlled setting with constant speed. Some studies in dogs have used a treadmill to record walking kinematics in healthy dogs [14, 15], as well as in dogs with different orthopaedic conditions [16–22].

The rationale behind using a treadmill is based on the assumption that its use induces a stable, repeatable gait. This is well established for humans, horses and

*Correspondence: pia.gustas@slu.se
[1] Department of Clinical Sciences, Faculty of Veterinary Medicine and Animal Husbandry, Swedish University of Agricultural Sciences, Box 7054, 750 07 Uppsala, Sweden
Full list of author information is available at the end of the article

dogs. On the other hand, for subjects unfamiliar with the treadmill it is known that their gait is characterised by both divergent mean values and increased between-stride variability [11, 23–25]. To obtain reliable data, it is therefore important to give new subjects enough time to become accustomed to a treadmill [11, 23, 26, 27]. This presents a challenge for measurements of dogs at walk because no studies have described the process of adaptation in dogs. Treadmill training of dogs in trot has been described [24, 25, 28–30] but because a study in horses showed that longer training time was needed to achieve habituation in walk compared to trot [23], recommendations for trotting dogs cannot safely be applied to walk.

This study aimed to describe the pattern of gait adaptation in naïve Labrador retrievers when trained to walk on a treadmill, and to determine the training time needed for them to become accustomed to treadmill walking. It was hypothesized that being unfamiliar with treadmill walking would change kinematic and spatiotemporal variables and increase the between-stride variability, and that these changes would decrease with time and evolve into a regular, repeatable walking pattern in six sessions of training during two days, similar to observations in our previous study on treadmill training of naïve Labrador retrievers in trot [25].

Methods

Data were collected in connection with our earlier study on treadmill habituation in trot [25]. The experimental setup has been described in detail earlier [25] and is therefore only summarized here.

Animals

Twenty-five healthy privately owned Labrador Retrievers (22–34 kg) aged 22–36 months were used. All dogs passed an orthopaedic examination on entering the study. No dog had previous experience of treadmill exercise. Informed consent was obtained from the owners, in accordance with the ethical guidelines for the study, approved by the Uppsala Animal Ethics Committee, Sweden and Swedish Board of Agriculture (No. C32/7).

Data collection

A rubber-belt treadmill (Rodby, Vänge, Sweden) with a 1.44 × 0.54-m running area was used. Dogs were always handled by the same person, held on a leash in the same manner. A motion analysis system with six infrared light emitting video cameras (Proreflex, Qualisys, Gothenburg, Sweden) was used to record three-dimensional kinematic data (240 Hz) using the proprietary camera software (Qualisys Track Manager, Qualisys, Gothenburg, Sweden).

A total of 26 spherical reflective markers, diameter 12 mm, were attached to each dog's skin by the same person, with double-sided adhesive tape and glue over specific anatomical landmarks. Marker positions for the forelimbs were as follows: the distal end of the fifth metacarpal bone, the lateral styloid process, the lateral epicondyle of the humerus and the acromion; and for the hind limbs: the distal end of the fifth metatarsal bone, the lateral malleolus, the lateral epicondyle of the femur and the greater trochanter of the femur.

Each dog performed six sessions on the treadmill, three on each day on two consecutive days. Between sessions dogs rested for 30 min. Each session lasted 8–10 min and was divided into four consecutive 2-min trials at different treadmill speeds. In session 1 the dogs only walked: in trial 1 at 0.78 m/s, in trial 2 at 0.96 m/s, in trial 3 at 0.78 m/s and in trial 4 at 0.96 m/s. For session 2 to 6, dogs first walked and then trotted: trial 1 was walk at 0.78 m/s; trial 2 was walk at 0.96 m/s; trial 3 was trot at 1.81 m/s and trial 4 was trot at 2.06 m/s. The walking speeds were aimed to be a slow walk and a normal-to-fast walk. Kinematic data were recorded for 10 s every 30 s, i.e. four 10-s motion data capture periods were recorded at each speed. The first motion capture period started as soon as the treadmill reached the predetermined speed for the specific trial. For each walking speed, the 10-s motion capture periods from each session were termed 1.1–1.4 and 1.5–1.8 (for session 1), 2.1–2.4 (for session 2) and so on up to 6.1–6.4 (for session 6). The number of strides recorded in each motion capture period ranged from 8 to 10.

The data from each motion capture period was divided into strides using a custom written program (MathWorks Inc, Natick, Mass). First contact and toe-off for each limb were determined from the vertical and horizontal velocity of the marker of the distal fifth metacarpal or metatarsal bone, respectively, in a semi-automatic procedure adapted from a method previously used for equine treadmill trotting [31].

To quantify the basic gait characteristics a selection of spatiotemporal and kinematic variables were calculated: Spatiotemporal variables were stride time (time between two consecutive first contacts of the left hind limb), and stance time (time between first contact and toe-off) and relative stance time (stance time divided by stride time) for each limb. The kinematic variables calculated were total angular displacement, i.e. the difference between stride maximum and minimum joint angles, for the carpal, elbow, tarsal and stifle joints, respectively.

Statistical methods

For all variables, mean and standard deviation (SD) were calculated for each dog and 10-s motion capture period.

Group mean and a 95% confidence interval (CI) were then calculated for each motion capture period, and these values were plotted for each walking speed and variable to visualize overlaps and differences between the consecutive motion capture periods.

For each speed and variable, the distribution of dog mean values across motion data capture periods were evaluated by the study of overlaps between the 95% CIs, and with paired *t* test of the respective periods with that of the last motion capture period (6.4). Further, differences in the distribution of SDs (used as a measure of between-stride variability) between the last motion capture period and the previous periods were compared using a Wilcoxon signed rank test (a non-parametric test was chosen because the SDs were not normally distributed).

Results

Total angular displacements remained largely unchanged during the study (Figs. 1, 2). Significant differences compared to the final motion capture period (6.4) were observed during the first 4 min of walking on the treadmill, i.e. the trial 1 at each speed in the first session. During motion capture periods 1.1–1.4 the total angular displacements were significantly larger for all evaluated joints, except for the elbow and carpus at the slower walking speed (0.78 m/s). At the faster walking speed (0.96 m/s) the carpus total angular displacement also tended to be larger during the second session and in the first motion capture period of the third session.

The spatiotemporal variables followed a similar pattern as the angular displacements (Figs. 3, 4); significant differences compared to the final motion capture period (6.4) were observed in motion capture periods 1.1–1.4 at each speed, and were more prominent at the slower walking speed (0.78 m/s). Both stride and stance times were shorter during the first session on the treadmill, and combined with the increased angular displacements this gave the walk an abnormal visual appearance. At 0.95 m/s stride time was shorter also in the second session, while at the slower walking speed (0.78 m/s) both stride and stance times tended to be shorter during the first two motion capture periods in each of the following sessions (Fig. 4), i.e. during the dogs' first minute on the treadmill after a rest period.

The intra-individual between-stride variability at the walk, measured as the intra-individual SD for each variable, changed for longer than the stride mean values (Table 1). At the higher walking speed (0.96 m/s) the SDs for stride time and elbow and carpal total angular displacements were significantly larger compared with the last motion capture period (6.4) even at the end of the 5th session (5.4). At the slower walking speed (0.78 m/s) the intra-individual variability decreased faster during

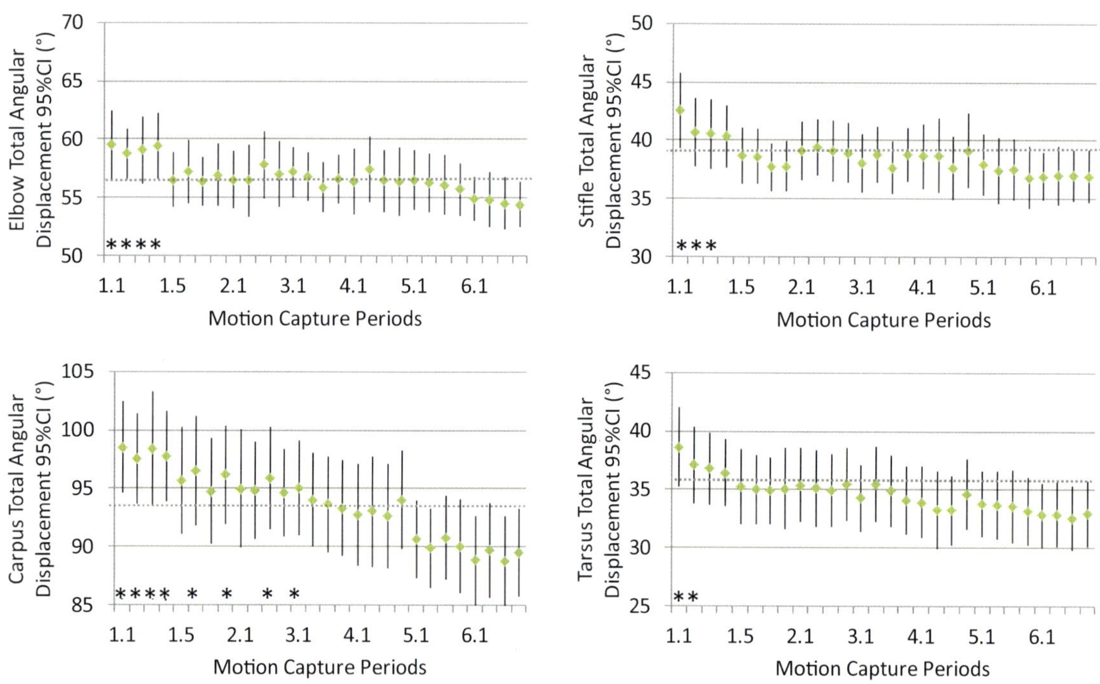

Fig. 1 Group mean values (*dot*) and 95% confidence intervals (*error bars*) for the total angular displacement of the elbow, carpus, stifle and tarsus in dogs (n = 25) walking on a treadmill at 0.96 m/s. Motion capture periods deviating significantly ($P < 0.05$) from the final motion capture period (6.4) are marked "*"

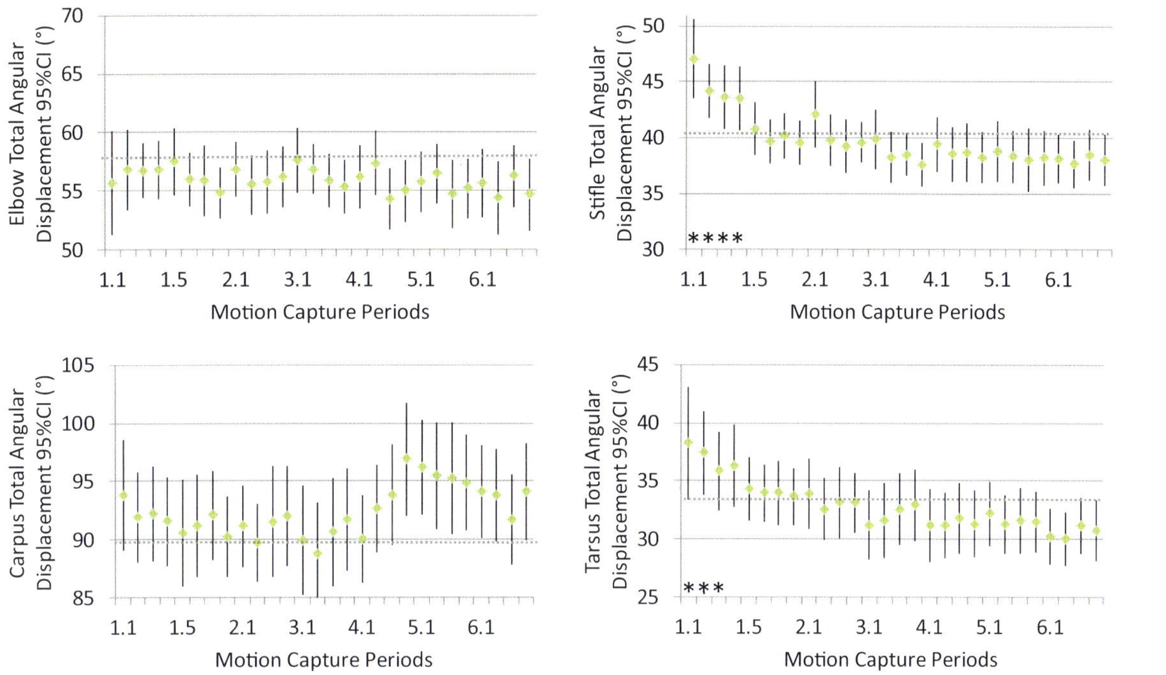

Fig. 2 Group mean values (*dot*) and 95% confidence intervals (*error bars*) for the total angular displacement of the elbow, carpus, stifle and tarsus in dogs (n = 25) walking on a treadmill at 0.78 m/s. Motion capture periods deviating significantly ($P < 0.05$) from the final motion capture period (6.4) are marked "*"

the habituation: already in the second motion capture period of the fourth session (4.2) the SDs did not differ significantly from the SDs of the last motion capture period (6.4) for any variable, with stride time and stifle total angular displacement being the last variables to stabilize. Further, if the first two motion capture periods in each session were excluded as time to acclimate after a rest period or change in speed, then the second motion capture period of the third session (3.2) became the last session at slow walk (0.78 m/s) for which the SDs for any variable were significantly larger compared with the final motion capture period (6.4). In contrast, at the higher walking speed (0.96 m/s) exclusion of the first minute in each session only slightly influenced the results: the only change in time of stabilization was for the total angular displacement of the stifle (Table 2).

Discussion

Dogs on their first encounter with the treadmill showed a clearly aberrant gait pattern: during the first 4 min the stride mean angular displacements of the joints were significantly larger, mean stance and stride times were significantly shorter, and the between-stride variability was significantly higher compared with in the final session. This is in accordance with findings in previous studies on walking humans [26, 32] and horses [23] and trotting dogs [24, 25]; it has been found that the gait of subjects unfamiliar with the treadmill is characterized by an altered movement pattern and increased between-stride variability. Further, in the current study the initial divergences in mean values were larger in walk compared with the same dogs in trot [25]. This could be related to the study design: all dogs performed their very first training session on the treadmill in walk only and trot was not included until the second session. However, a study in horses also found that individuals needed longer training time to become fully accustomed to treadmill walking compared with treadmill trotting [23]. Based on the latter finding, it can be speculated whether the longer training time for walk might be related to the differences in limb coordination and pattern of mechanical work that exist between walk and trot because these differences are common to both dogs and horses [33, 34].

As the training of the dogs progressed, the mean total angular displacement and stride and stance times soon stabilised at values not significantly different from those obtained in the final session (Figs. 1, 2, 3 and 4). This indicates that a marked gait adaptation occurred already during the initial walking sessions. However, the between-stride variability of the same variables, quantified as the intra-individual standard deviation over all strides recorded during a 10-s motion capture period, continued to decrease over a longer time before non-significant levels were reached (Tables 1, 2). This is in

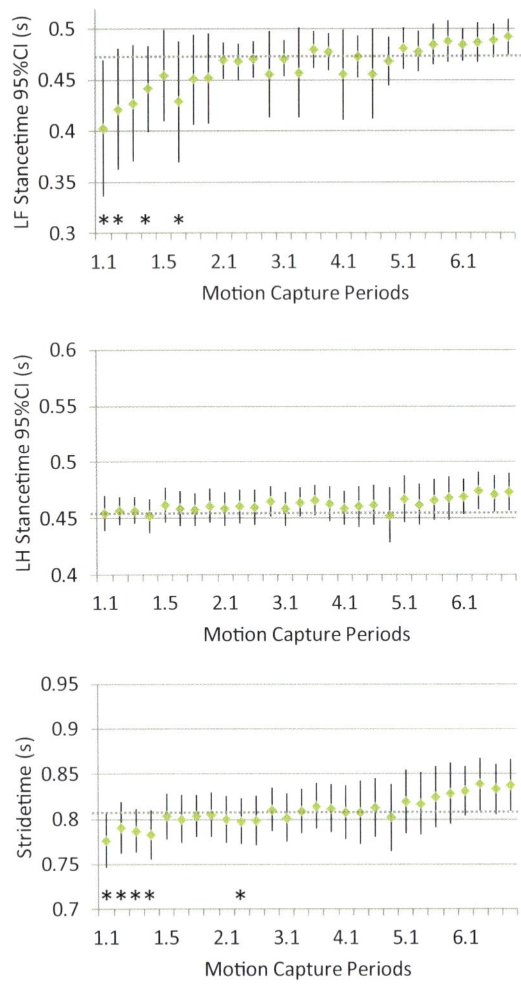

Fig. 3 Group mean values (*dot*) and the 95% confidence intervals (*error bars*) for the stride time, left forelimb (LF) and left hind limb (LH) stance in dogs (n = 25) walking on a treadmill at 0.96 m/s. Motion capture periods deviating significantly ($P < 0.05$) from the final motion capture period (6.4) are marked "*"

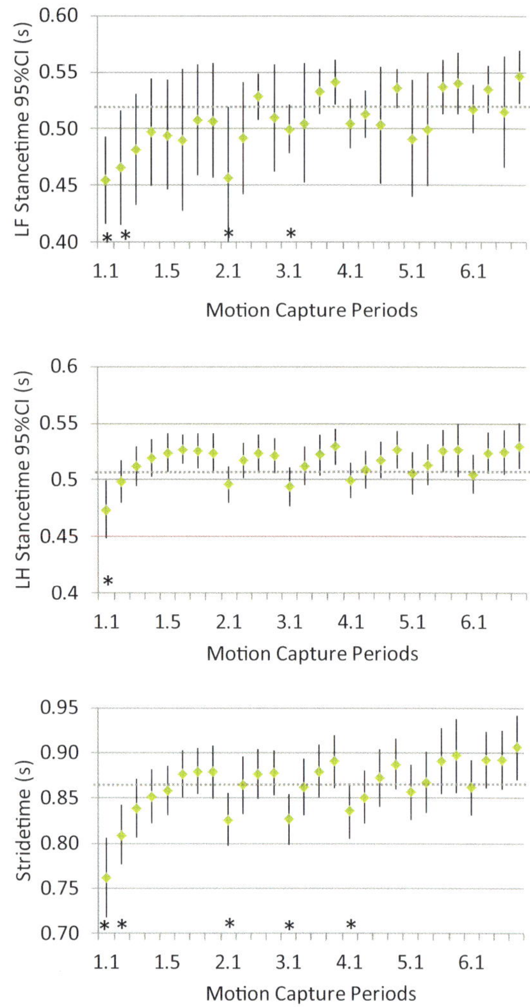

Fig. 4 Group mean values (*dot*) and the 95% confidence intervals (*error bars*) for the stride time, left forelimb (LF) and left hind limb (LH) stance in dogs (n = 25) walking on a treadmill at 0.78 m/s. Motion capture periods deviating significantly ($P < 0.05$) from the final motion capture period (6.4) are marked "*"

accordance with previous studies in humans [11, 35] and horses [23] and in trotting dogs [25]. Thus, the general pattern for treadmill gait adaptation appears to be that a longer training time is required to reduce variability of the gait variables, compared with the time needed for the gait to be just on average similar to the subject's gait when fully accustomed [23, 25, 35]. This stresses the need to not only assess mean values but also variability to determine whether a subject is fully accustomed to treadmill locomotion at a particular gait.

When comparing the literature on treadmill training of humans and horses at walk, it can be noted that the criteria for when a subject is considered sufficiently accustomed to treadmill locomotion varies somewhat between studies. In both an early human study and an equine study, full habituation was considered to have occurred when a consistent gait pattern was re-established in less than 1 or 2 min when returning to the treadmill for a new session [11, 23]. However, in later human studies, the subjects were considered to be sufficiently accustomed when a stable gait pattern was observed after 5 to 10 min [26, 27, 32, 35]. The current study therefore assessed how time to habituation was affected if a 1-min acclimatization period was allowed for at the beginning of each session. Dogs were fully habituated to treadmill walking in the fifth session at the slower speed (0.78 m/s) and in the sixth session at the higher speed (0.96 m/s). In these respective sessions none of the measured variables, neither mean values nor SDs, differed significantly from the last motion capture

Table 1 Spatiotemporal variables

Speed	0.78 m/s				0.96 m/s			
P-level	<0.001	<0.01	<0.05	<0.05#	<0.001	<0.01	<0.05	<0.05#
Stride time	1.2	3.1	4.1	2.4	2.1	4.2	5.4	5.4
Stance time LF	1.1	1.2	1.3	1.3	1.2	1.8	2.4	2.4
Stance time LH	1.3	2.1	3.1	2.4	2.1	4.1	4.4	4.4
Relative stance time LF	n/a	n/a	n/a	n/a	n/a	n/a	n/a	n/a
Relative stance time LH	1.2	1.5	2.1	1.7	1.1	1.1	1.3	1.3

Between-stride variability decrease for stride and stance times during treadmill training of dogs (n = 25) in walk at 0.78 and 0.96 m/s, respectively. Table values represent the last 10-s motion capture period during which the intra-individual SDs were significantly higher compared with the final motion capture period (6.4), determined from a paired Wilcoxon sign rank test

First two motion capture periods in each session excluded

Table 2 Angular displacements

Speed	0.78 m/s				0.96 m/s			
P-level	<0.001	<0.01	<0.05	<0.05#	<0.001	<0.01	<0.05	<0.05#
Elbow	1.5	2.1	2.3	2.3	3.3	5.2	5.4	5.4
Carpus	n/a	n/a	n/a	n/a	5.1	5.1	5.4	5.4
Stifle	1.2	3.1	4.1	2.4	1.8	3.2	5.1	4.3
Tarsus	1.4	2.1	3.1	1.8	3.2	5.1	5.1	4.4

Between-stride variability decrease for the stride total angular displacement of the elbow, carpus, stifle and tarsus during treadmill training of dogs (n = 25) in walk at 0.78 and 0.96 m/s, respectively. Table values represent the last 10-s motion capture period during which the intra-individual SDs were significantly higher compared with the final motion capture period (6.4), determined from a paired Wilcoxon sign rank test

First two motion capture periods in each session excluded

period (6.4), not even during the first minute of the session (motion capture periods 5.1–2 and 6.1–2, respectively). If the first minute of treadmill walking at each speed (motion capture period X.1 and X.2) are excluded and referred to as acclimatization period, then habituation was achieved already in the third session at the slower speed (0.78 m/s). At the higher speed (0.96 m/s), however, time to habituation did not differ depending on whether a 1-min acclimatization was allowed for or not; at this speed significant differences compared with the last motion capture period (6.4) were found even in the last motion capture period of the fifth session. A change in speed within the same gait thus seems to be equivalent to a break because the slower walk always preceded the faster walk in each session and yet the dogs required more training time to habituate in the faster walking speed. One reason habituation was achieved with less training time at the slower speed may be that this speed better matched the dogs' preferred walking speed, and that it was therefore relatively more demanding for the dogs to adapt to treadmill walking at the faster speed.

An important aim of the current study was to evaluate the training time needed for dogs to get accustomed to treadmill walking. Our results suggest that five 8- to 10-min sessions during two consecutive days is sufficient to ensure full habituation to treadmill walking, and that two training sessions on a single day may be sufficient if the dogs are allowed a 1-min acclimatisation period after a break or change in speed. However, some limitations must be considered if our findings are to be applied as guidelines for treadmill training of dogs in future studies. One limitation is the duration of the training period. Two days of training is still a relatively short period and possibly additional more subtle adaptations may have continued if the training had continued. The time to full habituation would then have been longer, if variable values had been compared to values obtained after e.g. 2 weeks of daily training. Another limitation is the observed variation in required training time between speeds, and also between individuals. The fact that between-stride variability at group level did not decrease significantly after the fifth session does not imply that every single individual had reached minimum between-stride variability at that point. Finally, the systematic difference between the two speeds, as discussed above, indicates that the choice of walking speed influences the training time needed. Because of these limitations it is advisable that a margin of safety is applied if training time is scheduled based on the results of the current study to ensure that a particular dog is fully accustomed to treadmill walking in an arbitrary speed.

Conclusions

Being unfamiliar with treadmill walking significantly affects kinematic and spatiotemporal variables, initially both measurement mean values and between-stride variability. Longer treadmill training is needed to achieve low-normal between-stride variability, compared with the time needed to obtain stable measurement mean values. To obtain reliable data for gait analysis, it must therefore be ensured that participating dogs are fully accustomed to treadmill walking. The current study provides some guidance to the training time needed, but variation between individuals and the difference found between a slower and faster walking speed indicates that generalising the guidance to other groups of walking dogs should be done with caution.

Authors' contributions

PG contributed on conception and design of the study, acquisition, tracking, analysis and interpretation of data and writing the article. KP and SH contributed on conception and design of the study, acquisition and tracking of data and drafting the manuscript. ASL contributed on conception and design of the study, drafting and critically revising the manuscript. AB contributed on conception and design of the study, analysis and interpretation of data and writing and revising the manuscript. All authors read and approved the final manuscript.

Author details

[1] Department of Clinical Sciences, Faculty of Veterinary Medicine and Animal Husbandry, Swedish University of Agricultural Sciences, Box 7054, 750 07 Uppsala, Sweden. [2] University Animal Hospital, Swedish University of Agricultural Sciences, Box 7040, 750 07 Uppsala, Sweden. [3] Department of Anatomy, Physiology and Biochemistry, Faculty of Veterinary Medicine and Animal Husbandry, Swedish University of Agricultural Sciences, Box 7011, 750 07 Uppsala, Sweden. [4] Present Address: Evidensia Specialistdjursjukhuset Helsingborg, Bergavägen 3, 250 23 Helsingborg, Sweden.

Acknowledgements

This study was supported with funds provided by Agria Animal Insurance and the Swedish Kennel Club's Foundation for Research. The authors thank Sophia Alanko, University Animal Hospital, SLU, for excellent dog handling during the treadmill sessions.

Competing interests

The authors declare that they have no competing interests.

References

1. Drevemo S, Dalin G, Fredricson I, Hjerthén G. Equine locomotion 1. The analysis of linear and temporal stride characteristics of trotting standardbreds. Equine Vet J. 1980;12:60–5.
2. Budsberg SC, Verstraete MC, Soutas-Little RW. Force plate analysis of the walking gait in healthy dogs. Am J Vet Res. 1987;48:915–8.
3. DeCamp CE, Soutas-Little RW, Hauptman J, Olivier B, Braden T, Walton A. Kinematic gait analysis of the trot in healthy greyhounds. Am J Vet Res. 1993;54:627–34.
4. Allen K, Decamp CE, Braden TD, Bahns M. Kinematic gait analysis of the trot in healthy mixed breed dogs. Vet Comp Orthop Traumatol. 1994;7:148–53.
5. Hottinger HA, DeCamp CE, Olivier NB, Hauptman JG, SoutasLittle RW. Noninvasive kinematic analysis of the walk in healthy large-breed dogs. Am J Vet Res. 1996;57:381–8.
6. Jevens DJ, Hauptman JG, DeCamp CE, Budsberg SC, Soutas-Little RW. Contributions to variance in force-plate analysis of gait in dogs. Am J Vet Res. 1993;54:612–5.
7. Roush JK, McLaughlin RM Jr. Effects of subject stance time and velocity on ground reaction forces in clinically normal greyhounds at the walk. Am J Vet Res. 1994;12:1672–6.
8. Bennett RL, DeCamp CE, Flo GL, Hauptman JG, Stajich M. Kinematic gait analysis in dogs with hip dysplasia. Am J Vet Res. 1996;57:966–71.
9. Lee DV, Bertram JE, Todhunter RJ. Acceleration and balance in trotting dogs. J Exp Biol. 1999;202:3565–73.
10. Bertram JEA, Lee DV, Case HN, Todhunter RJ. Comparison of the trotting gaits of labrador retrievers and greyhounds. Am J Vet Res. 2000;61:832–8.
11. Wall JC, Charteris J. A kinematic study of long-term habituation to treadmill walking. Ergonomics. 1981;24:531–42.
12. Fredricson I, Drevemo S, Dalin G, Hjertén G, Björne K, Rynde R, et al. Treadmill for equine locomotion analysis. Equine Vet J. 1983;15:111–5.
13. Vilensky JA, O'Connor BL, Brandt KD, Dunn EA, Rogers PI, DeLong CA. Serial kinematic analysis of the unstable knee after transection of the anterior cruciate ligament: temporal and angular changes in a canine model of osteoarthritis. J Orthop Res. 1994;12:229–37.
14. Bockstahler B, Muller M, Henninger W, Mayrhofer E, Peham C, Podbregar I. Kinetic and kinematic motion analysis of the forelimbs in sound Malinois dogs—sampling of basic values. Wien Tierärztl Monatschr. 2008;95:127–38.
15. Holler PJ, Brazda V, Dal-Bianco B, Lewy E, Mueller MC, Peham C, et al. Kinematic motion analysis of the joints of the forelimbs and hind limbs of dogs during walking exercise regimens. Am J Vet Res. 2010;71:734–40.
16. Marsolais GS, McLean S, Derrick T, Conzemius MG. Kinematic analysis of the hind limb during swimming and walking in healthy dogs and dogs with surgically corrected cranial cruciate ligament rupture. J Am Vet Med Assoc. 2003;222:739–43.
17. Tashman S, Anderst W, Kolowich P, Havstad S, Arnoczky S. Kinematics of the ACL-deficient canine knee during gait: serial changes over two years. J Orthop Res. 2004;22:931–41.
18. Bockstahler BA, Henninger W, Muller M, Mayrhofer E, Peham C, Podbregar I. Influence of borderline hip dysplasia on joint kinematics of clinically sound Belgian shepherd dogs. Am J Vet Res. 2007;68:271–6.
19. Sanchez-Bustinduy M, de Medeiros MA, Radke H, Langley-Hobbs S, McKinley T, Jeffery N. Comparison of kinematic variables in defining lameness caused by naturally occurring rupture of the cranial cruciate ligament in dogs. Vet Surg. 2010;39:523–30.
20. de Medeiros M, Bustinduy MS, Radke H, Langley-Hobbs S, Jeffery N. Early kinematic outcome after treatment of cranial cruciate ligament rupture by tibial plateau levelling osteotomy in the dog. Vet Comp Orthop Traumatol. 2011;24:178–84.
21. Abdelhadi J, Wefstaedt P, Nolte I, Schilling N. Fore-aft ground force adaptations to induced forelimb lameness in walking and trotting dogs. PLoS ONE. 2012;7:e52202.
22. Fischer S, Anders A, Nolte I, Schilling N. Compensatory load redistribution in walking and trotting dogs with limb lameness. Vet J. 2013;197:746–52.
23. Buchner HHF, Savelberg HHCM, Schamhardt HC, Merkens HW, Barneveld A. Habituation of horses to treadmill locomotion. Equine Vet J. 1994;26(Suppl 17):13–5.
24. Clements DN, Owen MR, Carmichael S, Reid SWJ. Kinematic analysis of the gait of 10 Labrador retrievers during treadmill locomotion. Vet Rec. 2005;156:478–81.
25. Gustås P, Pettersson K, Honkavaara S, Lagerstedt AS, Byström A. Kinematic and temporospatial assessment of habituation of Labrador retrievers to treadmill trotting. Vet J. 2013;198:114–9.

26. Matsas A, Taylor N, McBurney H. Knee joint kinematics from familiarised treadmill walking can be generalised to overground walking in young unimpaired subjects. Gait Posture. 2000;11:46–53.
27. Van de Putte M, Hagemeister N, St Onge N, Parent G, de Guise JA. Habituation to treadmill walking. Biomed Mater Eng. 2006;16:43–52.
28. Owen MR, Richards J, Clements DN, Drew ST, Bennett D, Carmichael S. Kinematics of the elbow and stifle joints in greyhounds during treadmill trotting—an investigation of familiarisation. Vet Comp Orthop Traumatol. 2004;17:141–5.
29. Fanchon L, Valette JP, Sanaa M, Grandjean D. The measurement of ground reaction force in dogs trotting on a treadmill: an investigation of habituation. Vet Comp Orthop Traumatol. 2006;19:81–6.
30. Fanchon L, Grandjean D. Habituation of healthy dogs to treadmill trotting: repeatability assessment of vertical ground reaction force. Res Vet Sci. 2009;87:135–9.
31. Faber M, Johnston C, van Weeren PR, Barneveld A. Repeatability of back kinematics in horses during treadmill locomotion. Equine Vet J. 2002;34:235–41.
32. Taylor NF, Evans OM, Goldie PA. Angular movements of the lumbar spine and pelvis can be reliably measured after 4 minutes of treadmill walking. Clin Biomech. 1996;11:484–6.
33. Cavagna GA, Heglund NC, Taylor CR. Mechanical work in terrestrial locomotion: two basic mechanisms for minimizing energy expenditure. Am J Physiol. 1977;233:243–61.
34. Biewener AA. Patterns of mechanical energy change in tetrapod gait: pendula, springs and work. J Exp Zool A Comp Exp Biol. 2006;305:899–911.
35. Zeni JA, Higginson JS. Gait parameters and stride-to-stride variability during familiarization to walking on a split-belt treadmill. Clin Biomech. 2010;25:383–6.

5

Identification and characterization of cancer stem cells in canine mammary tumors

Agata Rybicka* and Magdalena Król

Abstract

Cancer stem cells (CSC) represent a small subpopulation of cells in malignant tumors that possess the unique ability to self-renew, differentiate and resist chemo- and radiotherapy. These cells have been postulated to be the basis for some of the difficulties in treating cancer, and therefore, numerous approaches have been developed to specifically target and eliminate CSC in diverse types of cancer, including breast cancer. Spontaneously occurring mammary tumors in canines share clinical and molecular similarities with the human counterpart, making the dog a potentially powerful model for the study of human breast cancer and clinical trials. Studies focused on canine mammary CSC might therefore enhance our understanding of the biology and possible treatment of the disease in both dogs and humans. In this review, we discuss various approaches currently in use to isolate and characterize canine mammary CSC.

Keywords: Cancer stem cells, Canine mammary tumor, Translational medicine

Background

Canine mammary tumors (CMT) remain some of the most common neoplasms affecting female dogs. Approximately 200–250 new diagnoses of CMT per 100,000 bitches are reported annually [1, 2], and of these cases, ~50% are malignant [3, 4]. Surgical removal of the tumor is a standard treatment for CMT, but in many cases, the procedure alone is ineffective due to existing micro-metastases [3]. Moreover, lack of effective chemo- and radiotherapy following mastectomy excludes possible alternative treatment strategies.

Recently, it has been hypothesized that a small subpopulation of cells, cancer stem cells (CSC), underlies tumor initiation, progression and metastasis. CSC are thought to share similar properties with normal stem cells, such as the ability to self-renew and differentiate into various cell types. High expression of adenosine triphosphate (ATP)-binding cassette transporters, quiescence and specific DNA repair abilities also make them remarkably drug resistant [5]. Therefore, understanding the biology of CSC and critical pathways involved in their maintenance might lead us to the discovery of novel compounds for breast cancer therapy.

Interestingly, CMT shares many clinical and molecular similarities with human breast cancer. Epidemiology and tumor behaviour follow the same pattern as in humans, rendering spontaneously occurring CMT an interesting model for breast cancer preclinical studies. Thus, close cooperation between human and veterinary medicine in breast cancer studies is likely to be of mutual benefit for treatment of the disease in both humans and dogs.

This review summarizes current knowledge regarding canine mammary CSC. Various techniques used for CSC isolation, the signaling pathways involved in tumor development, and studies regarding drug resistance and targeted treatment are presented. In addition, current challenges and future perspectives in the study of CMT are discussed.

Search strategy

A literature search was performed in PubMed (http://www.ncbi.nlm.nih.gov/pubmed) using the terms "canine mammary tumor" OR "canine neoplasms" AND "cancer stem cells" OR "canine mammary cancer stem cells". Only papers written in English and published within the last 25 years through November 2016 were included. All

*Correspondence: rybicka.agt@gmail.com
Department of Physiological Sciences, Faculty of Veterinary Medicine, Warsaw University of Life Sciences, Warsaw, Poland

articles based on cancer stem-like cells isolated from tumor samples and canine mammary tumor cell lines were incorporated. Studies employing immunohistochemistry as a method for the identification of cancer stem-like cells in situ were evaluated, and the most relevant to our review were selected. An additional resource was our own data from the isolation and identification of canine cancer stem-like cells [6, 7].

Canine model for breast cancer studies

Breast cancer is the second leading cause of death in women worldwide [8]. The International Agency for Research on Cancer (IARC) estimated in 2012 that approximately 1.67 million women were diagnosed with breast cancer globally, and 522,000 died from the disease or related complications. At present, a murine model with inducible or implanted mammary tumors is used in the majority of human breast cancer studies. Despite the broad capability to investigate complex mechanisms of cancer pathways, tumor progression and therapeutic agents, genetically engineered mice possess limitations in modeling human cancer. Alterations in the immune system of certain mouse strains, inbreeding and homogeneity of experimental cells implanted into mice all lead to a limited picture of tumor biology. In this regard, the dog might be a unique alternative for breast cancer research for a number of reasons. First, the disease in dogs is pathologically similar to that in humans, and importantly, exhibits the heterogeneity that is observed in human tumors [9]. Second, the dog is one of the few species in which mammary gland neoplasms occur spontaneously with almost 3 times the incidence in humans [10]. The highest incidence occurs in intact, older bitches in the age range of 8–12 years [11]. Third, the clinical course and tumor progression of CMT is comparable to breast cancer in women. In both, for example, larger size and metastasis detected in adjacent lymph nodes or distant organs are correlated with higher tumor grade and poorer prognosis [12]. Fourth, shorter overall lifespan than human and larger size compared to mouse enables the possibility of monitoring tumor progression and treatment outcomes in a shorter period of time. Fifth, close similarity to the human genome and comparable kinetics regarding drug metabolism indicates that the canine might be an invaluable model bridging clinical trials between mouse and human (Fig. 1). Finally, environmental factors, including diet, lifestyle, and UV and chemical exposure, are similar between dogs and humans [9].

Cancer stem cells

A solid tumor is a heterogeneous mass made up of a variety of cell types, including cancer cells, cells in the tumor microenvironment and the extracellular matrix. CSC make up a small subpopulation of the cancer cells that are thought to play a major role in tumor initiation and progression. Unique properties of the CSC, such as self-renewal, differentiation and drug resistance, determine both long-term survival as well as the ability to escape chemotherapy.

Although the initial evidence that cancer might arise from a population of stem-like cells dates as far back as the nineteenth century, improved technology in basic cancer research enabled comprehensive studies in this field [13]. The development of flow cytometry together with discovery of cell surface markers and the increased

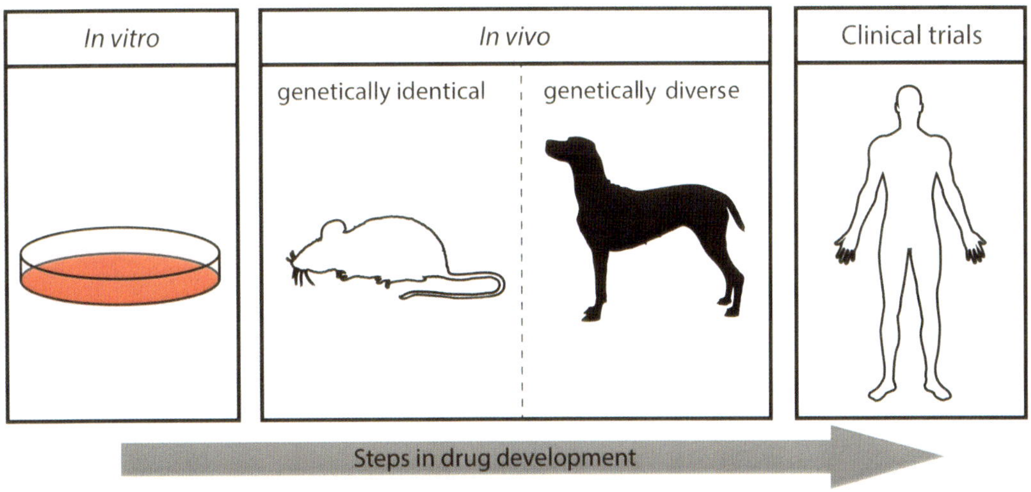

Fig. 1 The canine model provides an invaluable model bridging murine in vivo studies and clinical trials to the study and drug development for human breast cancer

availability of xenograft mouse models for human cancer have enabled the isolation and characterization of human CSC. A study conducted by Bonnet and Dick in 1997 was the first to show that within a cancer only a certain population of cells possessed the unique potential for self-renewal [14]. They demonstrated that only the $CD34^{+}CD38^{-}$ fraction of cells isolated from human acute myeloid leukemia had the ability to initiate hematopoietic malignancy in non-obese diabetic/severe combined immunodeficiency (NOD/SCID) mice during serial transplantations. Interestingly, because of the presence of the same surface markers on normal stem cells, the authors proposed that CSC might originate from normal primitive cells rather than committed progenitor cells. Six years later, Al-Hajj et al. [15] identified cells with stem cell-like properties in solid tumors. Using the combination of anti-CD24, anti-CD44 and anti-epithelial-specific antigen (ESA) antibodies, the authors dissociated nine primary or metastatic human breast cancer samples. The cells were sorted, and 10 serial dilutions were injected into the mammary gland of NOD/SCID mice. This study revealed the explicit tumorigenic potential of selected $ESA^{+}CD44^{+}CD24^{-/low}$ $Lineage^{-}$ cells. As few as only 100 cells were able to initiate tumor growth. Furthermore, intra tumor heterogeneity was present in the xenografts, paralleling the cellular diversity observed in the primary counterparts. Thus, CSC not only self-renew but also differentiate into phenol typically diverse cells of a particular tumor. To date, stem-like cancer cells have been identified in numerous solid tumors including lung, prostate, brain, melanoma and ovarian cancer [16–19].

Metastasis, the development of secondary tumors in adjacent or distant organs, is estimated to be responsible for 90% of cancer related deaths [20]. It is believed to take place in part through the corruption of a normal cellular process, the epithelial-mesenchymal transition (EMT), which is observed in normal tissue development and wound healing. Reversible transformation of a polarized epithelial cell into a motile mesenchymal type enables cells to migrate to distant regions, invade tissues and generate metastases. Cells undergoing EMT are characterized by a reduced expression of E-cadherin-mediated intercellular junctions and keratin rich intermediate filaments with a concurrent increase in mesenchymal markers including vimentin and fibronectin. Recently, several studies suggested that there is a link between CSC and EMT. For instance, a study by Mani et al. [21] revealed that induction of the EMT program through SNAIL, TWIST or TGF-β1 in immortalized human mammary epithelial cells led to the generation of $CD44^{+}/CD24^{-}$ cells with stemness properties.

Treatment regimens for human breast cancer today often include chemo- and radiotherapy. However, despite these aggressive approaches, many patients experience tumor recurrence possibly due to the presence of dormant cancer cells [22]. It has been hypothesized that CSC with their multiple defense mechanisms largely make up this population of tumor cells. Chemotherapy is generally most effective against rapidly proliferating cancer cells; thus, the low proliferation rate and increased number of ATP-driven efflux transporters allow stem-like cells to escape the cytotoxic effects of multiple compounds [5]. Moreover, the over expression of anti-apoptotic proteins, such as B-cell lymphoma 2 (BCL2), and increased resistance to DNA damage make them highly resistant to radiotherapy [23]. Failure of chemo- and radiotherapy in breast cancer treatment has stimulated research for novel compounds that might selectively target those remaining CSC.

Isolation of canine mammary cancer stem cells

The discovery of CSC in human breast cancer triggered investigation of a similar subpopulation in canine mammary tumors. Based on their characteristic features, namely, sphere-forming ability under non-adherent conditions, expression of specific surface markers and high expression of ATP-binding cassette (ABC) transporters, several methods have been proposed for CSC isolation (Fig. 2).

Somatic mammalian cells have limited replicative potential and undergo cell senescence. Stem cells differ in that they possess the unique ability to self-renew and to perpetuate their pool throughout the life span of an organism. In cancer, CSC exhibit these same properties driving tumor progression and recurrence. Thus methods to enrich for more undifferentiated cell types from normal mammary gland tissue, such as the system developed by Dontu et al. [24], have been important for the functional and molecular characterization of CSC. These authors generated more favorable conditions for the proliferation of progenitor cells by culturing cells dissociated from tissue on low attachment plates in serum-free medium supplemented with B27, epidermal growth factor (EGF), basic fibroblast growth factor (bFGF) and heparin. More cells within floating spherical colonies expressed a high level of ABC transporters compared to the parental cell line (27 vs 1%, non adherent vs adherent culture, respectively). Moreover, only cells within the floating spheres were able to regenerate colonies and possessed multi lineage differentiation potential.

Using this method, Cocola et al. [25] isolated the first canine mammary CSC in 2009. Serially dissociated spheroids obtained from eight CMT samples were able to regenerate for up to 5 passages and displayed similar morphology to mammospheres obtained from normal tissue. In a 3D assay in vitro, the canine CSC cultured

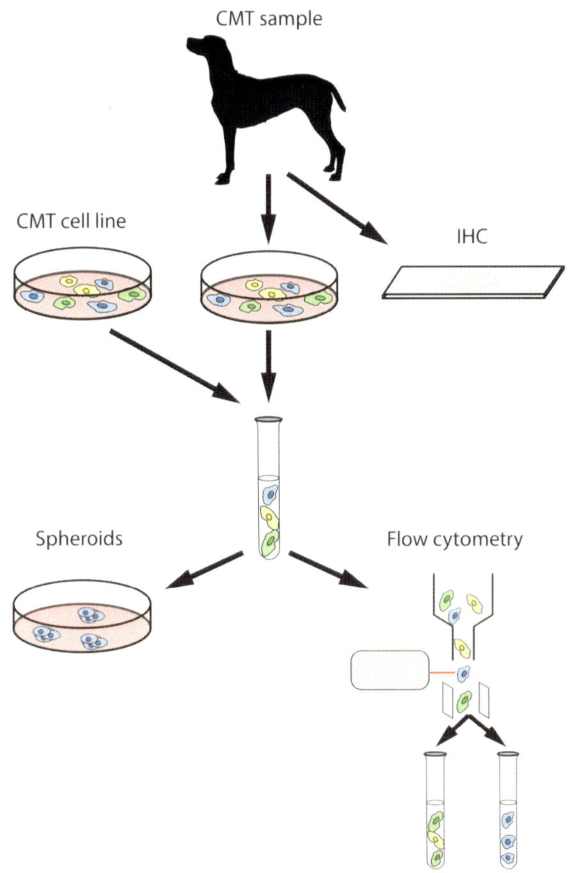

Fig. 2 Methods used for the identification and isolation of canine mammary cancer stem cells

on collagen gels generated branching structures reminiscent of primitive tubes of the mammary gland, and when implanted into the fat pads of NOD/SCID mice, induced tumor growth. The regeneration potential as well as the number of spheroids varied in subsequent studies [25–33]. Cells isolated from the REM134 canine mammary carcinoma cell line formed spheres 16 times in long-term serial passaging. These cells were cultured under analogous conditions but were additionally supplemented with progesterone, putrescine, sodium selenite, transferrin and insulin [29]. Differences in sphere culturing media however have also been shown to influence the regeneration potential of CSC from CMT. The results of these experiments revealed that in contrast to stem cells isolated from normal mammary gland tissue, self-renewal of CSC was repressed by increased concentrations of EGF and FGF2 rather than promoted [33]. In another study, cells obtained from four canine mammary gland adenoma cell lines (1×10^4) formed between 45 and 273 spheres demonstrating the existence of different percentages of progenitor cells among samples [27].

The self-renewing, sphere culturing system is a useful and easy method for the isolation of CSC; however, some limitations do exist. First, the in vitro environment may not fully reflect in vivo conditions and may lead to the selection of a specific group of cells that might vary from putative CSC. Second, calculations for sphere formation might be sometimes highly inaccurate, as so-called larger spheres are often the result of the aggregation of smaller spheres [34]. Finally, technical difficulties in obtaining single-cell suspensions might lead to biases and chimerism in the formation of spheres.

One of the most common methods currently used to isolate CSC from human breast cancer samples is flow cytometry. Based on the expression of specific cell surface markers or functional properties, CSC can be easily and quickly identified. Using multiple parameters simultaneously, flow cytometry enables the isolation of this very rare subpopulation of cells depending on set criteria. Human breast CSC have been previously characterized as $CD44^+/CD24^{-/low}$ [15]. Detection of $CD44^+/CD24^{-/low}$ cells has also been reported in CMT [27, 30, 35]. A study by Michishita et al. [27] demonstrated that 85% of cells were $CD44^+/CD24^{-/low}$ in spheres derived from a canine mammary adenocarcinoma cell line. Surprisingly, the authors also observed that 45.3–91.7% of cells were $CD44^+/CD24^{-/low}$ in the four parental cell lines analyzed. Such high levels of CD44 positive cells might however be associated with proliferation status rather than stem cell phenotype as the proportion of cells in G0/G1 that are $CD44^{-/low}$ has been shown to be higher than in G2/M where the majority are $CD44^+$ [36]. Therefore, isolation of CSCs should be performed with a combination of cell surface markers.

Ferletta et al. [30] detected canine mammary CSC using the marker stem cell antigen (Sca-1; also known as mouse mammary progenitor cell marker) and additional antibodies against CD10, CD34, CD44, CD24 and CD49f surface markers. In these experiments, the Sca-1^+ side population from the atypical benign mixed mammary tumor line CMT-U229 expressed a $CD10^{low}/CD34^+/CD44^+/CD24^{low}$ and $CD49f^+$ antigenic profile. Moreover, $CD133^+$ cells sorted from the same Sca-1^+ side population formed spheroids on low-attachment plates. These observations suggested that CD133 and Sca-1 might be relevant markers for canine mammary CSC isolation. Data from our own studies corroborate these results [6]. The Sca-1^+ cells isolated from three CMT cell lines (CMT-U27, CMT-U309 and P114) formed colonies with an undifferentiated morphology and expressed CD44 and epithelial cell adhesion molecule (EpCAM) genes at significantly higher levels. However, in contrast to the results of Michishita et al. [27], only between 0.2 and 1.2% of cells in these canine mammary neoplastic cell lines were characterized with progenitor features and a Sca-1^+ phenotype.

Immunohistochemistry (IHC) is a second method used for the identification and quantification of CSC within tumor specimens. A few groups have presented promising results using this technique [28, 37–40]. In a large study conducted by Magalhaes et al. [39], 130 CMT samples, including benign, malignant and lymph node metastases, were analyzed for CD44 and CD24 expression. The $CD44^+/CD24^-$ phenotype, which is characteristic of CSC, was detected more frequently in higher-grade tumors and lymph node metastases, while the $CD24^+$ phenotype was identified more frequently in lower grade samples (grade I) compared to the other pathologies. Similar results were also demonstrated by other groups concluding that a higher frequency of $CD44^+/CD24^-$ cells is associated with poorer prognosis [37–39]. However, results might be often underestimated due to non-homogenous expression of CD44 within tissue, uneven localization of putative cells and difficulties with serial sectioning of samples [41].

Based on current knowledge, there is no single method for CSC isolation that is necessarily superior to others. The choice of sample type as well as isolation technique have certain limitations that should be considered when analyzing data. Optimization of the protocol in the future might therefore be beneficial in order to more clearly define a set of conditions that will lead to consistent and comparable results.

Functional characterization of canine mammary cancer stem cells

Several groups have analyzed the effect of chemo- and radiotherapy on isolated canine mammary CSC. Doxorubicin is a widely used anti-tumor agent that causes DNA damage and inhibits cell proliferation. Spheres isolated from the canine mammary carcinoma cell line REM134 cultured with increasing concentrations of doxorubicin exhibited higher resistance compared to the parental, adherent cells [29]. The cytotoxic effect was almost twofold less in these cells. The doses 0.001, 0.01 and 0.05 μM left 80, 60 and 30% viable cells, respectively. The same cells were resistant to radiation doses of 1–5 Gy and exhibited a reduced loss of colony formation ability. Increased resistance to doxorubicin and no response to paclitaxel treatment were also observed by three other groups [27, 31, 35]. Barbieri et al. [31] did not observe any reduction in cell viability, even at the highest concentrations (5–10 μM) of the drugs. Discordance between results obtained using cell lines and spheres derived from tumor samples might be explained by possible different gene expressions and cellular properties that occur during the process of immortalization [24].

Recently, the effect of three alternative drugs has been investigated in the treatment of canine mammary tumors. In one study, the anti-diabetic drug metformin was shown to specifically inhibit the viability of CSC [31]. The IC_{50} concentration after treatment for 48 h varied between samples, resulting in a mean value of ~10 mM. In an in vivo study in NOD/SCID mice, a 62% reduction in tumor growth was observed in animals receiving metformin in the drinking water. In culture, only 2% of cells dissociated from tumor samples obtained from treated animals were able to form spheres compared to 13% of cells derived from the untreated group. The significantly lower clonogenic potential of CSC observed in the ex vivo assay, and the high safety of the drug make metformin a promising agent for combined anti-tumor therapy [31].

In a second study, simvastatin, a cholesterol-decreasing therapeutic used for the prevention of myocardial infarction, was tested as a potential agent to target CSC [35]. Although the drug is known to competitively inhibit 3-hydroxy-3-methylglutaryl coenzyme A reductase which is involved in cholesterol synthesis, it also reduces expression of CD44, a CSC surface marker. The effect of simvastatin on sphere forming capacity was therefore investigated in the canine mammary cancer cell line, CF41 Mg, which is enriched for $CD44^+/CD24^{-/low}$ cells. The number and size of colonies generated in the presence of the drug was significantly decreased in a dose-dependent manner. At the molecular level, simvastatin led to the reduction of β-catenin in the plasma membrane of cells within spheres and activation of caspase 3/7 which increased DNA fragmentation in CSC. Moreover, spheres were more sensitive to combination treatment with doxorubicin compared to spheres treated with 10 μM simvastatin alone [35].

In a third potential therapeutic strategy, melatonin, a hormone synthesized by the pineal gland, was shown to suppress properties of EMT in CSC. Under treatment with the hormone (1 mM), the expression levels of OCT4, N-cadherin and vimentin were significantly decreased in CSC isolated from the cell line CMT-U229 whereas E-cadherin levels were increased. Migration and invasion potential of treated cells was also found to be reduced, by 40% compared to controls, indicating a potential anti-metastatic role for melatonin in CMT [42].

According to Skidan and Steininger [43], anti-CSC drugs can be divided into three main categories: chemical compounds, small molecules targeting CSC and therapeutic biological agents including microRNA (miRNA) based drugs. A family of endogenous, non-coding RNAs (ncRNA) regulates ~30% of genes, and altered expression of miRNA has been associated with cancer development [44, 45]. Our group was the first to study miRNA expression in canine CSC isolated from three different CMT cell lines [6]. Comparison of miRNA profiles using a custom-designed canine miRNA microarray revealed significant deregulation of 33 miRNAs in CSC relative to differentiated tumor cells. Interestingly, genes targeted by the down regulated miRNAs were mostly involved in the TGF-β signaling pathway. Similarly, Pang et al. [29] observed that REM134 cells treated with TGF-β led to enrichment in the number of sphere-derived cells and induced EMT. Therefore, it is possible that regulation of the expression of some miRNAs might control EMT and deplete the CSC subpopulation.

It has also been recently demonstrated that non-neoplastic cell types within the tumor microenvironment influence biological properties of CSC isolated from CMT [7]. Tumor-associated macrophages (TAMs), the most abundant population of immune cells infiltrating solid tumors, have been shown to promote over expression of the monocyte chemo attractant CCL2 in CSC, which led to enhanced TAM infiltration [46]. Moreover, co-culturing with TAMs yielded CSC with higher invasive potential and elevated pro-angiogenic properties. These results corroborate previous findings associating TAMs with tumor progression and metastasis in human breast cancer [47, 48].

Conclusions and perspectives

Studies performed in recent decades indicate that the mechanism of tumor initiation, progression and recurrence might be driven by rare subpopulation of cells called cancer stem cells. These cells possess the unique ability to self-renew and differentiate into a variety of cell types. While CSC have been previously characterized in numerous human cancers, they have only recently been identified in canine neoplasms, including mammary tumors. Interestingly, studies have demonstrated that canine mammary CSC not only express similar surface markers to human CSC but are also resistant to chemo- and radiotherapy. These results highlight the value of comparative oncology and the possible utility of the canine model in breast cancer research.

Abbreviations

ABC: ATP binding cassette; ATP: adenosine triphosphate; BCL2: B cell lymphoma 2; bFGF: basic fibroblast growth factor; CMT: canine mammary tumor; CSC: cancer stem cells; EGF: epidermal growth factor; EMT: epithelial-mesenchymal transition; EpCAM: epithelial cell adhesion molecule; ESA: epithelial specific antigen; IHC: immunohistochemistry; NOD/SCID: non-obese diabetic/severe combined immunodeficiency; Sca-1: stem cells antigen 1; TAMs: tumor-associated macrophages; TGF-β: transforming growth factor beta.

Authors' contributions

AR reviewed the literature and wrote the main body of the manuscript. MK critically reviewed and substantially contributed to the final draft of the manuscript. Both authors read and approved the final manuscript.

Authors' information

MK is a Professor in Veterinary Physiology investigating canine mammary cancer with particular focus on cancer metastasis and tumour microenvironment. AR is a Ph.D. candidate and together with MK an author of two original publications in canine mammary cancer stem-like cells.

Acknowledgements

The authors would like to thank Dr. Cedric Hamelin for assistance in the preparation of figures.

Competing interests

The authors declare that they have no competing interests.

References

1. Dorn CR, Taylor DO, Schneider R, Hibbard HH, Klauber MR. Survey of animal neoplasms in Alameda and Contra Costa counties, California. II. Cancer morbidity in dogs and cats from Alameda county. J Natl Cancer Inst. 1968;40:307–18.
2. Dobson JM, Samuel S, Milstein H, Rogers K, Wood JL. Canine neoplasia in the UK: estimates of incidence rates from a population of insured dogs. J Small Anim Pract. 2002;43:240–6.
3. Misdorp W. Tumors of the mammary gland. 4th ed. Meuten DJ, editor. Ames, Iwona: Iowa State Press 2002. pp. 575–606.
4. Sorenmo K. Canine mammary gland tumors. Vet Clin North Am Small Anim Pract. 2003;33:573–96.
5. Chen K, Huang Y, Chen J. Understanding and targeting cancer stem cells: therapeutic implications and challenges. Acta Pharmacol Sin. 2013;34:732–40.
6. Rybicka A, Mucha J, Majchrzak K, Taciak B, Hellmen E, Motyl T, et al. Analysis of microRNA expression in canine mammary cancer stem-like cells indicates epigenetic regulation of transforming growth factor-beta signaling. J Physiol Pharmacol. 2015;66:29–37.
7. Rybicka A, Eyileten C, Taciak B, Mucha J, Majchrzak K, Hellmen E, et al. Tumour-associated macrophages influence canine mammary cancer stem-like cells enhancing their pro-angiogenic properties. J Physiol Pharmacol. 2016;67:491–500.
8. Ferlay J, Soerjomataram I, Ervik M, Dikshit R, Eser S, Mathers C, Rebelo M, Parkin DM, Forman D, Bray, F. GLOBOCAN 2012 v1.0, Cancer incidence and mortality worldwide: IARC CancerBase No. 11 [Internet]. Lyon: International Agency for Research on Cancer; 2013. http://globocan.iarc.fr. Accessed 1 Aug 2015.
9. Cheon DJ, Orsulic S. Mouse models of cancer. Annu Rev Pathol. 2011;6:95–119.
10. MacEwen EG. Spontaneous tumors in dogs and cats: models for the study of cancer biology and treatment. Cancer Metastasis Rev. 1990;9:125–36.
11. Chang SC, Chang CC, Chang TJ, Wong ML. Prognostic factors associated with survival two years after surgery in dogs with malignant mammary tumors: 79 cases (1998–2002). J Am Vet Med Assoc. 2005;227:1625–9.
12. Misdorp W, Hart AA. Prognostic factors in canine mammary cancer. J Natl Cancer Inst. 1976;56:779–86.
13. Dalerba P, Cho RW, Clarke MF. Cancer stem cells: models and concepts. Annu Rev Med. 2007;58:267–84.
14. Bonnet D, Dick JE. Human acute myeloid leukemia is organized as a hierarchy that originates from a primitive hematopoietic cell. Nat Med. 1997;3:730–7.
15. Al-Hajj M, Wicha MS, Benito-Hernandez A, Morrison SJ, Clarke MF. Prospective identification of tumorigenic breast cancer cells. Proc Natl Acad Sci USA. 2003;100:3983–8.
16. Kim CF, Jackson EL, Woolfenden AE, Lawrence S, Babar I, Vogel S, et al. Identification of bronchioalveolar stem cells in normal lung and lung cancer. Cell. 2005;121:823–35.

17. Collins AT, Berry PA, Hyde C, Stower MJ, Maitland NJ. Prospective identification of tumorigenic prostate cancer stem cells. Cancer Res. 2005;65:10946–51.
18. Fang D, Nguyen TK, Leishear K, Finko R, Kulp AN, Hotz S, et al. A tumorigenic subpopulation with stem cell properties in melanomas. Cancer Res. 2005;65:9328–37.
19. Szotek PP, Pieretti-Vanmarcke R, Masiakos PT, Dinulescu DM, Connolly D, Foster R, et al. Ovarian cancer side population defines cells with stem cell-like characteristics and mullerian inhibiting substance responsiveness. Proc Natl Acad Sci USA. 2006;103:11154–9.
20. Chaffer CL, Weinberg RA. A perspective on cancer cell metastasis. Science. 2011;331:1559–64.
21. Mani SA, Guo W, Liao MJ, Eaton EN, Ayyanan A, Zhou AY, et al. The epithelial-mesenchymal transition generates cells with properties of stem cells. Cell. 2008;133:704–15.
22. Li X, Lewis MT, Huang J, Gutierrez C, Osborne CK, Wu MF, et al. Intrinsic resistance of tumorigenic breast cancer cells to chemotherapy. J Natl Cancer Inst. 2008;100:672–9.
23. Madjd Z, Mehrjerdi AZ, Sharifi AM, Molanaei S, Shahzadi SZ, Asadi-Lari M. CD44 + cancer cells express higher levels of the anti-apoptotic protein Bcl-2 in breast tumours. Cancer Immun. 2009;9:4.
24. Dontu G, Abdallah WM, Foley JM, Jackson KW, Clarke MF, Kawamura MJ, et al. In vitro propagation and transcriptional profiling of human mammary stem/progenitor cells. Genes Dev. 2003;17:1253–70.
25. Cocola C, Anastasi P, Astigiano S, Piscitelli E, Pelucchi P, Vilardo L, et al. Isolation of canine mammary cells with stem cell properties and tumour-initiating potential. Reprod Domest Anim. 2009;44(Suppl 2):214–7.
26. Michishita M, Akiyoshi R, Suemizu H, Nakagawa T, Sasaki N, Takemitsu H, et al. Aldehyde dehydrogenase activity in cancer stem cells from canine mammary carcinoma cell lines. Vet J. 2012;193:508–13.
27. Michishita M, Akiyoshi R, Yoshimura H, Katsumoto T, Ichikawa H, Ohkusu-Tsukada K, et al. Characterization of spheres derived from canine mammary gland adenocarcinoma cell lines. Res Vet Sci. 2011;91:254–60.
28. Huang J, Zhang D, Xie F, Lin D. The potential role of COX-2 in cancer stem cell-mediated canine mammary tumor initiation: an immunohistochemical study. J Vet Sci. 2015;16:225–31.
29. Pang LY, Cervantes-Arias A, Else RW, Argyle DJ. Canine mammary cancer stem cells are radio- and chemo-resistant and exhibit an epithelial-mesenchymal transition phenotype. Cancers (Basel). 2011;3:1744–62.
30. Ferletta M, Grawe J, Hellmen E. Canine mammary tumors contain cancer stem-like cells and form spheroids with an embryonic stem cell signature. Int J Dev Biol. 2011;55:791–9.
31. Barbieri F, Thellung S, Ratto A, Carra E, Marini V, Fucile C, et al. In vitro and in vivo antiproliferative activity of metformin on stem-like cells isolated from spontaneous canine mammary carcinomas: translational implications for human tumors. BMC Cancer. 2015;15:228.
32. Caceres S, Peña L, Lacerda L, Illera MJ, de Andres PJ, Larson RA, et al. Canine cell line, IPC-366, as a good model for the study of inflammatory breast cancer. Vet Comp Oncol. 2016. doi:10.1111/vco.12238.
33. Cocola C, Molgora S, Veronesi MC, Greco M, Bragato C, Moro M, et al. FGF2 and EGF is required for self-renewal of canine normal and tumor breast stem/progenitor cells that have organoid formation potential. J Cell Biochem. 2016. doi:10.1002/jcb.25737
34. Singec I, Knoth R, Meyer RP, Maciaczyk J, Volk B, Nikkhah G, et al. Defining the actual sensitivity and specificity of the neurosphere assay in stem cell biology. Nat Methods. 2006;3:801–6.
35. Torres CG, Olivares A, Stoore C. Simvastatin exhibits antiproliferative effects on spheres derived from canine mammary carcinoma cells. Oncol Rep. 2015;33:2235–44.
36. Blacking TM, Waterfall M, Argyle DJ. CD44 is associated with proliferation, rather than a specific cancer stem cell population, in cultured canine cancer cells. Vet Immunol Immunopathol. 2011;141:46–57.
37. Im KS, Jang YG, Shin JI, Kim NH, Lim HY, Lee SM, et al. CD44 +/CD24 − cancer stem cells are associated with higher grade of canine mammary carcinomas. Vet Pathol. 2015;52:1041–4.
38. Figueroa FC, Zanetti JS, Ribeiro-Silva A, Fonseca-Alves CE, Rocha NS. Association of CD44 +/CD24 − cells to more agressive molecular phenotypes in canine mammary carcinomas. Int J of Cancer Res. 2015;11(3):119–27.
39. Magalhaes GM, Terra EM, de Oliveira Vasconcelos R, de Barros Bandarra M, Moreira PR, Rosolem MC, et al. Immunodetection of cells with a CD44 +/CD24 − phenotype in canine mammary neoplasms. BMC Vet Res. 2013;9:205.
40. Webster JD, Yuzbasiyan-Gurkan V, Trosko JE, Chang CC, Kiupel M. Expression of the embryonic transcription factor Oct4 in canine neoplasms: a potential marker for stem cell subpopulations in neoplasia. Vet Pathol. 2007;44:893–900.
41. Barbieri F, Wurth R, Ratto A, Campanella C, Vito G, Thellung S, et al. Isolation of stem-like cells from spontaneous feline mammary carcinomas: phenotypic characterization and tumorigenic potential. Exp Cell Res. 2012;318:847–60.
42. Goncalves Ndo N, Colombo J, Lopes JR, Gelaleti GB, Moschetta MG, Sonehara NM, et al. Effect of melatonin in epithelial mesenchymal transition markers and invasive properties of breast cancer stem cells of canine and human cell lines. PLoS ONE. 2016;11:e0150407.
43. Skidan I, Steiniger SC. In vivo models for cancer stem cell research: a practical guide for frequently used animal models and available biomarkers. J Physiol Pharmacol. 2014;65:157–69.
44. Calin GA, Croce CM. MicroRNA signatures in human cancers. Nat Rev Cancer. 2006;6:857–66.
45. Lewis BP, Burge CB, Bartel DP. Conserved seed pairing, often flanked by adenosines, indicates that thousands of human genes are microRNA targets. Cell. 2005;120:15–20.
46. Noy R, Pollard JW. Tumor-associated macrophages: from mechanisms to therapy. Immunity. 2014;41:49–61.
47. Obeid E, Nanda R, Fu YX, Olopade OI. The role of tumor-associated macrophages in breast cancer progression (review). Int J Oncol. 2013;43:5–12.
48. Jinushi M, Chiba S, Yoshiyama H, Masutomi K, Kinoshita I, Dosaka-Akita H, et al. Tumor-associated macrophages regulate tumorigenicity and anticancer drug responses of cancer stem/initiating cells. Proc Natl Acad Sci USA. 2011;108:12425–30.

6

Correlations between cresty neck scores and post-mortem nape fat measurements in horses, obtained after photographic image analysis

Severiano R. Silva[1], Rita Payan-Carreira[1*], Cristina M. Guedes[1], Simão Coelho[1] and Ana Sofia Santos[2,3]

Abstract

Background: Obesity and emaciation in horses have major detrimental effects on health and morbidity, reproductive failure, work performance or carcass quality. Scoring is a current management tool used to assess and monitor equine body condition due to its simplicity and low cost. However, accurate assessment of obesity remains a challenge, even though a number of approaches have been tested, particularly for research purposes on adiposity. Their merit is usually validated by comparison with standard scoring methods. The overall aim of this study was to establish the correlation between post-mortem nape fat measurements obtained after photographic image analysis and cresty neck score (CNS) in horses. Data were collected from seventeen horses with a hot carcass weight of 165 ± 51 kg. Pre-slaughter CNS measurements were obtained using a six-point scale (from 0 to 5). Image capture was performed post-mortem, in the slaughter line; for each carcass, images of the dorsal and medial views were collected and afterwards transferred to a computer for analysis. After outlining the cresty neck fat, its area, major axis and thickness were determined. Correlation coefficients between nape fat measurements, CNS and carcass fatness were determined.

Results: The horses in the study show similar variation for CNS and hot carcass weight [Coefficient of variation (CV) = 32 and 31 %, respectively], but a high variation for carcass fattening (CV = 41 %). The nape fat area measurement was the parameter exhibiting the greatest variation (CV = 50 %). Correlations established between CNS and the variables tested revealed the existence of moderate to strong correlations among CNS, nape fat measurements, and carcass fatness. The highest correlation coefficients were found between CNS and nape fat thickness ($r = 0.882$; $P < 0.01$). The linear regression between CNS and nape fat thickness accounted for 77 % of the recorded variation for nape fat thickness.

Conclusions: The present study showed that there is a strong correlation between horse CNS and post-mortem nape fat measurements or carcass fatness.

Keywords: Adiposity, Cresty neck score, Image analysis, Body condition, Obesity, Horses

*Correspondence: rtpayan@gmail.com
[1] Zootecnia Department, Centro de Ciência Animal E Veterinária, Universidade de Trás-os-Montes e Alto Douro, 5000-801 Vila Real, Portugal
Full list of author information is available at the end of the article

Background

Obesity and emaciation pose significant problems in horses and have been associated with an increased risk of health and morbidity, reproductive failure, and poor work performance or carcass quality [1–3]. The ability to quantify and monitor animal body condition is a key issue for successful equine production and may also contribute to animal welfare [4, 5].

Body condition scoring (BCS) is currently the most common management tool for assessing and monitoring body condition in horses. Henneke's nine-point scale [6] is probably the most widely used scoring system, outlining the analysis of fat deposition over diverse body regions. Recently, a new 5-point scoring system was developed, focused on grading neck crest fatness [7]. Increased adiposity in specific locations, namely the fat deposits along the crest of the neck, has been associated with disequilibrium in the metabolic state and with an increased risk of metabolic disorders and inflammatory states [8]. Although body condition scoring (BCS) systems are useful to assess equine obesity, cresty neck scores (CNS) are a better predictor of the risk of metabolic diseases [8]. Therefore, CNS may be highly beneficial in screening levels of neck crest adiposity and recognising animals at an increased risk of obesity-related diseases [9].

Developed by experienced observers, scoring methods depend on a subjective score supported by a range of classified anatomical descriptors focused on a horse's external form/frame [6, 7]. These scoring systems are currently applied to horses and ponies due to their simplicity and reduced cost, although they require the operator to be experienced in judging condition as well as sufficiently practised in obtaining consistency of scores. More objective morphometric measurements (such as the girth-height ratio or the neck circumference) are, nonetheless, available to assess adiposity in particular body regions [7, 10, 11]. However, assessing obesity remains a challenge, due both to under-recognition of obesity by owners and the limitations in available scoring and measurement systems [11].

In an attempt to avoid these constraints, in particular for research purposes on horse adiposity, several methods and techniques have been tested to determine body condition in horses. These include tracer dilution methodologies, such as deuterium oxide [12], bioelectrical impedance analysis [13] or image techniques, which include real-time ultrasonography [14–16]. The merits of all these techniques are usually validated by comparison to matched BCS [6] or CNS [7], which have recognised limitations, including the influence of breed or body size on scoring measurements or lack of knowledge about their relationship with the actual content of body fat [17]. CNS being a subjective method, small variations may remain undetected even if good inter-observer reliability has been established [8].

Although CNS is a commonly used method to assess nuchal crest adiposity, it has not been formally validated using post-mortem methods, as recognised by Giles et al. [8]. Therefore, the overall aim of this study was to establish the correlation between nape fat measurements obtained in carcass after photographic image analysis and CNS in horses.

Methods

Animals

Data were collected in a national abattoir from 17 horses aged 3–9 years old, with a hot carcass weight of 165 ± 51 kg. No account was taken of nutritional history or of the breed of the horses. All horses slaughtered were approved for meat consumption; only animals with non-existing metabolic disease or signs of trauma (according to sanitary inspection documents) were used. For data collection prior to slaughter, animals were handled in accordance with International Ethical standards. The official entities regulating meat inspection and the management of the industrial facilities gave their permission to conduct the study within the abattoir and for data collection on carcasses, as required by national laws.

Collection of data

Cresty neck scores measurements were obtained before slaughter by two skilled evaluators (SC and SRS) while animals were in the lairage. CNS was assigned on a six-point scale (from 0—no palpable crest to 5—enormous crest), with half-score increments, according to the system described by Carter et al. [7].

The capture of carcass images was performed in an efficient manner so as to avoid any disturbances to workflow in the slaughter line. Images of dorsal and medial views were collected for each carcass (Fig. 1). Images representing the dorsal nuchal view were taken before the longitudinal section of the carcass, whereas the images corresponding to the medial side view were captured in the resulting hemi-carcasses, before weighing. Care was taken to completely immobilize the (hemi-) carcasses before capturing images. Images were captured using a digital camera (Nikon Coolpix S210) featuring an 8 Megapixel sensor. The camera was set as follows: shutter speed 1/10 s; manual operation mode; aperture Av F/4.6; ISO velocity 200; flash off; focal distance 74 mm; f 3.3. Captured images were saved as 3264 × 2448 pixel JPEG format photographs. The camera was placed 4 m from the carcasses, under standard artificial light. In addition, during the capture of images from the medial view of hemi-carcasses, two red laser dots were projected on

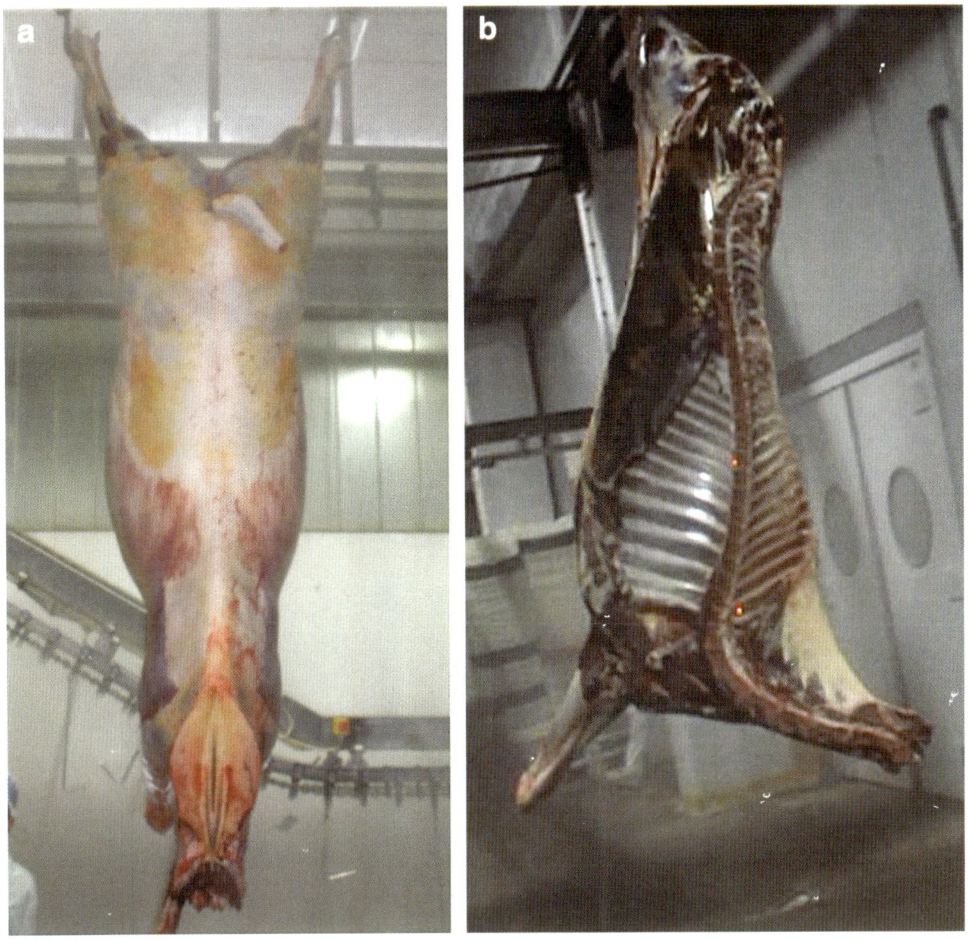

Fig. 1 Collection of images at the abattoir. Example of the dorsal side (**a**) and the medial side (**b**) images taken at the slaughter-line

the carcass (Fig. 2a), for scale-bar purposes; the two red lasers, each with a 650 nm wavelength, were mounted on a frame, held in a position parallel to the shot area, with a predetermined distance between the two lasers of 32 cm.

Carcass fatness was graded using an adapted 15 point scale described by Bohuslávek [17], derived from fat cover classification developed for adult bovine carcasses, and proposed for horses by Sarriés and Beriain [18]. Grading of carcass fatness was performed from its dorsal view, by a researcher (SC).

Image analysis and nape fat measurements

Captured images were transferred to a computer for analysis and a new identity code was randomly attributed, for blind assessment. A single operator performed the image analysis, using ImageJ software (version 1.38×, NIH, USA). To perform the measurements, the neck crest fat was outlined by means of ImageJ's freehand area tool, using the nuchae ligament as an anatomical reference point (Fig. 2b, c). The major axis and the minor axis, representing the thickness of nape fat, were automatically determined after setting the area measurement selection (Fig. 2c). The distance between the two red laser dots (32 cm) was used in ImageJ to give pixels real dimension; the result in pixels was entered in the software's set scale box.

Statistical analyses

All statistical tests were analysed using JMP software (version 7, SAS Institute, Cary, NC, USA). After testing data normality, simple descriptive statistical analyses were performed. Results are presented herein as mean ± standard deviation, minimum and maximum values and coefficient of variation (CV). The correlation coefficient (r) between nape fat measurements, CNS, and carcass fatness were determined after correlation analysis. A linear regression between the CNS scores and the thickness of nape fat was also performed. The coefficient of determination (R^2) was used to evaluate the ability of the prediction equation.

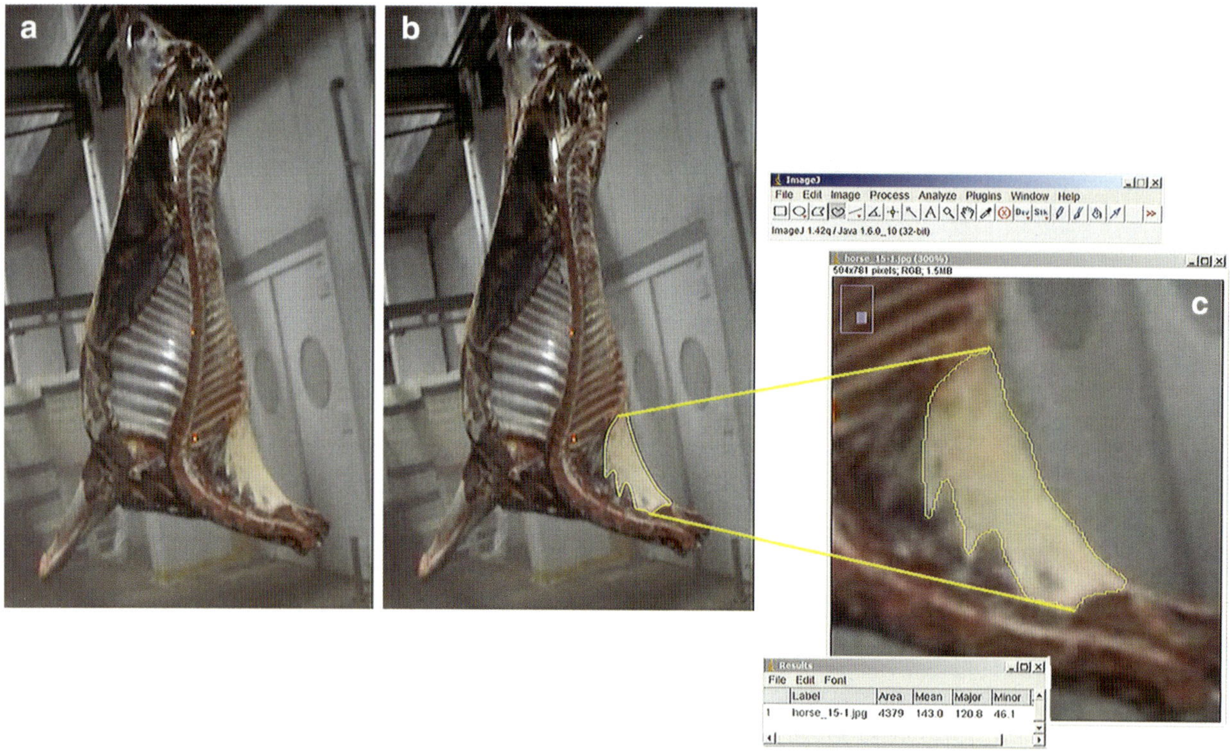

Fig. 2 Nape fat evaluation in carcasses at the abattoir. A medial view of hemi-carcass showing the two red laser points used as scale (**a**); outline of the nape fat using the *ligamentum nuchae* as reference (**b**) and a detail of ImageJ application to obtain the nape fat measurements (i.e., area, major axis and the minor axis (thickness of the nape fat) (**c**)

Results

Table 1 summarises the results for hot carcass weight, CNS, fat carcass level and nape fat measurements of the horses studied.

The 17 horses showed similar variation for CNS and hot carcass weight (CV of 32 and 31 %, for CNS and hot carcass, respectively; Table 1). However, they exhibited greater variation with respect to carcass fattening than CNS (CV = 41 vs. 32 %, for carcass fattening and CNS, respectively). Interestingly, the nape fat area measurement was the parameter showing the greatest variation (CV = 50 %), while the other two nape fat measurements revealed a CV of 25 and 34 % for major axis and nape fat thickness, respectively, which was in line with the variation observed in CNS.

The correlations established between the CNS and the other variables tested in the present study are presented in Table 2. The data showed that moderate to strong correlations existed among CNS, nape fat measurements, and carcass fatness. There were strong correlations between CNS and nape fat variables, with higher correlation coefficients within nape fat thickness ($r = 0.882$; $P < 0.01$). The

Table 1 Hot carcass weight, cresty neck scores (CNS), carcass fat and nape fat measured in horses (n = 17)

Parameter	Mean	SD	Min.	Max	CV (%)
Hot carcass weight, kg	164.6	50.7	105	272	30.8
CNS, 1–5	2.35	0.745	1.00	3.00	31.7
Carcass fat level, 1–15	7.24	2.93	3.00	13.0	40.5
Nape fat measurements					
Major axis (cm)	17.1	4.34	11.0	26.3	25.3
Area (cm^2)	310.5	156.3	120.5	691.8	50.3
Thickness (cm)	8.99	3.07	3.30	14.2	34.1

SD standard deviation; *Min.* minimum values; *Max.* maximum values; *CV* coefficient of variation

Table 2 Correlation among cresty neck scores (CNS), nape fat measurements and carcass fatness in horses (n = 17)

Nape fat measurements	Major axis	Area	Thickness	Carcass fatness
CNS	0.737	0.691	0.882	0.760
Major axis		0.991	0.840	0.596
Area			0.827	0.558
Thickness				0.734

All correlation coefficients are significantly ($P < 0.01$) different from zero correlation coefficients were similar between CNS and the other nape fat variables (r = 0.737 and r = 0.691 for the nape fat major axis and area, respectively; and 0.760 for carcass fatness; $P < 0.01$). Additionally, a strong correlation also existed between the various measurements taken for nape fat (r between 0.827 and 0.991, $P < 0.01$).

The linear regressions explaining the relationship between CNS and nape fat thickness or CNS and carcass fatness are presented in Figs. 3, 4, respectively. CNS explains 77 and 58 % of the observed variation of nape fat thickness and carcass fatness, respectively.

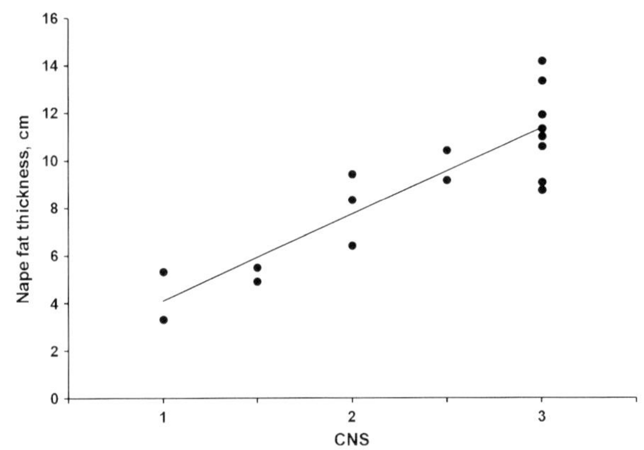

Fig. 3 Linear relationship ($y = 3.612x + 0.5011$; $R^2 = 0.774$) of nape fat thickness and cresty neck score (CNS) in horses

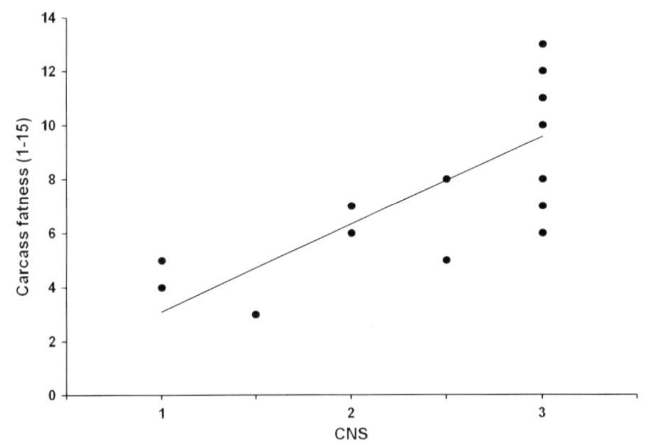

Fig. 4 Linear relationship ($y = 3.229x - 0.1258$; $R^2 = 0.578$) of carcass fatness and cresty neck score (CNS) in horses

Discussion

This study details the relationship between CNS and matching nape fat measurements. Typically, to establish a relationship between fat scores (e.g. CNS) and other body composition traits, the use of the widest range of variables is sought. In the present study, CNS ranges from 1 to 3, with no values of 0 and 0.5 or between 3.5 and 5. Nevertheless, the variation of the fattening traits assessed here (CV between 25 and 50 %) is comparable to that presented in other studies using horses with a carcass weight range of 105–418 kg [14, 19–21]. These studies showed that fat was the most variable component of the body (CV between 18 and 43 %) [14, 20] and in carcasses (CV between 33 and 73 %) [19, 21]. More recently, Verhees [22] confirmed that horses displaying a CV of 22 % for live weight showed higher variations for CNS and BCS (CV 45 vs. 38 %, for CNS and BCS, respectively).

Results from the present study also demonstrated the existence of a significant correlation between CNS and fat measurements or carcass fatness. This is an interesting result that may allow further research to address issues regarding adiposity and adiposity variation in horses. Giles et al. [23] recently showed that seasonal changes of neck crest adiposity differ from those of overall adiposity, suggesting that the importance of adiposity may differ in different regions, even if both parameters are commonly associated. Carter et al. [7] point out two main limitations for CNS: the fact that it only assesses visibly apparent or appreciable neck crest adiposity, and the lack of breed or size references for horses. Therefore, CNS would only really be useful when used as a ratio to neck length [23]. However, the use of image-based neck crest parameters may attract additional interest, particularly for research on horse nutrition, adiposity, and metabolic disease risk factors. Further studies should seek to address the relation between nape fat measurements and nape fat thickness and features as measured by ultrasound in a larger cohort of animals, covering a wider range of CNS in different periods of the year. Recent studies by Giles et al. [8] report the existence of an apparently opposite pattern in the seasonal variation of CNS, compared to general obesity in domestic horses and ponies: CNS values were higher in winter compared to summer. Whether or not this difference reflects a real winter increase in regional fat deposition or whether it results in differences in the risk of metabolic stress still needs to be ascertained.

The present study also establishes a strong correlation between CNS and carcass fatness, which is supported by findings from other authors, who have found a strong relationship between nape fat and body or carcass adiposity [21, 24], and it supports a broader understanding of the mechanism of body adiposity in horses through the use of indicators based on nape fat.

Despite the lack of breed or size references, regarded by Giles et al. [23] as a significant pitfall for CNS in practice, Morrison et al. [24] argue that the strong relationship between nape fat and BCS is not confounded by an animal's phenotype. It is noteworthy that the present study revealed that nape fat thickness showed the best correlation with CNS.

Conclusions

Our results have revealed the existence of a significant correlation between CNS and nape fat measurements in horse obtained after image analysis, in particular with nape fat thickness. The present study has, moreover, established a strong correlation between CNS and carcass fatness. In future research, a sample with a wider range of body weights and sizes would be beneficial to get a better understanding of the relationship between CNS and carcass fatness in horses.

Abbreviations

BCS: body condition scoring; CNS: cresty neck scores; CV: coefficient of variation; r: coefficient of correlation; R^2: coefficient of determination.

Authors' contributions

SRS and ASS conceived and designed the experiments. SRS, ASS and SC were involved in data acquisition. SRS performed the image analysis; SRS and CMG analysed the data. SRS, SC and RP-C contributed to materials and analysis tools or technical assistance. SRS, CMG, RP-C and ASS contributed to the manuscript writing and the reviewing of the literature. All authors read and approved the final manuscript.

Author details

[1] Zootecnia Department, Centro de Ciência Animal E Veterinária, Universidade de Trás-os-Montes e Alto Douro, 5000-801 Vila Real, Portugal. [2] EUVG-Escola Universitária Vasco da Gama, Campus Universitário, Bloco B, Lordemão, 3020-210 Coimbra, Portugal. [3] CITAB, Universidade de Trás-os-Montes e Alto Douro, Quinta de Prados, 5000-801 Vila Real, Portugal.

Acknowledgements

This work was supported by the Portuguese Science and Technology Foundation (FCT) under Project PEst-OE/AGR/UI0772/2014.

Competing interests

The authors declare that they have no competing interests.

Declaration

Publication charges for this article were funded by the research platform Future Animal Health and Welfare at the Swedish University of Agricultural Sciences.

References

1. Argo CM. Feeding thin and starved horses. In: Geor RJ, Harris PA, Coenen M, editors. Equine applied and clinical nutrition. Amsterdam: Elsevier Ltd; 2013. p. 503–11.
2. Argo CM, Dugdale AHA, Curtis GC, Morrison PK. Evaluating body composition in living horses: where are we up to? In: Craigie C, Bunger L, editors. Maltin CA. Farm Animal imaging. Copenhagen. Quality Meat Scotland: Ingliston, UK; 2014. p. 12–7.
3. Robin CA, Ireland JL, Wylie CE, Collins SN, Verheyen KLP, Newton JR. Prevalence of and risk factors for equine obesity in Great Britain based on owner-reported body condition scores. Equine Vet J. 2015;47:196–201.
4. Argo CM. Appraising the portly pony: body condition and adiposity. Vet J. 2009;179:158–60.
5. Dugdale AHA, Curtis G, Cripps P. Effect of dietary restriction on body condition, composition and welfare of overweight and obese pony mares and welfare of overweight and obese pony mares. Equine Vet J. 2010;42:600–10.
6. Henneke D, Potter G, Kreider J, Yeates B. Relationship between condition score, physical measurements and body fat percentage in mares. Equine Vet J. 1983;15:371–2.
7. Carter RA, Geor RJ, Staniar WB, Cubitt TA, Harris PA. Apparent adiposity assessed by standardised scoring systems and morphometric measurements in horses and ponies. Vet J. 2009;179:204–10.
8. Giles SL, Nicol CJ, Rands SA, Harris PA. Assessing the seasonal prevalence and risk factors for nuchal crest adiposity in domestic horses and ponies using the cresty neck score. BMC Vet Res. 2015;11:13.
9. Morgan R, Keen J, McGowan C. Equine metabolic syndrome. Vet Rec. 2015;177:173–9.
10. Carroll C, Huntington P. Body condition scoring and weight estimation of horses. Equine Vet J. 1988;20:41–5.
11. Fernandes KA, Rogers CW, Gee EK, Bolwell CF, Thomas DG. Body condition and morphometric measures of adiposity in a cohort of pony club horses and ponies in New Zealand. Proc New Zeal Soc Anim Prod. 2015;75:195–9.
12. Dugdale AHA, Curtis GC, Harris PA, Argo CM. Assessment of body fat in the pony: part I. Relationships between the anatomical distribution of adipose tissue, body composition and body condition. Equine Vet J. 2011;43:552–61.
13. Gee EK, Fennessy PF, Morel PCH, Grace ND, Firth EC, Mogg TD. Chemical body composition of 20 thoroughbred foals at 160 days of age, and preliminary investigation of techniques used to predict body fatness. N Z Vet J. 2003;51:125–31.
14. Westervelt R, Stouffer JR, Hintz HF, Schryver HF. Estimating fatness in horses and ponies. J Anim Sci. 1976;43:781–5.
15. Gentry LR, Thompson DL, Gentry GT. The relationship between body condition score and ultrasonic fat measurements in mares of high versus low body condition. J Equine Vet Sci. 2004;24:198–203.
16. Quaresma M, Payan-Carreira R, Silva SR. Relationship between ultrasound measurements of body fat reserves and body condition score in female donkeys. Vet J. 2013;197:329–34.
17. Dugdale AHA, Grove-white D, Curtis GC, Harris PA, Argo CMC. Body condition scoring as a predictor of body fat in horses and ponies. Vet J. 2012;194:173–8.
18. Bohuslávek Z. Analysis of the commercial grades for beef carcasses. Czech J Anim Sci. 2002;2002:112–8.
19. Sarrie MV, Beriain MJ. Carcass characteristics and meat quality of male and female foals. Meat Sci. 2005;70:141–52.
20. Mazan MR, Deveney EF, Dewitt S, Bedenice D, Hoffman A. Energetic cost of breathing, body composition, and pulmonary function in horses with recurrent airway obstruction. J Appl Physiol. 2004;97:91–7.
21. Znamirowska A. Prediction of horse carcass composition using linear measurements. Meat Sci. 2005;69:567–70.
22. Verhees E. The relationship between body condition score and real time ultrasound measurements in different horse types and an inventory of data of ultrasound, body condition and morphological body measurements from Garrano horses in northern Portugal. Universidade de Trás-os-Montes e Alto Douro and Wageningen University; 2008.
23. Giles SL, Rands SA, Nicol CJ, Harris PA. Obesity prevalence and associated risk factors in outdoor living domestic horses and ponies. PeerJ. 2014;2:e299.
24. Morrinson P, Harris P, Maltin CA, Grove-White D, Argo CMC. Relationships between body condition score and regional adipose depots in the horse. In: Maltin CA, Craigie C, Bunger L., editors. Farm Animal imaging. Kaposvar. Quality Meat Scotland, Ingliston, UK; 2013. p. 93.

7

Computed tomography of the thorax in rabbits: a prospective study in ten clinically healthy New Zealand White rabbits

Désirée Müllhaupt[1], Sandra Wenger[2], Patrick Kircher[1], Nadja Pfammatter[1], Jean-Michel Hatt[2] and Stefanie Ohlerth[1*]

Abstract

Background: Literature investigating the normal cross-sectional anatomy of rabbits with computed tomography (CT) is sparse and incomplete. The purpose of the present study was to investigate the normal thoracic structures, in particular the cranial thorax, with CT angiography in 10 clinically healthy New Zealand White (NZW) rabbits.

Results: Absolute and relative measurements of the trachea, heart, thoracic caudal vena cava and aorta, right and left principal bronchi, right and left caudal lobar bronchi and the accompanying branches of the right and left pulmonary artery and vein, right and left lung volume and lung density were taken. The three lobes of the thymus (right ventral, right dorsal and left thoracic lobes) were identified in all rabbits. Both the right dorsal and left thoracic lobes of the thymus extended between the heart and thoracic wall in all individuals with the left lobe reaching more caudally in seven animals. Consequently, the craniocaudal extension of the left lung was smaller than the right lung in these rabbits. Volume of the left lung was significantly smaller than the right ($P = 0.005$). The cranial mediastinal, right and left tracheobronchial and the aortic thoracic lymph nodes were very small and identified in four, four, seven and ten rabbits, respectively. The heart took up a median of 4.0 intercostal spaces, and in seven rabbits, it was located in the 2nd–5th intercostal space. Median relative cardiac height and width measured 74 and 88%, respectively. The median angle of the trachea to the spine was 5°. Median density between the right and left lung did not significantly differ (− 549 and − 583 Hounsfield units, respectively). In all but one rabbit, atelectasis was present and classified as mild, moderate or severe in six, two and one individuals, respectively. Mild subclinical bronchopneumonia was diagnosed in seven rabbits.

Conclusions: The present study provides species-specific anatomical CT information and reference values for structures in the thorax of the NZW rabbit. Subclinical bronchopneumonia appears to be a common CT finding.

Keywords: Computed tomography, Rabbit, Thorax, Thymus

Background

The number of rabbits held as pets in European households has been increasing over the last years and rabbits have become frequent patients at veterinary clinics [1]. At the Clinic of Zoo Animals, Exotic Pets and Wildlife at the University of Zurich, rabbits are now the species presented most often [2]. In addition, rabbits are frequently used as laboratory animals and represent a common animal model to study respiratory diseases in humans.

In rabbits, respiratory diseases are a major cause of morbidity and mortality. Pasteurellosis, essentially caused by *Pasteurella multocida*, is the primary respiratory disease; however, many other bacterial and viral pathogens play a role in the disease complex [3]. In pet rabbits, infections with *Bordetella bronchiseptica* or *Staphylococcus* species are more common than an infection caused by *P. multocida* in rabbits from rabbitries [3]. Depending on the causative agent, clinical signs include

*Correspondence: sohlerth@vetclinics.uzh.ch
[1] Clinic for Diagnostic Imaging, Vetsuisse Faculty, University of Zurich, Winterthurerstrasse 258c, 8057 Zurich, Switzerland
Full list of author information is available at the end of the article

upper respiratory disease (rhinitis, sinusitis, conjunctivitis, dacryocystitis), otitis, pleuropneumonia, bacteremia, pericarditis and abscesses in subcutaneous tissues, organs, bones, joints or genitalia [3]. Other reported thoracic diseases in the rabbit include bronchitis [4], thymoma [5], lymphoma [6], and metastatic pulmonary disease [7].

Because of its large availability, radiography represents the routine diagnostic imaging method in small animals to investigate abnormalities of the respiratory system, in particular the lower airway system. However, interpretation of thoracic radiographs in the rabbit presents several challenges. Among the intermediate-sized small companion mammals, the rabbit has a relatively small thoracic volume and the heart is located more cranially in the thorax. On latero-lateral radiographs, size of the retrosternal lucency, i.e. the cranial lung lobes is very small, making evaluation of the pulmonary opacity in the cranial thorax difficult. The accessory lobe of the right lung is also very small. Many rabbits have a large amount of subcutaneous and pericardial fat, further increasing overall thoracic opacity. Together, these species-specific features may simulate pulmonary disease or, on the contrary, mask true pulmonary changes [8, 9].

Computed tomography (CT) is considered the gold standard to evaluate thoracic disease in humans, and represents an increasingly available technology in veterinary medicine. Modern helical scanners allow very short scan times, thin slices, high resolution and post-processing software such as multiplanar reconstructions, making CT highly suitable for the examination of the thorax in small companion mammals. So far, CT has been reported to be superior to conventional radiographs in rabbits for the diagnosis of intrapulmonary disease such as abscesses or lung metastases [10]. So far, there is only a single report including an atlas comparing CT and cross-sectional cadaver anatomy of the rabbit's neck and thorax. However, the study lacks measurements and information on the topical relationship of normal structures [11]. Another recent study evaluated in detail the normal CT anatomy and dimensions of the larynx and upper trachea in rabbits for the establishment of an animal model [12]. However, detailed cross-sectional studies of the normal lower airways in rabbits have not yet been performed. Therefore, the purpose of the present study was to use CT to investigate the normal thoracic structures, particularly the cranial thorax, in clinically healthy New Zealand White rabbits.

Methods

Animals

Ten clinically healthy 7-month-old intact female New Zealand White rabbits with a median body weight of 5.0 kg (SE 0.15 kg; range 4.4–6.0 kg) were included in the study. Animals were obtained from a wholesale source with annual hygiene monitoring and allowed to acclimatize to the new environment for 1 week. Rabbits were not fasted before CT.

Anaesthesia

All rabbits were judged to be healthy based on a physical examination. Then, animals were sedated with a combination of fentanyl citrate 0.0473 mg/kg body weight (BW) and fluanisone 1.5 mg/kg BW (Hypnorm; Veta-Pharma Ltd, Leeds, UK) administered intramuscularly. Twenty minutes after the injection, they were placed and kept in sternal recumbency until the end of the CT scan. First, a venous catheter was placed in the external ear vein. Then, rabbits were pre-oxygenated for 2 min prior to induction of anaesthesia with propofol (Propofol 1% MCT; Fresenius Kabi AG, Oberdorf, Switzerland) given intravenously to effect, starting with a dose of 1 mg/kg BW over 20 s. Anaesthesia was maintained with a constant rate infusion of propofol (0.2–0.6 mg/kg BW/min). Oxygen was provided by a tight-fitting facemask. After the CT scan, animals received Ringer's lactate solution 10 ml/kg BW (Ringer Lactat Fresenius; Fresenius Kabi AG, Oberdorf, Switzerland) intravenously over 30 min and were returned to the group when fully awake.

Computed tomography

Examination of the thorax was performed in sternal recumbency using a 40-slice scanner (SOMATOM Sensation Open, Siemens Schweiz AG, Zurich, Switzerland). Images were acquired from the caudal cervical spine to the mid-abdomen (slice thickness 2 mm, increment 0.7 mm, pitch 1.2, 120 kVp, 120 mA, rotation time 1 s). To improve identification of cardiovascular structures, the thymus and lymph nodes, CT angiography was performed subsequently. Iodinated contrast agent (Ultravist®-370, Bayer AG, Zurich, Switzerland) was given intravenously as a manual bolus (dose 2 ml/kg BW). Bolus tracking was performed in the pulmonary outflow tract (threshold 100 Hounsfield units (HU)) with a subsequent caudocranial thoracic scan using a slice thickness of 2 mm. CT data was reconstructed to images with 0.75 mm slice thickness using a medium-frequency (soft tissue) and a high-frequency image reconstruction algorithm (lung, bone), respectively.

Analysis of computed tomographic images

Image interpretation and all measurements were done with dedicated software using multiplanar reconstruction (MPR) images and electronic callipers integral to the software system (OsiriX Open Source™ 5.0.2, OsiriX Foundation, Geneva). Measurements were performed once and by the same author (DM). Bony structures, soft tissues and the lungs were evaluated in a bone (window width (WW) 1500 HU, window level (WL) 300 HU), soft tissue (WW 350 HU, WL 40 HU) and lung window (WW 1400 HU, WL– 500), respectively. Mediastinal, cardiovascular and bronchial structures were identified and measured on post-contrast images in an analogous manner to radiographs. If indicated, ratios were calculated to compensate for differences in size and body weight. Anatomic structures were identified based on standard literature [13–15]. The anatomical nomenclature used in this study followed the format of the Nomina Anatomica Veterinaria [16].

Measurements—mediastinal structures

In the sagittal plane, the maximal height of the caudal vena cava and the descending thoracic aorta were measured along their course. The length of the thoracic vertebra at the level of the tracheal bifurcation was determined along its mid-ventral surface to calculate ratios of the maximal height of the large vessels.

Location of the heart in relation to the intercostal spaces and number of intercostal spaces (ICS) determining cardiac width was determined subjectively based on MPR images. In the dorsal plane, the relative cardiac width was calculated as a ratio of the maximal cardiac width to the thoracic width at the same level. Relative cardiac height was calculated on sagittal images as the ratio of the maximal cardiac height measured along the ribs to the thoracic height at the same level. In the mid-sagittal plane of the caudal vena cava, the short axis of the heart was measured along the atrioventricular valves. Perpendicular to it, the long axis of the heart was measured from the ventral border of the tracheal bifurcation to the cardiac apex. The long and short axis dimensions were added, transposed onto the vertebral column and recorded as the number of vertebrae starting at the cranial edge of the 4th thoracic vertebra. The given distance along the vertebral column to the caudal point was estimated as the number of vertebrae resulting in a vertebral heart score [17, 18]. In the same plane, the cardiac angle was determined between the heart base and the apex, along the lumen of the left ventricle.

Measurements—airways, lungs

In the bone window, thoracic height was measured in the transverse plane at the level of and parallel to the 1st ribs between the ventral aspect of the 1st thoracic vertebra and the manubrium. At the same level, but in a lung window, the maximal luminal tracheal height and width were measured. A ratio of tracheal height to thoracic height at the thoracic inlet was calculated electronically. The cross-sectional area (CSA) of the tracheal lumen was measured just cranial to the tracheal bifurcation. Caudal to the tracheal bifurcation, the CSA of the lumen of the right and left principal bronchus were evaluated. At the level of the 6th rib, the CSA of the lumen of the caudal lobar bronchus and the accompanying branch of the pulmonary artery and vein were calculated on the right and left. In the dorsal plane, the interbronchial angle between the mid-axis of both principal bronchi was assessed. Lung density (HU) was determined on native images in a defined area of 50 mm^2 dorsolateral to the right and left caudal lobar bronchi avoiding the inclusion of vessels. The tracheal angle was determined between the dorsal wall of the trachea and the spine in the sagittal plane.

The maximal cranial and caudal extent of the left and right lungs was determined. The volume of the right and left lungs was assessed delineating their cross-sectional areas on 8–11 transverse images at intervals of 1 cm from the cranial to the caudal thorax; volumes were calculated electronically.

Subjective evaluation of lung changes

Lung atelectasis was defined as loss of lung volume in combination with various degrees of increased attenuation in the ventral lung aspects. Atelectasis was classified subjectively in four grades for the right and left lung: no atelectasis; mild atelectasis: increased attenuation, ventral aspect of the lung partially aerated; moderate atelectasis: complete attenuation, less than to the level of the heart base; severe atelectasis: complete attenuation $\geq$ to the level of the heart base. Total grade of atelectasis referred to the most severely affected side.

Lung changes in the dorsal regions were classified according to a system described for the assessment of high-resolution CT findings in the dog [19]. Lung abnormalities were finally categorized subjectively in four grades: normal lung, mild (< 1/3 of the lung affected), moderate (1/3–2/3 affected), and severe ($\geq$ 2/3 affected).

Data analysis

Descriptive statistics and ratios were calculated electronically. Due to the small sample size, the nonparametric Wilcoxon signed rank test was used for the comparison of two related samples (SPSS statistics, release 23.0.0.2, IBM Corporation, Armonk, New York). A P value < 0.05 was considered significant.

Results

Image quality was considered good to excellent in all rabbits despite minor motion artefacts due to spontaneous breathing. Branches of the lobar bronchi and the accompanying pulmonary vessels could always be identified up to the 3rd generation. Major abnormalities or pathologies were not detected in any animal. Therefore, all datasets were included in the study.

In eight and two rabbits, respectively, 12 and 13 thoracic vertebrae with an equivalent number of rib pairs were present; transitional vertebrae were not identified. The 1st to 9th rib pair was connected to the sternum whereas the 10th to 12th or 13th rib pair ended free and separately. The cartilages of the 7th to 9th rib were fused and joined uniformly the xyphoid process. The sternum was composed of the large manubrium cranially, the body including four vertebrae, and the xyphoid process caudally with a thin but broad cartilaginous process.

The thymus was visible pre- and postcontrast in the cranial and middle mediastinum in all rabbits (Fig. 1). All three lobes were identified: (1) the right dorsal thoracic lobe was seen dorsal to the right cranial vena cava; (2) the right ventral thoracic lobe was located ventral to the right cranial vena cava with two parts, cranial and caudal to the right internal thoracic artery, respectively; and (3) the left thoracic lobe was identified ventral to the left cranial vena cava with two parts, cranial and caudal to the left internal thoracic artery, respectively. Whereas the right dorsal thoracic lobe represented the most enhancing, homogeneous and compact lobe, which was easily identified in all rabbits, the right ventral and left thoracic lobes, in particular the caudal parts, subjectively demonstrated less enhancement, were less well marginated and more heterogeneous due to a loose structure and a mixed density composed of fat and soft tissue. The right dorsal lobe was of a round shape in the transverse plane and of an elliptical shape in the sagittal plane. It was clearly separated from the right ventral lobe. Both ventral lobes had a multilobulated appearance and extended caudally in between the heart and the thoracic wall. The cranial part of the left thoracic lobe was the smallest and most difficult lobe to visualize in all rabbits. However, the left lobe reached more caudally than the right lobe in seven animals (Fig. 1). In two rabbits, the caudal extent of the right and left thoracic lobe was at a similar level whereas the right thoracic lobe extended more caudally in one rabbit only. Multiple efforts were undertaken by the authors (DM, SO) to determine the total volume of the thoracic thymus and its lobes. However, due to its incoherent structure and very small caudal extensions in between the heart and the thoracic wall, reliable measurements could not be achieved.

The cranial mediastinal lymph node was identified caudomedial to the right dorsal thoracic lobe of the thymus in four individuals (Fig. 1b); it was very small in three of those four rabbits. The right and left tracheobronchial lymph nodes, located to either side of the caudal trachea just cranial to the bifurcation, were found in four and seven rabbits, respectively (Fig. 2); the left node was constantly larger than the right node and therefore easier to recognize. The dorsal thoracic lymph centrum i.e. the cranial and caudal aortic thoracic lymph nodes, was depicted in all rabbits lateral to the ascending and descending aorta comprising a single to multiple nodes of varying size (Fig. 2). In general, lymph nodes were round to slender in transverse and fusiform in sagittal images.

The oesophagus was identified on the left of the trachea at the thoracic inlet, then coursing dorsally to the trachea through the mediastinum, finally passing the diaphragm in the midline in all animals. It contained little to moderate amount of gas in six rabbits.

The trachea was mildly mineralized and coursed almost parallel to the spine in all rabbits (Fig. 3). At the thoracic

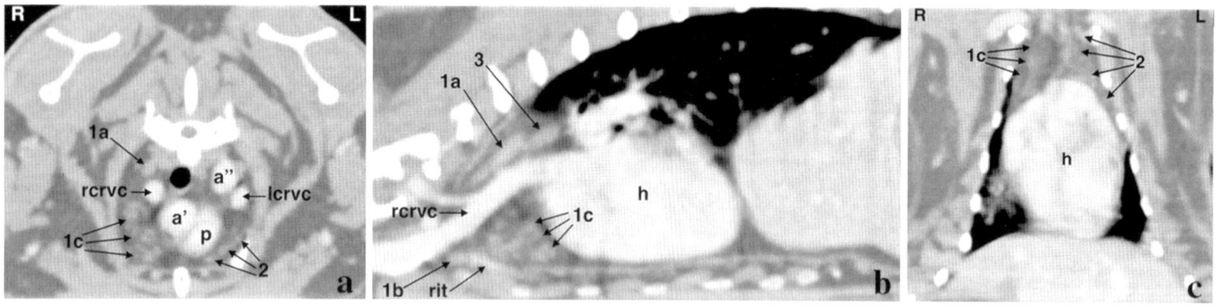

Fig. 1 Post-contrast computed tomographic appearance of the thoracic thymus in a rabbit. **a** On a transverse image at the cranial border of the heart, the right dorsal thoracic thymus lobe (1a) is clearly isolated from the right ventral lobe (1c). The multilobulated heterogeneous structure of the caudal parts of the right ventral (1c) and left thoracic thymus lobes (2) is noted. A right (rcrvc) and left cranial vena cava (lcrvc) is present (ascending (a') and descending thoracic aorta (a"), pulmonary trunk (p)). **b** On a right sagittal image at the level of the right cranial vena cava (rcrvc), the separated right dorsal thoracic thymus lobe (1a) shows a round to ovoid shape with a compact structure. The right ventral thoracic thymus lobe has a small cranial (1b) and larger caudal (1c) part separated by the right internal thoracic artery (rit). Caudal to the right dorsal thoracic thymus lobe, the mediastinal lymph node (3) is seen (heart (h)). **c** On the dorsal plane, the left thoracic thymus lobe (2) extends more caudally in between the heart and the thoracic wall in comparison to the right ventral thoracic thymus lobe (1c). Cranial to the heart, only little lung tissue is seen on the right. Note the wide cardiac size in relation to the thoracic width (heart (h))

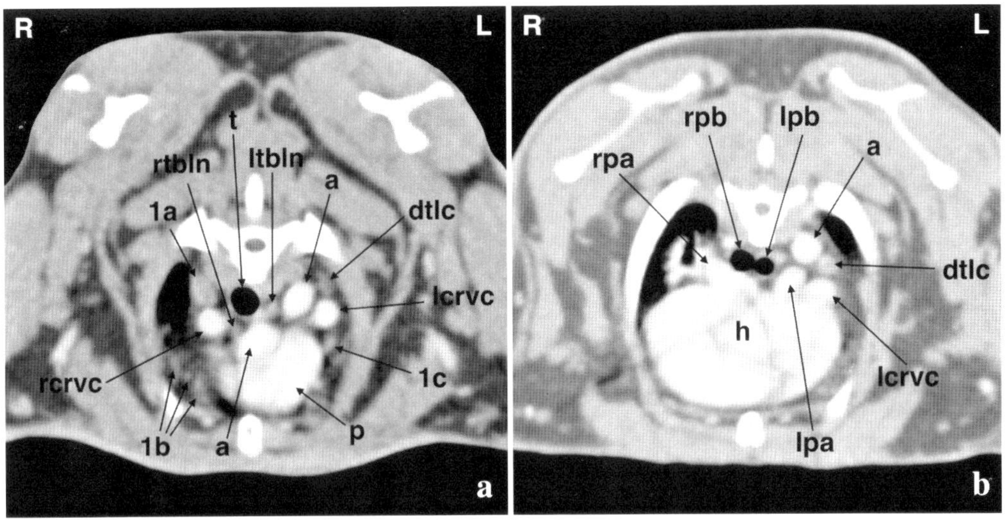

Fig. 2 Post-contrast transverse computed tomographic images at the level of the pulmonary trunk (**a**) and the tracheal bifurcation (**b**) in a rabbit. The right (rtbln) and left tracheobronchial lymph nodes (ltbln) and one of the lymph nodes of the dorsal thoracic lymph centrum (dtlc) are shown (right dorsal thoracic thymus lobe (1a), right ventral thoracic thymus lobe (1b), left thoracic thymus lobe (1c), aorta (a), heart (h), trachea (t), pulmo nary trunk (p), right (rpa) and left pulmonary artery (lpa), right (rpb) and left principal bronchus (lpb), right (rcrvc) and left (lcrvc) cranial vena cava)

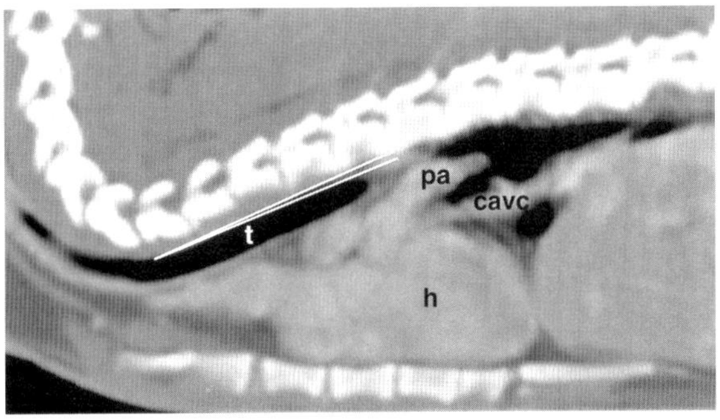

Fig. 3 Post-contrast sagittal computed tomographic image in a rabbit (bone window): the tracheal angle between the dorsal wall of the trachea (t) and the thoracic spine is very small (white lines). Cardiac height in relation to the thoracic height is large (heart (h), caudal vena cava (cavc), pulmonary artery (pa))

inlet, the tracheal cross section area was almost round. The tracheal bifurcation was located at the level of the 3rd or 4th thoracic vertebra in two and eight animals, respectively.

The absolute and relative height of the aorta was significantly smaller than for the caudal vena cava ($P = 0.03$). Subjectively, the heart appeared globoid and large (Fig. 1), which was reflected by a high number of ICS and relative cardiac height and width. The heart took a median of 4.0 ICS (SD 0.33; mean 3.8; min 3; max 4) and was located more commonly in the 2nd–5th ($n = 7$) than in the 3rd–6th ($n = 2$) or 3rd–5th ($n = 1$) ICS. In the sagittal plane, the cardiac axis was mildly oriented from craniodorsal to caudoventral in all rabbits. In the dorsal plane, the apex was located on the midline or to the left in six and four rabbits, respectively. In all rabbits, a left and right cranial vena cava was identified (Figs. 1, 2). Descriptive statistics of thoracic measurements are provided in Table 1. The CSA of the caudal lobar branch of the pulmonary artery was of a similar size as the accompanying vein bilaterally ($P = 0.2$ and 0.8); on the other hand, CSA of both, the lobar venous and arterial branch, was seven times the median CSA of the adjacent lobar bronchi (Fig. 4). Subjectively, CSA of the bronchial tree was constantly smaller than the accompanying vessels throughout the lungs of all rabbits.

In agreement with the commonly shorter right thoracic lobe of the thymus, the right lung field was markedly longer than the left in the dorsal plane (Table 2). The right lung expanded cranially to the 3rd or 4th thoracic vertebra (T3 or T4) and never to T5. In contrast, the cranial border of the left lung was most often seen at T4 or T5. Caudally, the right lung reached most commonly T11 whereas the left lung expanded most frequently to T10. Also, in the transverse image just cranial to the heart, only the right cranial lung lobe was identified dorsally in four rabbits. In the other six animals, no lung tissue was seen at all at this level. The median right lung volume was significantly larger than the left ($P = 0.005$). The visceral pleura i.e. pleural fissure lines were rarely visible and location of the lung lobes was only possible based on the course of the lobar bronchi and the accompanying pulmonary vessels.

Table 1 Descriptive statistics of thoracic computed tomographic measurements in 10 healthy New Zealand White rabbits

Variable	Median	Mean	SD	Min	Max
Cardiac angle (°)	35	35	2.5	30	38
Long axis of the heart (cm)	3.3	3.4	0.4	3	4
Short axis of the heart (cm)	3	3	0.2	2.7	3.2
Relative cardiac height (ratio maximal cardiac height/thoracic height) (%)	74	74	3.5	67	81
Relative cardiac width (ratio maximal cardiac width/thoracic width) (%)	88	88	4.9	81	95
Vertebral heart score	6.3	6.4	0.4	6	7.3
Maximal height of caudal vena cava (mm)	6.4	6.3	0.6	5	7.2
Maximal height of aorta (mm)	5.5	5.5	0.5	5	6.1
Ratio maximal height of caudal vena cava/length of thoracic vertebra at level of bifurcation (%)	73	71	5.9	57	76
Ratio maximal height of aorta/length of thoracic vertebra at level of bifurcation (%)	60	62	5.2	56	70
Angle of trachea to spine (°)	5	5	1.4	2	7
Tracheal height at thoracic inlet (mm)	5.4	5.1	1.1	2.4	6.2
Tracheal width at thoracic inlet (mm)	4.8	4.7	0.8	3.7	6.2
Ratio tracheal height/thoracic height at thoracic inlet (%)	26	25	5.5	10	30
CSA of tracheal lumen at bifurcation (mm^2)	28.3	27.8	3.4	21.9	32.2
Luminal CSA of right principal bronchus (mm^2)	15.5	15.4	2.4	11.1	18.8
Luminal CSA of left principal bronchus (mm^2)	12.7	12.4	1.8	9.9	15.4
Luminal CSA of right caudal lobar bronchus (mm^2)	1.7	2.0	0.6	1.3	2.9
Luminal CSA of left caudal lobar bronchus (mm^2)	1.7	1.7	0.4	1.1	2.4
CSA of caudal lobar branch of right pulmonary artery (mm^2)	14.8	14.4	4.9	7.7	22.3
CSA of caudal lobar branch of left pulmonary artery (mm^2)	11.9	11.8	2.1	9	15.3
CSA of caudal lobar branch of right pulmonary vein (mm^2)	15.8	15.1	4.7	7.7	22.5
CSA of caudal lobar branch of left pulmonary vein (mm^2)	10.9	11.8	3.8	7.4	18.4
Interbronchial angle (°)	54	55	4.9	50	65
Lung volume right (cm^3)	30.2	31.6	8.8	23.1	54
Lung volume left (cm^3)	20.7	22.2	7.2	14.8	40.4
Density of right caudal lung (HU)	− 549	− 573	92	− 783	− 447
Density of left caudal lung (HU)	− 583	− 587	98	− 774	− 425

SD standard deviation; *Min* minimum; *Max* maximum; *CSA* cross-sectional area; *HU* Hounsfield unit

In all rabbits, the branches of the pulmonary artery and vein were seen lateral and medial, respectively, and in close relationship to the corresponding principal bronchi (Fig. 4a). In contrast, the caudal lobar vessels were running parallel but with a certain distance to the lobar bronchi (Fig. 4b). Median luminal CSA of the right principal bronchus was significantly larger than on the left ($P = 0.005$). Although median CSAs of the caudal lobar branch of the right pulmonary artery and vein were larger than on the left, differences were not significant ($P = 0.074$ and 0.047, respectively). Otherwise, no significant differences were found between left and right measurements.

In all but one animal, atelectasis was present and classified as mild, moderate and severe in six, two and one subjects, respectively. In three animals, the dorsal lungs were considered normal on CT. In the other seven rabbits, mild lung changes were diagnosed including ground glass opacity, parenchymal bands, consolidation, peribronchovascular thickening and/or pleural thickening (Fig. 5).

Discussion

Although respiratory diseases are common in rabbits, clinical signs of lower respiratory diseases are often unspecific. The rabbit may present with anorexia, weight loss, depression and fatigue. Chronic infection in the thoracic cavity may be even subclinical long after the acute phase of the infection [3]. Low sensitivity of thoracic radiographs in rabbits further complicates the diagnosis for the treating veterinarian [3, 13]. Helical CT is considered highly superior to radiography for the evaluation of thoracic diseases, also in the small mammal patient. Rabbits also represent a common animal model to study respiratory diseases in humans. Due to a lack of pertinent data in the veterinary literature, the present study was performed to investigate the normal thoracic structures in clinically healthy New Zealand White rabbits using CT.

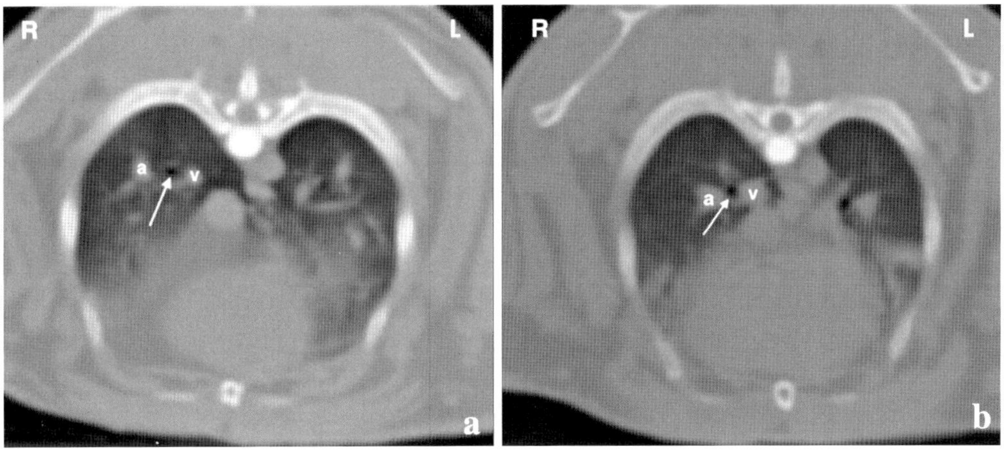

Fig. 4 Post-contrast transverse computed tomographic images of the caudal lung lobes in a rabbit. **a** The branches of the pulmonary artery (a) and vein (v) are seen lateral and medial, respectively, and in close relationship to the corresponding principal bronchi (arrow). **b** In contrast, the caudal lobar vessels are running parallel but with a certain distance to the lobar bronchi. The cross-sectional area of the bronchial tree is constantly smaller than the accompanying vessels throughout the lungs

Table 2 Lung extent in 10 healthy New Zealand White rabbits on multiplanar computed tomographic images

Extent of right lung	N	Extent of left lung	N
T3–T9	1	T3–T11	1
T3–T10	2	T4–T9	3
T3–T11	2	T4–T10	3
T3–T12	1	T5–T10	2
T4–T11	4	T5–T11	1

T thoracic vertebra, *N* number of rabbits

Radiographically, the craniocaudal dimension of the rabbit's thorax has been described to be short with a small thoracic lung volume and a small cranial lung field, with a cranially located, relatively large heart [8, 9]. This was confirmed and more precisely defined with CT in the present study. Whereas on radiographs of the dog and cat [20] the cranial lung lobes extend to the thoracic inlet at end inspiration, the rabbits' large cranial and middle mediastinum predominantly filled in the cranial thorax in the present study. However, the caudal extent of the lungs of the rabbits at the level of T9–T12 was similar or slightly less than that of the dog [21]. Relative cardiac height and in particular cardiac width and number of ICS were much higher in the rabbits than reported for dogs or cats [22]. This was also reflected in a small angle of the trachea to the spine in the present study. The more cranial location of the cardiac silhouette and the tracheal bifurcation in these rabbits is in contrast to a former radiographic report, where the carina lay more caudally, i.e. at the level of the 4th or 5th intercostal space [9].

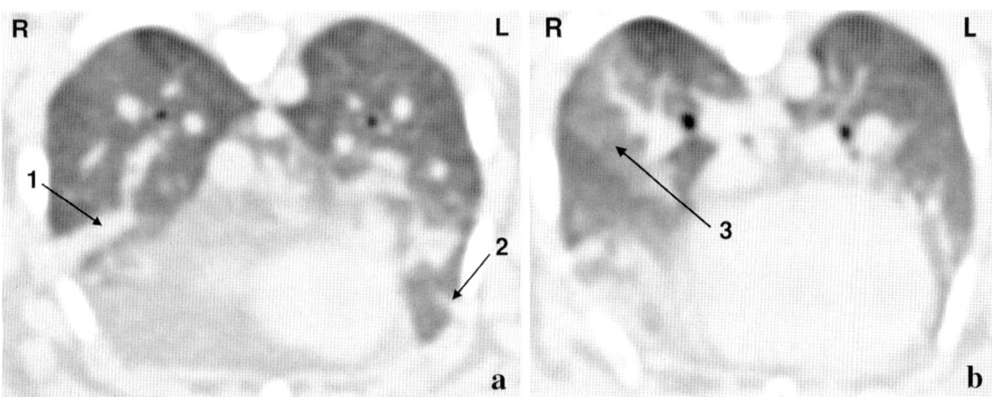

Fig. 5 Post-contrast transverse computed tomographic images of a rabbit showing consolidation (1), a parenchymal band (2) (**a**) and ground glass opacity (3) (**b**) in the lung

Whereas the normal position of the cardiac apex in the dog and cat is always on the left in the ventrodorsal view/plane [22], it was found more often on the midline than to the left in the present study and therefore, appears more variable in the rabbit.

In the adult rabbit, the thymus persists and consists of a right ventral and dorsal thoracic lobe and a left thoracic lobe. According to an anatomic atlas of the rabbit [16], the left lobe expands more caudoventrally around the heart, whereas the right lobe stretches out further dorsally. Cranially, both lobes extend into the thoracic inlet. In the present study, all lobes were identified in the described locations in all animals. However, identification was challenging. The right dorsal thoracic lobe was identified most easily in all rabbits whereas the boundaries of the right ventral and left thoracic lobes were indistinct due to a multilobulated architecture interspersed with fat.

Values for tracheal height in relation to the thoracic height at the thoracic inlet were similar to those reported in non-brachycephalic dogs [23]. Similar to other species [20], the volume of the left lung was significantly smaller than for the right lung in these rabbits. This was already described in an anatomical study of the rabbit at the end of the 19th century [15]. Larger absolute sizes of the right lung lobes, the existence of the accessory lobe as well as a relatively larger left lobe of the thymus [14] represent possible explanations. Moreover, rabbits were not fasted for the present study, since this is not necessary in this species. Therefore, the full stomach on the left might have displaced the diaphragm cranially decreasing the volume of the left lung. Interestingly, the median CSA of the right principal bronchus was significantly larger than the CSA of the left principal bronchus; the median CSAs of the accompanying artery and vein were also larger on the right although borderline not significant. These findings could support an anatomical difference between the right and left lung. However, due to the small size of the structures, measurement errors should also be considered.

The mean lung density measured in the present study is markedly higher compared to the dog, where mean values of − 713 to − 846 HU were reported [24]. Animals were always in sternal and never in lateral recumbency and therefore, haemostasis and hypoventilation can be ruled out. Spontaneous superficial breathing, differences in body condition or compression of the lung secondary to a large abdomen may have caused this finding. However, subclinical pulmonary disease cannot be ruled out, and unfortunately, necropsy was not available in the present study. Atelectasis in the ventral lung aspects was a common finding in the present study and was most likely caused by sternal recumbency. Lung changes were classified according to a system described previously for the assessment of high resolution CT findings in the dog [19]. This classification system applied very well in the rabbits of this study where all kinds of linear and reticular opacities as well as ground glass opacity were observed. However, the presence of subclinical respiratory changes in these rabbits limits the significance of the results of the present study. This is reinforced by the relatively high lung density measurements in the present study where values were significantly higher than reported values for the normal human or canine lung [24, 25]. On the other hand, clinically unapparent lung changes are rather common in rabbits, and therefore, the results of the present study might just reflect the situation in a normal population.

The pulmonary vessels could be followed to the 3rd-degree branch in the rabbits of this study whereas they can be followed to the 4th-degree branch in the normal lung of dogs and cats [26]. Authors of this study hypothesize that this finding is most likely due to the smaller size of the animals and smaller diameter of their peripheral pulmonary vessels and presumably this small size creates problems due to the limits of image resolution. The CSA of the caudal lobar branches of the pulmonary arteries and veins were of a similar size, but 7 times the median CSA of the adjacent lobar bronchi. In dogs, the pulmonary artery CSA should be between 0.4 and 0.6 of the external CSA of the adjacent bronchus measured at the level of the T8 vertebra [27]. In the present study, it was not possible to obtain measurements at the level of T8, because branching of the lobar vessels and bronchi took place more cranially in all rabbits. However, since the CSA of the bronchial tree was smaller than the accompanying vessels throughout the lungs of all rabbits, we hypothesize that this finding may represent a species-specific feature.

As reported previously, an average number of 12 thoracic vertebrae and a left and right cranial vena cava appear to be common and species-specific in rabbits [14].

A few limitations have to be considered regarding this study. Although image quality was considered satisfactory, it could have been improved by scanning during apnea similar to the standard practice in dogs and cats. Attempts to assess accuracy or intra-, interobserver reproducibility of measurements were not undertaken. A post mortem examination including macroscopic and histopathological evaluation of the major organs was not performed and animals were considered to be healthy on a clinical examination only. Additionally, only a small number of animals of a single breed were included. Therefore, subsequent CT studies should be performed in a larger cohort of animals of various breeds, including pet rabbits. Comparison to post-mortem findings would be preferable.

Conclusions

The present study provides preliminary species-specific computed tomographic anatomical information and reference values for structures in the thorax of the NZW rabbit. Subclinical bronchopneumonia appears a common CT finding.

Authors' contributions

SO, PK, NP, JMH and SW, in collaboration, conceived of and participated in the design of the study. SW and DM carried out general anesthesia in all animals. SO and DM analysed and interpreted the data, and drafted the manuscript with contributions from SW, JMH, PK and NP. SO was responsible for the statistical analysis. All authors read and approved the final manuscript.

Author details

[1] Clinic for Diagnostic Imaging, Vetsuisse Faculty, University of Zurich, Winterthurerstrasse 258c, 8057 Zurich, Switzerland. [2] Clinic for Zoo Animals, Exotic Pets and Wildlife, Vetsuisse Faculty, University of Zurich, Winterthurerstrasse 260, 8057 Zurich, Switzerland.

Acknowledgements

Not applicable.

Competing interests

The authors declare that they have no competing interests.

References

1. Kraft W. Heimtiere als Patienten in der tierärztlichen Praxis—Entwicklung seit 1967. Tierärztl Prax. 2005;3:221–6.
2. Langenecker M, Clauss M, Hässig M, Hatt JM. Comparative investigation on the distribution of diseases in rabbits, guinea pigs, rats, and ferrets. Tierärztl Prax. 2009;37:326–33.
3. Johnson-Delaney CA, Orosz SE. Rabbit respiratory system: clinical anatomy, physiology and disease. Vet Clin Exot Anim. 2011;14:257–66.
4. Deeb BJ. Respiratory disease and pasteurellosis. In: Quesenberry KE, Carpenter JW, editors. Ferrets, rabbits and rodents: clinical medicine and surgery. St. Louis: Saunders; 1997. p. 172–82.
5. Künzel F, Hittmair KM, Hassan J, Dupré G, Russold E, Guija de Arespachochaga A, Fuchs-Baumgartinger A, Bilek A. Thymomas in rabbits: clinical evaluation, diagnosis, and treatment. J Am Anim Hosp Assoc. 2012;48:97–104.
6. Gómez L, Gázquez A, Roncero V, Sánchez C, Durán ME. Lymphoma in a rabbit: histopathological and immunohistochemical findings. J Small Anim Pract. 2002;43:224–6.
7. Klaphake E, Paul-Murphy J. Disorders of the reproductive and urinary systems. In: Quesenberry KE, Carpenter JW, editors. Ferets, rabbits, and rodents: clinical medicine and surgery. St. Louis: Elsevier Saunders; 2012. p. 217–31.
8. Silverman S. Diagnostic imaging of exotic pets. Vet Clin North Am Small Anim Pract. 1993;23:1287–99.
9. Gibbs C, Hinton MH. Radiological examination of the rabbit. 1. The head, thorax and vertebral column. J Small Anim Pract. 1981;22:687–703.
10. Capello V, Lennox AM. Diagnostic imaging of the respiratory system in exotic companion mammals. Vet Clin North Am Exot Anim Pract. 2011;14:369–89.
11. Zotti A, Banzato T, Cozzi B. Cross-sectional anatomy of the rabbit neck and trunk: comparison of computed tomography and cadaver anatomy. Res Vet Sci. 2009;87:171–6.
12. Ajlan AM, Al-Khatib T, Al-Sheikah M, Jastaniah S, Salih A, Althubaiti A, et al. Helical computed tomography scanning of the larynx and upper trachea in rabbits. Acta Vet Scand. 2015;57:67.
13. Silverman S. Domestic rabbit. In: Silverman S, Tell LA, editors. Radiology of rodents, rabbits, and ferrets. An atlas of normal anatomy and positioning. St. Louis: Elsevier Saunders; 2005. p. 160–2.
14. Popesko P, Rajtova V, Horak J. Anatomy of small laboratory animals. Volume one: rabbit, guinea pig. London: Wolfe Publishing Ltd; 1990.
15. Lungen Krause W. In: Krause W, editor. Die Anatomie des Kaninchens in topographischer und operativer Rücksicht. Leipzig: Engelmann; 1884. p. 113–5.
16. International Committee on Veterinary Gross Anatomical Nomenclature. Nomina anatomica veterinaria. 5th ed. New York: Ithaca; 2012.
17. Buchanan JW, Bücheler J. Vertebral scale system to measure canine heart size in radiographs. J Am Vet Med Assoc. 1995;206:194–9.
18. Onuma M, Ono S, Ishida T, Shibuya H, Sato T. Radiographic measurement of cardiac size in 27 rabbits. J Vet Med Sci. 2010;72:529–31.
19. Johnson VS, Ramsey IK, Thompson H, Cave TA, Barr FJ, Rudorf H, Wiliams A, Sullivan M. Thoracic high resolution computed tomography in the diagnosis of metastatic carcinoma. J Small Anim Pract. 2004;45:134–43.
20. Mai W, O'Brien R, Scrivani P, Porat-Mosenco Y, Tobin E, Seiler G, McConnell F, Schwarz T, Zwingenberger A. The lung parenchyma. In: Schwarz T, Johnson V, editors. BSAVA manual of canine and feline thoracic imaging. Gloucester: BSAVA; 2008. p. 242–320.
21. Rudorf H, Taeymans O, Johnson V. Basics of thoracic radiography and radiology. In: Schwarz T, Johnson V, editors. BSAVA manual of canine and feline thoracic imaging. Gloucester: BSAVA; 2008. p. 1–19.
22. Johnson V, Hansson K, Mai W, Dukes-McEwan J, Lester N, Schwarz T, Chapman P, Morandi F. The heart and major vessels. In: Schwarz T, Johnson V, editors. BSAVA manual of canine and feline thoracic imaging. Gloucester: BSAVA; 2008. p. 86–176.
23. Harvey CE, Fink EA. Tracheal diameter: analysis of radiographic measurements in brachycephalic and non-brachycephalic dogs. J Am Anim Hosp Assoc. 1982;18:570–4.
24. Morandi F, Mattoon JS, Lakritz J, Turk JR, Wisner ER. Correlation of helical and incremental high-resolution thin-section computed tomographic imaging with histomorphometric quantitative evaluation of lungs in dogs. Am J Vet Res. 2003;64:935–44.
25. Griffin CB, Primack SL. High-resolution CT: normal anatomy, techniques, and pitfalls. Radiol Clin North Am. 2001;39:1073–90.
26. Schwarz T, Johnson V. Lungs and bronchi. In: Schwarz T, Saunders J, editors. Veterinary computed tomography. UK: Wiley-Blackwell; 2011. p. 261–78.
27. D'Anjou MA, Schwarz T. Hearts and vessels. In: Schwarz T, Saunders J, editors. Veterinary computed tomography. UK: Wiley-Blackwell; 2011. p. 229–42.

8

A survey of straw use and tail biting in Swedish pig farms rearing undocked pigs

Torun Wallgren*, Rebecka Westin and Stefan Gunnarsson

Abstract

Background: Tail biting is a common problem in intensive pig farming, affecting both welfare and production. Although routine tail docking is banned within the EU, it remains a common practice to prevent tail biting. Straw as environmental enrichment has been proposed as an alternative to tail docking, but its effectiveness against tail biting and function in manure handling systems have to be considered. The aim of the study was to survey how pigs with intact tails are raised and how tail biting is handled in Sweden, where tail docking is banned through national legislation. The study emphasises straw usage and its association with tail biting pigs and problems in the manure handling system. The expectation is that this information could be conveyed to the rest of the EU to reduce the need for tail docking.

Results: In a telephone survey of randomly selected Swedish pig farmers (46 nursery and 43 finishing pig units) with at least 50 sows or 300 finishing places, it was found that straw was used by 98% of the farmers. The median daily straw ration provided was 29 g/pig for nursery and 50 g/pig for finishing pigs in systems with partly slatted flooring. The reported prevalence of tail biting was 1.6% at slaughter. The majority of farmers reported that they never had manure handling problems caused by straw (56% of nursery units and 81% of finishing pig units). A proportion of farmers (37%) also provided with additional material apart from straw on some occasions, which may have affected tail biting prevalence and manure handling problems.

Conclusions: Swedish farmers rear undocked pigs without large problems with tail biting. Straw is the main manipulable material used, and additional manipulable material is used to various extents. The low incidence of straw obstructing the manure handling systems implies that it is indeed possible to use straw in partly slatted flooring systems, reducing the need for tail docking. The impact of using additional manipulable material is unknown and requires more investigation to separate the impact of such material from the impact of straw.

Keywords: Intact tail, Manure handling system, Farmer survey, Nursery herd, Finishing herd, Growing pigs, Fattening pigs, Tail docking, Enrichment, Manipulable material

Background

Tail biting is a common problem in pig production, affecting animal health and welfare, as well as production and profitability [1–4]. In housing systems where pigs have no or limited access to manipulable material, exploratory behaviour can be redirected towards tails, and tail biting may occur [2, 5]. This behaviour can lead to the development of lesions and cause infections so severe that subjected pigs must be prior to slaughter [6, 7]. Reduced welfare caused by tail biting is hence not only attributed to the bitten pig but also to the biting pig, as the behaviour may arise when behavioural needs are unfulfilled [8].

The cause of tail biting is multifactorial, and outbreaks often affect several pigs in the same batch [4, 9]. Identification of specific factors triggering tail biting can be difficult, as triggering factors may differ between outbreaks both within and between farms [4]. However, outbreaks often seem to be associated with housing or management changes such as a new shipment of feed, inadequate

*Correspondence: torun.wallgren@slu.se
Department of Animal Environment and Health, Swedish University of Agricultural Sciences, PO-Box 234, 532 23 Skara, Sweden

indoor climate, season, disease outbreaks or lack of rooting material [1, 3, 9, 10].

Previous studies have shown that providing manipulable material such as straw to growing pigs reduces the incidence of tail biting [2]. Few studies have investigated the amount of straw needed to reduce tail biting. One study showed that pigs provided with more than 100 g straw/pig per day spent less than 5% of their time in redirected behaviours (nibbling another pig; ear- or tail-biting) [11]. Another study suggested that a straw ration exceeding 400 g/pig per day was required to meet the pigs' need to explore and to reduce oral manipulation of pen mates to a minimum [2]. It is possible that there is a difference between a straw ration that fulfils the pigs' behavioural need and a straw ration that keeps oral manipulation, such as tail biting behaviour, at an acceptable level.

The EU Council Directive 2008/120/EC, which establishes minimum standards for the protection of pigs, states that "pigs must have permanent access to a sufficient quantity of material to enable proper investigation and manipulation activities, such as straw, hay, wood, sawdust, mushroom compost, peat or a mixture of such [...]". However, the EU directive does not offer any guidance as to how the manipulable materials should be provided to the pigs (i.e., how much or how frequently) and a large variation can therefore be expected. Furthermore, knowledge of how much straw is needed to fulfil the legislative requirements concerning proper investigation or manipulation activities is limited.

Routine tail docking is banned within the EU according to The EU Council Directive 2008/120/EC. Still, over 90% of pigs in the EU are tail docked, especially pigs raised on slatted flooring [12]. Sweden, as well as Finland and Lithuania, is an exception; 100% of the pigs are reared with intact tails due to a total ban on tail docking by national legislation [12, 13].

In addition, the space allowance in Swedish pig farms is higher compared to the minimum requirements of the EU directive. For example, the space requirements per nursery pig of 20 kg live weight (LW) are 0.32 m^2 in Sweden compared to 0.20 m^2 according to the EU legislation. For a finishing pig of 110 kg LW, the space requirement is 1.02 m^2 in Sweden and 0.65 m^2 according to the EU legislation [11, 13]. The maximum amount of slatted floor is weight dependent in Sweden. Maximum amount of slatted flooring range from 32 to 25% for pigs between 20 and 110 kg, e.g. 32% for 20 kg LW pigs and 25% for 110 kg LW, while there is no ban on fully slatted floors for growing pigs in the EU. The maximum widths of slat openings are 14 mm for nursery pigs (9–25 kg LW) and 18 mm for finishing pigs (>25 kg LW); the minimum slat widths are 50 mm for nursery and 80 mm for finishing pigs according to both Swedish and EU legislation [13, 14].

Swedish pig farmers may possess valuable information regarding the rearing of undocked pigs and how to use straw in partly slatted flooring systems. As far as we know, this information has not yet been systematically documented in Sweden. The expectation is that this information could be conveyed to the rest of the EU to reduce the need for tail docking.

The aim of this study was to describe the main management factors in rearing undocked pigs in Sweden and how tail biting is handled. The study emphasises straw usage and how straw is associated with bitten pigs and problems in the manure handling systems.

Methods

Farmers and data records

A telephone survey of commercial pig farmers in Sweden was conducted from July to November 2014. Their contact information was supplied in January 2014 by the Swedish Board of Agriculture. To be included on the contact list, farms had to have at minimum 50 sows or 300 finishing pig places. The farms were categorised as nursery farms (keeping nursery pigs approximately 5–12 weeks of age; 10–30 kg LW), finishing pig farms (keeping growing pigs from approximately 12 weeks of age until slaughter around 6 months of age; 30–120 kg LW) or integrated farms keeping both nursery and finishing pigs. The final contact list consisted of 747 nursery farms, 892 finishing pig farms and 4618 integrated farms. Farmers were called in a random order generated by a computer.

All telephone calls were conducted by a single person according to the randomised list. The farmers were informed of the purpose of the survey and told it was being conducted on behalf of the Swedish University of Agricultural Sciences. Participation was voluntary, and reasons for not participating were recorded. Each farmer not answering the phone was called a maximum of three times before being excluded as "unable to reach".

The survey

The survey consisted of two general questions, 60 questions (35 multiple-choice, 25 open-ended) related to nursery pigs and 28 questions (29 multiple-choice, 29 open-ended) related to finishing pigs. Farmers with integrated farms answered questions concerning nursery and finishing pigs separately. The complete survey is presented in the Additional file 1, and the layout of the survey was as follows:

- General questions—e.g. type of production (conventional or organic) and breed.

- Production information—number of pig places and growth rate.
- Tail biting—e.g. occurrence of bites (frequency, amount), suspected causes.
- Straw usage—e.g. species, ration, frequency of straw and/or other manipulable material provision.
- Pen conformation—e.g. pen size, type of flooring.
- Feeding system—e.g. type of feed, feeding system.
- Manure handling—e.g. type of manure handling system, occurrence of problems related to straw usage.

Calculation of straw usage

A majority of farmers (72%) reported straw usage as the number of bales used in a week or in a year combined with bale weight. The amount of straw provided per pig/day in kg could hence be calculated according to the following equations:

$$\frac{\left(\frac{\text{straw usage per week(kg)}}{\text{number of nursery piglet places in the herd}}\right)}{7} = \text{straw ration/nursery pig per day (kg)}$$

$$\frac{\left(\frac{\text{straw usage per week (kg)}*52\text{ weeks}}{\text{number of produced finishing pigs per year}}\right)}{99^{a}} = \text{straw ration/finishing pig per day (kg)}$$

According to the Swedish national herd monitoring database (PigWin Slakt), the average number of days[a]in the finishing pig unit for rearing a finishing pig was 99 days in Sweden in 2014 [15].

Integrated farms were divided into nursery and finishing units. The survey contained no information regarding the number of batches or pens per unit. Thus, to acquire a relevant estimation of straw use, the calculations of straw use were based on the total number of nursery pig places or finishing pigs produced per year.

Statistical analysis

The information obtained in the survey was recorded in Microsoft Excel and transferred to SAS software ver. 9.4 (SAS Inst. Inc., Cary, NC, USA) for statistical analysis. Descriptive statistics were calculated and presented as frequencies, and mean and median values. Because data were not normally distributed, median values were preferred over mean values.

Outcomes from the questions in the survey were classified as either continuous (e.g., straw usage), ordinal (possible to rank; e.g., frequency of tail biting estimated by the farmer) or categorical (not possible to rank, e.g., strategies for avoiding outbreaks of tail biting). Categorical data were solely presented as frequencies and median/mean when feasible.

Correlations between continuous and ordinal outcomes were analysed with Spearman's rank correlation, as the data were not normally distributed. Correlations were calculated for variables where there was information about both parts of the investigated correlations, namely:

- Straw ration and frequency of problems in the manure handling systems (including and excluding deep litter systems).
- Frequency of tail biting and affected pens/outbreak, percentage of bitten pigs/batch at slaughter, number of slaughtered pigs per year and straw ration.

Results

Response rate and general information about participating farms

A total of 139 farmers were called. Out of these farmers, 60 participated in the survey (43% response rate); 28 (20%) could not be reached; six (4%) did not have the time to participate; six (4%) were unwilling to participate and 38 (28%) did not have pigs anymore or did not have pigs according to the inclusion criteria of the study. The participating farmers included 29 integrated farms, indicating that in total, 46 farmers answered the nursery pig part of the survey and 43 farmers answered the finishing pig questions. Seven of the participating farms produced organic pigs. One survey was excluded because it was incomplete due to technical problems.

Detailed information about participating farms is found in Table 1. The breeds used were Landrace (L)*Yorkshire(Y)*Hampshire crosses (35), L*Y*Duroc-crosses (24), L sows (3), Y sows (3), LY sows (2), and Linderödsvin (Swedish native breed) (1). Eight farmers kept several breeds within the same farm.

Occurrence of bitten pigs and suspected causes

Bitten pigs were reported in 50% of the nurseries and 88% of the finishing pig units. In affected nursery units ($n = 23$), 78.3% of farmers observed bitten pigs less than two times/year, 17.4% 3–6 times/year and 4.3% at least every month (tail-biting frequency). In affected finishing pig units ($n = 38$), 21% observed bitten pigs less than two times/year, 37% 3–6 times/year, 34% at least every month and 8% every week (tail-biting frequency).

Farmers reported observing bitten pigs in on average 1.6 pens (median 1, range 1–5) during the last tail biting outbreak in nursery units and in on average 1.5 pens (median 1, range 1–4) in finishing pig units. The finishing pig units had on average 1.6% bitten pigs in each batch at slaughter (range 0.1–6.5%). The number of affected pens per outbreak was positively correlated to the tail-biting frequency ($r = 0.33$, $P = 0.04$, $n = 38$) in finishing pig

Table 1 General information of participating pig farms, reported by farmers

Parameter	Nursery units						Finishing pig units					
	n	Median	Mean	SD	Min	Max	n	Median	Mean	SD	Min	Max
Total number of pig places	46	815	1088	894	126	4000	43	1200	1434	1164	132	6500
Number of produced pigs/year	–	–	–	–	–	–	43	3600	4484	3795	350	20,000
Age at entry (days)	35	35	37.9	8.9	31	84	42	84	84	8.7	63	105
Weight at entry (kg)	35	10.5	11.4	5.1	9	40	43	30	31	2.8	25	37
Number of pigs/pen	45	11	24	43	10	300	43	10	15	17	7	100
Size of pen (m^2)	45	6	21	49	3	300	43	9.6	19	40	7	250
Space allowance/pig (m^2)	44	0.5	0.53	0.13	0.3	1.9	43	1	0.96	0.08	0.8	2.5

n is number of farmers answering the question. Eleven of the farmers did not move nursery pigs into a new stable after weaning, which is why age and weight at entry to the nursery unit was only answered by 35 farmers

units. The tail-biting frequency was also positively correlated to the percentage of bitten pigs (r = 0.55, $P < 0.001$, n = 38) and to the number of slaughtered pigs/year of the farm (r = 0.32, $P = 0.05$, n = 38), in finishing pig units.

The most commonly reported causes attributed to tail biting outbreaks by farmers were stocking density in nursery farms and stocking density and salt deficiency in finishing pig units (Table 2).

Prevention of outbreaks and treatment of bitten pigs

All farmers except in one nursery and two finishing pig units (95%) reported that they took measures to prevent outbreaks after observing bitten pigs. The most common preventive action reported to mitigate an ongoing outbreak was to identify and separate the biting pig (Table 3). Bitten pigs were treated with antibiotics in 76% of the nurseries and 92% of the finishing pig units, while one farmer provided analgesia (Table 4). Farmers in two nursery (4.3%) and four (9.3%) finishing pig units reported that they would have wanted to dock tails if it were legal in Sweden.

Usage of straw and other manipulable materials

All farmers except two (in one nursery and one finishing pig unit), i.e., 99%, stated that they provided pigs with straw (Table 5). These two farmers reported using sawdust or wood shavings instead, as they believed that straw made pens slippery and caused blockages in the manure handling system. Among farmers that used straw, chopped straw was used in 77% (n = 44) of nursery and 74% (n = 42) of finishing pig units. Straw was the only manipulable material used in 60.9% (n = 46) of nursery and 67.4% (n = 43) of finishing pig units, while the remaining farmers provided additional manipulable material. Usage of additional manipulable material was used to keep pens dry (11), when moving piglets into the nursery unit (3), when it was hot outside (2), to create a light environment (2) and when there was not enough straw (1) in

Table 2 Suspected causes for tail biting in Swedish pig farms, reported by farmers

	Nursery units n = 23		Finishing pig units n = 38	
	During the last outbreak	Overall on the farm	During the last outbreak	Overall on the farm
Coincidence	8	5	1	0
Do not know	5	3	11	10
Feed composition/feed equipment	0	0	12	15
Genetics/nervous pigs	4	2	8	7
Insufficient feeding space	0	0	0	5
Insufficient ventilation/high temperature	0	0	4	7
Lack of occupation	1	1	0	0
Salt deficiency	0	7	0	0
Stable/climate	0	1	0	0
Stocking density/overcrowding	6	6	2	5

n is number of farmers answering the question

Coincidence: e.g. a pig escaping into the wrong pen

Only farmers that had observed tail biting on their farm (23 nursery farmers and 38 finishing pig farmers) answered the questions about causes for tail biting outbreaks. Each farmer could give several causes for tail biting outbreaks, which is why the number of causes could exceed the number of respondents

Table 3 Measures for preventing tail biting outbreaks after observed tail wounds in Swedish pig farms, reported by farmers

	Nursery units n = 21	Finishing pig units n = 38
Addition of extra manipulable material or "toys"	5	5
Checking ventilation/feeding system	5	7
Increasing of straw ration	6	11
Nothing	1	2
Other	4	0
Separation of biter	12	20
Separation of bitten pigs	6	14

n is number of farmers answering the question

Only farmers that had observed tail biting on their farm (23 nursery and 38 finishing pig units) could answer the questions about causes for tail biting outbreaks. Each farmer could give several causes for tail biting outbreaks, which is why the number of causes could exceed the number of respondents

Table 4 Treatments of tail bitten pigs in Swedish pig farms, reported by farmers

	Nursery units n = 23	Finishing pig units n = 38
Analgesia/pain killers	1	0
Antibiotics, kept in original pen	13	21
Antibiotics, moved to sick pen	3	14
Moved to sick pen without antibiotics if pig look healthy	0	2
Nothing	3	3
Other	6	4

n is number of farmers answering the question

Only farmers that had observed tail biting on their farm (23 nursery farmers and 38 finishing pig units) could answer the questions about causes for tail biting outbreaks. Each farmer could give several causes for tail biting outbreaks, which is why the number of causes could exceed the number of respondents

Table 5 Type of manipulable materials used in Swedish pig farms, reported by farmers

	Nursery units n = 46 n (%)	Finishing pig units n = 38 n (%)
Straw only	28 (60.9)	24 (63.2)
Straw + saw dust	0 (0)	2 (5.3)
Straw + wood shavings	16 (34.8)	9 (23.7)
Straw + meal	0 (0)	1 (2.6)
Straw + peat + wood shavings	1 (2.2)	1 (2.6)
Saw dust only	1 (2.2)	0 (0)
Sawdust + wood shavings	0 (0)	1 (2.6)

n is number of farmers answering the question

nursery units. In finishing pig units, additional material was used when moving pigs into the finishing unit (7), if pens were wet/dirty (4), to create a light environment (1), to provide enrichment to the pigs (1), when there was not enough straw (1) and because additional straw would cause blockages in the manure handling system (1). Each farmer could give several reasons for using additional material, which is why the number of answers exceeds the number of respondents. Hence, straw was commonly the only provided manipulable material; additional manipulable material was mainly used at special occasions.

The calculated daily straw rations in systems with partly slatted floorings were median 35 g/pig per day for nursery pigs and 50 g/pig per day for finishing pigs (Table 6). Six nursery and four finishing pig units had deep litter systems, which are very straw intensive. When farms with deep litter systems were excluded, the median straw ratio decreased (Table 6).

A proportion of farmers (24%) reported that they would like to increase the straw ration unless it was limited by other factors. The most commonly reported limiting factor preventing farmers from increasing straw rations was that it was thought to block the manure handling system (Table 7).

Objects other than manipulable materials were provided in 13% (n = 46) of the nursery and 16% (n = 43) of the finishing pig units. These other objects were balls (2), rope (3), silage/hay (1), newspapers (1), sacks (6), chains (1), wood logs (5) and salt stones (5). However, in 69% of the units, pigs had access to the additional objects only when bitten pigs had been observed to prevent tail biting and fighting between pigs at certain occasions, such as when pig groups were mixed.

The majority of farmers provided new straw daily (76% of nursery and 83% of finishing pig units) (Table 8). Straw was distributed evenly on the pen floor (41% of nursery and 38% of finishing pig units) or in a pile on the pen floor (59% of nursery and 62% of finishing pig units).

The ration of manipulable material was modified by farmers depending on the health status in the pen in 35% (n = 46) of the nursery and 33% (n = 42) of the finishing pig units. Some nursery units were given more straw if pigs seemed cold or dirty (5), switched to wood shavings when pigs were sick (7) or switched to peat when pigs had diarrhoea (3). One farmer reported providing less straw when pigs were sick. In finishing pig units, straw rations were increased when bitten pigs were observed (9), when pigs had diarrhoea or it was wet in the pen (3) or when the animals were sick (2). One farmer decreased the ration if it was hot outside. Farmers could give several reasons for altering the manipulable material ration, which is why the amount of answers exceeds the number of responding farmers.

Table 6 Straw ration and straw length of provided straw in Swedish pig farms

	Nursery units						Finishing pig units					
	n	Median	Mean	SD	Min	Max	n	Median	Mean	SD	Min	Max
All farms (including deep straw bedding)												
Straw length, cm	35	5	6.3	2.6	1	10	31	8	8.2	4.1	1	20
Straw ration, g/pig per day	29	45	99	149	8	714	35	53	130	225	9	1156
Excluding farms with deep straw bedding												
Straw length, cm	35	5	6.3	2.6	1	10	28	6.5	7.8	4.1	1	20
Straw ration, g/pig per day	22	29	35	24	8	85	28	50	62	45.5	9	225

n is number of farmers answering the question

The straw ration per pig was calculated from the farms straw consumption. Farms that were unable to provide such information was excluded from the calculations and hence the number of farms were reduced from 43 to 35 nursery units and 43–31 finishing pig units

The straw ration and straw length was also calculated excluding farms with deep litter systems (removing 6 nursery units, 4 finishing pig units) since deep litter systems are uncommon in European pig production

Table 7 Reported limitations to increase straw rations in Swedish pig farms, reported by farmers

	Nursery units, n n = 13	Finishing pig units, n n = 8
Would be too costly	1	1
Would be too dirty	3	2
Would block manure handling system	5	6
Would block slats	5	1
Would require too much work	2	0

n is number of farmers answering the question. Only farmers reporting that they would have wanted to increase the straw ration if possible answered this question and gave reasons for why an increase of the straw ration was impossible

Each farmer could give several causes limiting an increased straw ration, which is why the number of causes could exceed the number of respondents

Table 8 Frequencies of new straw allocation in Swedish pig farms, reported by farmers

	Nursery units, n (%) n = 45	Finishing pig units, n (%) n = 41
Deep straw bedding, never adding new straw	2 (4.4)	0 (0)
Every second week	0 (0)	1 (2.4)
Once/week	2 (4.4)	1 (2.4)
Twice/week	1 (2.2)	0 (0)
Every second day	1 (2.2)	0 (0)
Once/day	34 (75.6)	34 (82.9)
Twice/day	5 (11.1)	5 (12.2)

n is number of farmers answering the question. Only farmers that reported using straw could answer this question

Straw usage and tail biting

In finishing pig units, the reported occurrence of bitten pigs had a negative rank correlation with deep straw systems ($r = -0.42$, $P < 0.01$, $n = 38$) compared to systems that had partly slatted flooring, and there was a negative rank correlation between size of straw ration and tail-biting frequency ($r = -0.32$, $P < 0.05$, $n = 37$). In nursery units, the coefficient of correlation between reported tail-biting frequency and straw ration was $r = -0.328$ ($P < 0.01$, $n = 38$).

Manure handling systems

The most common manure handling system reported was rope/cable and arm scrapers (Table 9). When asked how frequently straw caused blockages or other problems with the manure handling system, 56% nursery and 81% finishing pig units had never experienced problems in the manure handling system caused by straw. No farmer reported problems in manure handling more often than once a month. There was a negative rank correlation between frequency of manure handling problems and straw ration in nursery units ($r = -0.44$, $P = 0.02$, $n = 28$), but not in finishing pig units ($r = 0.16$, $P = 0.35$, $n = 35$). When farms with deep straw bedding were excluded, there was no correlation in nursery units ($r = -0.33$, $P = 0.12$, $n = 22$), but a tendency was found in finishing pig units ($r = 0.31$, $P = 0.09$, $n = 31$).

Discussion

Response rate and farmer self-reporting

According to the Swedish agricultural statistical compilation 2016 [16], there were 1228 pig businesses in

Table 9 Frequencies of problems caused by straw in manure handling systems used, reported by Swedish pig farmers

	Nursery units, n (%) n = 45					Finishing pig units, n (%) n = 43				
	Total	Never	Few times/year	At least monthly	At least weekly	Total	Never	Few times/year	At least monthly	At least weekly
Rope/cable with arm scraper(s)	23 (51.1)	12 (52.3)	8 (34.8)	3 (13)	0 (0)	25 (58.1)	22 (88)	2 (8)	1 (4)	0 (0)
Rope/cable with box scraper	6 (13.3)	2 (33.3)	3 (50)	1 (16.7)	0 (0)	9 (20.9)	6 (66.7)	3 (33.3)	0	0 (0)
Hydraulic scraper	4 (8.9)	3 (75)	1 (25)	0	0 (0)	1 (2.3)	1 (100)	0	0	0 (0)
Shallow pit with pull-plugs	6 (13.3)	3 (50)	2 (33.3)	1 (16.7)	0 (0)	3 (6.9)	1 (33.3)	2 (66.7)	0	0 (0)
Deep straw bedding	6 (13.3)	5 (83.3)	1 (16.7)	0	0 (0)	4 (9.3)	4 (100)	0	0	0 (0)
Slurry	0 (0)	0	0	0	0 (0)	1 (2.3)	1 (100)	0	0	0 (0)

n is number of farmers answering the question

Sweden in 2015, meaning that 5% of Swedish pig farms are included in this study. All farmers were called in a randomised order. The vast majority of reached farmers that fit into the inclusion criteria (84%) wanted to participate in the study, which indicates that we have a representative sample of Swedish farmers.

The results from this study are based on farmers answering questions and reporting about how pigs with intact tails are reared. Self-reporting of routines and how often bitten pigs are seen is not exact. Farmers report their perceptions, but reality may differ for different reasons such as the farmer not being aware of the *true* prevalence of tail biting outbreaks and reporting only detected outbreaks. The aim of this study was to investigate how undocked pigs are reared, how farmers handle bitten pigs, how straw is managed and how its use is linked to tail biting and manure handling problems. Due to the nature of the aims, a survey in which farmers report their experiences gives more information in this stage than a controlled on-farm study would. The fact that farmers reported similarly (e.g., similar causes of tail biting outbreaks, similar frequency of tail biting outbreaks) indicates that the results are reliable. Furthermore, the results of this study are in accordance with those of previous studies (e.g., number of bitten pigs/batch and that tail biting increases with increased age), which also indicates that the results from this study are reliable. However, the results of this study should be considered for what they are: farmers' opinions and not absolute facts.

Occurrence of bitten pigs and suspected causes

In the present study, suspected causes of tail biting varied between farms and pig age groups (nursery or finishing pigs), which is in accordance with previous studies concluding that different production systems have different risks for developing tail biting [9, 10]. Previous findings show that pigs with permanent access to straw are mainly exposed to climatic risk factors for tail biting (e.g., temperature and air humidity), whereas pigs with restricted access to manipulable material were mainly exposed to the risk factor "strawless system" [10].

In the present study, farmers suggested stocking density as the main risk factor in nursery units and feed composition/feed equipment as the main risk factor in finishing pig units and did not suggest factors related to the housing climate, which have also previously been considered less important [10]. This finding is partly in accordance with a survey showing that pig farmers in The Netherlands (rearing docked pigs) consider stocking density to be the main risk factor for tail biting, along with stable climate [17]. Stocking density has been considered to be one of the most common risks associated with tail biting in pigs reared in partly slatted systems with straw, as seen in previous studies [12]. Although the maximum stocking density in Sweden is lower than specified in the EU directive, stocking density was considered the most common cause of tail biting outbreaks in nursery pig units in this study and was also highly ranked in finishing pig units. It has been shown that tail biting significantly increases when the feeding space decreases in nursery units [4] and as the pen facilities remain unchanged, the stocking density will increase in the pens, decreasing feeding space per pig. Therefore, increased stocking density is associated with an increase in other pen-related risk factors. Stocking density and not only provision of additional manipulable material may be an important preventive factor for rearing undocked pigs with low incidences of tail biting.

Only one nursery farmer thought that observed tail biting outbreaks were caused by boredom. This result could indicate that farmers are satisfied with the provided straw ration and outcome. Dutch farmers report similar a prevalence of problems with tail biting (approximately 50% have tail biting problems, ranging from 1 to 6% in docked pigs) but consider provision of manipulable material to be less efficient than docking for preventing tail biting [17]. The manipulable materials used in the Dutch non-organic farms were mainly objects such as chains and ropes, while straw, sawdust or wood shavings were used by only 2–3% of participating farms. Similarly, in a survey of Finnish farmers rearing undocked pigs, manipulable material was considered less important than feeding space, animal health and indoor climate [18], but there was no information about what type of manipulable material was provided daily to the pigs in that study.

It is difficult to evaluate and compare the percentage of bitten pigs between countries and studies due to the different scoring criteria used. A review comparing the prevalence of tail biting from different sources found a wide range both within and between countries depending on data source [19]. This variation may partially be attributed to differences in definition, as definitions range from swollen tails to tissue loss [19, 20]. In this survey, the "bitten" was not defined in the protocol or by surveyed farmers. According to finishing pig farmers, the percentage of bitten pigs was on average 1.6% at slaughter, which is in agreement with tail biting recorded by National Food Agency standards in two Swedish abattoirs (1.5–1.9%) [20]. In addition, the finding that tail biting increases with age is in agreement with the findings of previous studies [3, 21]. We therefore argue that the farmers' definition of bitten was similar to that used by the National Food Agency: "evident biting damage" or "at least half the tail missing" [22]. According to this definition, only severely bitten pigs were recorded; milder tail lesions without blood that are not easy to detect when looking at the pig from outside the pen were excluded from this study. Both abattoir and farmer scoring may therefore be under-reporting tail lesions compared to a scoring scheme that includes a swollen tail or superficial scratches as the lower limit for bitten [20, 23]. However, according to Swedish regulations, pigs with swollen tails or unhealed tail wounds are not allowed to be transported to the abattoir, which is why these types of injuries might not appear in slaughterhouse data even if the criteria were altered. Also, less severe wounds may be of less importance when investigating the current aim (i.e. how pigs with intact tails are reared and managed). Tail docking is conducted to reduce the problems with injured pigs and carcass losses due to more severe tail wounds. Hence, the lack of information about tail lesions that are less severe than those reported at the abattoir is of less importance for investigating whether or not it is possible to rear pigs with intact tails although less severe wounds may also affect the production and welfare of the pigs [e.g. 12].

Usage of straw and other manipulable materials

All participating farmers reported providing access to manipulable material; of these farmers, 99% provided straw in various amounts. The wide usage of straw in this study indicates that straw usage is considered feasible and functional under commercial conditions in Sweden.

Permanent access to straw has previously been defined as the permanent presence of more than one litre of unsoiled straw in the pen before new straw allocation [2]. Permanent straw access was achieved at 80–290 g straw/pig per day for 30–80 kg LW pigs at a stocking density of 0.7 m^2 per pig according to a Danish study [2]. According to this definition, many Swedish farmers do not provide permanent access, as the reported median straw ration was 29 g/pig per day for nurseries and 50 g/pig per day in partly slatted flooring systems.

In this study, however, all calculations regarding daily ration were based only upon the amount of straw, even though 37% of the farmers also provided additional material to various extents. Therefore, the actual ration of accessible manipulable material may be underestimated here. A more detailed analysis of the other manipulable material was not possible because the survey did not request further information on this matter. When developing the survey and collecting experiences from researchers and the Swedish trade organisation for pigs, the wide use of additional material was not foreseen. However, it was shown that provision of additional material was common only during certain periods of time, such as when pigs are newly moved into the stable or due to poor pen hygiene, while straw was given on a daily basis. Additional material may therefore have been of less importance in preventing tail biting outbreaks on participating farms.

If the provided additional material is of high value for the pig, it may affect tail biting behaviour. High-value materials that stimulate pig exploratory behaviour are destructible, manipulable, changeable and complex [7]. Furthermore, the most used objects during the first 24 h after presentation are odorous, deformable, rootable, unattached and chewable according to previous studies [24]. The most used objects 5 days after presentation are ingestible, destructible, contained (e.g., straw provided in a box as opposed to directly on the floor as in this study), particulate and rootable [24]. In this study, sawdust and wood shavings were the most commonly provided complements to straw and they may possess the previously identified characteristics. Additionally, the pigs' usage of sawdust or wood shavings is reduced when they are combined with another material with greater manipulative value [25], and both chopped and long straw are used more than sawdust [24]. The effect of adding sawdust or wood shavings to straw is therefore limited, and the usage of additional material along with the straw could be considered to have a limited effect on tail biting behaviour.

Straw length has, however, been suggested to affect its investigative value for the pigs, as reduced straw length decreases the diversity of behaviours [26]. The majority of farmers in this study used chopped straw, with a mean length of 5 cm in nursery and 6.5 cm in finishing pig units. This straw is considerably longer and therefore possibly of higher value than the chopped straw of 1–4 cm used in the previously mentioned study [26]. The straw on Swedish farms may still be long enough to be of high investigative value to the pigs and seems efficient in preventing tail biting behaviour.

Straw usage and tail biting

The amount of straw needed to reduce the prevalence of tail biting behaviour by satisfying the need to explore has previously been determined to be approximately 400 g straw/pig per day for 30–80 kg LW pigs and 400 g/pig per day for what the author describes as nursery-finishing pigs [2, 11]. Again, this ration is far greater than most of the straw rations reported in this study (median 45–53 g/pig per day). However, the reported rates of bitten pigs at slaughter (average 1.6% at slaughter) and tail biting were low, and no bitten pigs were ever seen in 50% of the nursery and 12% of the finishing pig units. Furthermore, the number of affected pens during an outbreak was reported to be low in both nursery and finishing pig units (on average 1 pen/outbreak), indicating that few pigs are affected in each outbreak and thus that the environment is overall sufficient. The use of additional material along with straw and its effect on tail biting was not assessed in this study.

Straw usage and manure handling

Straw provision in pig pens has been suggested to cause blockage of the slatted floor and to cause obstructions in the manure handling system [6, 27]. However, chopped straw reduces the need for manual cleaning of the pen compared to long straw [25]. Previous studies have shown that provision of large amounts of straw in partly slatted farrowing pens does not cause blockage of slats if straw chop length is adjusted to the type and design of the slatted flooring [28]. The results of this study show that the frequencies of reported problems in the manure handling system were low. The majority of farmers (76%) provided chopped straw, which could explain the low frequency of problems caused by straw in manure handling systems.

The main reported restriction on increasing the straw ration was that straw was thought to cause blockages in the manure handling system or the slatted floor, although most farmers reported never having experienced these problems. This finding implies that the argument that straw would be unusable with current manure handling systems is not correct and shows a gap in knowledge where future research is needed. Straw could also be used in fully slatted flooring systems given that the pigs can make use of the straw before it passes through the slats.

It is reasonable to believe that the pipe diameter of the manure handling systems has an impact on the frequency of obstruction. Pipe diameter is not regulated in the EU Directive or in the Swedish national legislation and could therefore not be assessed in this study, but it could be an interesting area of new research.

Conclusion

This study surveyed straw usage and tail biting on Swedish pig farms. All interviewed farmers reported supplying pigs with manipulable material. The majority of farmers (99%) used straw in various amounts, and 37% also supplied other materials along with the straw (e.g., wood shavings) on certain occasions. Even though the straw rations were restricted (approx. 50 g/pig per day), the percentage of bitten pigs at slaughter (1.6%) and the tail-biting frequency were low (twice yearly in nursery units and 3–6 times/year in finishing pig units). Straw was commonly provided daily, but the farmers reported limited problems in the manure handling systems. We conclude that tail biting can be prevented by straw access in undocked pig populations and that daily straw usage is possible in commercial pig production.

Authors' contributions

TW carried out the analyses and completed the manuscript. RW planned the project, participated in the analyses and commented on the manuscript. SG applied for funding, planned the project, took part in the analyses and commented on the manuscript. All authors read and approved the final manuscript.

Acknowledgements

The authors thank Beth Young for help with designing the questionnaire and Karin Olsson and Barbro Mattsson at Svenska Pig (currently Farm and Animal Health) for commenting on the questionnaire. We also thank Karin Olsson for performing the telephone interviews and data recording. We would also like to thank the anonymous reviewers for valuable comments on the manuscript.

Competing interests

The authors declare that they have no competing interests.

Funding

This study was conducted within the FareWellDock project. FareWellDock is funded by the European Health and Welfare ERA-net (ANIHWA) and the Swedish Research Council for Environment, Agricultural Sciences and Spatial Planning (Formas).

References

1. Wallgren P, Lindahl E. The influence of tail biting on performance of fattening pigs. Acta Vet Scand. 1996;37:453–60.
2. Pedersen LJ, Herskin MS, Forkman B, Halekoh U, Kristensen KM, Jensen MB. How much is enough? The amount of straw necessary to satisfy pigs' need to perform exploratory behaviour. Appl Anim Behav Sci. 2014;160:46–55.
3. Schroder-Petersen DL, Simonsen HB. Tail biting in pigs. Vet J. 2001;162:196–210.
4. Smulders D, Hautekiet V, Verbeke G, Geerst R. Tail and ear biting lesions in pigs: an epidemiological study. Anim Welfare. 2008;17:61–9.
5. Day JEL, Kyriazakis I, Lawrence AB. An investigation into the causation of chewing behaviour in growing pigs: the role of exploration and feeding motivation. Appl Anim Behav Sci. 1996;48:47–59.
6. Sutherland MA, Tucker CB. The long and short of it: a review of tail docking in farm animals. Appl Anim Behav Sci. 2011;135:179–91.
7. Ursinus WW, Van Reenen CG, Kemp B, Bolhuis JE. Tail biting behaviour and tail damage in pigs and the relationship with general behaviour: predicting the inevitable? Appl Anim Behav Sci. 2014;156:22–36.
8. Brunberg E, Jensen P, Isaksson A, Keeling LJ. Behavioural and brain gene expression profiling in pigs during tail biting outbreaks—evidence of a tail biting resistant phenotype. PLoS ONE. 2013;8:e66513. doi:10.1371/journal.pone.0066513.
9. D'Eath RB, Arnott G, Turner SP, Jensen T, Lahrmann HP, Busch ME, et al. Injurious tail biting in pigs: how can it be controlled in existing systems without tail docking? Animal. 2014;8:1479–97.
10. Taylor NR, Parker RMA, Mendl M, Edwards SA, Main DCJ. Prevalence of risk factors for tail biting on commercial farms and intervention strategies. Vet J. 2012;194:77–83.
11. Bodin L, Algers B, Andersson M, Olsson AC, Botermans J. The amount of straw for growing-finishing pigs considering the reduction of time spent in manipulative behavior. SOJ Vet Sci. 2015;1:105.
12. Scientific Opinion of the Panel on Animal Health and Welfare on a request from Commission on the risks associated with tail biting in pigs and possible means to reduce the need for tail docking considering the different housing and husbandry systems. EFSA J. 2007. https://www.efsa.europa.eu/en/efsajournal/pub/611.
13. SJVFS. Statens jordbruksverks föreskrifter och allmänna råd om djurhållning inom lantbruket m.m. [The Swedish Board of Agriculture's regulations and general recommendations on animal husbandry in agriculture]. Case No L 100. Jönköping: Swedish board of Agriculture. 2010:15.
14. Mul M, Vermeij I, Hindle V, Spoolder H. EU-welfare legislation on pigs. In: Wageningen UR Livestock Research; 2010. https://www.researchgate.net/publication/46386577_EU-welfare_legislation_on_pigs. Accessed 15 Aug 2016.
15. Slaktgrisar årsmedeltal-samtiliga anslutna [Yearly production averages for finishing pigs in Sweden]. 2015. http://www.gardochdjurhalsan.se/upload/documents/Dokument/Startsida_Gris/WinPig/Medeltal_o_topplistor/Medeltal_slakt/Slaktgris_medel_2014.pdf. Accessed 15 Aug 2016.

16. Doe J. Företag och företagare. In: Jordbruksstatistisk sammanställning 2016. Business' and entrepeneurs. In: Swedish agricultural statistical compilation 2016; 2016. http://www.jordbruksverket.se/download/18.4a82b0a7155953b608a99d94/1467198318281/Kapitel+2+F%C3%B6retag+och+f%C3%B6retagare.pdf. Accessed 5 Oct 2016.
17. Bracke MBM, De Lauwere CC, Wind SMM, Zonerland JJ. Attitudes of Dutch pig farmers towards tail biting and tail docking. J Agr Environ Ethic. 2013;26:847–68.
18. Valros A, Munsterhjelm C, Hänninen L, Kauppinen T, Heinonen M. Managing undocked pigs- on-farm prevention of tail biting and attitudes towards tail biting and docking. PHM. 2016;2:2.
19. Taylor NR, Main DCJ, Mendl M, Edwards SA. Tail-biting A new perspective. Vet J. 2010;186:137–47.
20. Keeling LJ, Wallenbeck A, Larsen A, Holmgren N. Scoring tail damage in pigs: an evaluation based on recordings at Swedish slaughterhouses. Acta Vet Scand. 2012;54:32.
21. Camerlink I, Ursinus WW, Bijma P, Kemp B, Bolhuis JE. Indirect genetic effects for growth rate in domestic pigs alter aggressive and manipulative biting behaviour. Behav Genet. 2015;45:117–26.
22. Livsmedelsverket. Vägledning för genomförande av offentliga kontroller vid slakt av tama hov- och klövdjur [Guidance for the implementation of official controls on the slaughter of domestic ungiulates and hoofed animals]. Livsmedelsverket: Enheten för Kötttilssyn; 2006.
23. Nannoni E, Valsami T, Sardi L, Martelli G. Tail docking in pigs: a review on its short- and long-term consequences and effectiveness in preventing tail biting. Ital J Anim Sci. 2014;13:98–106.
24. Van de Weerd HA, Docking CM, Day JEL, Avery PJ, Edwards SA. A systematic approach towards developing environmental enrichment for pigs. Appl Anim Behav Sci. 2003;84:101–18.
25. Guy JH, Meads ZA, Shiel RS, Edwards SA. The effect of combining different environmental enrichment materials on enrichment use by growing pigs. Appl Anim Behav Sci. 2013;144:102–7.
26. Day JEL, Van de Weerd HA, Edwards SA. The effect of varying lenghts of straw bedding on the behaviour of growing pigs. Appl Anim Behav Sci. 2008;109:249–60.
27. Lahrmann HP, Oxholm LC, Steinmetz H, Nielsen MBF, D'Eath RB. The effect of long or chopped straw on pig behaviour. Animal. 2015;9:862–70.
28. Westin R, Holmgren N, Mattsson B, Algers B. Throughput capacity of large quantities of chopped straw in partly slatted farrowing pens for loose housed sows. Acta Agric Scand A. 2013;63:18–27.

In vitro investigations on extracellular proteins secreted by *Aphanomyces invadans*, the causative agent of epizootic ulcerative syndrome

Muhammad Majeed[1], Gokhlesh Kumar[1], Sarah Schlosser[2], Mansour El-Matbouli[1*] and Mona Saleh[1]

Abstract

Background: Proteases produced by many microorganisms, including oomycetes, are crucial for their growth and development. They may also play a critical role in disease manifestation. Epizootic ulcerative syndrome is one of the most destructive fish diseases known. It is caused by the oomycete *Aphanomyces invadans* and leads to mass mortalities of cultured and wild fish in many countries. The areas of concern are Australia, China, Japan, South and Southeast Asian countries and the USA. Extracellular proteases produced by this oomycete are believed to trigger EUS pathogenesis in fish. To address this activity, we collected the extracellular products (ECP) of *A. invadans* and identified the secreted proteins using SDS-PAGE and mass spectrometery. *A. invadans* was cultivated in liquid Glucose-Peptone-Yeats media. The culture media was ultra-filtered through 10 kDa filters and analysed using SDS-PAGE. Three prominent protein bands from the SDS gel were excised and identified by mass spectrometery. Furthermore, we assessed their proteolytic effect on casein and immunoglobulin M (IgM) of rainbow trout (*Oncorhynchus mykiss*) and giant gourami (*Osphronemus goramy*). Antiprotease activity of the fish serum was also investigated.

Results: BLASTp analysis revealed that the prominent secreted proteins were proteases, mainly of the serine and cysteine types. Proteins containing fascin-like domain and bromodomain were also identified. We could demonstrate that the secreted proteases showed proteolytic activity against the casein and the IgM of both fish species. The antiprotease activity experiment showed that the percent inhibition of the common carp serum was 94.2% while that of rainbow trout and giant gourami serum was 7.7 and 12.9%, respectively.

Conclusions: The identified proteases, especially serine proteases, could be the potential virulence factors in *A. invadans* and, hence, are candidates for further functional and host–pathogen interaction studies. The role of identified structural proteins in *A. invadans* also needs to be investigated further.

Keywords: *Aphanomyces invadans*, Epizootic ulcerative syndrome, LC–MS/MS, Oomycetes, Proteases, Virulence

Background

Infection with *Aphanomyces invadans*, also known as epizootic ulcerative syndrome (EUS), is an OIE-listed disease [1]. It has historically caused mass mortalities in cultured and wild fish in Asia and Oceania and recently in North America and Africa. An EUS-like condition was first reported from Japan in farmed Ayu (*Plecoglossus altivelis*) [2, 3] and later from Australia. Initial symptoms are described as focal haemorrhages on fish skin with variable size of ulcerative lesions that may progress to necrotizing dermatitis resulting in deep dermal ulcer [4, 5]. The economic impact of this disease is huge. It has caused an estimated loss of US $110 million only in few countries of Asia–Pacific region during late 80's and early 90's [6]. Clinical EUS has not been reported from Europe so far, but *A. invadans* has been detected in imported

*Correspondence: Mansour.El-Matbouli@vetmeduni.ac.at
[1] Clinical Division of Fish Medicine, University of Veterinary Medicine, Veterinärplatz 1, 1210 Vienna, Austria
Full list of author information is available at the end of the article

ornamental fish species from different non-European countries [7].

EUS is a water-borne disease caused by *A. invadans*. It is a slow growing, thermolabile [8] and non-septate microorganism [9]. It lacks reproductive structures and belongs to the class Oomycota (water moulds) and order Saprolegniales [6, 10]. Oomycetes, including *Aphanomyces* and *Saprolegnia* species, have caused some of the most devastating fish diseases [11]. About 125 fish species have been confirmed to be affected by *A. invadans* [12] and the number is gradually increasing [13]. Recently, the mitochondrial genomes of *A. invadans* and *Aphanomyces astaci* were assembled and annotated, which provides good basis for further functional studies and development of diagnostic methods [14].

Proteases are vital for fungal physiology and development and digesting external proteins required for fungal growth [15]. However, many infectious microorganisms, including fungi and oomycetes, produce extracellular proteases or effector proteins that initiate the disease process [15].

Involvement of microbial proteases in disease development in humans and using these proteases as targets for development of therapeutic agents against such diseases has also been reported [16]. An important strategy in drug development is to focus on natural inhibitors of disease-involved proteases to counter their effects. Although natural antiproteases are present in every organism, they can be repressed by the pathogens, hence triggering disease development.

Extracellular proteases produced by the oomycete *A. invadans* have been suggested to play a part in EUS pathogenesis. Proteases have also been reported to affect the immune response of the host and support the invasion of the hyphae in host musculature [17]. In this study, we aimed at identifying *A. invadans*' secreted proteases using SDS-PAGE and mass spectrometery and investigating their proteolytic activity against casein and fish immunoglobulin M (IgM). The results of this study suggest that the secreted proteases may be considered as potential virulence factors of *A. invadans* in EUS.

Methods

Oomycete culture and zoospore production

Aphanomyces invadans NJM 9701 was cultured on peptone glucose-1 (PG-1) agar (Fig. 1). Fungal plugs (6–7 cm^2) were cut and placed on new PG-1 plates every 6–7 days as subculture and maintained at 25 °C. In parallel, the fungal plugs were grown at 25 °C for 6–7 days in glucose-peptone-yeast (GPY) broth. These fungal plugs were collected and placed in filtered autoclaved pond water (FAPW) pH 7.2 for 12–24 h at 22 °C for zoospore production [6]. Zoospores were observed under light microscope.

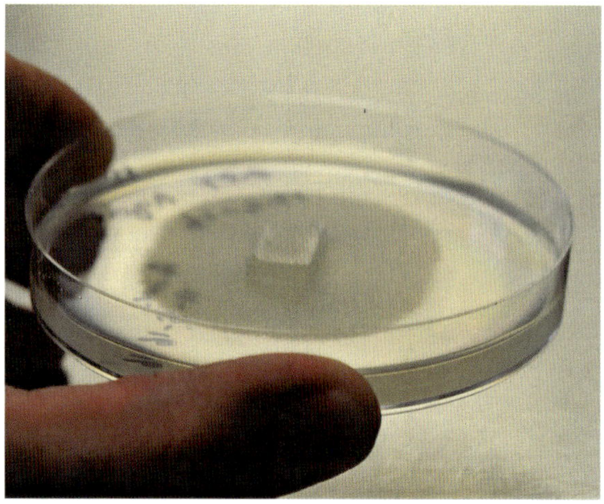

Fig. 1 *Aphanomyces invadans* culture. The PG-1 agar plate shows the growth of *Aphanomyces invadans*

Germination of zoospores and isolation of extracellular products

FAPW suspension containing zoospores was transferred to double strength GPY broth in 1:1 ratio and placed at 25 °C for 6–7 days for the germination of zoospores [6]. The contents of the plates were then pooled into a 50 mL tube and centrifuged to remove the fungal hyphae. The soluble fraction as a source of extracellular products was collected and subsequently filtered using 10 kDa Amicon Ultra-15 filters (Sigma, Germany) at 3220 g for 15 min. Retentate was collected as final extracellular product (hereafter referred as ECP).

SDS-PAGE

ECP samples (10 μL) in triplicate were subjected to 12% SDS-PAGE as described by Laemmli [18] and Kumar et al. [19] with some modifications. Samples were mixed with 2 × SDS gel-loading buffer and heated at 100 °C for 5 min. Electrophoresis was carried out at 60 V for 4 h (BIO-RAD). The gel was stained with Coomassie blue G-250. Three bands of interest were excised manually from the gel. After washing and destaining with methanol: acetic acid mixture, the proteins were reduced with dithiothreitol and alkylated with iodoacetamide [20]. In-gel digestion was performed with trypsin (Promega) for 8 h at 37 °C [21]. Peptides were extracted, dried and redissolved in 0.1% aqueous TFA prior to LC–MS injection.

nanoLC-MS/MS analysis

Sample pre-concentration and desalting was accomplished with a 5 mm Acclaim PepMap μ-Precolumn (300 μm inner diameter, 5 μm particle size, and 100 Å pore size, Dionex). For sample loading and desalting 2% ACN in ultra pure water with 0.05% TFA was used as a mobile phase with a flow rate of 5 μL/min.

Separation of peptides was performed on a 25 cm Acclaim PepMap C18 column (75 μm inner diameter, 3 μm particle size, and 100 Å pore size) with a flow rate of 300 nL/min. The gradient started with 4% B (80% ACN with 0.1% formic acid) and increased to 35% B in 120 min. It was followed by a washing step with 90% B. Mobile Phase A consisted of ultra pure water with 0.1% formic acid. For mass spectrometric analysis the LC was directly coupled to a high resolution quadrupole time of flight mass spectrometer (Triple TOF 5600 + , Sciex) via nano electrospray source.

For information dependent data acquisition (IDA runs) MS1 spectra were collected in the range of 400–1500 *m/z*. The 25 most intense precursors with charge state 2–4, which exceeded 100 counts per second, were selected for fragmentation for 250 ms. MS2 spectra were collected in the range 100–1800 *m/z* for 110 ms. Precursor ions were dynamically excluded from reselection for 12 s. The nano-HPLC system was operated by Chromeleon 6.8 (Dionex) and the MS by Analyst Software 1.6 (Sciex). Database searches of raw files were processed with ProteinPilot Software version 5.0 (Sciex). The UniProt and NCBI database (Release 08_2016) was restricted to *A. invadans*. After having the result of mass spectrometer analysis, a BLASTp analysis was done using Uniprot and NCBI database.

Protease activity experiment using casein as substrate

To confirm the protease activity of the ECP, caseinolytic activity was assessed according to the method described by Cupp-Enyard [22]. Briefly, reaction mixture containing 0.5 mL ECP was added to 5 mL 0.65% casein solution in PBS pH 7.5 and incubated for 10 min at 37 °C. The reaction was stopped by adding 5 mL trichloroacetic acid (TCA). A blank tube was run in parallel. Appropriate volume of ECP was then added in both tubes to bring the final volume to 1 mL, incubated for 30 min at 37 °C and filtered afterwards. 2 mL filtrate was mixed with 5 mL Na_2CO_3 solution (500 mM) followed by the addition of 1 mL Folins-Ciocalteu's (FC) reagent and incubated for 30 min at 37 °C. Tyrosine standard vials were also prepared side by side. The contents of these tubes were then filtered, the amount of tyrosine released was measured at 660 nm and protease activity in units/mL was calculated according to the formula by Cupp-Enyard [22].

Protease activity experiment using IgM as substrate

Rainbow trout (*Oncorhynchus mykiss*) and giant gourami (*Osphronemus goramy*) were anaesthetized using ethyl 3-aminobenzoate methanesulfonate (Sigma, Darmstadt, Germany) (MS-222; 100 mg/L) and their blood was collected through caudal vein puncture using non-heparinized sterile syringe with 23G needle (B|Braun, Maria Enzersdorf, Austria). Serum was obtained by spinning the blood at 2000 g for 10 min. IgM precipitation was performed using ammonium sulfate as per the protocol described by Hay and Westwood [23]. Further, the activity of extracellular proteases was tested against fish IgM using dot blot analysis as per the protocol described by Jiang et al. [24] with slight modification. Briefly, 20 μL ECP as a source of secreted proteases were incubated overnight at 10 °C with 20 μL IgM (400 ng) from both fish species separately. EDTA (metalloproteinase inhibitor, 10 mM), E-64 (a cysteine protease inhibitor, 10 μM) and phenylmethanesulfonyl fluoride (PMSF) (serine protease inhibitor, 1 mM) were used to confirm that the proteases in the ECP were responsible for the observed proteolytic activity and to identify the classes of proteases. IgM with GPY broth and with water were separately incubated as negative controls. After overnight incubation, 2.5 μL sample volume from each reaction was spotted onto nitrocellulose membranes, dried for 45–50 min at room temperature and blocked with 5% dry milk for 30–40 min. Membranes were then accordingly dipped in anti-rainbow trout and anti-giant gourami monoclonal antibodies (Aquatic Diagnostics) for 10 min and washed four times with PBS for 15 min. Remaining IgM was detected using goat-anti-mouse HRP conjugated antibody (BIO-RAD).

Antiprotease activity of fish serum

The capacity of the fish serum to degrade the proteases was tested according to the method described by Zuo and Woo [25] with slight modifications. Briefly, sera from rainbow trout, giant gourami and common carp (*Cyprinus carpio*) were collected as described above. 10 μL test serum from each fish species was incubated with 100 μL trypsin (100 μg/mL) (bovine pancrease type I, Sigma, Germany) at 25 °C along with 110 μL PBS as negative control, 10 μL PBS and 100 μL trypsin as positive control and 10 μL serum and 100 μL PBS as serum blank. After 30 min incubation 1 mL 0.25% casein was added and incubated for 15 min at 25 °C. The reaction was stopped by adding 500 μL 10% TCA. Samples were then centrifuged to remove the precipitates. The absorbance (optical density; OD) of the supernatant was measured at 280 nm and anti-protease activity was calculated [17, 25]: Reference value (RV) = Absorbance of the positive control − Absorbance of the negative control Test value

(TV) = Absorbance of the test sample − Absorbance of the serum blank Percent inhibition = ((RV − TV)/RV) × 100.

Results

Zoospores, proteases and the ECP

Thick-walled zoospores were observed under microscope (Fig. 2). Germinating zoospores produced hyphae that covered the entire surface area of the plate in 7–8 days. Filtering the soluble fraction using 10 kDa filters yielded 200–250 μL ECP.

Identified proteins

SDS-PAGE showed three prominently expressed protein bands (Fig. 3). Using nano LC-MS/MS and subsequent BLASTp analyses, a total of 5, 13 and 12 proteins were identified in bands a, b and c, respectively (Table 1). These proteins were identified mainly as proteases including serine and cysteine. Proteins containing fascin-like domain and bromodomain were also identified.

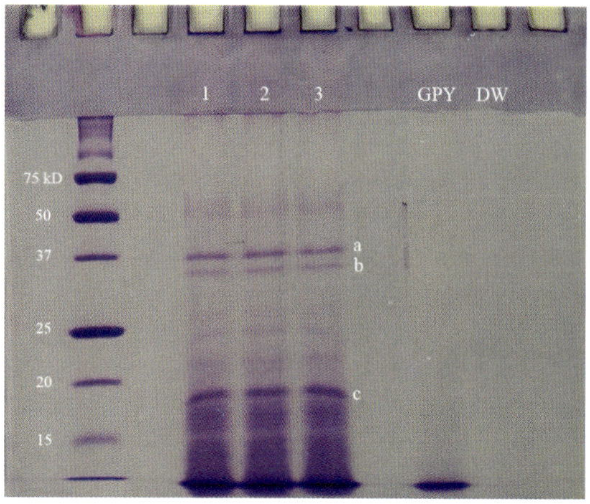

Fig. 3 SDS-PAGE profile of extracellular products of *Aphanomyces invadans*. Lane 1, 2 and 3: Triplicate ECP samples showing three prominent protein bands (a, b and c). These protein bands were identified as proteases by mass spectrometer and subsequent BLASTp analysis. GPY broth and distilled water (DW) were used as negative controls

Protease activity experiments

Activity of protease sample using casein as substrate was calculated which was found to be 0.206 units/mL. Dot blot results showed that the proteases were able to degrade the IgM of both fish species (Fig. 4 spot-1) however inactivated proteases were unable to proteolyze the IgM (Fig. 4 spot-2). No color was seen when both IgM and proteases were heat inactivated (Fig. 4 spot-3). IgM in GPY and distilled water were used as positive controls (Fig. 4 spots-4 and 5, respectively). The protease inhibitors EDTA, E-64 and PMSF inhibited the protease activity (Fig. 4 spots-6, 7 and 8, respectively).

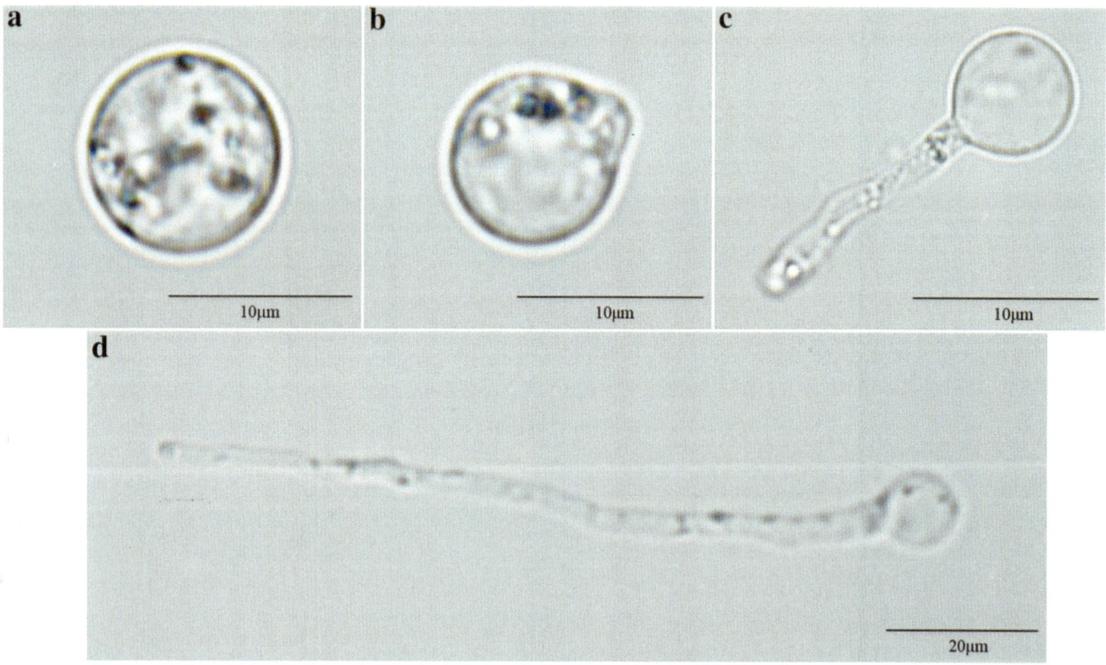

Fig. 2 Different phases of germinating spores of *Aphanomyces invadans*. **a** Spore having thick cell wall. **b** Spore starts to germinate as the development of a small outgrowth (a bud-like structure) is seen. **c** Newly-formed small hyphae. **d** A long thread like structure (hyphae)

Table 1 List of hypothetical proteins identified in extracellular product of *Aphanomyces invadans*

Band	NCBI accession	Total ProtScore	Sequence coverage (%)	Confident peptides/protein	Conserved domain
a	gi|673043857	24	28.6	22	Peptidase_S8_S53 super family
	gi|673054889	20.96	21.6	15	Fascin super family
	gi|673023204	6	8.6	3	Trypsin_2
	gi|673025822	4	4.6	2	Peptidase_S8_S53 super family
	gi|673031752	2.04	7.5	6	Peptidase_S8_S53 super family
b	gi|673043857	17.69	25.8	22	Peptidase_S8_S53 super family
	gi|673054889	15.29	19.1	9	Fascin super family
	gi|673031752	14	20.6	10	Peptidase_S8_S53 super family
	gi|673040359	9.29	27.5	5	Trypsin_2
	gi|673039729	7.19	9.00	4	Peptidase_S8_S53 super family
	gi|673049945	6	8.5	4	Glyco_hydro_1 super family
	gi|673023204	6	8.6	3	Trypsin_2
	gi|673036800	4	5.3	2	Peptidase_C1A
	gi|673036298	4	8.1	3	—[a]
	gi|673036612	3	4.9	2	Peptidase_C1 super family
	gi|673033024	2	0.3	2	Bromodomain super family
	gi|673022270	2	2.5	2	S1-P1_nuclease
	gi|673021356	2	2.5	3	Peptidase_C1
c	gi|673054889	28	39.8	35	Fascin super family
	gi|673038963	14.04	15.3	8	Beta-lactamase
	gi|673043857	14	15.2	11	Peptidase_S8_S53 super family
	gi|673039719	8	13.5	4	Peptidase_S8_S53 super family
	gi|673050561	6	5.3	3	Peptidase_C1
	gi|673040359	4.03	12.3	2	Trypsin_2
	gi|673050209	4	13.1	2	—[a]
	gi|673028596	4	13.8	2	—[a]
	gi|673025822	4	4.6	2	Peptidase_S8_S53 super family
	gi|673039729	6	4.2	3	Peptidase_S8_S53 super family
	gi|673051517	2	2.8	2	Peptidase_C1A
	gi|673033024	2	0.3	2	Bromodomain super family

Conserved domain of each protein was identified using NCBI database. No conserved domain was found against the proteins/proteases marked with[a]

Total anti-protease activity

Total anti-protease activity assay showed that the percent inhibition of the carp serum was 94.2% while that of rainbow trout and giant gourami serum was 7.7 and 12.9%, respectively.

Discussion

Aphanomyces were initially known as parasites of plants, small invertebrates and crustaceans. Probably the first case reported of fish being infected by *Aphanomyces* species was from guppy (*Poecilia reticulata*), Maxican blind cave (*Astyanax mexicanus*), a hybrid of platy (*Platypoecilus maculatus*) and swordtail (*Xiphophorus hellerii*) [26]. *Aphanomyces*, along with other oomycetes, e.g. *Saprolegnia* species have caused severe losses to aquaculture industry till to-date. From an evolutionary point of view it seems that the pathogenesis of plant oomycetes is mediated by effectors, while host invasion by animal pathogenic oomycetes is facilitated by expansion of proteases [24]. Many infectious microorganisms require proteases for replication or use proteases as virulence factors to cross proteinaceous barrier within the host. Proteases secreted by the fish oomycete *Saprolegnia parasitica* are suggested to be involved in attacking the host tissue and paving the way for further penetration of the fungus into the fish [24]. In the present study, we investigated *A. invadans*' secreted proteases using SDS-PAGE and mass spectrometery followed by BLASTp analysis. 30 peptides belonging to eight major protein domains have been identified (Table 1). Identified proteases containing Trypsin_2 domain (gi|673023204 and gi|673040359) show sequence similarity to *Aphanomyces astaci*, *Saprolegnia parasitica*,

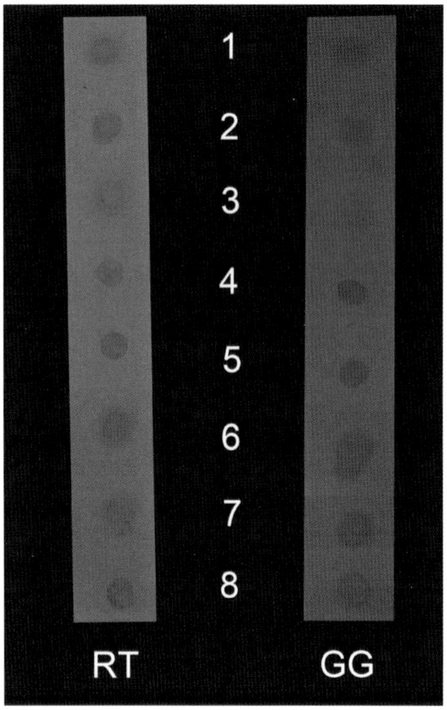

Fig. 4 Protease activity of *Aphanomyces invadans* secreted proteases against IgM of rainbow trout (RT) and giant gourami (GG). Spot 1: IgM was degraded by proteases as no dark spot is seen. Spot 2: IgM was intact when proteases were heat inactivated and upon addition of anti-antibodies and the substrate produced a dark spot. 3: ECP and IgM both were heat inactivated hence produced no dark spot. Spots 4 and 5: IgM was intact in GPY media and distilled water respectively hence produced dark spots. Spot 6: EDTA, Spot 7: E-64 protease inhibitor and Spot 8: phenylmethanesulfonyl fluoride inhibited the proteases hence dark spots are seen

Saprolegnia diclina, *Achlya hypogyna* and *Thraustotheca clavata*. Dubovenko et al. [27] have reported that most of the fungal species that have trypsin or similar-to-trypsin peptidases genes are pathogenic to animals, plant and fungi and suggested them as possible markers of pathogenicity. Extracellularly secreted trypsin-like proteases of *A. invadans* might have a similar role.

Identified protein with fascin-like domain (gi|673054889) was found in all three bands. Members of fascin-like domain are actin bundling proteins required for motility and invasion in *Rickettsia conorii* and *Listeria* [28, 29]. Actin polymerization is the main driving force for cell locomotion. It is used by the bacteria e.g. *Listeria* sp. and *Shigella* sp., and viruses e.g. vaccinia for intracellular and intercellular movements [30, 31]. We suggest that this protein may also be required for actin-bundling in *A. invadans* and has a conserved role in adhesion, mobility and invasion in oomycetes as in other pathogens [28–31]. However, the functional mechanisms of protein members of the fascin-like domain and their role in adhesion, motility and invasion remain largely unknown in oomycetes.

Bromodomains are chromatin-associated proteins and are important mediators of gene expression. Such proteins are reported to be crucial in viability and virulence of protozoan parasites [32] and are reported to be essential in the pathogenesis of *Plasmodium falciparum* [33]. S1–P1 nucleases have been reported to be involved in the degradation of the genetic material in programmed cell death in plants [34]. In our study, the identified proteases that belong to bromodomain (gi|673033024) and S1–P1_ nuclease domain (gi|673022270) might also have pathogenic as well as structural role in *A. invadans* as in other pathogens [32, 33]. Beta-lactamase, mostly produced by bacteria, have an indirect role in infection. These are mostly used against the broad-spectrum beta-lactam antibiotics and provide resistance [35]. Beta-lactamase (gi|673038963) identified in the ECP of *A. invadans* suggests that these proteins might have a similar role against beta-lactam broad-spectrum antibiotics and may promote resistance.

Glycoside hydrolase (GH) enzymes are one of the largest families of enzymes produced by the fungi to break down plant cell wall [36]. One GH enzyme, XEG1, from plant pathogenic oomycete *Phytophthora sojae* has been reported as a major virulence factor in soybean [37]. As animals, including fish, do not contain large amounts of cellulose on their skin, extracellular secretion of GH domain enzyme (gi|673049945) from an animal pathogen, *A. invadans*, mainly reflects the adaptation to nutrient supply [38].

The C1 group of peptidases belongs to the papain-like cysteine proteases. This type of proteases is important for parasites for their virulence and tissue and cell invasion [39]. Many plant pathogenic bacteria produce cysteine effectors to proteolyze the host substrate to alter the plant physiology [40]. Fish parasitic oomycete, *S. parasitica*, has been reported to secrete cysteine proteases, among others, that could function in virulence [41]. Cystein proteases identified in our study (gi|673036800, gi|673036612, gi|673021356, gi|673050561 and gi|673051517) may also be important in *A. invadans* virulence.

However, the most prominent identified protein in our results is the serine type peptidase as 10 out of 30 identified peptides belong to Peptidase_S8 domain with active serine motif. The S8 family has a catalytic triad similar to that found in trypsin-like proteases. BLASTp analysis against NCBI database suggested that the identified hypothetical proteins gi|673043857, gi|673025822, gi|673031752, gi|673039729 and gi|673039719 have significant sequence similarity to peptidase_S8 domain from a range of animal and plant parasitic oomycetes including *A. astaci, S. parasitica, S. diclina, P. sojae, P. parasitica, Plasmopara halstedii* and *A. hypogyna* and nonpathogenic saprophytic oomycete *Teinoptila clavata*. One of the important classes of this protease domain is subtilisin-like serine protease. These proteases have long been implicated as virulence factor in bacteria and true fungi [11]. A serine protease, SPRG_14567, secreted by oomycete *S. parasitica* has been reported to be able to degrade the rainbow trout IgM [24]. Our results suggest that at least one of these identified serine type proteases is also involved in degradation of rainbow trout and giant gourami's IgM.

Involvement of extracellular serine protease of a nematophagous fungus *Lecanicillium psalliotae* in degradation of casein has been reported [42]. We found that the extracellular proteases secreted by *A. invadans* have actively degraded the casein. Consequently, we were encouraged to also investigate the proteolytic activity of these proteases against fish IgM. Fish depends mainly on its innate immunity as fundamental defense against antigens [43, 44]. IgM is the first antibody to be produced after an antigen attacks the host. These are also the natural antibodies of the innate immune system presented as an initial defense component. These immunoglobulins immediately recognize the invading pathogens and aim to destruct them [45, 46]. Banfield and Kamoun [47] have reported that degradation of IgM of rainbow trout by the proteases of *S. parasitica* is critical in order to cause the disease saprolegniasis. Jiang et al. [24] have also reported that at least one of the proteases produced by *S. parasitica* has the ability to degrade the IgM of rainbow trout, which suggests that the oomycete has the ability to manipulate and conquer the initial immune response of the fish.

We tested the secreted proteases of *A. invadans* against IgM of rainbow trout (*Oncorhynchus mykiss*) and giant gourami (*Osphronemus goramy*) and found that the proteases were able to degrade the IgM of both fish species. These are involved in competing against the initial immune defense of the fish thus enables the oomycete to invade the host and play a part in EUS pathogenesis. Lilley et al. [48] suggested that the virulence of pathogenic *A. invadans* may be attributed to production of proteolytic enzymes.

Dot blot results showed that EDTA, PMSF and E-64 inhibited the protease activity of ECP suggesting that metalloproteinase, cysteine and serine proteases were secreted by *A. invadans*. These findings are in agreement with the results obtained by mass spectrometery and BLASTp analysis.

Fish plasma contains enzymes, or antiproteases, that play important role in degrading the proteases of invading pathogens. These are mainly α-1 antiprotease, α-2 antiplasmin and α-2 macroglobulin [25, 49]. These antiproteases have the ability to degrade the extracellular proteases secreted by pathogens hence restricting the entry of the pathogen. Results of our antiprotease activity experiment showed that common carp had the highest protease inhibition capacity as compared to rainbow trout and giant gourami. These findings could explain the resistance of common carp to infection with *A. invadans* [50, 51] and the susceptibility of the other two species tested. Consequently, the virulence of *A. invadans* could be reduced if protease secretion is affected or strong antiproteases are used.

Our findings offer a baseline for further investigations on the role of the secreted proteases in EUS pathogenesis using genome editing tools, such as CRISPR/Cas9 system, and pave the way for the development of novel drugs to control the disease.

Conclusions

The ECP of *A. invadans* was collected and secreted proteins were identified using SDS-PAGE and mass spectrometery. BLASTp analysis revealed that the prominent secreted proteins were proteases, mainly the serine and cysteine type. These secreted proteases degraded the casein and the initial defense component (IgM) of rainbow trout and giant gourami. Dot blot results showed that inhibition of these proteases using various protease inhibitors resulted in reduced proteolytic activity. Our findings suggest that these extracellular proteases could potentially be involved in EUS virulence mechanisms. Hence, they may experimentally be targeted and explored for development of novel controlling methods and therapeutics for EUS.

Authors' contributions

MS and MEL designed the study and supervised the project. MM and GK performed the experiments and prepared the first draft. GK, MS and SS analysed and interpreted the results. MS, GK and MEL revised the manuscript. All authors read and approved the final manuscript.

Author details

[1] Clinical Division of Fish Medicine, University of Veterinary Medicine, Veterinärplatz 1, 1210 Vienna, Austria. [2] VetCore Facility for Research, University of Veterinary Medicine, Vienna, Austria.

Acknowledgements

MM thanks the Higher Education Commission of Pakistan for providing the scholarship to study abroad and Österreichische Austauschdienst for their institutional support and guidance. The authors thank Dr. med vet. Eva Lewisch and Dr. Simon Menanteau-Ledouble for their help in obtaining the fish blood and Dr. med. vet. Andrea Dressler for maintaining *A. invadans* cultures.

Competing interests

The authors declare that they have no competing interests.

Funding
This study was funded by the Austrian Science Fund (FWF) Project No. P29294-B25 and the University of Veterinary Medicine, Vienna (PP291-ELM).

References

1. OIE (World Organisation for Animal Health) Listed Diseases. 2017. http://www.oie.int/en/animal-health-in-the-world/oie-listed-diseases-2017/. Accessed Oct 31 2017.
2. Egusa S, Masuda N. A new fungal disease of *Plecoglossus altivelis*. Fish Pathol. 1971;6:41–6.
3. Kar D, Singha R, Das BK, John R, George R, Mansoor M, et al. Preliminary epidemiological studies on epizootic ulcerative syndrome (EUS) in fresh-water fishes of Assam. Int J Sci Res Sci Eng Tech. 2015;1:256–63.
4. Lilley JH, Roberts RJ. Pathogenicity and culture studies comparing the *Aphanomyces* involved in epizootic ulcerative syndrome (EUS) with other similar fungi. J Fish Dis. 1997;20:135–44.
5. Khoo L. Fungal diseases in fish. J Exot Pet Med. 2000;9(2):102–11.
6. Lilley JH, Callinan RB, Chinabut S, Kanchanakhan S, Macrae IH, Phillips MJ. Epizootic ulcerative syndrome (EUS) technical handbook. Bangkok: Aquatic Animal Health Research Institute; 1998.
7. El-Matbouli M, Saleh M, Soliman H. Biosecurity risks associated with epizootic ulcerative syndrome and iridovirus in ornamental fish imported into the European Union. Vet Rec. 2014;174:1–2.
8. Lilley JH, Roberts RJ. Pathogenicity and culture studies comparing the *Aphanomyces* involved in epizootic ulcerative syndrome (EUS) with other similar fungi. J Fish Dis. 1997;20:135–44.
9. Chinabut S. Epizootic ulcerative syndrome: information up to 1997. Fish Pathol. 1998;33:321–6.
10. Kiryu Y, Blazer VS, Vogelbein WK, Kator H, Shields JD. Factors influencing the sporulation and cyst formation of *Aphanomyces invadans*, etiological agent of ulcerative mycosis in Atlantic menhaden. Brevoortia Tyrannus. 2005;97:569–75.
11. Minor KL, Anderson VL, Davis KS, Van Den Berg AH, Christie JS, Lobach L, et al. A putative serine protease, SpSsp1, from *Saprolegnia parasitica* is recognised by sera of rainbow trout, *Oncorhynchus mykiss*. Fungal Biol. 2014;118:630–9.
12. Kamilya D, Baruah A. Epizootic ulcerative syndrome (EUS) in fish: history and current status of understanding. Rev Fish Biol Fish. 2014;24:369–80.
13. Pradhan PK, Rathore G, Sood N, Swaminathan TR, Yadav MK, Verma DK, et al. Emergence of epizootic ulcerative syndrome: large-scale mortalities of cultured and wild fish species in Uttar Pradesh, India. Curr Sci. 2014;106:1711–8.
14. Makkonen J, Vesterbacka A, Martin F, Jussila J, Diéguez-Uribeondo J, Kortet R, Kokko H. Mitochondrial genomes and comparative genomics of *Aphanomyces astaci* and *Aphanomyces invadans*. Sci Rep. 2016;6:36089. https://doi.org/10.1038/srep36089.
15. Yike I. Fungal proteases and their pathophysiological effects. Mycopathologia. 2011;171(5):299–323.
16. Rao MB, Tanksale AM, Ghatge MS, Deshpande VV. Molecular and biotechnological aspects of microbial proteases. Miocrobiol Mol Bio Rev. 1998;62:597–635.
17. Yadav MK, Pradhan PK, Sood N, Chaudhary DK, Verma DK, Debnath C, et al. Innate immune response of Indian major carp, *Labeo rohita* infected with oomycete pathogen *Aphanomyces invadans*. Fish Shellfish Immunol. 2014;39:524–31.
18. Laemmli UK. Cleavage of structural proteins during assembly of the head of bacteriophage T4. Nature. 1970;227:680–5.
19. Kumar G, Rathore G, Sengupta U, Singh V, Kapoor D, Lakra WS. Isolation and characterization of outer membrane proteins of *Edwardsiella tarda* and its application in immunoassays. Aquaculture. 2007;272:98–104.
20. Jiménez CR, Huang L, Qiu Y, Burlingame AL. In-gel digestion of proteins for MALDI-MS fingerprint mapping. Curr Protoc Protein Sci. 2001;14:16–24.
21. Shevchenko A, Wilm M, Vorm O, Mann M. Mass spectrometric sequencing of proteins from silver-stained polyacrylamide gels. Anal Chem. 1996;68:850–8.
22. Cupp-Enyard C. Sigma's non-specific protease activity assay-casein as a substrate. J Vis Exp. 2008;19:1–2.
23. Hay FC, Westwood OMR. Practical immunology. 4th ed. London: Blackwell Science; 2002.
24. Jiang RHY, de Bruijn I, Haas BJ, Belmonte R, Lobach L, Christie J, et al. Distinctive expansion of potential virulence genes in the genome of the oomycete fish pathogen *Saprolegnia parasitica*. PLoS Genet. 2013;9:e1003272.
25. Zuo X, Woo PTK. Natural anti-proteases in rainbow trout, *Oncorhynchus mykiss* and brook charr, *Salvelinus fontinalis* and the in vitro neutralization of fish α2-macroglobulin by the metalloprotease from the pathogenic haemoflagellate, Cryptobia salmonicita. Parasitology. 1998;114:375–81.
26. Shanor L, Saslow HB. Aphanomyces as a fish parasite. Mycologia. 1944;36:413–5.
27. Dubovenko AG, Dunaevsky YE, Belozersky MA, Oppert B, Lord JC, Elpidina EN. Trypsin-like proteins of the fungi as possible markers of pathogenicity. Fungal Biol. 2010;114:151–9.
28. Gouin E, Egile C, Dehoux P, Villeirs V, Adams J, Gertler F, et al. The RickA protein of *Rickettsia conorii* activates theArp2/3 complex. Nature. 2004;427:457–61.
29. Brieher WM, Coughlin M, Mitchison TJ. Fascin-mediated propulsion of *Listeria monocytogenes* independent of frequent nucleation by the Arp2/3 complex. J Cell Biol. 2004;165:233–42.
30. Frischknecht F, Way M. Surfing pathogens and the lessons learned for actin polymerization. Trends Cell Biol. 2001;11:30–8.
31. Pollard TD, Borisy GG. Cellular motility driven by assembly and disassembly of actin filaments. Cell. 2003;112:453–65.
32. Jeffers V, Yang C, Huang S, Sullivan WJ Jr. Bromodomains in protozoan parasites: evolution, function, and opportunities for drug development. Microbiol Mol Biol Rev. 2017;81(1):e00047–116.
33. Josling GA, Petter M, Oehring SC, Gupta AP, Dietz O, Wilson DW, et al. A Plasmodium *falciparum bromodomain* protein regulates invasion gene expression. Cell Host Microbe. 2015;17:741–51.
34. Mochizuki-Kawai H, Niki T, Shibuya K, Ichimura K. Programmed cell death progresses differentially in epidermal and mesophyll cells of lily petals. PLoS ONE. 2015;. https://doi.org/10.1371/journal.pone.0143502.
35. Brook I. β-Lactamase-producing bacteria in mixed infections. Clin Microbiol Infect. 2004;10(9):777–84.
36. Murphy C, Powlowski J, Wu M, Butler G, Tsang A. Curation of characterized glycoside hydrolases of fungal origin. Database. 2011. https://doi.org/10.1093/database/bar020.
37. Ma Z, Song T, Zhu L, Ye W, Wang Y, Shao Y, et al. A *Phytophthora sojae* glycoside hydrolase 12 protein is a major virulence factor during soybean infection and is recognized as a PAMP. Plant Cell. 2015;27:2057–72.
38. Berlemont R, Martiny AC. Glycoside hydrolases across environmental microbial communities. PLoS Comput Biol. 2016. https://doi.org/10.1371/journal.pcbi.1005300.
39. Sajid M, McKerrow JH. Cysteine proteases of parasitic organisms. Mol Biochem Parasitol. 2002;120:1–21.
40. Hotson A, Mudgett MB. Cysteine proteases in phytopathogenic bacteria: identification of plant targets and activation of innate immunity. Curr Opin Plant Biol. 2004;7:384–90.
41. Torto-Alalibo T, Tian M, Gajendran K, Waugh ME, van West P, Kamoun S. Expressed sequence tags from the oomycete fish pathogen *Saprolegnia parasitica* reveal putative virulence factors. BMC Microbiol. 2005;5:46.
42. Yang J, Huang X, Tian B, Wang M, Niu Q, Zhang K. Isolation and characterization of a serine protease from the nematophagous fungus, *Lecanicillium psalliotae*, displaying nematicidal activity. Biotechnol Lett. 2005;27:1123–8.
43. Magnadottir B. Innate immunity of fish (overview). Fish Shellfish Immunol. 2006;20:137–51.
44. Uribe C, Folch H, Enriquez R, Moran G. Innate and adaptive immunity in teleost fish: a review. Vet Med. 2011;56(10):486–503.
45. Boes M. Role of natural and immune IgM antibodies in immune responses. Mol Immunol. 2000;37:1141–9.
46. Panda S, Ding JL. Natural antibodies bridge innate and adaptive immunity. J Immunol. 2015;194(1):13–20.
47. Banfield MJ, Kamoun S. Hooked and cooked: a fish killer genome exposed. PLoS Genet. 2013;9(6):e1003590.
48. Lilley JH, Thompson KD, Adams A. Characterization of *Aphanomyces invadans* by electrophoresis and western blot analysis. Dis Aquat Org. 1997;30:187–97.

Blood pressure and heart rate during ovariohysterectomy in pyometra and control dogs: a preliminary investigation

Odd Viking Höglund[1*], Johanna Lövebrant[2], Ulf Olsson[3] and Katja Höglund[4]

Abstract

Background: Surgery causes a stress response, a physiologic response to trauma. The intraoperative surgical stress response in dogs diagnosed with pyometra has not previously been described. The aim of this study was to investigate the intraoperative surgical stress response, assessed by blood pressure and heart rate measurements, in dogs diagnosed with pyometra and healthy controls. All dogs were premedicated with acepromazine and methadone, anaesthesia was induced with propofol and maintained with isoflurane, where after the dogs were subjected to ovariohysterectomy.

Results: Eight dogs diagnosed with pyometra and eight healthy controls were used. Systolic blood pressure and heart rate were measured to assess the surgical stress response. Additionally propofol dosage at induction of anaesthesia and the end-tidal isoflurane concentration were investigated. The surgery was split into four phases. Phase 0 was the period 10 min before the skin incision, phase 1 was skin incision and opening of abdomen, phase 2 was manipulation of uterine horns, lifting of the ovary with stretching of the mesovarium, ligation and transection of mesovarium and phase 3 was ligation and transection of cervix, removal of organs and closing of the abdomen. Dosage of propofol at induction of anaesthesia was 3.6 ± 1 mg/kg in dogs with pyometra and 4.1 ± 1 in healthy controls ($P = 0.37$). In both groups, systolic blood pressure increased between phase 1 and 2, from 87 ± 15 to 114 ± 19 mmHg in dogs with pyometra, and from 88 ± 18 to 106 ± 20 mmHg in healthy controls, (both $P < 0.0001$). Systolic blood pressure did not differ significantly between groups in any of the phases. Heart rate and end-tidal concentration of isoflurane did not differ significantly between phases or between groups.

Conclusions: The increased blood pressure at removal of ovaries during ovariohysterectomy suggests a pronounced noxious stimulus at this part of the procedure. In principle, the study parameters and response to surgery did not differ significantly between dogs with pyometra and healthy controls.

Keywords: Surgical stress, Blood pressure, Heart rate, Canine, Pyometra, Isoflurane, Acepromazine, Methadone

Background

Pyometra is a common disease in intact bitches. In a study of insured dogs in Sweden approximately 25% of females were affected by pyometra before 10 years of age [1]. Protective and risk-factors may vary between breeds as there are differences in incidence rates between breeds [2–5]. Surgery is curative of the disease. In animals subjected to surgery, the noxious stimuli caused by the procedure triggers a stress response [6–8] which can be used for assessment and evaluation of surgical methods and anaesthetic protocols [9–14]. The stress response is a physiological response to trauma or surgery and is generally considered to be proportional to the degree of surgical trauma [15–18]. Physiological parameters such as heart rate and blood pressure can be used as surrogate measure of the stress response and there are studies of the perioperative surgical stress response in healthy female dogs subjected to neutering [11, 19–27]. However, the effect of pyometra on the intraoperative surgical

*Correspondence: Odd.Hoglund@slu.se
[1] Department of Clinical Sciences, Box 7054, 750 07 Uppsala, Sweden
Full list of author information is available at the end of the article

stress response is not known. It may be expected that patients affected by pyometra and endotoxemia [28–33] will differ in intraoperative hemodynamic response compared to healthy dogs due to the effects on circulation of the endotoxins [34–36]. Based on previous studies, we hypothesized that noxious stimuli at removal of ovaries would cause systolic blood pressure to peak, regardless if pyometra was diagnosed or not. The aim of this study was to investigate the intraoperative surgical stress response, assessed by blood pressure and heart rate measurements, in dogs diagnosed with pyometra and healthy controls, all of which were subjected to ovariohysterectomy (OHE).

Methods

Animals

The study population consisted of female privately owned dogs admitted to the University animal hospital for surgical treatment, OHE, due to pyometra. Dogs of different breeds and ages were included (Table 1). All dogs were examined by an experienced veterinarian and diagnosis was confirmed with ultrasound and/or radiographs. The control group consisted of eight female privately owned dogs that were confirmed healthy by owner interview and clinical examination and that were admitted for elective OHE at the owners' request (Table 1). The Uppsala Animal Ethics Committee, Sweden and Swedish Board of Agriculture approved the study (C 127/10).

Anaesthesia

Acepromazine and methadone were used for sedative premedication (Table 2). Carprofen was given preoperatively or immediately at end of surgery. Postoperatively, methadone hydrochloride was administered subcutaneously every 6 h for the first 24 h.

Anaesthesia was induced by intravenous administration of propofol (PropoVet Multidose, 10 mg/ml, Orion Pharma Animal Health) given to effect at approximately 4 mg/kg and maintained with inhalation of isoflurane mixed in air at 2–3%. Oxygen and air mixture at approximately 50% was used at a flow of approximately 20–40 ml/kg/min in a circle breathing system. The dosage of isoflurane was controlled by an experienced and qualified veterinary nurse who monitored the anaesthesia. All dogs breathed spontaneously. The setting of the vaporizer was aimed at maintaining the dog anesthetized at surgical plane of anaesthesia (stage 3, plane 2). Depth of anaesthesia was judged by subjective assessment of the muscular tonus of the jaw, position of the eyeballs, dilation of the pupils, and the response to surgery.

The end-tidal isoflurane concentration heart rate and blood pressure were recorded using a multi-parameter anaesthetic monitoring device (LifeWindow 6000, Digicare Biomedical Technology, Boynton Beach, FL, USA). Non-invasive arterial blood pressure and heart rate were monitored by use of an oscillometric method. An automatic pneumatic cuff, with a width to circumference ratio of approximately 0.4, was wrapped around the distal forelimb and connected to the monitoring device. Data were registered once per minute following induction of anaesthesia until completion of surgery. Data was transferred to an Excel file (Microsoft Office) and all data points were included in the analysis.

Surgery

The dog was placed in dorsal recumbency and the animal´s abdomen was clipped and scrubbed. A ventral midline incision 2–3 cm cranial to the umbilicus was made and extended caudally and the abdomen was opened. The uterus was located, the ovaries were identified and a hole

Table 1 The age and body weight of the 16 dogs included in the study and duration of phases (mean ± standard deviation)

Dogs	n	Age (years)	Weight (kg)	Phase 0 (min)	Phase 1 (min)	Phase 2 (min)	Phase 3 (min)
Pyometra	8	5.4 ± 2	22.7 ± 13	10 ± 0	6.9 ± 5	14.0 ± 6	16.6 ± 6
Controls	8	4.7 ± 2	17.5 ± 7	10 ± 0	7.8 ± 4	12.9 ± 4	20.0 ± 8

Age, bodyweight and duration of phases did not differ between groups (Student's *t* test, $P > 0.05$)

Table 2 Drugs used for premedication and anesthesia of the 16 dogs included in the study

Drug	Indication	Dosage	Trade name	Route
Acepromazine	Sedative	0.03 mg/kg	Plegicil vet, Vericore Ltd	Intramuscular
Carprofen	Analgesic	4 mg/kg	Rimadyl vet, Pfizer ApS	Subcutaneous
Methadone hydrochloride	Analgesic	0.2 mg/kg	Metadon Recip, Recip AB	Subcutaneous
Propofol	General anesthesia	To effect	PropoVet Multidose, Orion Pharma Animal Health	Intravenous
Isoflurane	General anesthesia	To effect	Isoba vet, Schering-Plough A/S	Inhalation

was made in the mesovarium. Haemostat forceps were placed across the ovarian pedicle. Forceps were repositioned distally (closer to the ovary) to expose the compressed mesovarial tissue and one or two ligatures were placed and tied. An absorbable suture size 2–0 or 3–0 was used for ligation. The ovarian pedicle was cut between the distal ligature and the forceps. A ligature was also placed over the broad ligament. The procedure was repeated on the contralateral side. The uterine body was ligated at the cranial tip of the cervix, the tissue was transected and the uterus was removed. The ligated tissue was observed and verified for hemostasis. The abdominal wall was closed in three layers (*linea alba*, subcutaneous tissue and skin).

Protocol for data analysis

A protocol was designed for analysis of the different parts of the surgery. For comparison and evaluation of the cardiovascular response the surgery was split into four phases: 10 min immediately before skin incision (phase 0), skin incision and opening of abdomen (phase 1), manipulation of uterine horns, ligation and transection of mesovarium (phase 2), ligation of cervix, removal of organs and closing (phase 3). Other actions by the surgeon that could affect the surgical stress response were noted in the protocol, i.e. application of forceps or diathermy. The exact time when all parts of the surgical procedures that represented each phase were performed were noted in the protocol. The recorded data was thus labelled by phase.

Statistics

Student's t test (two-sided, unequal variance) was used (Excel, Microsoft Office) for comparison of age, body weight, dosage of propofol and duration of phases between the groups (Tables 1, 5). Remaining statistical analysis was performed with the statistical program SAS (Cary, NC, USA). No serious deviations from normality were detected. The effects of surgery on heart rate, systolic blood pressure and end-tidal concentration of isoflurane in each phase were analysed using mixed linear models for repeated measures data [37, 38]. The least square means (LSMean) and standard error of least square means were computed and compared within and between groups (Procedure mixed) for each phase. Significant differences were calculated comparing LSMean with Tukey–Kramer's adjustment for multiplicity. Results are reported as mean and standard deviation (SD) of each phase (Tables 3, 4, 5). $P < 0.05$ was considered significant for the analyses.

Results

Age and body weight (Table 1) did not differ significantly between the groups ($P = 0.6$ and 0.3, respectively). There were no significant differences between the groups' corresponding phases in systolic blood pressure, heart rate or concentration of anaesthetic gas. Duration of phases 0–3 for pyometra and control dogs did not differ significantly between groups ($P = 1.0$, 0.7, 0.7 and 0.3 respectively; Table 1).

Table 3 Systolic blood pressure (Mean ± standard deviation, mmHg) in control dogs and dogs diagnosed with pyometra that were subjected to ovariohysterectomy

Diagnosis	n	Phase 0	Phase 1	Phase 2	Phase 3
Pyometra	8	87.1 ± 17	86.8 ± 15	114.5[a,b] ± 19	101.2 ± 17
Control	8	77.6 ± 12	88.5 ± 18	105.6[a,b] ± 20	98.8[a] ± 21

Data was compared by the mixed procedure (SAS) with Tukey–Kramer's adjustment ($P < 0.05$). There were no significant differences between the groups' corresponding phases

[a] Differ significantly compared with phase 0

[b] Differ significantly compared with previous phase

Table 4 Heart rate (Mean ± standard deviation, beats per minute) in control dogs and dogs diagnosed with pyometra that were subjected to ovariohysterectomy

Diagnosis	n	Phase 0	Phase 1	Phase 2	Phase 3
Pyometra	8	95.3 ± 18	91.8 ± 17	106.8 ± 15	106.5 ± 15
Control	8	89.5 ± 22	91.5 ± 22	89.6 ± 20	95.2 ± 19

Data was compared by the mixed procedure (SAS) with Tukey–Kramer's adjustment ($P < 0.05$). There were no significant differences compared to previous phase or between the groups' corresponding phases

The values for systolic blood pressure, heart rate and end-tidal concentration of isoflurane are given in Tables 3, 4 and 5, respectively. In both groups the systolic blood pressure (Table 3) did not change significantly at opening of the abdomen (phase 0–1) but increased between phase 1 and 2 (both $P < 0.0001$). Neither heart rate, nor end-tidal concentration of isoflurane, changed significantly during the procedures in any of the groups (Tables 4, 5). Dosage of propofol was 10% below the manufacturer's recommended dosage (4 mg/kg) in the dogs with pyometra. The dosage did not differ significantly between the groups ($P = 0.37$; Table 5).

The surgeries were performed in total by seven different surgeons whereof two surgeons were involved in the control group and six in the pyometra group. In both groups, the ovarian pedicle was single ligated in six dogs and was double ligated in two dogs at removal of ovaries.

One dog in the pyometra group was given carprofen before surgery whereas six dogs were given carprofen immediately at end of the surgery. Of the control dogs seven dogs were given carprofen before surgery whereas one dog was given carprofen immediately at end of surgery. One dog in the pyometra group was on meloxicam treatment, no NSAID was given to that dog at day of surgery.

Table 5 Dosage of propofol (mg/kg) and end-tidal concentration of isoflurane, % (Mean ± standard deviation) in control dogs and dogs diagnosed with pyometra that were subjected to ovariohysterectomy

Diagnosis	n	Propofol induction	Isoflurane phase 0	Isoflurane phase 1	Isoflurane phase 2	Isoflurane phase 3
Pyometra	8	3.6 ± 1	1.9 ± 0.3	1.8 ± 0.3	2.1 ± 0.3	2.0 ± 0.2
Control	8	4.1 ± 1	2.2 ± 0.3	2.0 ± 0.2	2.1 ± 0.2	1.9 ± 0.2

Dosage of propofol was compared between groups with student's *t* test ($P = 0.37$). Data for end-tidal concentration of isoflurane was compared by the mixed procedure (SAS) with Tukey-Kramer's adjustment ($P < 0.05$). There were no significant differences compared to previous phase or between the groups' corresponding phases

Complications

In one dog in the control group an intraoperative haemorrhage from a single ligated ovarian pedicle was observed. The ovarian pedicle was swiftly re-ligated, haemostasis was confirmed and blood loss was not considered significant.

In another control dog a postoperative haemorrhage was suspected. The dog was re-anesthetized, the abdomen was opened and haemorrhage was observed from the left ovarian pedicle which had been single ligated. The ovarian pedicle was re-ligated, the abdomen closed and the dog recovered uneventfully.

One dog in the control group developed diarrhoea after 2 days on carprofen and the drug was discontinued. In another dog in the control group a wound infection was suspected. Antibiotics were prescribed and the dog recovered uneventfully. All dogs in the pyometra group recovered uneventfully.

Discussion

In this study, the intraoperative surgical stress response in dogs diagnosed with pyometra and controls was assessed by measurements of systolic blood pressure and heart rate. The response did not differ significantly between groups. In both groups there was a peak of blood pressure at removal of ovaries which is in agreement with other studies of surgical stress in dogs subjected to OHE [11, 19, 25–27]. This part of the procedure, ligation of the mesovarium and removal of ovaries, caused a significant increase in blood pressure, regardless if the dogs were diagnosed with pyometra or not. Removal of ovaries is considered maximum noxious stimuli during a bitch spay [11, 25]. Attempts to reduce the noxious stimuli at removal of the ovaries by adding local anaesthetic to the mesovarium has been investigated with no proven benefit in dogs [21], while a positive effect was reported in a study in cats [39]. As results of these previous studies on local anaesthesia of the mesovarium are in conflict, further studies on targeted analgesia are needed. Less surgical stress at ovary removal has been reported in healthy dogs with a laparoscopic technique compared to the traditional open abdomen technique [11] and a laparoscopic-assisted technique for pyometra is described [40–42]. Furthermore, development of a new method for ligation of the mesovarium may enable a more standardized technique with potentially less noxious stimuli [43–45].

Most drugs used in the present study, except carprofen, may cause hypotension [46–48] and dogs of both groups could be considered hypotensive [49]. Acepromazine is a neuroleptic substance that blocks the post-synaptic dopamine receptors in the central nervous system (CNS). Methadone is an opiate agonist (μ-receptor agonist) and one of the potential adverse effects of methadone is bradycardia, which was an unlikely side effect at the dosage used and was not observed in the present study. The half-life of methadone is 10.7 ± 4.3 h following subcutaneous (s.c.) administration, and half-life of acepromazine is 7.1 ± 1.3 h following intravenous (i.v.) administration [50, 51]. There may have been some variation in time between premedication and induction of anaesthesia, but this variation was assumed to be small in comparison to the half-lives of the drugs. It can therefore be assumed that the intraoperative effects of the drugs were similar in both groups considering the half-lives of these drugs. The end-tidal concentration of isoflurane was stable throughout the procedures but could be considered high. A high or low isoflurane concentration has not been shown to have any effect on magnitude of blood pressure increase after stimuli in humans [47]. In another study on people, different concentrations of desflurane did not influence the endocrine response to surgery [52]. In the present study the end-tidal isoflurane concentration did not differ significantly between phases or the groups' corresponding phases.

Carprofen is a weak cyclo-oxygenase (COX) inhibitor and the mechanism behind its main anti-inflammatory effect is unknown. No perioperative adverse effects on the cardiovascular system have been reported at recommended dosages [53, 54]. The usual procedure at the University animal hospital is to administer NSAID to patients affected by pyometra immediately after surgery, and not before. In contrast, the majority of the control dogs were administered NSAID before surgery. The treatment of the two groups with carprofen therefore differed and comparison between the two groups should be made cautiously.

In a previous study where markers of surgical stress in dogs subjected to OHE were measured, the heart rate increased at ligation of mesovarium and removal of the ovary [25]. The same anaesthetic protocol was used in the two studies but heart rate did not increase in the present study. However, the phases were defined differently and comparisons should be made with care. In the previous study removal of one ovary represented one phase, whereas in the present study removal of both ovaries represented one phase. Removal of ovaries in the present study caused blood pressure to increase, however, the longer duration for removal of both ovaries may have allowed the baroreceptor reflex to normalise a possible initial increase in heart rate.

In one dog an intraoperative haemorrhage was observed after single ligation of the ovarian pedicle. In addition one dog was re-operated due to haemorrhage from a single ligated ovarian pedicle. The complications described in this study confirm the current recommendation that the ovarian pedicle should be double ligated [55].

There were study limitations. One limitation was the use of non-invasive blood pressure measurements. An invasive technique is considered gold standard, but with repeated measurements a reliable average of a series of systolic blood pressure readings can be obtained. Systolic blood pressure values are given as the non-invasive method may be less accurate at lower pressures [56–58]. The use of systolic blood pressure values therefore lowers the risk of measurement errors. The number of dogs used in this study was low, individual variations may have affected the results, and therefore the results should be interpreted cautiously. Another variable that could have influenced the results was the dogs' general condition. Possible endotoxemia was not investigated. Dogs with pyometra may have been affected by endotoxins which have effect on circulation [34–36]. The dogs' status of pain, their blood pressure or the possible influence of endotoxins before surgery may have varied between dogs. No measurements of heart rate or blood pressure or scoring of pain were made before or after surgery. However, there were no significant differences between the groups' intraoperative study parameters at corresponding phases and duration of phases did not differ between groups. Furthermore, pyometra dogs may have been given crystalloid fluids i.v. preoperatively and the exact timing is not known, which is an additional study limitation. However, if fluids were administered preoperatively, the effect on study parameters was considered to be minor as administration of isotonic fluids has little effect on arterial blood pressure according to a study on healthy dogs [59]. Extrapolation of results to dogs with concurrent disease should be done cautiously. There were seven different surgeons involved, which may have caused disparity in tissue handling and surgical technique. However, in a previous study no effect was seen on blood pressure changes of covariate surgeon [11]. This was considered to be in agreement with a study which demonstrated no effect of surgeon experience and duration of surgery on post-operative pain [60]. The person handling the anaesthesia was not aware of study aim or study parameters, but was not blinded to diagnosis, which may be considered a study limitation. The judgment of depth of anesthesia is partly subjective and deep planes of anesthesia may have been a reason for the observed low blood pressure. End-tidal concentration of isoflurane did not change significantly and did not differ between groups, but dosage requirements of end-tidal isoflurane concentration may differ between individuals. Furthermore, variations in carbon dioxide levels and body temperatures may affect the cardiovascular system. Neither of these parameters were evaluated, which is another study limitation.

Conclusions

In principle, the study parameters and the response to surgery did not differ significantly between corresponding phases of the groups. Blood pressure increased at removal of the ovaries, both in dogs diagnosed with pyometra and healthy controls that were subjected to OHE under isoflurane anaesthesia and premedicated with acepromazine and methadone. Blood pressure did not differ significantly between the groups' corresponding phases. Heart rate and end-tidal concentration of isoflurane did not change significantly during the procedure and did not differ significantly between groups.

Authors' contributions

OVH performed several of the surgeries and was involved in the design of the study. JL recorded and managed data for statistical analysis. UO was responsible for statistical analysis. KH was involved in data analysis. All authors were involved in writing of the manuscript. All authors read and approved the final manuscript.

Author details

[1] Department of Clinical Sciences, Box 7054, 750 07 Uppsala, Sweden.
[2] Alingsås Veterinärstuga AB, Björkekärrsvägen 26, 441 91 Alingsås, Sweden.
[3] Unit of Applied Statistics and Mathematics, Swedish University of Agricultural Sciences, Box 7032, 750 07 Uppsala, Sweden. [4] Department of Anatomy, Physiology and Biochemistry, Swedish University of Agricultural Sciences, Box 7011, 750 07 Uppsala, Sweden.

Acknowledgements

We would like to thank Ragnvi Hagman and Supranee Jitpean at Swedish University of Agricultural Sciences for valuable comments on this work.

Competing interests

OVH has invented, developed and patented [61, 62] an implant for surgical ligation, the LigaTie®, which has been tested for ligation of the ovarian pedicle. The implant was not used in this study. The other authors declare that they have no competing interests.

References

1. Egenvall A, Hagman R, Bonnett BN, Hedhammar A, Olson P, Lagerstedt AS. Breed risk of pyometra in insured dogs in Sweden. J Vet Intern Med. 2001;15:530–8. doi:10.1111/j.1939-1676.2001.tb01587.x.
2. Jitpean S, Hagman R, Ström Holst B, Höglund OV, Pettersson A, Egenvall A. Breed variations in the incidence of pyometra and mammary tumours in Swedish dogs. Reprod Domest Anim. 2012;47(Suppl 6):347–50. doi:10.1111/rda.12103.
3. Gibson A, Dean R, Yates D, Stavisky J. A retrospective study of pyometra at five RSPCA hospitals in the UK: 1728 cases from 2006 to 2011. Vet Rec. 2013;173:396. doi:10.1136/vr.101514.
4. Niskanen M, Thrusfield MV. Associations between age, parity, hormonal therapy and breed, and pyometra in Finnish dogs. Vet Rec. 1998;143:493–8. doi:10.1136/vr.143.18.493.
5. Hagman R, Lagerstedt AS, Hedhammar A, Egenvall A. A breed-matched case-control study of potential risk-factors for canine pyometra. Theriogenology. 2011;75:1251–7. doi:10.1016/j.theriogenology.2010.11.038.
6. Desborough JP. The stress response to trauma and surgery. Br J Anaesth. 2000;85:109–17.
7. Giannoudis PV, Dinopoulos H, Chalidis B, Hall GM. Surgical stress response. Injury. 2006;37(Suppl 5):S3–9. doi:10.1016/S0020-1383(07)70005-0.
8. Weissman C. The metabolic response to stress: an overview and update. Anesthesiology. 1990;73:308–27.
9. Kataja J, Chrapek W, Kaukinen S, Pimenoff G, Salenius JP. Hormonal stress response and hemodynamic stability in patients undergoing endovascular vs. conventional abdominal aortic aneurysm repair. Scand J Surg. 2007;96:236–42.
10. Yoo KY, Lee MK, Jeong CW, Kim SJ, Jeong ST, Shin MH, et al. Anaesthetic requirement and stress hormone responses in patients undergoing lumbar spine surgery: anterior vs. posterior approach. Acta Anaesthesiol Scand. 2009;53:1012–7. doi:10.1111/j.1399-6576.2009.01993.x.
11. Höglund OV, Olsson K, Hagman R, Ohlund M, Olsson U, Lagerstedt AS. Comparison of haemodynamic changes during two surgical methods for neutering female dogs. Res Vet Sci. 2011;91:159–63. doi:10.1016/j.rvsc.2010.08.013.
12. Freeman LJ, Rahmani EY, Al-Haddad M, Sherman S, Chiorean MV, Selzer DJ, et al. Comparison of pain and postoperative stress in dogs undergoing natural orifice transluminal endoscopic surgery, laparoscopic, and open oophorectomy. Gastrointest Endosc. 2010;72:373–80. doi:10.1016/j.gie.2010.01.066.
13. Yoder B, Wolf JS Jr. Canine model of surgical stress response comparing standard laparoscopic, microlaparoscopic, and hand-assisted laparoscopic nephrectomy. Urology. 2005;65:600–3. doi:10.1016/j.urology.2004.10.021.
14. Ledowski T, Bein B, Hanss R, Paris A, Fudickar W, Scholz J, et al. Neuroendocrine stress response and heart rate variability: a comparison of total intravenous versus balanced anesthesia. Anesth Analg. 2005;101:1700–5. doi:10.1213/01.ane.0000184041.32175.14.
15. Marana E, Scambia G, Maussier ML, Parpaglioni R, Ferrandina G, Meo F, et al. Neuroendocrine stress response in patients undergoing benign ovarian cyst surgery by laparoscopy, minilaparotomy, and laparotomy. J Am Assoc Gynecol Laparosc. 2003;10:159–65. doi:10.1016/S1074-3804(05)60291-5.
16. Chernow B, Alexander HR, Smallridge RC, Thompson WR, Cook D, Beardsley D, et al. Hormonal responses to graded surgical stress. Arch Intern Med. 1987;147:1273–8. doi:10.1001/archinte.1987.00370070087013.
17. Naitoh T, Garcia-Ruiz A, Vladisavljevic A, Matsuno S, Gagner M. Gastrointestinal transit and stress response after laparoscopic vs conventional distal pancreatectomy in the canine model. Surg Endosc. 2002;16:1627–30. doi:10.1007/s00464-002-0007-0.
18. Horta RS, Figueiredo MS, Lavalle GE, Costa MP, Cunha RM, Araujo RB. Surgical stress and postoperative complications related to regional and radical mastectomy in dogs. Acta Vet Scand. 2015;57:34. doi:10.1186/s13028-015-0121-3.
19. Väisänen M, Raekallio M, Kuusela E, Huttunen P, Leppäluoto J, Kirves P, et al. Evaluation of the perioperative stress response in dogs administered medetomidine or acepromazine as part of the preanesthetic medication. Am J Vet Res. 2002;63:969–75. doi:10.2460/ajvr.2002.63.969.
20. Benson GJ, Grubb TL, Neff-Davis C, Olson WA, Thurmon JC, Lindner DL, et al. Perioperative stress response in the dog: effect of preemptive administration of medetomidine. Vet Surg. 2000;29:85–91. doi:10.1111/j.1532-950X.2000.00085.x.
21. Bubalo V, Moens YP, Holzmann A, Coppens P. Anaesthetic sparing effect of local anaesthesia of the ovarian pedicle during ovariohysterectomy in dogs. Vet Anaesth Analg. 2008;35:537–42. doi:10.1111/j.1467-2995.2008.00421.x.
22. Van Goethem B, Van Nimwegen SA, Murell JC, Kirpensteijn J. The effect of neuromuscular blockade on canine laparoscopic ovariectomy: a double-blinded, prospective clinical trial. Vet Surg. 2012;41:374–80. doi:10.1111/j.1532-950X.2011.00962.x.
23. Fox SM, Mellor DJ, Firth EC, Hodge H, Lawoko CR. Changes in plasma cortisol concentrations before, during and after analgesia, anaesthesia and anaesthesia plus ovariohysterectomy in bitches. Res Vet Sci. 1994;57:110–8.
24. Moldal ER, Kristensen AT, Peeters ME, Nodtvedt A, Kirpensteijn J. Hemostatic response to surgical neutering via ovariectomy and ovariohysterectomy in dogs. Am J Vet Res. 2012;73:1469–76. doi:10.2460/ajvr.73.9.1469.
25. Höglund OV, Hagman R, Olsson K, Olsson U, Lagerstedt A-S. Intraoperative changes in blood pressure, heart rate, plasma vasopressin, and urinary noradrenalin during elective ovariohysterectomy in dogs: repeatability at removal of the 1st and 2nd ovary. Vet Surg. 2014;43:852–9. doi:10.1111/j.1532-950X.2014.12264.x.
26. Höglund OV, Hagman R, Stridsberg M. Chromogranin A and cortisol at intraoperative repeated noxious stimuli: surgical stress in a dog model. SAGE Open Med. 2015;3:1–6. doi:10.1177/2050312115576432.
27. Tallant A, Ambros B, Freire C, Sakals S. Comparison of intraoperative and postoperative pain during canine ovariohysterectomy and ovariectomy. Can Vet J. 2016;57:741–6.
28. Hagman R, Reezigt BJ, Bergstrom Ledin H, Karlstam E. Blood lactate levels in 31 female dogs with pyometra. Acta Vet Scand. 2009;51:2. doi:10.1186/1751-0147-51-2.
29. Hagman R, Kindahl H, Lagerstedt AS. Pyometra in bitches induces elevated plasma endotoxin and prostaglandin F2α metabolite levels. Acta Vet Scand. 2006;47:55–67. doi:10.1186/1751-0147-47-55.
30. Fransson BA, Lagerstedt AS, Bergstrom A, Hagman R, Park JS, Chew BP, et al. C-reactive protein, tumor necrosis factor alpha, and interleukin-6 in dogs with pyometra and SIRS. J Vet Emerg Crit Care. 2007;17:373–81. doi:10.1111/j.1476-4431.2006.00203.x.
31. Jitpean S, Holst BS, Höglund OV, Pettersson A, Olsson U, Strage E, et al. Serum insulin-like growth factor-I, iron, C-reactive protein, and serum amyloid A for prediction of outcome in dogs with pyometra. Theriogenology. 2014;82:43–8. doi:10.1016/j.theriogenology.2014.02.014.
32. Jitpean S, Pettersson A, Höglund OV, Holst BS, Olsson U, Hagman R. Increased concentrations of serum amyloid A in dogs with sepsis caused by pyometra. BMC Vet Res. 2014;10:273. doi:10.1186/s12917-014-0273-9.
33. Jitpean S, Ström-Holst B, Emanuelson U, Höglund OV, Pettersson A, Alneryd-Bull C, et al. Outcome of pyometra in female dogs and predictors of peritonitis and prolonged postoperative hospitalization in surgically treated cases. BMC Vet Res. 2014;10:6. doi:10.1186/1746-6148-10-6.
34. Kuida H, Gilbert RP, Hinshaw LB, Brunson JG, Visscher MB. Species differences in effect of gram-negative endotoxin on circulation. Am J Physiol. 1961;200:1197–202.
35. Maclean LD, Spink WW, Visscher MB, Weil MH. Studies on the circulatory changes in the dog produced by endotoxin from gram-negative microorganisms. J Clin Invest. 1956;35:1191–8. doi:10.1172/JCI103373.
36. Parratt JR. Myocardial and circulatory effects of *E. coli* endotoxin; modification of responses to catecholamines. Br J Pharmacol. 1973;47:12–25. doi:10.1111/j.1476-5381.1973.tb08154.x.
37. Fitzmaurice GM, Laird NM, Ware JH. Applied longitudinal analysis. New York: Wiley; 2004.
38. Littell RC, Milliken GA, Stroup WW, Wolfinger RD, Schabenberger O. SAS for mixed models. 2nd ed. Cary: SAS Institute; 2006.
39. Zilberstein LF, Moens YP, Leterrier E. The effect of local anaesthesia on anaesthetic requirements for feline ovariectomy. Vet J. 2008;178:214–8. doi:10.1016/j.tvjl.2007.10.011.
40. Wallace ML, Case JB, Singh A, Ellison GW, Monnet E. Single incision, laparoscopic-assisted ovariohysterectomy for mucometra and pyometra in dogs. Vet Surg. 2015;44(Suppl 1):66–70. doi:10.1111/vsu.12344.
41. Adamovich-Rippe KN, Mayhew PD, Runge JJ, Culp WT, Steffey MA, Mayhew KN, et al. Evaluation of laparoscopic-assisted ovariohysterectomy for treatment of canine pyometra. Vet Surg. 2013;42:572–8. doi:10.1111/j.1532-950X.2013.12012.x.

42. Minami S, Okamoto Y, Eguchi H, Kato K. Successful laparoscopy assisted ovariohysterectomy in two dogs with pyometra. J Vet Med Sci. 1997;59:845–7. doi:10.1292/jvms.59.845.
43. Aminlashgari N, Höglund OV, Borg N, Hakkarainen M. Degradation profile and preliminary clinical testing of a resorbable device for ligation of blood vessels. Acta Biomater. 2013;9:6898–904. doi:10.1016/j.actbio.2013.02.018.
44. Höglund OV, Ingman J, Södersten F, Hansson K, Borg N, Lagerstedt AS. Ligation of the spermatic cord in dogs with a self-locking device of a resorbable polyglycolic based co-polymer—feasibility and long-term follow-up study. BMC Res Notes. 2014;7:1–7. doi:10.1186/1756-0500-7-825.
45. da Mota Costa MR, de Abreu Oliveira AL, Ramos RM, de Moura Vidal LW, Borg N, Höglund OV. Ligation of the mesovarium in dogs with a self-locking implant of a resorbable polyglycolic based co-polymer—a study of feasibility and comparison to suture ligation. BMC Res Notes. 2016;9:1–6. doi:10.1186/s13104-016-2042-2.
46. Merin RG, Bernard JM, Doursout MF, Cohen M, Chelly JE. Comparison of the effects of isoflurane and desflurane on cardiovascular dynamics and regional blood flow in the chronically instrumented dog. Anesthesiology. 1991;74:568–74.
47. Zbinden AM, Petersen-Felix S, Thomson DA. Anesthetic depth defined using multiple noxious stimuli during isoflurane/oxygen anesthesia. II. Hemodynamic responses. Anesthesiology. 1994;80:261–7.
48. Brearley JC, Heath SE, Jones RS, Skerritt GC. Drugs acting on the nervous system. In: Bishop Y, editor. The veterinary formulary. 5th ed. Cambridge: Pharmaceutical press; 2001. p. 361–414.
49. Ruffato M, Novello L, Clark L. What is the definition of intraoperative hypotension in dogs? Results from a survey of diplomates of the ACVAA and ECVAA. Vet Anaesth Analg. 2015;42:55–64. doi:10.1111/vaa.12169.
50. Ingvast-Larsson C, Holgersson A, Bondesson U, Lagerstedt AS, Olsson K. Clinical pharmacology of methadone in dogs. Vet Anaesth Analg. 2010;37:48–56. doi:10.1111/j.1467-2995.2009.00476.x.
51. Hashem A, Kietzmann M, Scherkl R. The pharmacokinetics and bioavailability of acepromazine in the plasma of dogs. Deutsch Tierarztl Wochenschr. 1992;99:396–8.
52. Baldini G, Bagry H, Carli F. Depth of anesthesia with desflurane does not influence the endocrine-metabolic response to pelvic surgery. Acta Anaesthesiol Scand. 2008;52:99–105. doi:10.1111/j.1399-6576.2007.01470.x.
53. Boström IM, Nyman GC, Lord PE, Häggström J, Jones BE, Bohlin HP. Effects of carprofen on renal function and results of serum biochemical and hematologic analyses in anesthetized dogs that had low blood pressure during anesthesia. Am J Vet Res. 2002;63:712–21. doi:10.2460/ajvr.2002.63.712.
54. Frendin JH, Boström IM, Kampa N, Eksell P, Häggström JU, Nyman GC. Effects of carprofen on renal function during medetomidine-propofol-isoflurane anesthesia in dogs. Am J Vet Res. 2006;67:1967–73. doi:10.2460/ajvr.67.12.1967.
55. Howe LM. Surgical methods of contraception and sterilization. Theriogenology. 2006;66:500–9. doi:10.1016/j.theriogenology.2006.04.005.
56. Meurs KM, Miller MW, Slater MR. Comparison of the indirect oscillometric and direct arterial methods for blood pressure measurements in anesthetized dogs. J Am Anim Hosp Assoc. 1996;32:471–5. doi:10.5326/15473317-32-6-471.
57. Sawyer DC, Brown M, Striler EL, Durham RA, Langham MA, Rech RH. Comparison of direct and indirect blood pressure measurement in anesthetized dogs. Lab Anim Sci. 1991;41:134–8.
58. Bodey AR, Michell AR, Bovee KC, Buranakurl C, Garg T. Comparison of direct and indirect (oscillometric) measurements of arterial blood pressure in conscious dogs. Res Vet Sci. 1996;61:17–21. doi:10.1016/S0034-5288(96)90104-6.
59. Valverde A, Gianotti G, Rioja-Garcia E, Hathway A. Effects of high-volume, rapid-fluid therapy on cardiovascular function and hematological values during isoflurane-induced hypotension in healthy dogs. Can J Vet Res. 2012;76:99–108.
60. Wagner AE, Worland GA, Glawe JC, Hellyer PW. Multicenter, randomized controlled trial of pain-related behaviors following routine neutering in dogs. J Am Vet Med Assoc. 2008;233:109–15. doi:10.2460/javma.233.1.109.
61. Höglund OV. Inventor Tissue ligation device. US patent 8696692; 2014.
62. Höglund OV. Inventor device and method for tissue ligation—patent application. US patent 20150157327; 2015.

Ability of vaccine strain induced antibodies to neutralize field isolates of caliciviruses from Swedish cats

Jonas Johansson Wensman[1*], Ayman Samman[2], Anna Lindhe[3], Jean-Christophe Thibault[4], Louise Treiberg Berndtsson[3] and Margaret J. Hosie[2]

Abstract

Background: Feline calicivirus (FCV) is a common cause of upper respiratory tract disease in cats worldwide. Its characteristically high mutation rate leads to escape from the humoral immune response induced by natural infection and/or vaccination and consequently vaccines are not always effective against field isolates. Thus, there is a need to continuously investigate the ability of FCV vaccine strain-induced antibodies to neutralize field isolates.

Methods: Seventy-eight field isolates of FCV isolated during the years 2008–2012 from Swedish cats displaying clinical signs of upper respiratory tract disease were examined in this study. The field isolates were tested for cross-neutralization using a panel of eight anti-sera raised in four pairs of cats following infection with four vaccine strains (F9, 255, G1 and 431).

Results: The anti-sera raised against F9 and 255 neutralised 20.5 and 11.5 %, and 47.4 and 64.1 % of field isolates tested, respectively. The anti-sera against the more recently introduced vaccine strains G1 and 431 neutralized 33.3 and 70.5 % and 69.2 and 89.7 %, respectively. Dual vaccine strains displayed a higher cross-neutralization.

Conclusions: This study confirms previous observations that more recently introduced vaccine strains induce antibodies with a higher neutralizing capacity compared to vaccine strains that have been used extensively over a long period of time. This study also suggests that dual FCV vaccine strains might neutralize more field isolates compared to single vaccine strains. Vaccine strains should ideally be selected based on updated knowledge on the antigenic properties of field isolates in the local setting, and there is thus a need for continuously studying the evolution of FCV together with the neutralizing capacity of vaccine strain induced antibodies against field isolates at a national and/or regional level.

Keywords: Feline calicivirus, Vaccine, Virus neutralization, Feline upper respiratory tract disease

Background

Feline calicivirus (FCV) is one of the primary causes of infectious upper respiratory tract disease in cats, an important disease worldwide [1]. In addition to respiratory signs, FCV is frequently associated with chronic gingivostomatitis, and highly virulent strains have been associated with an acute systemic virulent disease with a high case fatality rate [2, 3].

Feline calicivirus is a single-stranded RNA-virus of positive sense genome with a high genetic and antigenic variability [4–6], associated with escape from the humoral immune response induced by natural infection and/or vaccination.

FCV is distributed world-wide in the cat population and is estimated to be the etiological cause of upper respiratory tract disease in 10–50 % of cases [1]. The prevalence of FCV varies depending on the management and number of cats in a household [7]. In multi-cat

*Correspondence: Jonas.Wensman@slu.se
[1] Department of Clinical Sciences, Swedish University of Agricultural Sciences, Uppsala, Sweden
Full list of author information is available at the end of the article

households, such as breeding catteries, cat shelters and cat colonies, FCV is more prevalent [8, 9]. In Sweden, 18 % of feline clinical samples submitted for virus isolation to the National Veterinary Institute during the year 2000 tested positive for FCV, while healthy carriers of FCV in Swedish catteries were estimated at 2.6 % [10].

Several commercial vaccines consisting of various vaccine strains are available, but due to the high mutation rate of FCV, vaccines are not always efficacious [11–13]. There is therefore a need to investigate and follow the ability of vaccine strain induced antibodies to neutralize field isolates of FCV, in order to evaluate and provide updated advice on vaccination strategies at local and/or regional levels.

In a previous study, the cross-neutralization of FCV field strains isolated in the UK by vaccine strain induced antibodies was examined [14]. Here, we used a similar approach to investigate whether comparable findings would apply in a different European country, namely Sweden.

Methods

FCV field isolates

A panel of 78 field isolates of FCV grown in vitro was selected from samples submitted between October 2008 and February 2012 to the National Veterinary Institute in Sweden. The samples were all collected from cats showing clinical signs compatible with FCV infection, although the clinical signs were not always stated in the referral form (Additional file 1), and FCV diagnosis had been confirmed by transmission electron microscopy (TEM).

Virus neutralization test

The isolated FCV isolates were expanded following the inoculation of 2×10^5 cell/mL of feline embryo A (FEA) cells [15] in T25 cm^2 flasks (Corning, NY). Cells were incubated at 37 °C in an atmosphere of 5 % CO_2. Cultures were observed for evidence of cytopathic effect (CPE) for up to 4 days post-infection. Once CPE became evident, culture fluids were harvested, passed through a 0.45 µm filter Minisart syringe filter (Sartorius, UK), aliquoted and stored at −80 °C prior to titration.

To titrate the virus isolates, fourfold dilutions of the viral stocks (starting at a dilution of 1/500) were prepared and then incubated (in quadruplicate, per dilution per isolate) in 96-well plates (Thermo scientific, NY) with 2×10^5 cells/mL of FEA cells in a total volume of 200 µl at 37 °C for 48 h. As previosuly, the $TCID_{50}$ was calculated as the reciprocal of the final dilution where CPE was evident in at least 50 % of the wells [14].

Virus isolates were tested for cross-neutralization using a panel of eight anti-sera, raised in four pairs of cats infected once by the oronasal route with 1 mL of each viral inoculum containing 10^6 $TCID_{50}$ of FCV strain F9, 255, G1 or 431 (one pair of cats was infected with each strain). Serial dilutions of anti-sera (threefold, starting from a 1/5 dilution) were incubated with 100 $TCID_{50}$ of each of the 78 field isolates in quadruplicate in 96-well plates in a total volume of 100 µl for 2 h at 37 °C. Next, 100 µl of FEA cells were added at a density of 2×10^5 cells/mL and the plates were incubated for 48 h. The neutralization titre was calculated as the reciprocal of the highest serum dilution where cells were free from CPE in at least two of four replicate wells.

Results and discussion

Virus neutralization of FCV field isolates

The FCV field isolates were analysed in a neutralization test using eight antisera raised against four commercially available FCV vaccine strains (G1, 431, 255 and F9). The same panel of paired anti-sera as had been used by Addie and co-workers [14] was used in this study, with the exception of the anti-sera raised against FCV G1. Fifteen of the field isolates were tested in parallel with the batch of anti-sera previously used [14] as well as the new pair of anti-sera raised against FCV G1, with similar results (Additional file 2). This comparison validated the use of the new batch of anti-sera, which was subsequently used to test all field isolates in this study. The paired anti-sera raised against vaccine strains 255 and F9, which have been used in vaccines for several decades, neutralized 47.4 and 64.1 % (strain 255) or 20.5 and 11.5 % (strain F9) of the field isolates with titres ≥ 5 (Table 1). The more recently introduced vaccine strains G1 and 431 [16] neutralized 33.3 and 70.5 % (strain G1) or 69.2 and 89.7 % (strain 431) of the field isolates with titres ≥ 5. In this study, similar differences in neutralizing capacity between paired anti-sera were observed, as had previously been recorded [14] (Table 1), consistent with inter-cat variation in humoral immune responses to FCV infection. As shown in Table 1, strain F9 neutralized few field isolates at titers greater than 45. Only one field isolate (isolated from cat no. 6 displaying upper respiratory signs; Additional files 1 and 2) was not neutralized by any of the anti-sera, and another field isolate (isolated from cat no. 75 with ulcerative stomatitis; Additional files 1 and 2) was neutralized at a titer of five by only one of the anti-sera raised against strain G1 (S2).

These results are in accordance with previous reports [11, 14, 17], indicating the poor ability of antibodies against FCV vaccine strain F9 to neutralize current field isolates. The reduced capacity of field isolate neutralization is driven by the high mutation rate of FCV to escape the host immune response leading to emergence of escape mutants [6, 18], whether the immunity is induced

Table 1 Results of virus neutralization tests

Titres	S1; G1	S2; G1	S3; 431	S4; 431	S5; 255	S6; 255	S7; F9	S8; F9
<5	52 (67)	35 (45)	24 (31)	8 (10)	41 (53)	28 (36)	62 (79)	69 (88)
5–15	20 (26)	22 (28)	39 (50)	32 (41)	28 (36)	19 (24)	12 (15)	7 (9)
45–1215	6 (8)	21 (27)	15 (19)	38 (49)	9 (12)	31 (40)	4 (5)	2 (3)

Antisera raised against four feline calicivirus vaccine strains (G1, 431, 255 and F9) were used in the neutralization tests of 78 Swedish field isolates. The number of field isolates neutralized by respective antiserum is indicated, with the proportion of neutralized strains shown as a percentage within parenthesis

by vaccination and/or natural infection. The likelihood of reduced protection increases when a vaccine strain has been extensively used for a long period of time. Antibodies raised against the more recently introduced vaccine strains (G1 and 431) demonstrated better neutralization of field isolates compared to those raised against strain F9 (Table 1); however, we observed no marked difference between antibodies raised against these strains compared to FCV vaccine strain 255. To our knowledge, vaccine strain 255 has not been extensively used in Sweden, although it was introduced a few decades ago; thus, it is likely that this strain has not contributed to the immune pressure driving FCV mutation.

Combining two vaccine strains increases the likelihood of neutralization

Currently, the vaccines registered and in use in Sweden contain either one single vaccine strain (either 255 or F9) or a combination of two vaccine strains (G1 and 431). Therefore, we compared the neutralizing capacity of the anti-sera raised against these vaccine strains as they are presented in current vaccine preparations. Only 10 % of the field isolates were neutralized by both paired anti-sera raised against strain F9, 44 % were neutralized by both paired anti-sera raised against strain 255, whereas 73 % of the field isolates were neutralized by combinations of the anti-sera against strains G1 and 431, where at least one of the paired anti-sera always was neutralizing (Table 2). These findings indicate that by combining two vaccine strains, the likelihood of neutralization of the field isolates increases. It is of interest to note that, by combining strains 431 and 255 in a putative vaccine preparation, an even broader neutralizing capacity (60/78; 77 %) would have been seen against this panel of field isolates (data not shown). This effect could be the result of the greater phylogenetic distance in amino acid sequence between isolates 431 and 255, compared to isolates 431 and G1 [16].

The combination of two antigenically distant vaccine strains has previously been proposed in order to achieve higher cross-neutralizing capacity [14]. When we examined data from a previous study of field isolates from the UK, a similar comparison (combining the results obtained for antisera raised against two vaccine strains available in one of the current vaccine preparations) gave comparable results; 72 % of the field isolates were neutralized by antibodies raised against strains G1 or 431, whereas antibodies raised against either strain 255 or F9 neutralized 34 or 15 %, respectively [14]. The use of dual vaccine strains has also been shown to be more effective in the protection against the virulent systemic (VS-) FCV strains [19], although the vaccine strains were not comparable to those used in the present study. Furthermore, there was no suggestion of VS-FCV strains being included among the field isolates used here (Additional file 1).

There is an ongoing discussion that FCV isolated from cats displaying clinical signs of chronic FCV infection are more often vaccine resistant [20, 21], and thus not as often neutralized by anti-sera raised against vaccine

Table 2 Virus neutralization tests interpreted by combining data from antisera raised against vaccine strains as currently presented in registered vaccine preparations

G1 and 431					255			F9		
G1 and 431 always neg.	G1 and 431 possibly neg.	G1 neg. or possibly neg. and 431 always pos.	G1 always pos. and 431 neg. or possibly neg.	G1 and 431 always pos.	Always neg.	Possibly neg.	Always pos.	Always neg.	Possibly neg.	Always pos.
2	19	34	4	19	25	19	34	61	9	8
3 %	24 %	44 %	5 %	24 %	32 %	24 %	44 %	78 %	12 %	10 %

Feline calicivirus (FCV) vaccines registered and used in Sweden either contain F9 or 255 only, or a combination of G1 and 431 vaccine strains. The cutoff for a positive neutralizing titer was set to ≥5. The result "possibly negative" indicates that one of the paired neutralizing sera was negative, while the other gave a positive (≥ 5) neutralization titer strains. Since this study was designed to investigate the capacity of different vaccine strains to neutralize field isolates from Swedish cats, it is not possible to draw any conclusions about the relation between clinical signs and virus neutralization based on the clinical information stated by the veterinary clinicians at submission of samples.

Conclusions

This study confirms previous observations that antibodies raised against more recently introduced vaccine FCV strains, or vaccine strains used less widely, cross neutralize a higher proportion of circulating field isolates than antibodies raised against strains that have been used in vaccines extensively for a long time. Moreover, we demonstrated higher cross-neutralization of field isolates when considering neutralization data for all of the antisera raised against two strains included in a dual FCV vaccine, compared to the neutralization observed by the antisera raised against single vaccine strains. Vaccine strains should ideally be selected based on updated knowledge on the antigenic properties of field isolates in the local setting, and there is thus a need to continuously study the evolution of FCV and the neutralizing capacity of vaccine strain-induced antibodies against field isolates at a national and/or regional level.

Additional files

Additional file 1: Clinical information about cats from which FCV was isolated. The table provides clinical information about the cats from which the field isolates originate, including year of isolation, breed, age, and clinical signs as stated on the referal form. DSH = domestic shorthair, ESH = European shorthair, y = years, m = months, w = weeks, - denotes information not available.

Additional file 2: Virus neutralization data. The Excel file lists the titers obtained in neutralization tests using vaccine strain induced anti-sera against the field isolates. Field isolates 64–78 were tested in parallel with the previously used batch of anti-sera (indicated S1§ and S2§) [14], and the new batch of anti-sera, with similar results.

Authors' contributions

JJW analysed and interpreted the data, and drafted the manuscript. AS performed the virus neutralization tests, analysed the data and helped to draft the manuscript. AL performed virus isolation, collected and compiled clinical data, and helped to draft the manuscript. JCT conceived and designed the study, analysed and interpreted the data, and helped to draft the manuscript. LTB participated in conceiving and designing the study, performed virus isolation, and helped to draft the manuscript. MJH conceived and designed the study, analysed and interpreted the data, and helped to draft the manuscript. All authors read and approved the final manuscript.

Author details

[1] Department of Clinical Sciences, Swedish University of Agricultural Sciences, Uppsala, Sweden. [2] MRC-University of Glasgow Centre for Virus Research, Glasgow, UK. [3] Department of Virology, Immune Biology and Parasitology, National Veterinary Institute, Uppsala, Sweden. [4] Global Technical Services, Merial, Lyon, France.

Acknowledgements

Samples were collected and selected by National Veterinary Institute (Uppsala, Sweden; SVA) independently and the serological testing was funded by Merial.

Competing interests

JCT is an employee of Merial. All of the authors had access to all of the data generated and contributed to the analyses and interpretation.

References

1. Sykes JE. Pediatric feline upper respiratory disease. Vet Clin Am Small Anim Pract. 2014;44:331–42.
2. Pedersen NC, Elliott JB, Glasgow A, Poland A, Keel K. An isolated epizootic of hemorrhagic-like fever in cats caused by a novel and highly virulent strain of feline calicivirus. Vet Microbiol. 2000;73:281–300.
3. Coyne KP, Jones BR, Kipar A, Chantrey J, Porter CJ, Barber PJ, et al. Lethal outbreak of disease associated with feline calicivirus infection in cats. Vet Rec. 2006;158:544–50.
4. Coyne KP, Edwards D, Radford AD, Cripps P, Jones D, Wood JL, et al. Longitudinal molecular epidemiological analysis of feline calicivirus infection in an animal shelter: a model for investigating calicivirus transmission within high-density, high-turnover populations. J Clin Microbiol. 2007;45:3239–44.
5. Coyne KP, Christley RM, Pybus OG, Dawson S, Gaskell RM, Radford AD. Large-scale spatial and temporal genetic diversity of feline calicivirus. J Virol. 2012;86:11356–67.
6. Radford AD, Dawson S, Ryvar R, Coyne K, Johnson DR, Cox MB, et al. High genetic diversity of the immunodominant region of the feline calicivirus capsid gene in endemically infected cat colonies. Virus Genes. 2003;27:145–55.
7. Radford AD, Coyne KP, Dawson S, Porter CJ, Gaskell RM. Feline calicivirus. Vet Res. 2007;38:319–35.
8. Polak KC, Levy JK, Crawford PC, Leutenegger CM, Moriello KA. Infectious diseases in large-scale cat hoarding investigations. Vet J. 2014;201:189–95.
9. Hellard E, Fouchet D, Santin-Janin H, Tarin B, Badol V, Coupier C, et al. When cats' ways of life interact with their viruses: a study in 15 natural populations of owned and unowned cats (Felis silvestris catus). Prev Vet Med. 2011;101:250–64.
10. Holst BS, Berndtsson LT, Englund L. Isolation of feline herpesvirus-1 and feline calicivirus from healthy cats in Swedish breeding catteries. J Feline Med Surg. 2005;7:325–31.
11. Lauritzen A, Jarrett O, Sabara M. Serological analysis of feline calicivirus isolates from the United States and United Kingdom. Vet Microbiol. 1997;56:55–63.
12. Radford AD, Bennett M, McArdle F, Dawson S, Turner PC, Glenn MA, et al. The use of sequence analysis of a feline calicivirus (FCV) hypervariable region in the epidemiological investigation of FCV related disease and vaccine failures. Vaccine. 1997;15:1451–8.
13. Radford AD, Dawson S, Coyne KP, Porter CJ, Gaskell RM. The challenge for the next generation of feline calicivirus vaccines. Vet Microbiol. 2006;117:14–8.
14. Addie D, Poulet H, Golder MC, McDonald M, Brunet S, Thibault JC, et al. Ability of antibodies to two new caliciviral vaccine strains to neutralise feline calicivirus isolates from the UK. Vet Rec. 2008;163:355–7.
15. Jarrett O, Laird HM, Hay D. Determinants of the host range of feline leukaemia viruses. J Gen Virol. 1973;20:169–75.
16. Poulet H, Jas D, Lemeter C, Coupier C, Brunet S. Efficacy of a bivalent inactivated non-adjuvanted feline calicivirus vaccine: relation between in vitro cross-neutralization and heterologous protection in vivo. Vaccine. 2008;26:3647–54.
17. Rinaldo D, Foti M, Bottari T, Fisichella V, Buonavoglia D. Feline calicivirus strains isolated in Italy. Pol J Vet Sci. 2008;11:359–61.
18. Radford AD, Turner PC, Bennett M, McArdle F, Dawson S, Glenn MA, et al. Quasispecies evolution of a hypervariable region of the feline calicivirus capsid gene in cell culture and in persistently infected cats. J Gen Virol. 1998;79:1–10.

Toxoplasma gondii seroprevalence in breeding pigs in Estonia

Azzurra Santoro[1†], Maarja Tagel[2*†], Kärt Must[2], Miia Laine[2], Brian Lassen[2,3] and Pikka Jokelainen[2,4,5]

Abstract

Background: *Toxoplasma gondii* is a widespread occurring parasite infecting warm-blooded animals, including pigs and humans. The aims of this study were to estimate the prevalence of anti-*T. gondii* antibodies and to evaluate risk factors for *T. gondii* seropositivity in breeding pigs raised in Estonia. Sera from 382 pigs were tested with a commercial direct agglutination test, using a cut-off titer of 40 for seropositivity, for the presence of anti-*T. gondii* immunoglobulin G antibodies.

Results: Twenty-two (5.8%) of the 382 pigs tested seropositive for *T. gondii*, and 6 of the 14 herds had at least one seropositive pig. The proportion of seropositive pigs within the herds ranged between 0 and 43%. Gender appeared as a significant factor, with sows having 5.6 times higher odds to be seropositive to *T. gondii* than boars. Seroprevalence did not increase with age.

Conclusions: Anti-*T. gondii* antibodies were present in a substantial proportion of breeding pig herds in Estonia. On the other hand, the presence of herds without seropositive pigs illustrates that porcine *T. gondii* infections can be avoided even in a country where the parasite is endemic and common in several other host species.

Keywords: Breeding herd, Epidemiology, Porcine, Serology, *Sus scrofa domesticus*, Swine, Toxoplasmosis, Zoonosis

Background

Toxoplasma gondii is a protozoan parasite with worldwide distribution. Recently, the Food and Agriculture Organization (FAO) and the World Health Organization (WHO) ranked it 4th among foodborne parasites causing the greatest global concern [1].

All warm-blooded animals, including humans and pigs, can host *T. gondii*. Both humans and pigs, being omnivores, can acquire the infection via ingestion of tissues of other hosts that carry the parasite, via ingestion of oocysts from a contaminated environment, or congenitally [2]. Infections with *T. gondii* can be subclinical, but toxoplasmosis can have severe consequences for both human and porcine health [3–5].

Pork is considered a major source of human *T. gondii* infections in Europe and the USA [2, 6]. Viable *T. gondii* parasites have been isolated from unprocessed tissues of infected pigs as well as from commercial cuts such as ham, bacon, and pork tenderloin [7, 8]. Possible sources of naturally-acquired porcine *T. gondii* infections have been investigated in studies evaluating different risk factors for porcine *T. gondii* infection [2, 4]. Some investigated risk factors, such as the age of the pigs and herd size, do not provide us with useful clues regarding the sources of infection, whereas others do. For example, the access of seropositive juvenile cats to areas where sows were housed [9], direct access of cats to pig feed [10], and a high density of cats at the farm [11] have been shown to be positively associated with *T. gondii* seropositivity in pigs, suggesting oocyst contamination of pig feed and the farm environment as possible sources of the infection. Inadequate rodent control has also been associated with *T. gondii* seropositivity in pigs, suggesting infected rodents as a possible source of *T. gondii* infection for pigs [12].

Toxoplasma gondii infection has been reported in humans and pigs worldwide [2, 4]. The European

*Correspondence: maarja.tagel@emu.ee
†Azzurra Santoro and Maarja Tagel contributed equally to this work
[2] Institute of Veterinary Medicine and Animal Sciences, Estonian University of Life Sciences, Kreutzwaldi 62, 51014 Tartu, Estonia
Full list of author information is available at the end of the article

Food Safety Authority (EFSA) has listed toxoplasmosis among the diseases to be reported by European Union (EU) member states according to their epidemiological situation and emphasized the lack of representative data for *T. gondii* in humans, animals, and food [13]. Moreover, EFSA has included *T. gondii* among the most relevant biological hazards in the context of meat inspection of swine and has pointed out that the current meat inspection is unable to detect the parasite [14].

In Estonia, a recent nationwide study estimated that *T. gondii* seroprevalence was 55.8% in the human population in general, and 74.4% in a separate group of animal caretakers [15]. Further epidemiological data from other host species, including domestic cats [16], cattle [17], and wild boars [18], indicate that *T. gondii* is endemic also in these populations, and present also in the environment. Based on a EU report from 2013, none of 20 pigs tested from Estonia were *T. gondii* seropositive [19]. While the consumption of pork has increased from 26.8 kg per person in 2002 to 44.2 kg per person in 2016 [20], there have been no studies with larger sample size on prevalence of subclinical *T. gondii* infection in domestic pigs in Estonia. Moreover, there are no reports of clinical porcine toxoplasmosis from Estonia.

The aims of our cross-sectional seroepidemiological study were to estimate *T. gondii* seroprevalence and to evaluate potential risk factors for *T. gondii* seropositivity in breeding pigs in Estonia. More specifically, we estimated the animal-level prevalence of anti-*T. gondii* immunoglobulin G (IgG) antibodies and evaluated both animal-level and farm-level risk factors for animal-level *T. gondii* seropositivity.

Methods

Study population and study design

The samples investigated were originally collected for national surveillance of other infectious diseases. The surplus of them were used in two other studies [21, 22] in addition to our study. Serology was performed blinded, and the data were coded and treated confidentially.

At the end of 2011, there were 365,700 pigs in Estonia [23]. This included 30 breeding herds with 15,337 animals, including boars used for insemination [24].

In this cross-sectional seroepidemiological study, we analyzed blood samples from breeding pigs in Estonia for evidence of naturally acquired *T. gondii* infections. The sample was a convenience sample.

Samples

The samples available for our study were sera from 382 domestic pigs from 14 breeding herds located in seven of the 15 counties in Estonia (Fig. 1). Information was not available for how the herds had been selected, but random sampling had been used at the animal-level. The number of pigs that had been sampled per herd was 5–52. The blood samples had been collected in 2012 by veterinarians of the Estonian Veterinary and Food Board. The samples had been collected on the farms, from the jugular vein of live pigs, into vacuum tubes without reagents. The sera had been separated by centrifugation and were stored at − 20 °C until analysis.

The sample size of 382 domestic pigs was evaluated to be sufficient for estimating the animal-level seroprevalence using the Epi Tools software calculator [25], with an expected seroprevalence range of 3.2–4.2% [26, 27], confidence level of 95%, and population size of 15,337 [24]. Ignoring clustering, the minimum required sample size would have been 48–62 samples. Clustering was expected, thus we did not settle for the minimum required sample size and included all the 382 samples that were available.

Background information

Background information for each pig was extracted from the registers of the Estonian Livestock Performance Recording Ltd and included gender, breed, and age in days and in years. Gender was unknown for 58 pigs, breed for 87 pigs, and age for 71 pigs. For each farm, we had information about herd size and farm location.

The sample consisted of breeding sows (66%) and boars (34%) (Table 1). Pigs that were crossbred Estonian Landrace breed and Estonian Large White breed were most common (36%), followed by pure Estonian Landrace breed (33%) and pure Estonian Large White breed (18%) (Table 1). The age of the pigs ranged from 178 to 2742 days (mean 726 days, median 651 days); that is, from 6 months to 7 years (mean 1.99 years, median 1.78 years). The herd size range was 58–11,295 (mean 3786, median 2366) pigs. Seven of the farms were located in the northern part of the country and seven of the farms were located in the southern part of the country (Fig. 1; divided as in [18]).

Serology

The serum samples were tested for the presence of specific IgG antibodies against *T. gondii* using a commercial direct agglutination test (Toxo-Screen DA, bioMérieux, Marcy-l'Étoile, France), according to the manufacturer's instructions. In this method, possible immunoglobulin M antibodies are denatured by 2-mercaptoethanol.

The dilution of the samples was 1:40 and pigs testing positive were defined as seropositive; that is, the cut-off for seropositivity was titer of 40 [18]. Only samples yielding clear positive results (an agglutination yielding a mat that covered at least half of the bottom of the well) were interpreted as positive, whereas borderline reactions

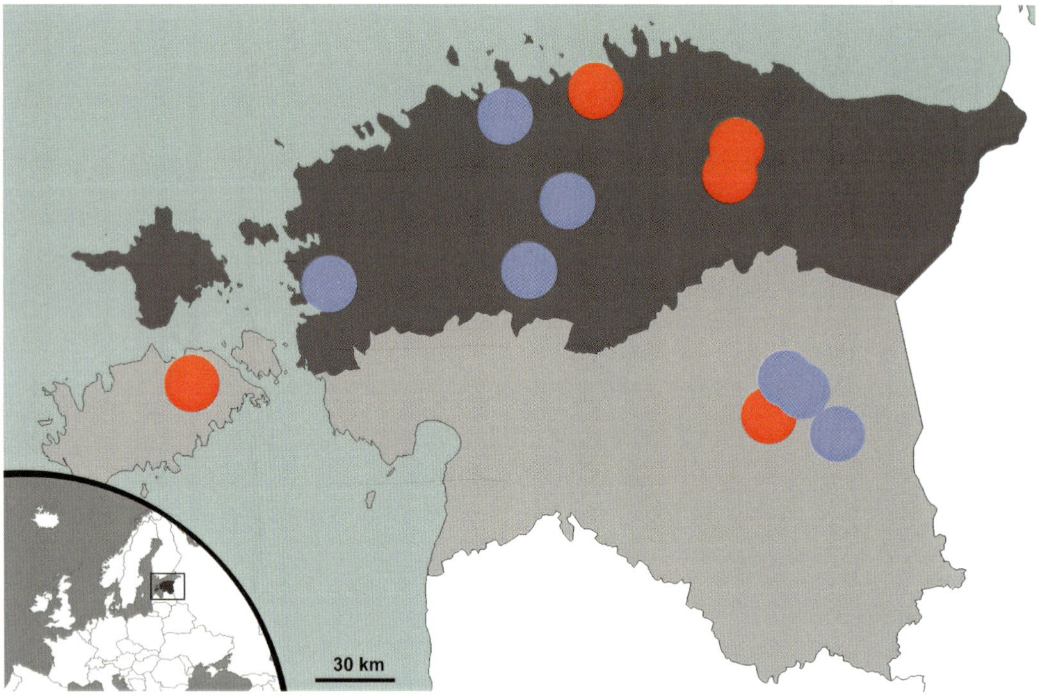

Fig. 1 A map of Estonia showing the geographical location of the farms included in this study. From each herd, 5–52 breeding pigs were tested for specific antibodies against *Toxoplasma gondii*. The herds with at least one *T. gondii* seropositive pig are marked with red dots and the herds with no *T. gondii* seropositive breeding pigs are marked with blue dots. The northern counties are shown with dark grey color, and the southern counties are shown with light grey color. The exact location of one herd with at least one *T. gondii* seropositive breeding pig and one herd with no *T. gondii* seropositive breeding pigs, both located in the southern part of the country, were unknown

were interpreted as negative. All plates contained the positive and negative controls provided in the kits, in two dilutions (1:40 and 1:4000), and an antigen control, as instructed by the manufacturer. The antigen control, consisting of all the reagents of the kit (i.e. no serum), confirmed that autoagglutination did not occur.

Statistical analyses

We estimated the seroprevalence (not adjusted, i.e. apparent seroprevalence) at animal-level and also report the proportion of herds that had at least one seropositive pig and the range of proportion of seropositive pigs within each herd. OpenEpi was used to calculate confidence intervals (CI, Mid-P exact) and to evaluate the differences using two by two Tables (2-tailed *P* values, Mid-P exact) [28]. Logistic regression analyses using Stata software 13.1 (StataCorp, College Station, TX, USA) were used to evaluate the potential risk factors. P values < 0.05 were considered statistically significant.

In the risk factor analyses, the outcome was a dichotomous animal-level outcome: each pig was either seronegative or seropositive. We evaluated five potential risk factors for seropositivity. The animal-level variables we evaluated were gender, breed and age. Breed was evaluated as a dichotomized variable: one group consisted of purebred Estonian Landrace pigs and crossbred Estonian Landrace pigs (Estonian Landrace breed crossed with Duroc, Estonian Large White, and Piétrain), while the other group consisted of pigs that had no Estonian Landrace breed in them (i.e. pigs that were purebred Piétrain, purebred Duroc, purebred Estonian Large White, or crosses of these three breeds). Age was evaluated in three ways: dichotomized as < 1 year vs. ≥ 1 year; as a continuous variable; and as different age categories based on the age distribution of the sample (dichotomized at 2 years, dichotomized at 3 years, categorized by every 3 months, categorized by every 6 months, categorized by every 12 months, categorized at quartiles, categorized at median, categorized at mean). The farm-level variables we evaluated were herd size (dichotomized: < 2000 vs. ≥ 2000 pigs) and location of the farm (dichotomized: the northern part of the country vs. the southern part of the country, as in [18]).

First, univariable logistic regression models were used to evaluate each potential risk factor separately. Multivariable logistic regression model building was then attempted by including all the variables, followed by backward elimination of those with *P* value ≥ 0.05 that

Table 1 Animal-level *Toxoplasma gondii* seroprevalence in breeding pigs in Estonia

	No. of pigs	No. of seropositive pigs	Seroprevalence (95% CI)
Gender[a]			
Sow	213	20	9.4** (6.0–13.9)
Boar	111	2	1.8** (0.3–5.8)
Breed[a]			
Landrace/Large White	106	8	7.5 (3.6–13.8)
Landrace	98	10	10.2* (5.3–17.4)
Large White	53	2	3.8 (0.6–11.9)
Other[b]	38	0	0.0* (0.0–7.6)
Age (year)[a]			
< 1	72	2	2.8 (0.5–8.9)
≥ 1	239	19	7.9 (5.0–11.9)
Herd size			
< 2000 pigs	170	6	3.5 (1.4–7.2)
≥ 2000 pigs	212	16	7.5 (4.5–11.7)
Location of the farm			
Northern part of the country	150	10	6.7 (3.4–11.6)
Southern part of the country	232	12	5.2 (2.8–8.6)
Total	382	22	5.8 (3.7–8.5)

CI confidence interval, Mid-P exact

* Significantly different seroprevalence (P < 0.05)

** Significantly different seroprevalence (P < 0.01)

[a] Some information unknown for some animals

[b] The other breeds were pure Piétrain, pure Duroc, Duroc/Landrace, Piétrain/Duroc, Piétrain/Landrace, and Piétrain/Landrace/Large White

did not act as confounders. We used > 20% change in the odds ratio as an indication of confounding. To account for clustering, the variable 'farm' was tried as a random factor in all the models.

Results

Seroprevalence

The overall *T. gondii* seroprevalence estimate in breeding pigs in Estonia was 5.8% (95% CI 3.7–8.5); 22 of 382 animals tested positive for anti-*T. gondii* IgG antibodies (Table 1). This estimate was not statistically significantly different from the earlier result of 20 pigs testing seronegative [19]. Six of the 14 herds (42.9%, 95% CI 19.6–68.9) had at least one seropositive pig. The proportion of seropositive pigs of pigs tested within each herd ranged between 0.00 and 42.9%, being ≥ 25% in two of the herds.

Risk factors

Toxoplasma gondii seroprevalence was significantly higher (P < 0.01) in sows than in boars (Table 1), and based on the univariable logistic regression model (without a random factor), sows had 5.65 (95% CI 1.3–24.6) times higher odds to test seropositive than boars. The seroprevalence was highest in the purebred Estonian Landrace pigs (Table 1). The two herds with ≥ 25% seropositive pigs of the pigs tested both included exclusively purebred or crossbred Estonian Landrace pigs. Age was not a significant factor in univariable analyses, neither as a dichotomized variable, as a continuous variable, nor as different age categories, and a histogram (Fig. 2) showed no obvious pattern for the seroprevalence by age. Seroprevalence in pigs from larger herds (≥ 2000

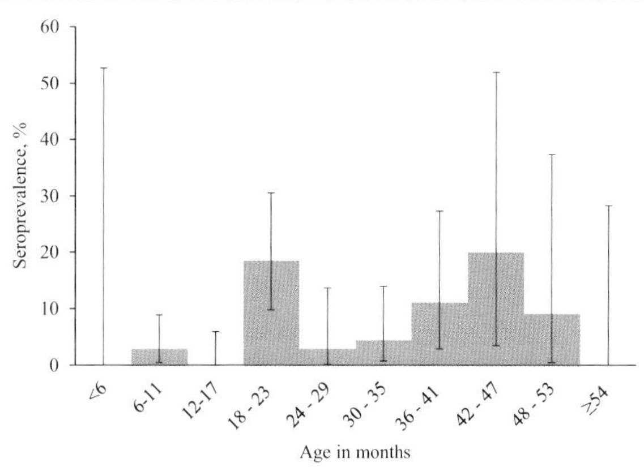

Fig. 2 *Toxoplasma gondii* seroprevalence in breeding pigs in Estonia, by age in months

pigs) did not differ significantly from the seroprevalence in pigs from smaller herds (< 2000 pigs) (Table 1). Three of the herds that had at least one seropositive pig were located in the northern part of the country and three were located in the southern part of the country (Fig. 1). None of the plausible risk factors were significant variables when tried in a multivariable model nor when 'farm' was included as a random factor in the models.

Discussion

In Europe, reports available show that animal-level *T. gondii* seroprevalence in domestic pigs ranges in the investigated regions from 0.4 to 64.4% [2, 29]; while looking at reports from northern European countries specifically, the range is from 3.2% in finishing pigs in Finland [26] to 33.7% in indoor sows in Denmark [30]. Seroprevalence estimates similar to the estimate obtained in breeding pigs in our study (5.8%) have been reported in pigs from Latvia (4.2%) [27] and Sweden (calculated from the numbers reported: 5.7%) [31].

It is important to note that, the estimates of *T. gondii* seroprevalence obtained in different studies are not directly comparable due to different study designs and methodology. The serology method used in our study to detect anti-*T. gondii* antibodies in breeding pigs is widely used [4, 32]. The seroprevalence in breeding pigs from Estonia did not differ significantly from estimates obtained using the same method and cut-off titer in pigs from Austria (6.5%) [33] and Portugal (7.1%) [34], but was significantly lower than *T. gondii* seroprevalence estimates obtained using the same method and cut-off in pigs from Canada (9.4%) [35] and Poland (26.4%) [36]. In Spain, *T. gondii* seroprevalence in pigs was 19.0% using 25 as the cut-off titer, while 5.8% tested positive when the cut-off titer was 50 (calculated from numbers reported) [37], which was similar to the seroprevalence estimate in breeding pigs in our study, obtained with 40 as the cut-off titer. Our study included pigs from breeding herds, whereas several of the other studies investigated samples collected from finisher pigs (i.e. pigs in the late stage of rearing, i.e. > 70 kg live weight). In Germany, the animal-level ELISA-based *T. gondii* seroprevalence estimate in breeding pigs was 18.5% [38], statistically significantly higher than our estimate from Estonia, while the proportion of herds with at least one seropositive animal, 69.1% [38], did not differ statistically from our result from Estonia.

Toxoplasma gondii seroprevalence differed significantly by gender, and sows had higher odds of testing seropositive than boars (univariable analysis). Possible explanations for this include differences in keeping sows and boars. For example, boars may be more likely kept in single pens and they may get different feed. If there are cats on the farm, they might be discouraged to approach the boars, and thus the immediate environment of the boars might be less likely to be contaminated with feline feces.

Some studies have shown an increase in *T. gondii* seroprevalence in pigs with age [39, 40], whereas others have not [41, 42]. No increase in *T. gondii* seroprevalence with age was observed in our study, despite the fact that we were able to evaluate a wide age range. Instead, we observed clustering of seropositive animals in specific age-groups (Fig. 2) and herds. A possible explanation for this observation could be focal feed- or waterborne outbreaks in the herds: a group of pigs of the same age on a farm were likely housed and fed together, and could have been given feed or water contaminated with infective *T. gondii*. Data on previous serostatus, direct detection of the parasites in feed or water, or genotyping the parasites could have confirmed the possible outbreaks.

Despite apparent differences in seroprevalence by pig breed (Table 1), being of the local Estonian Landrace breed did not appear as a risk factor for *T. gondii* seropositivity in further analyses. No statistical indication of herd size being associated with seropositivity was found, and no geographical pattern was evident. The latter result is in line with the quite even geographical distribution of seropositive wild boars in Estonia [18].

It should be noted that we used a single dilution of the samples and the titers were not evaluated. In addition, our cut-off titer for seropositivity of 40 can be considered high. Consequently, any pigs with low titers or recent infections (i.e. prior to antibody production), as well as undetected prozone phenomena (i.e. in case of too high antibody concentration for the test, few antibodies bind to more than one antigen and thus an agglutination mat is not formed, and a false negative result is seen), could contribute to an underestimation of the actual prevalence.

A concordance between *T. gondii* seropositivity and the presence of *T. gondii* in the tissues of pigs has been reported [43]. However, while serological screening is considered suitable for identifying high risk pig herds or individual pigs, serology is an indirect method and a negative result is not a guarantee of an uninfected pig or *T. gondii*-safe meat [43, 44]. All edible parts of a pig infected with *T. gondii* should be considered infectious since little variation in parasite load has been found between different skeletal muscles [44]. In Estonia, the amount of pork eaten per person has increased from 33.7 kg in 2012 to 41.8 kg in 2015 [20]. One single pig is estimated to be consumed by 300–400 people [45], thus even a low *T. gondii* prevalence must be considered an indication of food safety risk. However, meat from breeding pigs is generally processed in ways capable of inactivating viable stages of *T. gondii* [4]. Based on this, it has been suggested that meat from infected breeding pigs would be a minor source of infection in comparison with meat from infected finisher pigs [46]. A source attribution study could evaluate whether these assumptions are also true in Estonia.

Eating raw or undercooked meat of infected animals and eating food cross-contaminated with meat from infected animals are potential food safety risks not only for humans, but also for other host species, including cats. Our recent studies from Estonia and Finland revealed that a considerable proportion of domestic cats receive raw meat [16, 47, 48].

Both *T. gondii* and another tissue-dwelling zoonotic parasite group *Trichinella* spp. are endemic and common in Estonia in several of their host species; for example, the *T. gondii* seroprevalence was 24.0%, and the *Trichinella* seroprevalence was 42.1% in free-ranging wild boars [18, 22]. The *T. gondii* seroprevalence estimate in free-ranging wild boars [18] was obtained using the same serology method and cut-off that we used in this study, and it was significantly higher than our seroprevalence estimate in domestic pigs (24.0% vs. 5.8%; $P < 0.01$). This difference could be interpreted to exemplify the partial effectiveness of protecting Suidae from *T. gondii* by keeping pigs on farms, compared with free-ranging. Furthermore, *T. gondii* seropositive pigs could be seen as an indicator of unsuccessful biosafety measures on the farms—they have ingested tissues of infected animals or something contaminated with feces of infected felids that shed oocysts. Unfortunately, we did not have detailed information on the management and biosafety measures applied on the farms included in this study. Nevertheless, it should be noted that 374 of the pigs included in this study, including the 22 *T. gondii* seropositive pigs, were tested for antibodies against *Trichinella* spp. in our other study [22], and all tested negative. As the infection pressure of both parasites is high in Estonia, these results suggest that biosafety measures sufficient to stop *Trichinella* spp. infections are insufficient against *T. gondii*. *Trichinella* spp. infection can be acquired by carnivorism only, and the biosafety measures against *Trichinella* spp. infections target that. *Toxoplasma gondii* infection can be acquired by carnivorism or from oocysts, and thus biosafety measures targeting carnivorism only are insufficient. The EU-regulation on official control for *Trichinella* spp. infections in pigs focuses on carnivorism: the requirements for a farm to be recognized as applying controlled housing conditions include preventing mammals and carnivorous birds from having access to the buildings where pigs are kept, not allowing pigs access outdoors without specific risk analysis, and storing feed in closed containers that are impenetrable to rodents [49]. A previous national legal document on preventing *Trichinella* spp. infections in pigs listed e.g. regular rodent control, destroying of dead animals, and heat-treatment of animal-derived feed, while avoiding cats on the farms was also specifically mentioned [50]. While these measures that are targeted against *Trichinella* spp. infections can be expected to also have effect against *T. gondii*, they are not sufficient to avoid *T. gondii* infections: the prevention of oocyst-contamination, in particular of feed and water, has not been emphasized. A targeted *Toxoplasma*-control in domestic pigs would protect humans and other hosts that eat pork [2, 6], and porcine health and welfare [4].

Conclusions

Our results provide evidence that *T. gondii* infection was present in Estonian breeding pig herds, while being of the local Estonian Landrace breed did not appear to be a risk factor for *T. gondii* seropositivity. Sows had higher odds to test seropositive than boars, which could be due to their different management. The clustering of seropositive pigs in specific age groups and herds could be indicative of point sources of infection that were shared by the groups of pigs in the herds.

Authors' contributions

PJ and BL presented the idea and designed the study. ML performed the serology. AS, MT, KM and PJ analyzed the data and drafted the manuscript. All authors participated in the writing. All authors read and approved the final manuscript.

Author details

[1] Department of Veterinary Medicine, University of Perugia, Via San Costanzo 4, 06126 Perugia, Italy. [2] Institute of Veterinary Medicine and Animal Sciences, Estonian University of Life Sciences, Kreutzwaldi 62, 51014 Tartu, Estonia. [3] Department of Veterinary Disease Biology, Faculty of Health and Medical Sciences, University of Copenhagen, Grønnegårdsvej 15, 1870 Frederiksberg C, Denmark. [4] Faculty of Veterinary Medicine, University of Helsinki, P.O. Box 66, 00014 Helsinki, Finland. [5] Statens Serum Institut, Artillerivej 5, 2300 Copenhagen S, Denmark.

Acknowledgements

We thank the Veterinary and Food Board, Estonian Livestock Performance Recording Ltd, the veterinarians who collected the samples, and Diivi Põdersoo for their contributions to our study. We thank Lisa Thurston for providing language editing suggestions for the manuscript.

Competing interests

The authors declare that they have no competing interests.

Funding

Our study was supported financially by the Estonian Research Council health promotion research program TerVe 3.2.1002.11–0002 EKZE_SS and by Base Funding of Estonian University of Life Sciences 8P160014VLVP.

References

1. Food and Agriculture Organization (FAO) and World Health Organization (WHO). Multicriteria-based ranking for risk management of food-borne parasites. Microbiol Risk Assess. 2014;23:16.
2. Dubey JP. Toxoplasmosis of animals and humans. 2nd ed. Boca Raton: CRC Press; 2010.
3. Montoya JG, Liesenfeld O. Toxoplasmosis. Lancet. 2004;363:1965–76.
4. Dubey JP. Toxoplasmosis in pigs—the last 20 years. Vet Parasitol. 2009;164:89–103.
5. Kim JH, Kang KI, Kang WC, Sohn HJ, Jean YH, Park BK, Kim Y, Kim DY. Porcine abortion outbreak associated with *Toxoplasma gondii* in Jeju Island, Korea. J Vet Sci. 2009;10:147–51.
6. Tenter AM, Heckeroth AR, Weiss LM. *Toxoplasma gondii*: from animals to humans. Int J Parasitol. 2000;30:1217–58.
7. Dubey JP, Murrell KD, Fayer R, Schad GA. Distribution of *Toxoplasma gondii* tissue cysts in commercial cuts of pork. J Am Vet Med Assoc. 1986;188:1035–7.
8. Tsutsui VS, Freire RL, Garcia JL, Gennari SM, Vieira DP, Marana ERM, et al. Detection of *Toxoplasma gondii* by PCR and mouse bioassay in commercial cuts of pork from experimentally infected pigs. Arq Bras Med Vet Zootec. 2007;59:30–4.
9. Weigel RM, Dubey JP, Siegel AM, Kitron UD, Mannelli A, Mitchell MA, et al. Risk factors for transmission of *Toxoplasma gondii* on swine farms in Illinois. J Parasitol. 1995;81:736–41.
10. Limon G, Beauvais W, Dadios N, Villena I, Cockle C, Blaga R, Guitian J. Cross-sectional study of *Toxoplasma gondii* infection in pig farms in England. Foodborne Pathog Dis. 2017;14:269–81.
11. Ortega-Pacheco A, Acosta-Viana KY, Guzman-Marin E, Uitzil-Álvarez B, Rodríguez-Buenfil JC, Jimenez-Coello M. Infection dynamic of *Toxoplasma gondii* in two fattening pig farms exposed to high and low cat density in an endemic region. Vet Parasitol. 2011;175:367–71.
12. Kijlstra A, Meerburg B, Cornelissen J, De Craeye S, Vereijken P, Jongert E. The role of rodents and shrews in the transmission of *Toxoplasma gondii* to pigs. Vet Parasitol. 2008;156:183–90.
13. EFSA, European Food Safety Authority. Surveillance and monitoring of *Toxoplasma* in humans, food and animals. Scientific opinion of the panel on biological hazards. EFSA J. 2007;583:1–64.
14. EFSA, European Food Safety Authority. Scientific opinion on the public health hazards to be covered by inspection of meat (swine). EFSA J. 2011;9:2351.
15. Lassen B, Janson M, Viltrop A, Neare K, Hütt P, Golovljova I, et al. Serological evidence of exposure to globally relevant zoonotic parasites in the Estonian population. PLoS ONE. 2016;11:e0164142.
16. Must K, Lassen B, Jokelainen P. Seroprevalence of and risk factors for *Toxoplasma gondii* infection in cats in Estonia. Vector Borne Zoonotic Dis. 2015;15:597–601.
17. Jokelainen P, Tagel M, Mõtus K, Viltrop A, Lassen B. *Toxoplasma gondii* seroprevalence in dairy and beef cattle: large-scale epidemiological study in Estonia. Vet Parasitol. 2017;236:137–43.
18. Jokelainen P, Velström K, Lassen B. Seroprevalence of *Toxoplasma gondii* in free-ranging wild boars hunted for human consumption in Estonia. Acta Vet Scand. 2015;57:42.
19. EFSA, European Food Safety Authority. The European Union summary report on trends and sources of zoonoses, zoonotic agents and food-borne outbreaks in 2013. EFSA J. 2015;13:3991.
20. Statistics Estonia. AG42: supply balance for meat. http://pub.stat.ee/. Accessed 27 Nov 2017.
21. Ivanova A, Tefanova V, Reshetnjak I, Kuznetsova T, Geller J, Lundkvist Å, et al. Hepatitis E virus in domestic pigs, wild boars, pig farm workers, and hunters in Estonia. Food Environ Virol. 2015;7:403–12.
22. Kärssin A, Velström K, Gómez-Morales MA, Saar T, Jokelainen P, Lassen B. Cross-sectional study of anti-*Trichinella* antibody prevalence in domestic pigs and hunted wild boars in Estonia. Vector Borne Zoonotic Dis. 2016;16:604–10.
23. Statistics Estonia. AG170: livestock and poultry by county (quarters). http://pub.stat.ee/. Accessed 27 Nov 2017.
24. Estonian Livestock Performance Recording Ltd. 60. No. of pigs of different breeds in counties. https://www.jkkeskus.ee/assets/tekstid/aastaraamatud/aastaraamat_2012.pdf. Accessed 27 Nov 2017.
25. Sergeant, ESG. Epitools epidemiological calculators. Ausvet Pty Ltd; 2017. http://epitools.ausvet.com.au/. Accessed 27 Nov 2017.
26. Felin E, Jukola E, Raulo S, Fredriksson-Ahomaa M. Meat juice serology and improved food chain information as control tools for pork-related public health hazards. Zoonoses Public Health. 2015;62:456–64.
27. Deksne G, Kirjušina M. Seroprevalence of *Toxoplasma gondii* in domestic pigs (*Sus scrofa domestica*) and wild boars (*Sus scrofa*) in Latvia. J Parasitol. 2013;99:44–7.
28. Dean AG, Sullivan KM, Soe MM. OpenEpi: Open source epidemiologic statistics for public health. http://www.openepi.com/. Accessed 27 Nov 2017.
29. Bártová E, Sedlák K. Seroprevalence of *Toxoplasma gondii* and *Neospora caninum* in slaughtered pigs in the Czech Republic. Parasitology. 2011;138:1369–71.
30. Grønbech Kofoed K, Vorslund-Kiær M, Nielsen HV, Alban L, Johansen MV. Sero-prevalence of *Toxoplasma gondii* in Danish pigs. Vet Parasitol Reg Stud Rep. 2017;10:136–8.
31. Wallander C, Frössling J, Dórea FC, Uggla A, Vågsholm I, Lundén A. Pasture is a risk factor for *Toxoplasma gondii* infection in fattening pigs. Vet Parasitol. 2016;224:27–32.
32. Dubey JP. Validation of the specificity of the modified agglutination test for toxoplasmosis in pigs. Vet Parasitol. 1997;71:307–10.
33. Steinparzer R, Reisp K, Grünberger B, Köfer J, Schmoll F, Sattler T. Comparison of different commercial serological tests for the detection of *Toxoplasma gondii* antibodies in serum of naturally exposed pigs. Zoonoses Public Health. 2015;62:119–24.
34. Esteves F, Aquiar D, Rosado J, Costa ML, de Sousa B, Antunes F, Matos O. *Toxoplasma gondii* prevalence in cats from Lisbon and in pigs from centre and south of Portugal. Vet Parasitol. 2014;200:8–12.
35. Smith HJ. Seroprevalence of anti-*Toxoplasma* IgG in Canadian swine. Can J Vet Res. 1991;55:380–1.
36. Sroka J, Cencek T, Ziomko I, Karamon J, Zwoliński J. Preliminary assessment of ELISA, MAT, and LAT for detecting *Toxoplasma gondii* antibodies in pigs. Bull Vet Inst Pulawy. 2008;52:545–9.
37. García-Bocanegra I, Dubey JP, Simon-Grifé M, Cabezón O, Casal J, Allepuz A, et al. Seroprevalence and risk factors associated with *Toxoplasma gondii* infection in pig farms from Catalonia, north-eastern Spain. Res Vet Sci. 2010;89:85–7.
38. Damriyasa IM, Bauer C, Edelhofer R, Failing K, Lind P, Petersen E, et al. Cross-sectional survey in pig breeding farms in Hesse, Germany: seroprevalence and risk factors of infections with *Toxoplasma gondii*, *Sarcocystis* spp. and *Neospora caninum* in sows. Vet Parasitol. 2004;126:271–86.
39. Lundén A, Lind P, Engvall EO, Gustavsson K, Uggla A, Vågsholm I. Serological survey of *Toxoplasma gondii* infection in pigs slaughtered in Sweden. Scand J Infect Dis. 2002;34:362–5.
40. Klun I, Vujanić M, Yera H, Nikolić A, Ivović V, Bobić B, et al. *Toxoplasma gondii* infection in slaughter pigs in Serbia: seroprevalence and demonstration of parasites in blood. Vet Res. 2011;42:17.
41. Lopes AP, Dubey JP, Neto F, Rodrigues A, Martins T, Rodrigues M, Cardoso L. Seroprevalence of *Toxoplasma gondii* infection in cattle, sheep, goats and pigs from the North of Portugal for human consumption. Vet Parasitol. 2013;193:266–9.
42. Djokic V, Fablet C, Blaga R, Rose N, Perret C, Djurkovic-Djakovic O, et al. Factors associated with *Toxoplasma gondii* infection in confined farrow-to-finish pig herds in western France: an exploratory study in 60 herds. Parasit Vectors. 2016;9:466.
43. Opsteegh M, Maas M, Schares G, van der Giessen J. Relationship between seroprevalence in the main livestock species and presence of *Toxoplasma gondii* in meat (GP/EFSA/BIOHAZ/2013/01) an extensive literature review. Final report. EFSA Support Publ. 2016;13(2):996E.
44. Opsteegh M, Schares G, Blaga R, van der Giessen J. Experimental studies on *Toxoplasma gondii* in the main livestock species (GP/EFSA/BIOHAZ/2013/01) Final report. EFSA Support Publ. 2016;13(2):995E.
45. Kijlstra A, Eissen OA, Cornelissen J, Munniksma K, Eijck I, Kortbeek T. *Toxoplasma gondii* infection in animal-friendly pig production systems. Investig Ophthalmol Vis Sci. 2004;45:3165–9.
46. Jones JL, Dubey JP. Foodborne toxoplasmosis. Clin Infect Dis. 2012;55:845–51.
47. Jokelainen P, Simola O, Rantanen E, Näreaho A, Lohi H, Sukura A. Feline toxoplasmosis in Finland: cross-sectional epidemiological study and case series study. J Vet Diagn Investig. 2012;24:1115–24.
48. Must K, Hytönen MK, Orro T, Lohi H, Jokelainen P. *Toxoplasma gondii* seroprevalence varies by cat breed. PLoS ONE. 2017;12(9):e0184659.

Preventive measures aimed at minimizing the risk of African swine fever virus spread in pig farming systems

Silvia Bellini[1*], Domenico Rutili[2] and Vittorio Guberti[3]

Abstract

African swine fever (ASF) is one of the most severe diseases of pigs; it has a drastic impact on the pig industry, causing serious socio-economic consequences to pig farmers and pork producers. In Europe, there are currently two main clusters of infection; one in Sardinia caused by strains of African swine fever virus (ASFV) belonging to genotype I and another in Eastern Europe caused by strains of ASFV belonging to genotype II. The latter is inducing an acute form of ASF and it represents a serious threat to the pig sector. ASF is a disease for which there is no effective vaccine; therefore, prevention has a pivotal role in the control strategy of the disease. This review describes the main preventive measures to adopt to mitigate the risk of ASF spread in pig farming systems.

Keywords: African swine fever, ASF, Domestic pigs, Wild boar, Wildlife, Epidemiology, Prevention, Bio-security

Background

African swine fever (ASF) is a contagious and fatal disease of pigs caused by African swine fever virus (ASFV) currently classified as the only member of the *Asfarviridae* family. ASF is one of the most serious diseases of pigs; it can severely affect and disrupt regional and international trade with animals and animal products with a serious socio-economic impact on pig farming. The disease is mainly transmitted by direct contact between infected and susceptible pigs or through the ingestion of ASFV contaminated pork products [1, 2]. Wild boar (*Sus scrofa*) and feral pigs in general are also susceptible to ASFV and they show similar clinical signs and mortality rates as domestic pigs [3]. In certain areas, soft ticks of *Ornithodoros* genus can be involved in the epidemiology of the disease.

African swine fever is endemic in sub-Saharan Africa and on the Italian island of Sardinia. In 2007, the disease was reported in Georgia, most probably originating from Southeast Africa. From Georgia, the virus spread to Armenia and to Azerbaijan, meanwhile it crossed the Caucasus Mountains spreading into several states of the Russian Federation where, in certain areas, the disease became endemic representing a constant threat for the neighbouring countries [3]. In 2013, from the Russian Federation, the virus reached Belarus and Ukraine and later, in 2014, it was introduced into Lithuania, Poland, Latvia and Estonia affecting both domestic pigs and wild boar. Based on the characteristics of the virus and on the epidemiological findings, the introduction into the Baltic countries and into Poland was most probably from Belarus [4]. The ASFV strain that is currently circulating in the Eastern European countries and Baltic States is a highly virulent and highly lethal strain, belonging to genotype II which has 100% sequence homology with the ASFV identified in Belarus in June 2013 [5].

More than 1 year after its introduction into Poland and into the Baltic countries, ASF is still spreading in wild boar in the eastern member states of the European Union (EU) with few spill overs into the domestic pig population, while in Sardinia, Ukraine and in the Russian Federation the virus continues to spread in both wild boar and domestic pigs. The current epidemiological situation in the Eastern part of Europe represents a constant threat to the EU livestock sector, particularly if the infection

*Correspondence: silvia.bellini@izsler.it
[1] Istituto Zooprofilattico Sperimentale della Lombardia ed Emilia Romagna (IZSLER), Brescia, Italy
Full list of author information is available at the end of the article

pressure remains high at the eastern borders of the EU. The presence of ASF in Sardinia seems to pose a limited risk to the pig sector of the ASFV free territories of the EU. Indeed, in 38 years ASFV spread from the island of Sardinia only on one isolated occasion [6]. No vaccine or drugs are available to prevent ASFV infection. Therefore, it is particularly important to prevent the introduction of the disease in free areas and to reduce, as much as possible, the persistence of the virus in the infected ones.

Prevention and early detection play a key role in the control strategy for ASF and enhancing early detection would also improve the efficacy of the disease control measures. In the EU, the provisions to apply in case of infection are mainly targeted towards domestic pigs and are based on surveillance, epidemiological investigations, tracing of pigs and stamping out infected holdings [7]. However, in order to mitigate the risk of spread, such measures are to be applied in combination with strict preventive measures in domestic pig holdings. The basic elements of biosecurity derive from the knowledge of the epidemiology of the disease, the duration of pathogen excretion in infected animals, the main routes of excretion, survival of the pathogen in the environment and its routes of infection. Some basic principles of biosecurity apply to all farming systems and all diseases [8]. However, in order to better address preventive and control measures, the main practical biosecurity measures need to be tailored to the targeted disease and to the farming systems in which they are to be implemented [8]. Indeed, biosecurity measures are normally quite standardized in commercial holdings, whilst they are not well defined and of easy implementation in the backyard sector.

The aim of this paper is to define the main preventive measures to adopt to minimize the risk of ASF spread in the pig sector, including both industrial and backyard production systems. Indeed, backyard holdings with poor biosecurity in place are currently playing an important role in the maintenance and spread of ASFV in the infected eastern neighbouring countries of the EU [3]. Moreover, considering the significant involvement of wild boar in the current epidemic in the Eastern parts of Europe, we also take into account the role played by wild boar at the interface with domestic pigs and the measures to adopt to properly manage the hunting activities.

Search strategy

This critical review is based on a search in PubMed (http://www.ncbi.nlm.nih.gov/pubmed) using the terms African swine fever, ASF, domestic pigs, wild boar, wildlife, epidemiology, prevention and bio-security. Only articles in English were included in the text. EFSA Scientific Review and Opinions on ASF were used as source of additional information. Our experiences on ASF management and on the biological aspects of the disease were used to critically evaluate the articles and to identify the main preventive measures to be adopted against ASF. The EU legislation and OIE standards on ASF were consulted to ensure coherence with the proposed measures.

Review

African swine fever epidemiology

A range of wild and domestic pig species are susceptible to ASFV and different tick vector species, all belonging to *Ornithodoros* genus, can be involved in the epidemiology of the disease. Transmission and maintenance of ASF can occur in a sylvatic cycle and/or in a domestic pig cycle. Depending on the presence or absence of wild *Suidae* and arthropod vectors and on the type of pig production system, the epidemiology of the disease varies substantially between different habitats and regions. The African scenario includes the presence of ASFV-infected ticks, different species of wild suids acting as reservoirs for the disease, domestic pigs that have been exposed to ASFV for many years and partly ASF-resistant [9, 10]. These conditions do not exist in any European Country.

For the purpose of this review, we refer mainly to the epidemiological situation in Europe and to the domestic pig cycle. In Europe there are currently two main clusters of ASFV infection. One of them is in Sardinia where the disease was introduced in 1978, most probably from Iberian Peninsula [11], and it is caused by strains of ASFV belonging to genotype I [6]. The second is occurring in the eastern part of Europe and it is caused by strains of ASFV belonging to genotype II that has 100% sequence homology with the ASFV identified in Belarus in June 2013, a genetic variant of the virus introduced in Georgia in 2007 [5]. The latter is a highly virulent strain inducing an acute form of ASF that results in a mortality rate of 94.5–100% in both wild boar and domestic pigs [4, 12–15].

ASFV has a remarkable ability to survive for long periods in a protein rich environment and it remains stable at pH 4–10 [16]. The virus is not affected by meat maturation processes and meat from pigs slaughtered in the infective stages of ASF or that die spontaneously of the disease provides a good source of virus. ASFV persist in tissues for up to 6 months and can be infectious in susceptible animals fed with such meat [17]. The virus can also remain viable in the lymph nodes of the few survivors to the disease [18, 19] and, in such instance, the natural death of these animals can re-initiate a new epidemic cycle of ASF, if carcasses are not properly disposed and the virus gets in contact with a susceptible animal.

The virus is quite resistant to high temperatures and it requires exposure to a temperature of 60 °C for at least 20 min for inactivation [1]. Fresh and frozen pork, as well as smoked, salted and dried pork may contain infective quantities of ASFV [20, 21] whereas the virus is inactivated in heat-treated products [1]. Commercial processed products (such as ham or cured pork loin) contain no active virus 140 days after processing of the fresh meat started. ASFV is also able to survive for long periods in some tissues such as bone marrow, in spite of putrefaction [10]. This probably plays a role in infecting scavenging pigs in areas where the disease is endemic. The resistance of the virus to inactivation also means that transmission is possible via fomites such as contaminated clothing and shoes, equipment and vehicles.

Pigs are infected mainly through the oro-nasal route after contact with infected pigs or after feeding on virus-containing pork or contaminated products. All excretions and secretions of infected pigs such as blood, faeces, urine or saliva can contain virus, and ASFV may remain viable in blood and tissues for long periods [3, 5, 17, 19]. The onset of viremia is observed from 3 to 5 days post infection (DPI) and transmission via direct contact can occur for several weeks [22]. As regards ASFV genotype II, in pigs experimentally infected, it has been observed that the excretion of the virus started during the incubation period and lasted for the entire period of the disease. Hence, pigs were infectious from 4 to 10 DPI [23].

So far, with the strain circulating in the Baltic countries and in Poland there is no evidence that recovered pigs can become long-term carriers of the ASFV [2–4]. However, in large pig populations, ASF can be maintained for long periods in the area due to constant supply of susceptible pigs [10], illegal movements of infected pork meat, poor biosecurity in pig holdings, and aggregation of wild boar promoted by feeding [3].

The dynamic of the infection in the wild boar shows the same pattern observed in domestic pigs [24]. The role played by wild boar in the epidemiology of ASF is mainly determined by wild boar abundance and the geographical continuity of suitable habitats [25]. Indeed, it appears that in Sardinia wild boar have a limited role in the spread of the disease [26] whilst in the Baltic countries and Poland they are acting as reservoir [3, 4, 25].

Soft ticks of *Ornithodoros* species, in certain epidemiological contexts, can play a role in transmitting ASFV [19]. In Europe, only ticks of the *O. erraticus* complex have been reported in some countries around the Mediterranean Basin [27]. Ticks of the genus *Ornithodoros* are common in pig pens in many areas of Africa and in certain parts of the Iberian Peninsula, while the information available suggests that they are absent from Sardinia [28]. Knowledge on the occurrence of these ticks in other areas of Europe is rather incomplete. However, in the Baltic countries, in Poland and in Central Europe their presence seems unlikely, as their involvement in the epidemiological cycle of the disease [29]. Such ticks are able to retain ASFV for a long time, at least 5 years, and to transmit it to susceptible species [30, 31]. In addition, some of these ticks can transmit the virus from tick to tick through trans-stadial and trans-ovarian transmission [31]. *Ornithodoros* ticks mainly feed on animal species living in burrows or they are harboured inside pigsties in old buildings, where they hide in cracks and surfaces that provide sufficient humidity. Pigs are mostly accidental hosts, from which the ticks can be infected. Wild boar has never been found infested by *Ornithodoros* ticks, since wild boar normally rest on the surface, rarely on the same spot and never inside burrows. Therefore, such ticks can play an important role in maintaining local foci of infection, but not in the geographical spread of the virus [27].

ASF risk factors, pathways of transmission and preventive measures

Risk factors for the spreading of ASFV

Few analytical studies have been carried out to identify risk factors for ASF at farm level. Factors found to increase the risk of outbreak, include free range pig management system [11], the previous occurrence of a disease in the farm [32], the presence of an infected pig farm in the neighbourhood or of an abattoir in the community, and visits by veterinarians and para-veterinarians [33]. A spatial regression analysis found density of the road network, of water bodies and of the domestic swine population to be associated with outbreaks in Russia [34] and a spatial spread model found the movement of infected animals to be the most important factor in the spread of ASFV [35]. In the backyard sector the main risk factors are human induced, such as illegal movements of infected pork meat and swill feeding together with suspected cases underreporting and "emergency sales" [36]. The backyard sector commonly uses swill as supplementary feed, which may include untreated ASFV contaminated pork or pig products. Often, the contaminated meat may have been stored chilled, frozen or after treatment and kept over long periods, thus acting as the main mechanism for ASFV maintenance and re-introduction. Recent epidemiological investigations carried out in Lithuania and Latvia have suggested that fresh grass and seeds contaminated by secretions from infectious wild boar could be possible source of infection for backyards [2]. Virus re-introduction and amplification mainly takes place in the backyard pigs and then ASFV seasonally spills over first to small farms and then to commercial pig farms. Additionally, the interaction between wild boar and domestic pigs can prolong ASFV circulation in both swine populations, as observed in many outbreaks in Sardinia and in the Russian Federation [26, 37]. In Sardinia, the number of backyards together with the illegal free ranging of pigs is considered a main risk practice for the persistence of ASF in certain areas of the island [6]. Indeed, free-range pigs grazing on vast municipal owned lands have been strongly associated with the maintenance of ASFV infection in the endemic area of Nuoro, as demonstrated by the intense viral circulation amongst such pigs [11]. In a recent study carried out in Sardinia, also the number of closed farms, roads density and the mean altitude have been associated with an increased risk of ASFV introduction in pig holdings [38].

In the Baltic countries and in Poland, it was observed that wild boar habitat suitability, neighbouring distance from infected wild boar and domestic pigs were the main risk factors for the introduction into EU free areas through infected wild boar [39]. Different studies highlighted the continuity of the geographical distribution of wild boar, wild boar management (hunting system, winter feeding), local density and size of the infected population, direct contact with dead infected wild boar, as the most relevant risks for the spread and the persistence of the virus in wild boar populations [4, 25, 40].

ASF pathways of transmission and preventive measures

Preventive measures to apply to mitigate the risk of spread of a disease in the pig production system are to be targeted to the main potential routes of transmission of the pathogen. Some of them are applicable across all production systems, others are not [8].

Based on the epidemiological characteristics of ASF, the disease pathways of transmission [19] are:

- Direct pig-to-pig contact.
- Consumption of contaminated feed (swill feeding).
- Vehicles and other fomites, clothing, footwear, surgical equipment.
- Workers and visitors.
- Slurry.
- Genetic materials.
- Bites from ticks.

Direct pig-to-pig contact African swine fever virus is primarily transmitted by direct contact between infected and susceptible pigs. The spread of the virus from infected animals can start from the second DPI by means of saliva, ocular secretions and nasal discharges [17]. After a few days, the virus is shed via urine, faeces and semen. Aerosol can also transmit the virus over short distance [17, 22]. It is worth to be taken into consideration that infected pigs are most contagious during the incubation period of the disease, when they may shed virus for up to 48 h before showing clinical signs and during the clinical stage of disease, when a large amounts of virus is present in blood, secretions and excretions [23]. Given the characteristics of resistance of the virus, this pathway of transmission is extremely efficient both, locally (at farm level, village, and pasture) and long distance [4]. Therefore, in risk areas it is necessary to adopt specific measures to minimize the risk of introducing the disease into the herd by direct contact between infected and susceptible animals.

- Physical isolation of the herd

It is aimed at limiting the potential opportunities for a susceptible animal to get physically in contact with an infected one. Indeed, if a pathogen does not enter the holding no infection can take place. Depending on the pig production system, the local geographic and socio-economic conditions and the capacity to invest resources, isolation of the holding can be obtained by maintaining adequate distances between farms, by full fencing the herd and installing a closed entrance to the farm area [8]. There are simple measures such as permanent housing of pigs and closed entrance to the premise that achieve the same objective and can be implemented also in rural villages with very limited resources. For the holdings of new settlement, physical location of the premise should be carefully planned in the light of maintaining adequate distances from neighbouring farms, slaughterhouses, meat-processing establishments, animal markets and frequently used roads [8].

- Introduction of new pigs into the herd

No pigs should enter or leave the holding unless necessary and when necessary, adequate preventive measures shall be adopted to mitigate the risk. Pigs shall be introduced into the herd only from trusted and certified sources. To mitigate the risk of spread of pathogens, special attention shall be given to the management of animal transport and to the cleansing and disinfection procedures of the vehicles and the loading/unloading area. The number of suppliers for replacement stock should be limited and their health status carefully evaluated before purchase. Newly purchased pigs shall be maintained for a minimum of 30 days in quarantine or, at least, physically isolated from the rest of the herd. Frequency of introduction shall be limited too [8]. During the quarantine period the animals should be carefully checked to early detect the presence of conditions to avoid the introduction of diseased animals onto the herd. Clinical surveillance, is the most effective tool for early detection of ASF [4]. However, given the clinical similarity with other diseases of pigs, clinical surveillance should be supplemented, as appropriate, by serological and virological surveillance [41].

- Movement stand still

When pigs are for breeding and production and they are destined for another holding, pigs must have remained in the holding of origin for a period of 30 days prior to loading or since birth if less than 30 days old [42].

- Pig markets

In certain areas, live pig markets are extremely important for local trade. They are obvious mixing points and a potential source of disease. Pigs are brought to the market by owners or traders and they are a cross point where small and commercial producers, traders and butchers meet. Therefore, they are a crucial point for the spread of diseases. Once pigs are brought to the market, they comingle with other animals and they do not have any more the health status of the original herd. Therefore, to limit the risk of spread, pigs that have not been sold at market shall not be reintroduced into the original herd, unless they do not pass through an appropriate period of quarantine [8]. Pig markets should be kept under strict veterinary supervision and the animals are to be admitted to the market only if accompanied by a certificate attesting the favourable health status. However, in case ASF is confirmed in the area, live pig markets should be closed.

- Disposal of carcasses

Vehicles collecting dead animals represent a major risk for the transmission of the disease. They shall not enter into the farm and pig carcasses are to be collected outside the fence. Drivers have to strictly follow farm biosecurity protocols and they should not enter the holding. Carcasses of domestic pigs and wild boar found dead in the infected areas shall be processed under official supervision and they should be checked and tested to early detect the presence of ASFV. Carcasses, discarded parts from slaughtered pigs shall be disposed by incineration or burial in an authorized land fill. No part of any wild boar, whether shot or found dead, shall be brought into a pig holding.

- Natural mating

Natural mating provided by an external boar would also imply moving the boar or the sow for mating from one location to another. Such movements of pigs between herds are to be regarded as a dangerous practice. Therefore, in areas at risk such practice should not be conducted [8].

Consumption of contaminated feed (swill feeding) Feeding of catering waste is a high risk practice as several diseases, including ASF, can be introduced in a healthy population through such feeding. It is documented that the majority of the outbreaks occurred in ASFV-free zones were the result of feeding food waste products from infected pigs to susceptible animals [16, 19]. This risk is mitigated by observing the ban on feeding swill to pigs as foreseen by the EU legislation [43]. A proper implementation of the existing rules should be ensured and a communication campaign should be addressed to pig owners to make them understand the danger of that practice. In the absence of specific legislation and in areas in which swill feeding is practiced, treatment of swill at temperatures higher than 70 °C should be guaranteed [16, 19].

Vehicles and other fomites, clothing, footwear, surgical equipment African swine fever virus has a remarkable ability to survive in the environment for several days, especially if protected by organic material. The resistance of the virus to inactivation means that transmission is possible via contaminated clothing and shoes, equipment and vehicles.

Drivers and their vehicles transporting pigs to pig holdings, market or slaughterhouse, delivering feed, or collecting carcasses represent a major risk for the transmission of the disease. Vehicles used for transport of pigs shall be cleaned and disinfected immediately after every transport of animals, and if necessary before any new loading of animals using disinfectants officially authorized in cleaning and disinfection facilities approved by the competent authority, and provide documentary evidence that these operations have been performed. In cleaning and disinfecting the vehicles, special attention should be given to the truck body, the loading ramp, the equipment having been in contact with pigs, the driver's cabin and the protective clothes/boots used during unloading. Vehicles used for transport of animals shall keep a register containing place and date of disinfection [42]. Drivers should strictly follow farm biosecurity protocols when handling animals and, as a rule, they should not enter into pig holdings, at least the area where the animals are kept. Pig keepers should take precautions against contamination from vehicles by establishing a pig loading area and by not allowing drivers into pig area [8].

Sharing of equipment between holdings should be avoided. All instruments, equipment or tools that are likely to be in contact with pigs, also the ones to restrain animals, shall be assigned to the farm and kept clean. In case they have to be transported to other farms they have to be cleaned and disinfected, also when re-introduced into the farm [8].

Workers and visitors Visitors should be discouraged to enter pig holdings, both commercial and backyard. The role of people in transmitting pathogens is well documented. Appropriate hygiene measures have to be adopted by all persons entering into contact with pigs (domestic and/or feral). They can carry pathogens on clothing, footwear and hands. People entering the farm, including farmers and workers should not have been in contact with other pigs recently. In case they have, they should not be admitted to the farm.

Visitors, including farm workers, should be provided with specific clothes and footwear to be used and left into the farm. Workers, working with the herd should not have contact with other pigs and they shall not have pigs at their home. Pig workers must be well informed of their potential role in the spread of the disease.

On small farms, farmers shall avoid visiting other farms and also avoid allowing people to enter the premise. Farmers should have clothes and footwear to be worn and used when entering the pig stable [8].

Slurry Faeces from ASFV infected pigs contains large amount of virus [44]. Therefore, disposal of manure, bedding material and slurry have to be considered in areas at risk. Indeed, the dispersion of pig slurry on agricultural lands is a dangerous practice, the virus can be introduced into the environment infecting wild boar and free ranging pigs. The survival of ASFV in the environment depends also on the season, cold temperature facilitates the survival of the virus whereas sunlight and drying reduce its survival. Commercial pig holdings are normally provided with storage basins, which allow manure treatment with specific disinfectants [8, 16, 45].

Genetic materials There is not reliable evidence for ASFV transmission from sows to foetuses during pregnancy [46] as well as for sexual transmission in pigs. However, ASFV is shed in genital secretions and the virus was found in the semen of one boar experimentally infected [47]. Due to that, to ensure that semen is free from ASFV provisions and requirements are reported in the EU legislation [48] and by the OIE [49].

Bites from ticks *Ornithodoros* spp. ticks have been found infesting pig pens in Africa and Iberian Peninsula. As described previously, such ticks can maintain ASFV infection for several months or even years after feeding on viraemic animals and, at local level, they can be involved in the maintenance and long-term transmission of ASFV. In Madagascar, ASFV was isolated from ticks found on a farm where no pigs had been introduced for at least 4 years [50]. In Portugal an outbreak was determined by the presence of ticks that harboured the virus for more than 5 years [30]. Due to the ticks long life and ability to survive for a long time without feeding, eradication of ticks from the old pigsties is invariably unsuccessful. Therefore, in order to avoid contacts, pigs shall not be housed in infested premises. The premises should be isolated with fences to prevent the access of pigs or destroyed and then new premises rebuilt in another location.

In commercial pig holdings, the above-mentioned preventive measures can be adopted with different degrees of implementation. The level of implementation varies according to the size and profile of the holding, the existent infrastructure, the epidemiological situation and the capacity of the producer to invest resources [8].

In situation of risk, the farms bio-security plans have to be verified by veterinary services and because of the virus's ability to survive in the environment, the plans shall also include detailed procedures on cleaning and disinfection, which are an essential part of the farm biosecurity system. Lipidic solvents, which destroy the envelope of the virus and commercial disinfectants based on iodine and phenolic compounds, are effective in inactivating the ASFV [16, 19]. However, disinfectants should be officially authorized by the veterinary service and the conditions for their use strictly respected.

The situation is rather different for backyard holdings and for free-range pigs where, normally, the investment in infrastructures is minimal and few arrangements are made to provide the pigs with housing.

Preventive measures in backyard holdings

Backyard holdings with poor bio-security in place are currently playing an important role in the spread of ASFV in the Eastern part of Europe. Indeed, in this sector of the pig production system feeding pigs with kitchen waste is common practice and the main biosecurity measures are not easy to implement, due to the minimal investment in infrastructure typical for this type of pig production system. However, there is a set of basic preventive measures applicable also in backyard holdings and if they are properly and strictly implemented they are effective in minimizing the risk of ASFV spread. Such measures include:

- No swill feeding.
- Avoid feeding pigs with fresh fodder harvested in areas at risk for ASFV exposure.
- Buying pigs from trusted and certified sources (ASFV-free commercial holdings).
- Keeping pigs confined in stables.
- Restricting the access to pig's stable only to people in charge of taking care of the animals.
- People working in contact with pigs should wear clothes and footwear to be worn and used only when working in the stable and to be left in the stable after use.

- Workers cannot bring food onto the premise.
- People working in contact with pigs should wash hands with soap before entering and leaving the premise.
- Using effective disinfectants to be placed at the entrance of the stable.
- Proper disposal of dead animals or parts of dead animals to avoid the spread of infected material and also to attract wild animals.
- No wild boar or part of it, shall be brought onto the premise.
- In areas at risk for the presence of ASFV in wild boar, where the viral contamination of the environment can be high, effective disinfectants, such as calcium hydrate (slaked lime), should be spread and renewed, around pig's stable and at the entrance [51].
- Pig's owner and people in charge of pigs shall avoid visiting other farms.

Furthermore, to enhance ASFV early detection:

- Veterinary services should be informed in case of dead or sick pigs.
- Home slaughtering should be carried out under veterinary supervision.

Preventive measures in outdoor keeping practice and free-range pigs

Biosecurity in the free ranging system is almost impossible to apply, especially in endemic areas where common pasture is practiced (i.e. municipal pastures in Sardinia or in public forests as in Georgia/Armenia). Free ranging pigs is considered a dangerous practice for the persistence of ASFV in certain areas of endemicity. Indeed, animals belonging to different herds can share the same grazing areas, they can also comingle with wild boar facilitating the transmission of the virus [6]. In such circumstances, free ranging pigs should be forbidden.

In areas at risk, biosecurity in outdoor keeping system shall be focused on segregation and feed control. Fencing or double fencing is very difficult to implement, and also to maintain, but it is the only possible mean to try to mitigate the risk of pigs direct contact with infected animals and contaminated pasture.

Preventive measures during hunting

Hunting is allowed in the majority of the forested areas of North-East Europe and wild boar are one of the more intensively hunted ungulate species in Europe. Yet, wild boar has expanded throughout Europe during the last 40 years [52]. Indeed, they have a high reproductive rate, and populations can double in size after each reproduction season [53]. Wild boar are susceptible to ASFV and they show similar clinical signs and mortality to domestic pigs [12, 13] with similar virus elimination timing and concentration [24]. When wild boar die, infected carcasses, if not promptly removed, remain in the environment and they can, directly or indirectly, infect other susceptible pigs, continuing the epidemiological cycle of the disease. Wild boar can also contribute to spread the virus during the infectious period of the disease, since they eliminate the virus into the environment throughout their excretions and secretions [12, 24]. In 2015, in Poland and in the Baltic countries, 897 wild boar positive for ASFV have been hunted or found dead in the affected territories (data available at: http://www.efsa.europa.eu/it/events/event/151123). Most probably the reported figure is strongly underestimated, since it appears that only 10% of the positive dead wild boars are detected in the forest [4]. Considering that a large amount of ASFV is shed during the infectious period of the disease and that the virus is rather resistant in the environment, especially if protected by organic material, it can be expected that in the affected forests, the viral contamination of the environment to be rather high. Indeed, hunting wild boar implies blood contamination of the soil, transportation of dead animals to the dressing facility (when dressing is not performed directly on the field), dressing animals, offal discharge, meat dissection and its conservation. Therefore, in the light of a control strategy, the role of the wild boar and hunting cannot be underestimated and basic preventive measures are to be adopted to minimize the risk of spread of the disease.

Minimum biosecurity requirements to apply during hunting in the affected territories:

- Hunters shall be authorised to hunt in the area only after a specific training on basic hygiene and biosecurity practices;
- Hunted wild boar should never leave the hunting area unless checked and tested and the carcasses released only when resulted negative to ASFV.
- Transport of hunted animals to the dressing facility is carried out using dedicated vehicles. Private cars shall be parked outside the hunting house, possibly on the main road.
- The use of the dressing facilities should be authorised only in case it is available: tap water, electricity, waste water collection and freezers.
- Animal dressing should be performed using appropriate aprons which must remain in the facility. Working tools cannot be transported to other places.
- Hunting suits, including boots/shoes should be kept in specific bags. Boots are worn in the dressing room before hunting and re-placed in the same bag after hunting.

- Boots and apron shall be cleaned and disinfected after each use.
- Dressing rooms are to be equipped with effective disinfectants.
- Offals should be stored in proper containers inside the dressing areas and before storing, containers shall be cleaned and sprayed with effective disinfectants.
- Ground pits for offal disposal should be at least 1.5 m deep, fenced and closed with a locked closure. Pits should be located in close proximity to the dressing room.
- Wild boar carcasses shall be individually identified before storing. In case of ASFV positive outcome all stored carcasses have to be disposed under veterinary supervision and the whole dressing room cleaned and disinfected.

Conclusions

The current ASF situation in the East part of the EU is representing a constant threat to the EU livestock sector and the recent expansion of the disease has also demonstrated the ability of the virus to spread long distance. ASF is a disease for which there is no effective vaccine and its control relies on early detection followed by rapid eradication. Considering the epidemiological situation and the possible economic consequences of the introduction of ASF, it is extremely important that free territories are maintained free by preventing the introduction of the disease. For such purpose, bio security plays a key role in preventing ASF, and given its epidemiological cycle, simple measures may prove effective in mitigating the transmission pathways of the disease, also in the backyard sector. In certain countries, in case of occurrence of epidemic diseases, there is the attempt to try to decrease the local risk of further spread, by reducing the number of backyards, especially in the areas surrounding commercial holdings, and afterwards prohibiting this type of farming practice. Given the socio-economic relevance of the backyard sector, such discriminatory approach needs to be carefully evaluated since it might lead to poor compliance of the measures enforced to control the disease.

The final responsibility of controlling ASF belongs to the veterinary authorities. However, in risk areas, pig producers have to understand the risk posed by the presence of the disease and they have to adopt all the necessary precautionary measures to protect their own herds. To achieve this, veterinary services shall provide basic information to pig holders through appropriate communication campaigns and by promoting the adoption of preventive measures. The key for changing behaviours and practices lies in people's perception of the level of risk and in such situation, it is of crucial importance that all the elements of the pig production and marketing chain, including backyards, transporters, service providers and slaughterhouses, are involved in the implementation of the control strategy for the disease.

In adopting an eradication strategy against ASF, the role of wild boar cannot be underestimated and preventive measures need to be established also to control the possible pathways of ASFV transmission from wild to domestic pigs. Hunters may have an active role in preventing the spread of ASFV and they should be involved in the disease control strategy since the beginning.

Authors' contributions

SB conceived the idea of the review and coordinated the writing process. SB drafted the background, the parts on epidemiology and on domestic pigs. VG drafted the section on wild boar and participated in drafting the background. DR checked all the technical details related to the biological properties of the ASFV. All authors participated in the subsequent discussions and revisions of the entire text. All authors read and approved the final manuscript.

Author details

[1] Istituto Zooprofilattico Sperimentale della Lombardia ed Emilia Romagna (IZSLER), Brescia, Italy. [2] Private Consultant, Perugia, Italy. [3] Istituto Superiore per la Protezione e la Ricerca Ambientale (ISPRA), Ozzano Emilia, Bologna, Italy.

Competing interests

The authors declare that they have no competing interests.

References

1. Costard S, Mur L, Lubroth J, Sánchez-Vizcaíno JM, Pfeiffer DU. Epidemiology of African swine fever virus. Virus Res. 2013;173:191–7.
2. Guinat C, Gogin A, Blome S, Keil G, Pollin R, Pfeiffer DU, Dixon L. Transmission routes of African swine fever virus to domestic pigs: current knowledge and future research directions. Vet Rec. 2016;178:262–7.
3. EFSA. Scientific review on African swine fever. 2010. http://www.efsa.europa.eu/sites/default/files/scientific_output/files/main_documents/1556.pdf. Accessed 21 Mar 2016.
4. EFSA. Scientific opinion on African swine fever. 2015. http://www.efsa.europa.eu/sites/default/files/scientific_output/files/main_documents/4163.pdf Accessed 19 Apr 2015.
5. Gallardo C, Fernández-Pinero J, Pelayo V, Gazaev I, Markowska-Daniel I, Pridotkas G, et al. Genetic variation among African swine fever genotype II viruses, eastern and central Europe. Emerg Infect Diseases. 2014;20:1544–7.
6. Mur L, Atzeni M, Martinez-Lopez B, Feliziani F, Rolesu S, Sanchez-Vizcaino JM. Thirty-five year presence of African swine fever in Sardinia: history, evolution and risk factors for disease maintenance. Transboud Emerg Dis. 2014;63:e165–7.
7. Council Directive 2002/60/EC. Laying down specific provisions for the control of African swine fever and amending Directive 92/119/EEC as regard Teschen disease and African swine fever. http://eur-lex.europa.eu/LexUriServ/LexUriServ.do?uri=OJ:L:2002:192:0027:0046:EN:PDF. Accessed 18 Nov 2015.
8. Food and Agriculture Organization of the United Nation/World Organization for Animal Health/World Bank. 2010. Good practices for biosecurity in the pig sector—issues and options in developing and transition countries. FAO Animal Production and Health Paper N. 169. Rome, FAO. p. 69.
9. Penrith ML. History of "swine fever" in southern Africa. J S Afr Vet Assoc. 2013;84:1–6.
10. Penrith ML, Vosloo W. Review of African swine fever: transmission spread and control. J S Afric Vet Assoc. 2009;80:58–62.

11. Mannelli A, Sotgia S, Patta C, Sarria A, Madrau P, Sanna L, et al. Effect of husbandry methods on seropositivity to African swine fever in Sardinian swine herds. Pre Vet Med. 1997;32:235–41.
12. Gabriel C, Blome S, Malgolovkin A, Parilov S, Kolbasov D, Teifke JP, Beer M. Characterization of African swine fever Caucasus isolate in European wild boars. Emerg Infec Dis. 2011;17:2342–5.
13. Blome S, Gabriel C, Dietze K, Breithaupt A, Beer M. High virulence of African swine fever virus caucasus isolate in European wild boars of all ages. Emerg Infec Dis. 2012;18:708.
14. Gallardo C, Soler A, Nieto R, Cano C, Pelayo V, Sánchez MA, et al. Experimental infection of domestic pigs with African swine fever virus Lithuania 2014 genotype II field isolate. Transbound Emerg Dis. 2015. doi:10.1111/tbed.12346.
15. Vlasova NN, Varentsova AA, Shevchenko IV, Zhukov IY, Remyga SG, Gavrilova VL, et al. Comparative analysis of clinical and biological characteristics of African swine fever virus isolates from 2013 year in Russian Federation. Br Microbiol Res J. 2015;5:203–15.
16. Geering WA, Penrith ML, Nyakahuma D. Manual on procedures for disease eradication by stamping out. FAO Health Manual 12. Rome, 2001. http://www.fao.org/docrep/004/y0660e/Y0660E00.htm#TOC. p. 98. Accessed 19 Dec 2015.
17. Sánchez-Vizcaíno JL. Early detection and contingency plan for African swine fever. OIE conference 139–147; 2010. http://www.oie.int/doc/ged/D11831.PDF. Accessed 2 May 2016.
18. Wilkinson PJ. The persistence of African swine fever in Africa and the Mediterranean. Prev Vet Med. 1984;2:71–82.
19. Gallardo MC, de la Torre Reoyo A, Fernández-Pinero J, Iglesias I, Munoz MJ, Arias ML. African swine fever: a global view of the current challenge. PHM. 2015;1:21. doi:10.1186/s40813-015-0013-y.
20. McKercher PD, Yedloutschnig RJ, Callis JJ, Murphy R, Panina GF, Civardi A, et al. Survival of viruses in Prosciutto di Parma (Parma Ham). Can Inst Food Sci Technol J. 1987;20:267–72.
21. Mebus CA, Arias M, Pineda JM, Tapiador J, House C, Sanchez-Vizcaino JM. Survival of several porcine viruses in different Spanish dry-cured meat products. Food Chem. 1997;54:555–9.
22. Wilkinson PJ. African swine fever virus. In: Pensaert MB, editor. Virus infections of porcines. New York: Elsevier Science; 1989. p. 17–35.
23. Guinat C, Reis A, Netherton CL, Goatley L, Pfeiffer DU, Dixon L. Dynamics of African swine fever virus shedding and excretion in domestic pigs infected by intramuscular inoculation and contact transmission. Vet Res. 2014;45:93.
24. Pietschmann J, Guinat C, Beer M, Pronin V, Tauscher K, Petrov A, Blome S. Course and transmission characteristics of oral low-dose infection of domestic pigs and European wild boar with a Caucasian African swine fever virus isolate. Arch Virol. 2015;6:1–11.
25. EFSA. Evaluation of possible mitigation measures to prevent introduction and spread of African swine fever through wild boar. 2014. http://www.efsa.europa.eu/sites/default/files/scientific_output/files/main_documents/3616.pdf. Accessed 23 Mar 2015.
26. Iglesias I, Rodriguez A, Feliziani F, Rolesu S, de la Torre A. Spatio-temporal analysis of African swine fever in Sardinia (2012–2014): trends in domestic pigs and wild boar. Transbound Emerg Dis. 2015. doi:10.1111/tbed.12408.
27. EFSA. Scientific opinion on the role of tick vectors in the epidemiology of Crimean-Congo haemorrhagic fever and African swine fever in Eurasia. 2010. http://www.efsa.europa.eu/sites/default/files/scientific_output/files/main_documents/1703.pdf. Accessed 18 Nov 2015.
28. Mur L, Iscaro C, Cocco M, Jurado C, Rolesu S, De Mia GM, et al. Serological surveillance and direct filed searching reaffirm the absence of *Ornithodoros erraticus* ticks role in African swine fever cycle in Sardinia. Transbound Emerg Dis. 2016. doi:10.1111/tbed.12485.
29. Pietschmann J, Mur L, Blome S, Beer M, Pérez-Sanchez R, Oleaga A, Sánchez-Vizcaíno JM. African swine fever transmission cycles in Central Europe: evaluation of wild boar-soft ticks contacts through detection of antibodies against *Ornithodoros erraticus* saliva antigens. BMC Vet Res. 2016;12:1. doi:10.1186/s12917-015-0629-9.
30. Boinas F, Wilson JW, Hutchings GH, Martins C, Dixon JL. The persistence of African swine fever virus in field-infected *Ornithodoros erraticus* during the ASF endemic period in Portugal. PLoS ONE. 2011. doi:10.1371/journal.pone.0020383.
31. Ribeiro R, Otte J, Madeira S, Hutchings GH, Boinas F. Experimental infection of *Ornithodoros erraticus* sensu *stricto* with two Portuguese African swine fever strains. Study of factors involved in the dynamics of infection in ticks. PLoS ONE. 2015;14:20. doi:10.1371/journal.pone.0137718.
32. Randriamparany T, Grenier A, Tourette I, Maharavo Rahantamalala C, Rousset D, Lancelot R. Epidemiological situation of African swine fever in Lake Alaotra region (Madagascar) and possible consequences on the organization of the disease control and surveillance. Rev Elev Med Vet Pays Trop. 2005;58:15–20.
33. Fasina FO, Agbaje M, Ajani FL, Talabi OA, Lazarus DD, Gallardo C, Thompson PN, Bostos AD. Risk factors for farm-level African swine fever infection in major pig-producing areas in Nigeria, 1997–2011. Pre Vet Med. 2012;1:65–75.
34. Gulekin VM, Kerennoy FI, Karaulov AK, Dudnikov SA. Cartographical analysis of African swine fever outbreaks in the territory of the Russian Federation and computer modelling of the basic reproduction ratio. Pre Vet Med. 2011;102:167–74.
35. Olugasa BO, Ljagbone IF. Pattern of spread of African swine fever in south-western Nigeria, 1997–2005. Veterinaria Italiana. 2007;43:621–8.
36. Costard S, Zagmutt FJ, Porphyre T, Pfeiffer DU. Small-scale pig farmers' behaviour, silent release of African swine fever virus and consequences for disease spread. Sci Rep. 2015;5:17074. doi:10.1038/srep17074.
37. Lange M, Siemen H, Blome S, Tulke H-H. Analysis of spatio-temporal patterns of African swine fever cases in Russian wild boar does not reveal an endemic situation. Prev Vet Med. 2014;117:317–25.
38. Martínez-López B, Perez AM, Feliziani F, Rolesu S, Mur L, Sánchez-Vizcaíno JM. Evaluation of the risk factors contributing to the African swine fever occurrence in Sardinia, Italy. Front Microbiol. 2015;6:314. doi:10.3389/fmicb.2015.00314.
39. De la Torre A, Bosch J, Iglesias I, Muñoz MJ, Mur L, Martínez-López B, Sánchez-Vizcaíno JM. Assessing the risk of African swine fever introduction into the European Union by wild boar. Transbound Emerg Dis. 2015;62:272–9. doi:10.1111/tbed.12129.
40. Lange M. Alternative control strategies against ASF in wild boar populations. 2015. EFSA supporting publication. http://www.efsa.europa.eu/sites/default/files/scientific_output/files/main_documents/843e.pdf. Accessed 22 Mar 2015.
41. OIE. African swine fever. In: Manual of diagnostic tests and vaccines for terrestrial animals. Paris: Office International des Epizooties; 2016. http://www.oie.int/fileadmin/Home/eng/Health_standards/tahm/2.08.01_ASF.pdf. Accessed 3 May 2016.
42. Council Directive 64/432/EEC on animal health problems affecting intra-Community trade in bovine animals and swine. http://eur-lex.europa.eu/legal-content/EN/TXT/PDF/?uri=CELEX:31964L0432&from=en. Accessed 3 May 2016.
43. Regulation No 1069/2009 of the European Parliament and of the Council laying down health rules as regards animal by-products and derived products not intended for human consumption and repealing Regulation (EC) No 1774/2002 (Animal by-products Regulation). http://eur-lex.europa.eu/LexUriServ/LexUriServ.do?uri=OJ:L:2009:300:0001:0033:EN:PDF. Accessed 3 May 2016.
44. McVicar JW. Quantitative aspects of the transmission of African swine fever. Am J Vet Res. 1984;45:1535–41.
45. Turner C, Burton CH. The inactivation of viruses in pig slurries: a review. Biores Techn. 1997;61:9–20.
46. Penrith ML, Thomson GR, Bastos ADS. African swine fever. In: Coetzer JAW, Tustin RC, editors. Infectious diseases in livestock, vol. 2. 2nd ed. Cape Town: Oxford University Press; 2004. p. 1087–119.
47. Maes D, Van Soom A, Appletant R, Arsenakis I, Nauwynck H. Porcine semen as a vector for transmission of viral pathogens. Theriogenology. 2016;85:27–38.
48. Council Directive 90/429/EEC laying down the animal health requirements applicable to intra-Community trade in and imports of semen of domestic animals of the porcine species. http://eur-lex.europa.eu/legal-content/EN/TXT/PDF/?uri=CELEX:31990L0429&from=en. Accessed 3 May 2016.
49. OIE. African swine fever. In: Terrestrial Animal Health Code. 24th Edition. Paris: Office International des Epizooties; 2015. http://www.oie.int/index.php?id=169&L=0&htmfile=chapitre_asf.htm. Accessed 3 May 2015.
50. Ravaomanana J, Michaud V, Jori F, Andriatsimahavandy A, Roger F, Albina E, Vial L. First detection of African swine fever virus in *Ornithodoros porcinus* in Madagascar and new insights into tick distribution and taxonomy. Parasit Vectors. 2010;3:115.
51. Turner C, Williams SM. Laboratory-scale inactivation of African swine fever virus and swine vesicular disease virus in pig slurry. J Appl Microbiol. 1999;87:148–57. doi:10.1046/j.1365-2672.1999.00802.x.

Glycaemic and insulinemic response to dietary carbohydrates in horses

Christine Brøkner[1*†], Dag Austbø[2†], Jon A. Næsset[2†], Dominique Blache[3†], Knud Erik B. Knudsen[4†], Hanne H. Hansen[5†] and Anne-Helene Tauson[1,2†]

Abstract

Background: Dietary sugar and starch affect plasma glucose and insulin concentrations. Little information is available about the effect of dietary fibre on plasma glucose and insulin concentration. It is hypothesized that different dietary fibre compositions will alter post-prandial glycaemic- and insulinemic index of test meals. The objective was to measure postprandial glucose and insulin concentrations in horses fed meals of different fibre compositions.

Methods: Blood was drawn via jugular vein puncture and the glycaemic and insulinemic index were calculated.

Results: The meal effect on glycaemic and insulinemic response followed the expected pattern, where plasma concentrations increased after feeding and declined after peak concentration. Glycaemic index was 100 (H), 102 (OB), 102 (BB) and 106 (M) and did not differ significantly between meals. Insulinemic index was 100 (H), 140 (OB), 121 (BB) and 125 (M) and did not differ significantly between meals.

Conclusions: In conclusion, meals containing different fibre compositions did not affect the glycaemic- and insulinemic index in horses.

Keywords: Horses, Dietary fibre, Glucose, Insulin

Background

Horses are hindgut fermenting herbivores well adapted to a high carbohydrate diet consisting primarily of Gramineae (e.g. grasses and sedges) and some Leguminosae (e.g. herbaceous legumes), which both are rich in different plant fibre fractions [1]. The microbes of the equine hindgut produce fibre-fermenting enzymes, which are needed to degrade fibrous materials to monosaccharides. The microorganisms and the anaerobic environment of the hindgut prevent complete oxidation of the monosaccharides and instead short chain fatty acids (SCFA) are produced. The acids produced are mainly acetic acid, propionic acid and butyric acid, of which propionic acid is an important contributor to the blood plasma glucose concentration through hepatic gluconeogenesis. A systematic correlation between fibre fractions and hindgut propionic acid production was reported in horses [2], where more S-NCP resulted in higher production of propionic acid. Depending on growth rate, climate and time of harvest, grasses can contain up to 18 % non-structural carbohydrates (NSC; i.e. sugar, fructans and starch) [3].

A glycaemic index of human food was developed to classify sugar and starch containing foods based on their potential to raise post-prandial blood glucose concentrations, which could not be predicted by chemical food analysis [4]. A similar classification is relevant for horses, as starch and sugar digestion and glucose metabolism in the horse is similar as to human. Additionally, horses

*Correspondence: christine.broekner@sund.ku.dk
†All authors contributed equally to this work
[1] Department of Veterinary Clinical and Animal Sciences, Faculty of Health and Medical Sciences, University of Copenhagen, Grønnegaardsvej 3, 1870 Frederiksberg, Denmark
Full list of author information is available at the end of the article

have been shown to suffer some of the same health issues associated with high and fluctuating glucose and insulin concentrations as humans i.e. insulin resistance and obesity [5].

Forages therefore have gluconeogenic properties that contribute to a stable blood plasma glucose concentration. This occurs through either glucose absorption in the small intestine or a continuous supply of glucose through hepatic gluconeogenesis where propionic acid from hindgut fibre fermentation is metabolised into glucose. The objective of the present experiment was to measure postprandial glucose and insulin concentrations in horses fed meals of various carbohydrate compositions. It was hypothesized that the different fibre compositions will alter the post-prandial glycaemic and/or insulinemic index of the test meals.

Methods

Experimental procedure

A 4 × 4 Latin Square design was used to quantify the effect of four test meals on post prandial blood plasma glucose and insulin concentrations. This study was part of a main experiment where the horses were fed 1.6 kg dry matter hay 2½ h after the morning meals.

Within each experimental period, a sequence of 21 days adaptation to the diets was followed by four sampling days. On each of the four sampling days blood was collected from one horse, resulting in four replicates for each diet. On the blood collection day (day 22 through day 25), the horses were fed the test meal at 6 a.m. and given 30 min to finish the meal. The horses were fasted 8 h prior to the test meal.

Animals

Four geldings of Norwegian Cold-blooded Trotter horse (age 5–16 years) with an average body weight of 544 kg and a mean body condition score of 6 [6] were used in the experiment. The horses were housed under the same conditions in individual 3 × 3 m stalls on wood shavings. The horses were cared for according to laws and regulations controlling experimentation on live animals in Norway i.e. the Animal Protection Act of (December 20 1974) and the Animal Protection Ordinance concerning Experiments on Animals (December 15 1996).

Test meals

The composition and intake of carbohydrates of the test meals are shown in Table 1. A detailed description of the chemical composition of the individual ingredients is found in [3]. The test meals consisted of timothy hay (Phleum L.) (H), whole oats (Avena sativa L.) and soaked molassed sugar beet pulp (Beta vulgaris) (Betfor®) (OB), whole barley (*Hordeum vulgare* L.) and soaked Betfor® (BB), commercial muesli feed (Equigard®) (M). The test meals were formulated to provide the same amount of dry matter and to contain a maximum of 0.54 kg sugar and starch, equivalent to 1 g starch and sugar per kg BW per meal per horse.

Table 1 Dietary composition and intake of carbohydrates of the different test meals

	Test meals			
	H	OB	BB	M
Hay, kg DM	1.1			
Oats, kg DM		1.1		
Barley, kg DM			0.8	
Betfor®, kg DM		0.3	0.3	
Equigard®, kg DM				1.7
Feed intake, kg DM	1.1	1.4	1.1	1.7
Total carbohydrate intake, kg				
Sugar	0.12	0.09	0.08	0.27
Starch	–	0.42	0.42	0.08
Total NSP	0.57	0.43	0.26	0.61
-S-NCP	0.02	0.09	0.10	0.19
Fibre				
Dietary fibre	0.70	0.52	0.30	0.75
NDF	0.69	0.42	0.21	0.51

NSP non-starch polysaccharides, *S-NCP* soluble non-cellulosic polysaccharides, *H* Hay, *OB* Oats and Betfor®, *BB* Barley and Barley and Betfor®, *M* Equigard®

Sampling of blood

Blood was drawn via jugular vein puncture into heparinized vacutainer tubes at time 0 before the test meal and again at time (min) 30, 45, 60, 75, 90, 105, 120, 135, 150, 165, 180, 210, 240, 270, 330, 390, 450, 510, 570 post feeding. Immediately after sampling, the tubes were centrifuged at 2016×*g* at 4 °C for 10 min Plasma was harvested and stored in polypropylene micro tubes at −20 °C until analysis.

Chemical analyses of feedstuffs

All feed samples were analysed in duplicate and the obtained mean values reported. Dry matter was determined on original unprocessed feed samples, collected daily in the stall. NDF content with amylase pre-treatment and corrected for ash was analysed by the use of the Fibertec system (Fibertec™ 2010 Auto Fibre Analysis System, Hillerød, Denmark). Starch was analysed by an enzymatic-colorimetric method. Low molecular weight sugars (glucose, fructose and sucrose) were determined by use of two connected enzymatic reactions using hexokinase and glucose-6-phosphate dehydrogenase [3]. Total non-starch polysaccharides (NSP) consist of various fibre fractions of which the soluble non-cellulosic polysaccharides (S-NCP) were determined by gas–liquid chromatography for neutral sugars and by a colorimetric method for uronic acids in three parallel runs. Dietary fibre (DF) was calculated as described in details [3].

Analytical procedures for glucose and insulin

Blood plasma glucose was determined according to standard procedures (Siemens Diagnostics® Clinical Methods for ADVIA 1650). All analyses were performed using an auto-analyser, ADVIA 1650® Chemistry System (Siemens Medical Solutions, Tarrytown, NY 10591, USA). Intra- and inter assay precision were in all instances below 3 % (CV) and 5 %, respectively. The accuracy was within 4 %. Plasma insulin was assayed in duplicate by a double-antibody radioimmunoassay (RIA). The measurements were made using bovine insulin, the first antibody being raised in guinea pigs and the second in goats. All samples were processed in a single assay and the detection limit was 0.4 μU/ml. Six replicates of three control samples containing 2.19, 4.48, and 11.35 μU/ml were included in the assay and were used to estimate the intra-assay coefficients of variation of 5.5, 5.1 and 6.9 %, respectively. The assays were validated for horse: serial dilutions of horse plasma containing high concentrations of insulin produced curves parallel to the standard curve for the actual hormone [7].

Calculations

The glycaemic and insulinemic responses are defined by the increment area under the plasma vs. time curve (above pre-feeding plasma concentration) elicited by a meal. Area under the plasma glucose ($AUC_{glucose}$) and insulin ($AUC_{insulin}$) curve was calculated by the trapezoidal method of numerical integration [4]. Additionally the responses were grouped in time-interval in order to evaluate the dietary effect on glycaemic and insulinemic responses at different time points post-prandial.

The glycaemic (GI) and insulinemic (II) index were calculated according to the following equations:

$$GI = \frac{Area\ under\ 570\ \mathrm{min}\ plasma\ glucose\ curve\ for\ meals(OB, BB, M)}{Area\ under\ 570\ \mathrm{min}\ plasma\ glucose\ curve\ for\ H} \times 100$$

$$II = \frac{Area\ under\ 570\ \mathrm{min}\ plasma\ insulin\ curve\ for\ meals(OB, BB, M)}{Area\ under\ 570\ \mathrm{min}\ plasma\ insulin\ curve\ for\ H} \times 100$$

Statistical analyses

The effect of meals on post-prandial blood glucose and insulin concentrations were statistically evaluated as repeated measurements in a two-way ANOVA by use of the MIXED procedure in SAS. The calculated variables i.e. $AUC_{glucose/insulin}$, GI, II, $Peak_{glucose/insulin}$, Mean Time to Peak ($MTP_{glucose/insulin}$) were the within-subject factors and the between-subjects' factors were Meal and Time interval. Horse was included as random effect. The final model used was:

$$Y_{ij} = \mu + \alpha_i + \beta_j + \varepsilon_{ij}$$

where Y_{ij} is the ijth predicted values, μ is the overall mean, α_i is the fixed effect of test meals (i = H, OB, BB, M), β_j is the fixed Time interval (j = 1, 2, 3, 4, 5) and ε_{ij} is the residual error. Time measurements were aggregated into 5 intervals (1 = 0–60 min, 2 = 60–120 min, 3 = 120–180 min, 4 = 180–330 min and 5 = 330–570 min) to measure the meal effect on calculated variables within each interval using the same model.

Pearson correlation coefficients were calculated for selected traits by use of the CORR procedure in SAS. Results were considered significantly different when $P < 0.05$ and a tendency when $P < 0.10$. The SAS version 9.2 [8] was used for all analyses.

Results

General health

All horses remained healthy throughout the experiment and showed no signs of discomfort due to repeated blood sampling. During adaptation periods, the horses were let out daily for about 3 h on a dirt paddock in groups of four, in order to satisfy their need for social interaction.

Dietary composition and nutrient intake

Composition of meals and intake of carbohydrates are seen in Table 1. None of the meals exceeded the intended upper maximum limit of 540 g sugar and starch in total.

The effect of meals on plasma glucose (Table 2) and insulin (Table 3) concentration was measured and variables calculated. No significant difference was measured between these factors. Time to $peak_{glucose}$ occurred 2–3 h after feeding and was numerically faster for the OB, BB and M meals as compared to the H meal.

Table 2 LSMeans of area under the plasma glucose curve (AUC), LSMean of peak plasma glucose (mmol/L), LSMeans of time to peak plasma glucose (min) and LSMeans of glycaemic index (%) for the different test meals

Test meals	AUC	Peak glucose	Time to glucose peak	GI
H	3101	5.9	206	100
OB	3152	6.3	131	102
BB	3140	6.7	135	102
M	3275	6.4	169	106
SE	166	0.4	40	5.2
P value	>0.10	>0.10	>0.10	>0.10

LSMeans least squares means, *SE* standard error, *H* Hay, *OB* Oats and Betfor®, *BB* Barley and Betfor®, *M* Equigard®

Table 3 LSMeans of area under the plasma insulin curve (AUC), LSMeans of peak plasma insulin (μU/ml), LSMeans of time to peak plasma insulin (min) and LSMeans of insulinemic index (%) for the different test meals

Test meals	AUC	Peak insulin	Time to insulin peak	II
H	6670	15.5	350[a]	100
OB	9296	27.2	105[b]	140
BB	8055	22.9	98[b]	121
M	8334	19.5	188[b]	125
SE	1186	2.8	35	18
P value	>0.10	0.07	<0.01	>0.10

LSMeans least squares means, *SE* standard error, *H* Hay, *OB* Oats and Betfor®, *BB* Barley and Betfor®, *M* Equigard®. Within a column, means without a common superscript [a–b] differ (*P* value < 0.05)

As expected the plasma insulin concentration followed the increase in plasma glucose concentration, however, no significant differences between meals were measured. $Peak_{insulin}$ tended to differ significantly between meals, where the OB and BB meals resulted in the highest insulin concentration followed by the M meal. $Peak_{insulin}$ occurred between 1.5–3 h after feeding of the OB, BB and M meals, which was significantly ($P < 0.01$) faster as compared to the H meal.

A significant effect of meal on plasma glucose and insulin concentration was measured when grouping time into intervals (Table 4). Meals significantly affected plasma insulin concentration 60–120 min post prandial, where the OB meal had the highest concentration followed by the BB, M and H meals. During the same time interval, the glucose concentration remained unaffected by meals. During the 120–180 min interval, insulin concentration was significantly ($P < 0.01$) higher on the M and OB meals as compared to the BB and H meals. The insulin concentration had decreased in the 180–330 min interval; however, it was still significantly ($P = 0.01$) higher than the H meal.

No significant correlation was found between different carbohydrate fractions and glycaemic and insulinemic responses and calculated response variables in the horses.

Discussion

The focus of this study was to measure the postprandial effect of various dietary carbohydrate compositions on blood plasma glucose and insulin concentration in horses. The meal effect on glycaemic and insulinemic response followed the expected pattern, where plasma concentrations increased after feeding and declined after peak concentration in agreement with the 5–6 h [9]. This fluctuation demonstrates an effective down regulation of plasma glucose by insulin [10], which indicates normal regulating pathways in healthy horses [11].

Insulin secretion is a biphasic response. The first phase secretion is rapid and lasts for 3–4 min followed by a second phase, which develops slowly and lasts longer [10]. The first phase secretion most likely resembles the $peak_{insulin}$ response measured after 98–105 min (OB and BB meals) in the present experiment.

Several factors may affect and confound glycaemic and insulinemic responses in horses including rate of intake, meal size and feedstuff combination, absorption and perhaps gastro- intestinal passage rate [9]. No difference between test meals was measured on glycaemic and insulinemic responses in the present experiment. The sugar associated with the OB, BB and M meals was more easily accessible due to spray-on molasses, whereas sugar in hay is imbedded in the cell content [1] and therefore assumed less available for small intestine absorption. Additionally, the OB and BB meals contained pre-caecal digestible starch [2], which together with sugar is absorbed in the small intestine.

The M meal was associated with sugar intake but plasma glucose did not reach the highest level until the 120–180 min interval. This indicates a delayed glucose

Table 4 LSMeans of plasma glucose (GLU, mmol/L) and insulin (INS, μU/ml) concentrations at five different time intervals (min) post prandially for the different test meals

Test meals	Time intervals									
	0–60		60–120		120–180		180–330		330–570	
	GLU	INS	GLU	INS	GLU	INS	GLU	INS	GLU	INS
H	5.3	11.5	5.7	15.1[c]	5.2[b]	10.9[b]	5.3	14.6[b]	5.4	11.3
OB	5.6	15.9	6.0	26.4[a]	5.1[b]	20.6[a]	5.7	17.4[a]	5.2	12.1
BB	5.3	14.6	6.0	20.9[b]	4.7[b]	14.1[b]	5.4	15.8[ab]	5.2	9.9
M	5.8	15.1	6.3	16.4[c]	5.9[a]	19.3[a]	5.9	17.4[a]	5.6	12.2
SE	0.3	2.2	0.3	3.1	0.4	2.1	0.2	2.2	0.2	2.0
P value	>0.1	>0.1	>0.1	<0.01	0.05	<0.01	>0.1	0.01	>0.1	>0.1

LSMeans least squares means, *SE* standard error, *H* Hay, *OB* Oats and Betfor®, *BB* Barley and Betfor®, *M* Equigard®. Within a column, means without a common superscript [a–c] differ (*P* value < 0.05)

and subsequently insulin response perhaps due to slower gastric emptying leading to delayed glucose absorption. In other species diets high in soluble fibres have been shown to increase luminal viscosity [12] and thereby influencing the rate by which glucose is absorbed as well as the apparent insulin production. The viscosity of a product increases with increased molecular weight [13] and the luminal viscosity increases with increased intake of soluble NSP [14]. Caecal pH starts to decrease 3 h post prandially [2] due to starch reaching the hindgut when feeding the same meals as in the present study. This indicates that small intestine starch digestibility and glucose absorption takes place before 180 min post prandially in agreement with the present results. The horses in the present experiment were fed an additional hay meal 2½ h after the morning test meals, which presumably did not have had any negative effect on the post prandial metabolic responses as the small intestine absorption had already occurred. The blood plasma glucose response to all test meals was surprisingly low and resembled roughage only fed horses [15]. The M meal contained higher starch and sugar than the H meal, but less than BB or OB.

The GI and II predict the ranking of the glycaemic and insulinemic potential of different meals in horses. In the present study, the intention was to measure how various carbohydrates including fibre fractions affected the glycaemic and insulinemic responses. It therefore made sense to choose hay as reference when calculating the glycaemic and insulinemic indexes as hay or grass is the natural feed ingredient for horses [1] and then estimate the meal effect on GI and II in horses relative to hay. The method used in horses is not standardised and is therefore associated with errors [9] e.g. various length of the blood sampling interval, which consequently affects the calculation of the area under the glucose and insulin plasma curve. The GI and II are biased by long sampling intervals. It was not possible to determine, whether the effect on plasma glucose concentration was associated with absorption from the small intestine.

Conclusions

Meals with different fibre composition did not affect the glycaemic- and insulinemic index in horses when fed at the levels used in the present experiment.

Authors' contributions

Planning and conducting the practical experiment with the horses (CB, DA, JAN and AHT). The chemical analysis and other analytical work in the lab (CB, KEBK and DB). Statistical analysis and writing the manuscript (CB, HHH and AHT). All authors read and approved the final manuscript.

Author details

[1] Department of Veterinary Clinical and Animal Sciences, Faculty of Health and Medical Sciences, University of Copenhagen, Grønnegaardsvej 3, 1870 Frederiksberg, Denmark. [2] Department of Animal and Aquacultural Sciences, Norwegian University of Life Sciences, Box 5003, 1432 Ås, Norway. [3] School of Animal Biology, Faculty of Natural and Agricultural Sciences, University of Western Australia, 35 Stirling Highway, Crawley, Perth, WA 6009, Australia. [4] Department of Animal Science, Aarhus University, Blichers Allé 20, 8830 Tjele, Denmark. [5] Department of Large Animal Sciences, Faculty of Health and Medical Sciences, University of Copenhagen, Grønnegaardsvej 2, 1870 Frederiksberg, Denmark.

Acknowledgements

The authors would like to acknowledge Mette Henne for technical assistance during the practical part of the experiment and the Danish Directorate for Development for financial support, Nordic Sugar A/S and St. Hippolyt Denmark A/S.

Competing interests

None of the authors of this paper has financial or personal relationship with other people or companies that could inappropriately influence or bias the content of the paper.

Declarations

Publication charges for this article were funded by the research platform Future Animal Health and Welfare at the Swedish University of Agricultural Sciences.

References

1. Van Soest PJ. Nutritional ecology of the ruminants. 2nd ed. Ithaca: Comstock Publishing Associates, a division of Cornell University Press; 1994.
2. Brøkner C, Austbø D, Næsset JA, Bach Knudsen KE, Tauson AH. Equine pre-caecal and total tract digestibility of individual carbohydrate fractions and their effect on caecal pH response. Arch Anim Nutr. 2012;66:490–506.
3. Brøkner C, Bach Knudsen KE, Karaman I, Eybye KL, Tauson AH. Chemical and physicochemical characterisation of various horse feed ingredients. Anim Feed Sci Technol. 2012;177:86–97.
4. Wolever TMS, Jenkins DJA, Jenkins AL, Josse RG. The glycemic index: methodology and clinical implications. Am J Clin Nutr. 1991;54:846–54.
5. Rodiek AV, Stull CL. Glycemic index of ten common horse feeds. J Equine Vet Sci. 2007;27:205–11.
6. Henneke DR, Potter GD, Krieder JL, Yeates BF. Relationship between condition score, physical measurements and body fat percentage in mares. Equine Vet J. 1983;15:371–2.
7. Jensen RB, Austbø D, Blache D, Bach Knudsen KE, Tauson AH. The effect of feeding barley or hay alone or in combination with sugar beet pulp on the metabolic responses in plasma and caecum of horses. Anim Feed Sci Technol. 2016;214:53–65.
8. SAS Institute Inc. SAS/STAT user's guide, version 9.2. Cary: SAS Institute Inc.; 2008.
9. Bailey SR, Bamford NJ. Metabolic responses of horses and ponies to high and low glycaemic feeds: implications for laminitis. Anim Prod Sci. 2013;53:1182–7.
10. Schmidt SL, Hickey MS. Regulation of insulin action by diet and exercise. J Equine Vet Sci. 2009;29:274–84.
11. Frank N. Insulin resistance in horses. AAEP Proc Endocrinol. 2006;52:51–4.
12. Serena A, Jørgensen H, Bach Knudsen KE. Nutritional value of co-products from vegetable food industry. In: Wiseman J, Varley MA, McOrist S, Kemp B, editors. Paradigms in pig science. Nottingham: Nottingham University Press; 2007. p. 473–91.
13. Tosh MS, Wood PJ, Wang Q, Weisz J. Structural characteristics and rheological properties of partially hydrolyzed oat b-glucan: the effects of molecular weight and hydrolysis method. Carbohyd Polym. 2004;55:425–36.
14. Bach Knudsen KE, Lærke HL, Hedemann MS. The role of fibre in piglet gut health. In: Taulor-Pickard JA, Spring T, editors. Gut efficiency; the key ingredient in pig and poultry production. Wageningen: Wageningen Academic Publishers; 2008. p. 65–95.
15. Borgia L, Valberg S, McCue M, Watts K, Pagan J. Glycaemic and insulinaemic responses to feeding hay with different non-structural carbohydrate content in control and polysaccharide storage myopathy-affected horses. J Anim Physiol Anim Nutr. 2011;95:798–807.

Prevalence of subclinical mastitis in Finnish dairy cows: changes during recent decades and impact of cow and herd factors

Heidi Hiitiö[1], Johanna Vakkamäki[1*], Heli Simojoki[1], Tiina Autio[2], Jouni Junnila[3], Sinikka Pelkonen[2] and Satu Pyörälä[1]

Abstract

Background: The dairy industry has undergone substantial structural changes as intensive farming has developed during recent decades. Mastitis continues to be the most common production disease of dairy cows. Nationwide surveys of mastitis prevalence are useful in monitoring udder health of dairy herds and to study the impact of structural changes on the dairy industry. This survey on bovine subclinical mastitis was the first based on cow composite milk somatic cell count (SCC) data from the Finnish national health monitoring and milk recording database. A cow with composite milk SCC ≥200,000 cells/ml in at least one of the four test milkings during the year was considered to have subclinical mastitis and a cow with composite milk SCC ≥200,000 cells/ml in three or in all four test milkings during the year to have chronic subclinical mastitis. The aim of the study was to determine the prevalence of subclinical mastitis and chronic subclinical mastitis in Finland in 1991, 2001 and 2010 and to investigate cow and herd factors associated with elevated SCC.

Results: Prevalence of subclinical mastitis in Finland decreased over recent decades from 22.3% (1991) and 20.1% (2001) to 19.0% (2010). Prevalence of chronic subclinical mastitis was 20.4% in 1991, 15.5% in 2001 and 16.1% in 2010. The most significant cow and herd factors associated with subclinical mastitis or high milk SCC were increasing parity, Holstein breed, free-stalls with an automatic milking system and organic production. Milk SCC were highest from July to September. Main factors associated with chronic mastitis were increasing parity and Holstein breed.

Conclusions: Prevalence of subclinical mastitis in Finland decreased over recent decades, the greatest change taking place during the first decade of the study. Prevalence of chronic subclinical mastitis significantly decreased from 1991. The most significant factors associated with both types of mastitis were increasing parity and Holstein breed, and for subclinical mastitis also free-stalls with automatic milking. National surveys on mastitis prevalence should be carried out at regular intervals to monitor udder health of dairy cows and to study the impact of the ongoing structural changes in the dairy industry to enable interventions related to udder health to be made when needed.

Keywords: Prevalence, Bovine, Subclinical mastitis, SCC, Chronic subclinical mastitis

Background

The dairy industry has undergone structural changes during recent decades in many countries as the number of dairy herds has decreased but herd size substantially increased [1–3]. Simultaneously barn types and milking systems have changed, but nonetheless mastitis continues to be the most common and costly production disease of dairy cows [4]. In Finland, herd size and average milk yield have increased, while the number of dairy cows has declined [2]. The proportion of free-stalls has increased rapidly, especially those with automatic milking systems (AMS). The number of stalls with AMS (with one or more milking robots) increased from 0 in 1991 to near 600 in 2010 and continues to increase (currently about

*Correspondence: johanna.vakkamaki@helsinki.fi
[1] Department of Production Animal Medicine, Faculty of Veterinary Medicine, University of Helsinki, Paroninkuja 20, 04920 Saarentaus, Finland
Full list of author information is available at the end of the article

950, personal communication, Esa Manninen, Valio Ltd., January 2016). Larger herds kept in free-stalls instead of tie-stalls, in addition to new milking technology, represent challenges for udder health management and may increase the risk for high milk somatic cell counts (SCC), as previously recognized [5, 6]. Up-to-date information on milk SCC and mastitis prevalence, as well as on factors affecting them, are useful to increase the efficiency of udder health management. Knowledge of prevalence trends provides feedback on control measures taken and improves guidance for future strategies.

The Finnish national health monitoring and milk recording system of dairy herds was initiated in the late 1970s and was fully constituted in 1982 [7]. Finland has a long history of nationally organized mastitis control programs, which have included regular surveys on mastitis prevalence [8–11]. Finnish prevalence studies published to date have been based on quarter milk samples and have focused on bacteriology, using quarter milk SCC ≥300,000 cells/ml of milk at least in one quarter of the cow to define mastitis. According to the studies, mastitis prevalence in Finland decreased from 47.8% (1988) to 37.8% (1995) [10]. In the most recent survey (2001), mastitis prevalence was 30.6% [11]. All previous surveys cited here use the general term mastitis, but based on the accepted definitions the focus has been on subclinical mastitis (SCM).

For herds contributing data to the Finnish national health monitoring and milk recording system, milk characteristics, including cow composite SCC for every lactating cow of each herd, have been recorded at least four times a year. Currently, the data cover approximately 81% of Finnish dairy cows. To date, the Finnish national health monitoring and milk recording database has been exploited only for udder health management on farms, but not comprehensively at the national level. The aim of this study was to determine the prevalence of SCM and chronic subclinical mastitis (CSCM) in Finland in 1991, 2001 and 2010 by analyzing national cow composite SCC data and using a threshold of ≥200,000 cells/ml. Cow and herd factors affecting SCC and their associations with SCM and CSCM were studied.

Methods

Data collection

Somatic cell counts data were analyzed from the Finnish national health monitoring and milk recording database from 1991 (cows, n = 122,403, herds, n = 20,346), 2001 (cows, n = 337,335, herds, n = 13,749) and 2010 (cows, n = 273,012, herds, n = 7640). The proportion of herds in the system increased from 62% in 1991 to 81% 2010 (ProAgria Agricultural processing center). Sampling herds associated with the Finnish national health monitoring and milk recording database is carried out at least five times a year per herd and includes all lactating cows at least 2 days in milk (DIM). All samples were cow composite samples. In the study, the first sample result for each cow from each quartile (January–March, April–June, July–September, October–December) was selected (maximum of four results per cow) to maximize the number of cows, including from 1991, when sampling was not as frequent as now. If the cow was culled or otherwise removed from the herd or dried-off, those results available for the year were included.

Samples were collected in 30 ml plastic tubes with preservative (bronopol), using specific sampling devices during milking, or by automatic sampling devices on milking robots. The samples were sent to pre-assigned regional laboratories and SCC was determined with a fluoro-optical method using Fossomatic™ FC (FOSS Ltd., Hillerød, Denmark). Guidelines for sampling were similar over the years, but sampling has become automated in free-stalls with AMS. The gathered data included information for individual cows—breed, age, parity, cow composite SCC and total quantity of milk produced during the first 305 days lactation period for each cow. Herd level information was provided for each cow: production type, type of stall, herd size, milking system, and average annual milk SCC and milk yield of the herd (Table 1).

Cows with a cow composite milk SCC of ≥200,000 cells/ml in at least one of the four test milkings for the year were defined as having subclinical mastitis [13]. SCM refers to udder inflammation (increased milk SCC) that continues for some period of time but ceases by the next sampling. Cows with a cow composite milk SCC ≥200,000 cells/ml in three or all four test milkings during the year were recognized as having chronic subclinical mastitis. CSCM refers to udder inflammation (increased milk SCC) that continues for a long period of time. Only cows with test results from every quartile of the year were included in the analyses of CSCM (n = 100,261 cows in 1991, 220,354 in 2001 and 180,557 in 2010).

Descriptive analysis

First, the data were checked and evaluated for outliers and missing values (Microsoft Office, Excel 2010). The most frequent error was a letter or null instead of a consistent value. For some proportion of cows all information was not available, and the number of these cows for each variable is shown in the descriptive data (Tables 2, 3). The number and proportion of the cows with SCM were calculated for the year, annual quartile and for the following subgroups: parity (1 to ≥4), breed (Ayrshire

Table 1 Description of the variables used in the study

Analysis	Variable	Description of the variable
Prevalence of SCM (subclinical mastitis) and CSCM (chronic subclinical mastitis)		
	Breed	Holstein, Ayrshire, Other. Group "other breeds" includes Finncattle, Jerseys and their crossbreds and single cows of some other breeds
	Herd size	Average herd size *(continuous variable)*. The average herd size is calculated as follows: (Days in feeding$_{cow1}$ [a] + Days in feeding $_{cow2}$....) divided by 365 days (or 366 days if leap year) i.e. the total amount of days within the year of recording
	Milk yield	305 days milk yield from each cow primiparous period *(continuous variable)*
	Parity	Parity 1 to ≥4 *(categorical variable)*
	Production type	Organic, conventional
	Quartile[b]	Quartile of the year—Jan–Mar, Apr–Jun, Jul–Sept, Oct–Dec
	Region	Geographical region of Finland—South, West, North, East. Every herd belonged to one of the 22 regional ProAgria Agricultural units in study years of 1991, 2001 and 2010. These units were divided according to province borders (in 2012) into four geographic regions
	Type of the stall[c]	Tie-stall, free-stall, free-stall with AMS (automatic milking system)
	Year	Year of the data recording—1991, 2001, 2010
SCC		
Cow level	Breed	Holstein, Ayrshire, Other. Group "other breeds" includes Finncattle, Jerseys and their crossbreds and single cows of some other breeds
	Herd size	Average herd size *(continuous variable)*. The average herd size was calculated as follows: (Days in feeding$_{cow1}$ [a] + Days in feeding$_{cow2}$....) divided by 365 days (or 366 days if leap year) i.e. the total amount of days within the year of recording
	Milk yield	305 days milk yield from the first lactation period *(continuous variable)*
	Parity	Parity 1 to ≥4 *(continuous variable)*
	Production type	Organic, conventional
	Quartile	Quartile of the year—Jan–Mar, Apr–Jun, Jul–Sept, Oct–Dec
	Region	Geographical region of Finland—South, West, North, East. Every herd belonged to one of the 22 regional ProAgria Agricultural units in study years of 1991, 2001 and 2010. These units were divided according to province borders (in 2012) into four geographic regions
	Type of stall[b]	Tie-stall, free-stall, free-stall with AMS (automatic milking system)
	Year	Year of the data recording—1991, 2001, 2010
Herd level	Herd size	Average herd size *(continuous variable)*. The average herd size was calculated as follows: (Days in feeding[a] $_{cow1}$ + Days in feeding$_{cow2}$....) divided by 365 days (or 366 days if leap year) i.e. the total amount of days within the year of recording
	Herd milk yield	Average annual milk yield of the herd *(continuous variable)*. Milk yield of the herd was calculated as follows: (Milk kg of the year$_{cow\ 1}$ + Milk kg of the year$_{cow\ 2}$ + Milk kg of the year$_{cow\ 3}$ + Milk kg of the year cow 4..)/ average herd size
	Average parity, herd	Average parity of the cows in the herd *(continuous)*
	Region	Geographical region of Finland—South, West, North, East. Every herd belonged to one of the 22 regional ProAgria Agricultural units in study years of 1991, 2001 and 2010. These units were divided according province borders (in 2012) into four geographic regions
	Type of the stall[b]	Tie-stall, free-stall, free-stall with AMS (automatic milking system)
	Year	Year of the data recording—1991, 2001 and 2010

[a] Recording of feeding days starts from the first calving or the date that the cow enters the herd and ends when it is culled or otherwise removed from the herd. (Personal communication, specialist Juho Kyntäjä, ProAgria Agricultural processing center, August 2015)

[b] Not included in CSCM model

[c] Data available only for years 2001 and 2010

also known as Nordic Red, Holstein and others), type of the stall (tie-stall, free-stall or free-stall with AMS), herd size (<20, 20–60, > 60 cows), average annual milk yield of the herd (<7500, 7500–9500 and > 9500 kg), geographical region of Finland (South, West, North, East) and production type (organic or conventional). The numbers of Finncattle, Jerseys and other breeds were so low that they were grouped together as 'other breeds`. The cows with CSCM were assessed accordingly, except for annual quartile.

Table 2 Descriptive data of cows with subclinical mastitis in Finland in 1991, 2001 and 2010

	Year					
	1991		2001		2010	
	n, cows[a]	%, cows with SCM[b]	n, cows[a]	%, cows with SCM[b]	n, cows[a]	%, cows with SCM[b]
Parity						
1	24,791	12.2	104,995	16.2	85,532	14.3
2	25,896	14.5	89,197	17.1	75,156	15.4
3	25,737	23.8	61,749	22.2	52,769	21.8
4	19,642	28.6	37,919	25.4	31,082	25.9
5	11,539	31.9	20,405	27.4	15,833	28.2
6	6235	35.0	10,239	27.6	7110	29.3
7	3150	36.4	4669	30.6	3005	31.9
8	1544	37.7	2034	29.8	1329	31.2
≥9	1224	40.0	1495	31.7	1196	35.5
n/a[d]	2645		4633		0	
Breed						
Ayrshire	99,070	21.4	247,736	19.3	175,583	18.0
Holstein	21,776	26.3	85,704	22.3	93,644	20.8
Others[c]	1557	26.9	3872	21.7	3522	18.9
n/a[d]	0		23		263	
Type of the stall						
Tie-stall	0	0	82,688	20.5	108,824	18.7
Free-stall	0	0	9322	21.1	49,837	20.9
Free-stall (AMS)	0	0	0[e]	0[e]	21,712	22.6
N/a[d]	122,403		245,325		92,639	
Herd size, number of cows						
<20	99,832	22.0	150,611	19.8	49,446	17.5
20–60	21,504	23.6	174,433	20.1	158,661	18.6
>60	584	27.4	7532	23.5	59,430	21.4
n/a[d]	483		4759		5475	
Average milk yield (kg/year/herd)						
<7500	109,083	22.8	116,053	22.8	26,109	23.8
7500–9500	13,048	18.7	195,811	19.0	161,262	19.8
>9500	243	15.2	25,361	16.6	85,618	16.5
n/a[d]	29		110		23	
Production type						
Organic	15	13.3	6300	22.7	4300	22.2
Conventional	122,386	22.3	331,035	20.1	268,450	18.9
n/a[d]	2		0		262	
Total	122,403	22.3	337,335	20.1	273,012	19.0

[a] Total number of the cows of the study year

[b] Cows with a composite milk SCC ≥200,000 cells/ml in at least one of the four test milkings of the year

[c] Including Finncattle, Jerseys and other breeds

[d] Information not available

[e] Three AMS barns in 2001 were excluded from statistical calculations

Statistical methods

The associations of the SCC of the cows and explanatory factors were analyzed with linear mixed models. Logarithmic transformation was used to normalize the SCC-distribution, thus LnSCC was used as the response variable in the model. The factors (Table 1) were first modeled separately, so that only the year, quartile, the defined factor and the interaction between the factor and

Table 3 Descriptive data of cows with chronic subclinical mastitis in Finland in 1991, 2001 and 2010

	Year					
	1991		2001		2010	
	n, cows[a]	%, cows with CSCM[b]	n, cows[a]	%, cows with CSCM[b]	n, cows[a]	%, cows with CSCM[b]
Parity						
1	9676	7.8	41,444	11.3	39,148	10.5
2	24,582	12.2	73,130	13.3	59,752	13.0
3	24,041	20.3	47,476	16.7	39,401	18.2
4	18,206	25.4	27,959	19.3	22,286	21.9
5	10,538	29.5	14,563	20.9	11,136	24.2
6	5699	31.1	7190	21.6	4934	26.0
7	2857	32.6	3233	22.8	2112	27.9
8	1387	35.8	1421	22.4	886	26.1
≥9	1101	35.9	1063	25.3	843	33.9
N/a[d]	2174		2875		59	
Breed						
Ayrshire	81,185	19.1	162,484	14.5	116,443	14.6
Holstein	17,796	25.9	55,415	18.6	61,879	18.8
Others[c]	1280	24.4	2455	15.8	2235	15.3
N/a[d]	0		0		0	
Type of the stall						
Tie-stall	0	0	74,974	15.0	99,417	14.8
Free-stall	0	0	8444	16.1	45,098	16.6
Free-stall (AMS)	0	0	0[e]	0[e]	19,595	21.3
N/a[d]	100,261		136,936		16,447	
Herd size, cows						
<20	81,533	19.8	98,895	15.1	33,118	14.0
20–60	17,838	22.4	113,134	15.6	105,203	15.4
>60	508	32.1	4847	19.7	38,738	19.8
N/a[d]	382		3478		3498	
Average milk yield (kg/year/herd)						
<7500	89,100	20.9	73,763	18.0	14,635	19.5
7500–9500	10,954	16.5	129,343	14.4	105,937	16.4
>9500	207	15.5	17,248	13.1	59,985	14.6
N/a[d]	0		0		0	
Production type						
Organic	14	14.3	4028	18.8	2933	18.4
Conventional	100,247	20.4	216,326	15.5	177,624	16.0
N/a[d]	0		0		0	
Total	100,261	10.4	220,354	15.5	180,557	16.1

[a] Total number of the cows of the study year

[b] Cows with a composite milk SCC ≥200,000 cells/ml in three or all four of the test milkings of the year

[c] Including Finncattle, Jerseys and other breeds

[d] Information was not included to the original recording (missing value)

[e] Three AMS barns in 2001 were excluded from statistical calculations

year were included in the model as fixed factors, herd as a random effect and cow as a subject effect. Secondly, a multivariable mixed effects linear mixed model was fitted, where all statistically significant explanatory factors and their significant interactions with year were included in the same model. The statistical significance was determined based on Type III tests for fixed effects. This was done to assess all the factors simultaneously and to exclude possible confounding effects. The effects of the explanatory variables were quantified with least square means and

99.9% confidence limits (CL) (within and between group), calculated from the final multivariable model.

The effects of the variables presented in Table 1 on LnSCC of the herd were analyzed using ANOVA models. The fitted univariable models included the year, the defined factor and the interaction term of the factor and year as fixed factors. In addition, all significant explanatory factors were included in a multivariable ANOVA. The effects of the explanatory variables were quantified with least square means and 99% CL, calculated from the final multivariable model.

Effects of the same explanatory factors (Table 1) on the proportion of cows with SCC ≥200,000 cells/ml were studied with mixed effects logistic regression models, using data from all four quartiles. A similar analysis strategy (univariable and multivariable models), and the same fixed and random effects, were included as described for the mixed effects linear regression models. The statistical significance was determined based on Type III tests for fixed effects.

Similar mixed effects logistic regression models were constructed for the proportion of cows with CSCM. Explanatory factors (Table 1) were included in the model based on data from the first quartile. The definition of CSCM prohibits the possibility of studying effects of season, thus no seasonal effects were included in the models. Differences among the groups were quantified with odds ratios (OR) and their 99.9% CL.

Two different definitions of statistical significance were used. For herd level analyses, a probability level of <0.01 was considered statistically significant. In analyses based on individual cows, $p < 0.001$ was considered statistically significant. The significance limits were kept low because the datasets were large (they included data for most dairy cows in Finland). This led to very precise estimations of the effects and therefore the usual limits (e.g. $p < 0.05$) were not suitable for applying to the results. All p-values were 2-sided and not adjusted for multiple testing. Some of the investigated factors were only measured from the 2001 and 2010 data (see Table 1). Thus, the final statistical models were constructed both for the full data and for a subset of the data including only those for 2001 and 2010. The results of the models including years 2001 and 2010 are provided in the supplementary data.

All statistical analyses were done using SAS System for Windows, version 9.3 (SAS Institute Inc., Cary, NC, USA).

Results

The total number of cows included in the study and numbers in different subgroups for each study year, in addition to the proportion of cows with SCM, are presented in Table 2. The number of cows included in the CSCM investigation and the proportion (%) of cows with CSCM are presented in Table 3. The figures are given in total and in subgroups (Table 3).

Prevalence of SCM and associated factors

In 1991, the prevalence SCM (22.3%) was higher than in 2001 (20.1%) and in 2010 (19.0%, Fig. 1). The risk for SCM increased with increasing parity of the cow (Fig. 2), but in every parity group odds ratio (OR) for SCM was lower in 2010 than in 2001. Ayrshire cows, among other breeds, had a lower OR for SCM than Holsteins (Fig. 2). The milk yield from the first 305 days lactation for the primiparous cow did not affect the risk for SCM and was excluded from the final model.

According to the final model of logistic regression analyses, herd size had only a minimal increasing effect on SCM (Fig. 2). In 2001 and 2010 data, tie-stalls and free-stalls had lower OR for SCM than free-stalls with AMS (Additional file 1).

The risk for SCM was lower in East Finland compared with West (OR 0.863, CL 0.851–0.875) and South (OR 0.903, CL 0.887–0.918) and in North Finland compared with West (OR 0.860, CL 0.849–0.877) and South (OR 0.900, CL 0.886–0.913). The risk for SCM was lower during the first quartile, from January to March than during the other quartiles (Fig. 2). The highest risk for SCM was during July–September compared with the three other quartiles (Fig. 2).

Prevalence of CSCM and associated factors

The prevalence of CSCM was higher in 1991 (20.4%) than in 2001 (15.5%) and in 2010 (16.1%, Figs. 1, 3). The risk for CSCM in 2001 was higher than in 2010 (Fig. 3), despite that the proportion of cows with CSCM was

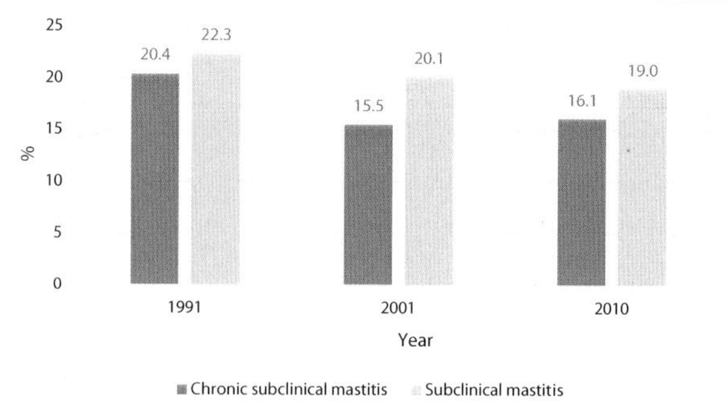

Fig. 1 Prevalence of subclinical mastitis (SCM) and chronic subclinical mastitis (CSCM) in years 1991, 2001 and 2010. Prevalence of subclinical mastitis (SCM) and chronic subclinical mastitis (CSCM) of dairy cows in the Finnish national health monitoring and milk recording system in 1991 (SCM n = 27,296 and CSCM n = 10,427), 2001 (SCM n = 67,804 and CSCM n = 34,155) and 2010 (SCM n = 51,872 and CSCM n = 29,070). A cow was assumed to have SCM in the study if it had a composite milk SCC ≥200,000 cells/ml in at least one of the four test milkings for each study year. A cow was assumed to have CSCM if it had a composite milk SCC ≥200,000 cells/ml in three or all four test milkings during the study year

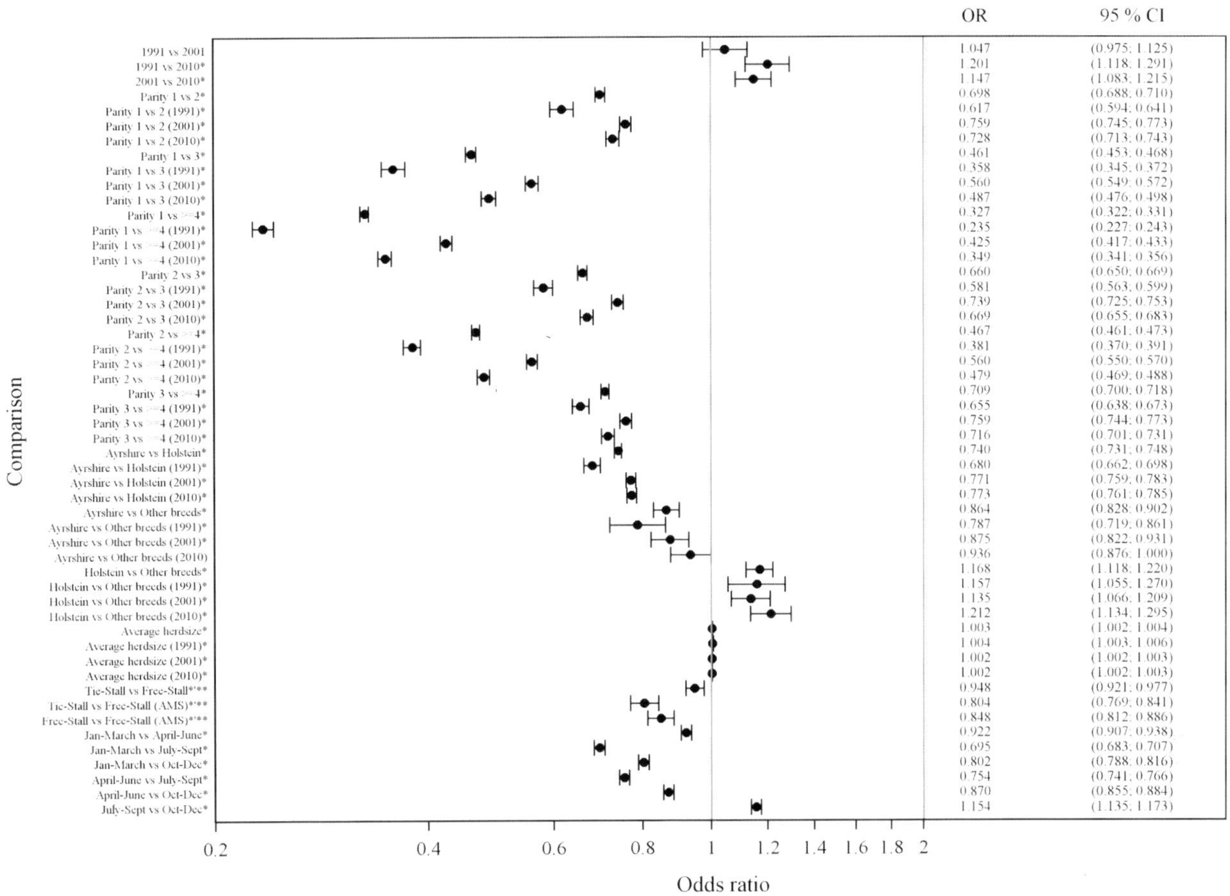

Fig. 2 Comparison of the impact of different factors on the prevalence of subclinical mastitis (SCM). Mixed effects logistic regression model of SCM and related factors. SCM was defined as cow composite milk SCC ≥200,000 cells/ml in one test milking of the year (observations used 2,050,362). Interactions between years and different variables are also presented. Results of the effect of different regions of Finland are described in the text. *OR* odds ratio, *95% CL* confidence limit. *Statistically significant. **Type of stall estimations only from years 2001 and 2010

slightly lower in 2001 compared with 2010. The OR for CSCM increased with increasing parity (Fig. 3). The effect of breed on CSCM was similar as on SCM: Ayrshire cows had lower OR for CSCM than Holstein cows (Fig. 3). Differences in ORs between these two breeds decreased over the two decades.

Herd size had only a minor increasing effect on CSCM (Fig. 3). The effect of different stall-types on the risk of having CSCM was similar than with SCM (Fig. 3). The regional associations with CSCM were included in the same mixed effects logistic regression model (Fig. 3). The OR for CSCM was lower in West compared with East (OR 0.872, CL 0.828–0.917) and North (OR 0.815, CL 0.783–0.847) of Finland.

SCC results at cow level

Average cow composite milk SCC values with standard deviations are presented in Table 4, grouped by breed, stall-type, production type and region. Average arithmetic milk SCC decreased from 209,200 cells/ml in 1991 to 192,500 cells/ml in 2001 and 192,000 cells/ml in 2010 (Table 4).

Average cow SCC values were lowest in primipara and increased with increasing parity (Table 5). Milk SCC of cows in each parity group increased during the study period (Table 5). Ayrshire cows had the lowest SCC and Holsteins the highest (Table 5), but SCC of all breed groups decreased from 2001 (Table 5).

Effect of the stall type was studied only in 2001 and 2010 because the number of free-stalls was marginal in 1991 (Additional file 2). Cows in tie stalls had the lowest SCC estimates (77.2; CI 76.2–78.1) and cows in free stalls with AMS the highest (94.5; CI 93.0–95.9); estimates for cows in free stalls with milking parlors were between the two other stall types (80.3; CI 79.3–81.4; Additional file 2).

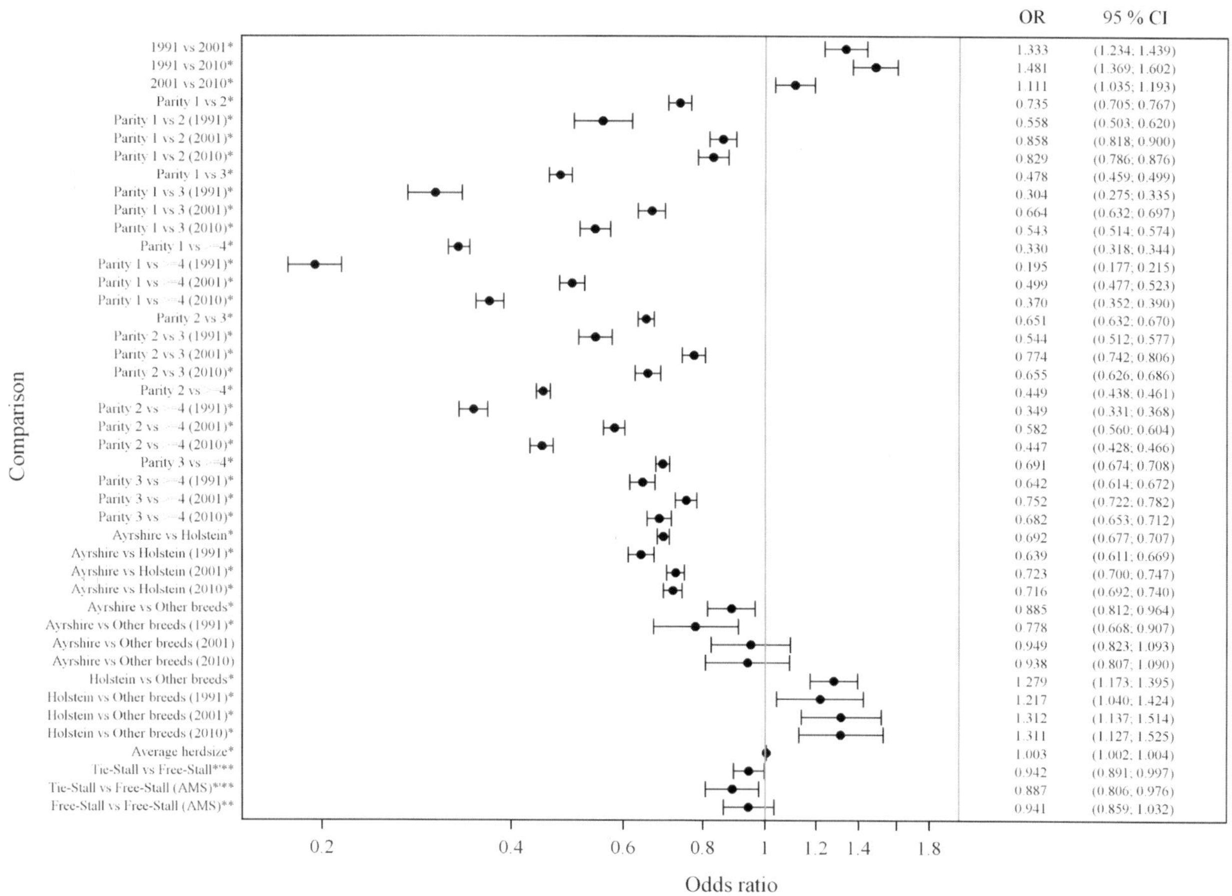

Fig. 3 Comparison of the impact of different factors on the prevalence of chronic subclinical mastitis (CSCM). Mixed effects logistic regression model of CSCM and related factors. CSCM was defined as cow composite milk SCC ≥200,000 cells/ml in three or four test milkings of the year (observations used 499,376). Interactions between years and different variables are also presented. Results of the effect of different regions of Finland are described in the text. *OR* odds ratio, *95% CL* confidence limit. *Statistically significant. **Type of stall estimations only from years 2001 and 2010

Cows in organic herds had higher SCC compared with cows in conventional production in years 2001 and 2010 (Additional file 2).

Milk yield of the first 305 days lactation period of the cow did not affect milk SCC and was excluded from the final model. The overall improvement of the cow composite milk SCC during the studied years can be calculated by summarizing the estimates. For example, a primiparous cow of Ayrshire breed from an organic herd in the West of Finland would have 26,400 cells/ml lower milk SCC in 2010 than in 1991. Similarly, a Holstein cow in her 4th lactation from a conventional herd in the West of Finland would have 14,900 cells/ml lower milk SCC in 2010 than in 1991.

SCC results on herd level

Average cow composite milk SCC of dairy herds in Finland was higher in 1991 than in 2001 and 2010 (Table 6). For every 100 kg of milk produced in the herd, a slight increase in the average milk SCC was noted and this increase was highest in 2010 (Table 6).

Average cow composite milk SCC for the herd increased with increasing herd size. According to our estimates, every cow added to the herd would increase milk SCC of the herd by approximately 1000 cells/ml. The effect of the increasing number of cows in the herd was smaller in 2010 than in 1991 or 2001 (Table 6).

Free-stall herds with or without AMS were associated with a higher average milk SCC than tie-stall herds (Additional file 3). Location of the herd in the South or West of Finland was also associated with a higher average milk SCC of the herd. Average parity of the herd did not affect milk SCC of the herd in the aggregated data, but average parity data only from 2001 and 2010 had a small effect (Additional file 3).

Table 4 Cow composite milk somatic cell count (SCC) (mean, SD) and related factors in Finland in 1991, 2001 and 2010

	1991		2001		2010	
	SCC x 10^3	SD	SCC x 10^3	SD	SCC x 10^3	SD
Ayrshire	201.8	425.3	186.6	467.8	182.0	472.8
Holstein	240.5	452.5	209.3	483.4	210.7	506.7
Others[a]	245.8	488.8	208.2	521.8	199.8	522.9
Tie-stall	n/a[b]	n/a[b]	186.5	457.3	179.1	450.9
Free-stall	n/a[b]	n/a[2]	197.8	488.1	200.2	499.2
Free-stall (AMS)	n/a[b]	n/a[b]	n/a[b]	n/a[b]	238.8	599.4
Organic production	n/a[b]	n/a[b]	n/a[b]	n/a[b]	213.9	539.9
Conventional production	209.2	431.4	192.0	471.0	191.7	484.5
South	217.9	460.6	206.6	510.9	204.5	526.4
West	219.8	456.0	206.2	508.4	200.2	499.8
East	194.9	393.5	177.7	425.1	180.4	455.2
North	202.6	411.7	178.0	432.2	182.9	463.4
Total	209.2	431.4	192.5	472.5	192.0	485.5

1991 n = 122,403, 2001 n = 337,335 and 2010 n = 273, 012

[a] Including Finncattle, Jerseys and other breeds

[b] Information not available

Table 5 Estimated effects of different factors on cow composite milk SCC (somatic cell count) in Finland

Factor				1991			2001			2010		
	99.9% CI			99.9% CI			99.9% CI			99.9% CI		
	Estimate	Lower	Upper	Estimate	Lower	Upper	Estimate	Lower	Upper	Estimate	Lower	Upper
Year				72.4	61.1	85.8	82.1	81.1	83.1	74.7	73.7	75.8
Number of parity												
1	53.1	50.1	56.2	46.1	38.9	54.7	53.3	52.5	54.1	73.8	72.9	74.7
2	66.4	62.7	70.3	61.2	51.7	72.6	64.8	63.9	65.7	93.0	91.8	94.2
3	88.3	83.4	93.5	86.4	72.8	102.4	85.6	84.3	86.9	112.6	95.0	133.6
≥4	108.9	102.9	115.3	60.9	60.1	61.7	108.9	107.5	110.4	105.3	103.8	106.9
Breed												
Ayrshire	69.3	65.4	73.3	63.8	53.8	75.6	76.1	75.3	76.8	68.5	67.7	69.3
Holstein	86.0	81.2	91.0	82.5	69.6	97.8	91.8	90.9	92.8	83.9	82.8	84.9
Other breeds	74.6	70.3	79.2	72.2	60.7	85.8	79.3	77.2	81.4	72.6	70.6	74.6
Type of production												
Organic production	74.2	66.2	83.1	61.3	43.6	86.0	87.1	85.3	88.8	76.4	74.7	78.3
Conventional production	78.5	78.0	79.0	85.6	84.3	86.8	77.5	76.8	78.1	73.0	72.4	73.7
Region												
East	72.6	68.5	76.8	67.0	56.5	79.4	79.7	78.7	80.8	71.6	70.5	72.6
North	72.3	68.3	76.5	72.2	60.9	85.6	75.0	74.0	76.0	69.8	68.8	70.8
South	78.9	74.5	83.6	73.9	62.4	87.7	85.8	84.6	87.0	77.4	76.2	78.6
West	81.9	77.3	86.7	76.9	64.8	91.1	88.6	87.5	89.8	80.5	79.4	81.7

The estimated effects (multivariate ANOVA model) of the different pre-determined factors on composite milk SCC of cows included in the Finnish National health monitoring and milk recording system in 1991, 2001 and 2010 (observations used 2,050,362). Interactions between years and variables are presented separately in the columns. All the included factors were tested statistically significant with Type III tests for fixed effects

Discussion

Prevalence of SCM

The prevalence of SCM based on cow composite milk SCC has decreased in Finland during the past two decades, in particular during the first decade from 1991 to 2001. This may be due to a long-term national strategy to manage mastitis. Indexes related to udder health were introduced in the breeding programs of dairy cows. A

Table 6 Estimated effects of different factors on average herd milk SCC (somatic cell count) in Finland

Comparison	99.9% CI			p value
	Estimate	Lower	Upper	
1991 vs. 2001	1.246	1.121	1.385	<0.001
1991 vs. 2010	1.630	1.437	1.849	<0.001
2001 vs. 2010	1.308	1.147	1.492	<0.001
Herd milk yield (100 kg)	0.990	0.989	0.990	<0.001
Herd milk yield (100 kg, 1991)	0.987	0.986	0.988	<0.001
Herd milk yield (100 kg, 2001)	0.989	0.988	0.990	<0.001
Herd milk yield (100 kg, 2010)	0.993	0.992	0.994	<0.001
Average herd size	1.007	1.006	1.008	<0.001
Average herd size (1991)	1.010	1.008	1.012	<0.001
Average herd size (2001)	1.007	1.006	1.009	<0.001
Average herd size (2010)	1.004	1.003	1.005	<0.001
South vs. West	1.011	0.987	1.035	0.236
South vs. North	1.118	1.089	1.148	<0.001
South vs. East	1.100	1.074	1.127	<0.001
West vs. North	1.106	1.083	1.129	<0.001
West vs. East	1.088	1.069	1.108	<0.001
North vs. East	0.984	0.964	1.005	0.051

The estimated effects (multivariate ANO VA model) of the dif ferent pre-determined factors on the average milk SCC of herds included in the Finnish national health monitoring and milk recording system in 1991, 2001 and 2010 (observations used 41,503). Interactions between years and variables are presented on separate lines. All the included factors were tested statistically significant with Type III tests for fixed effects

working group of the Finnish Ministry of Agriculture and Forestry established during the late 1980s initiated this activity. Advisory services and training were provided to dairy farmers, but probably the most effective measure was implementing quality-based milk pricing. Consequently, prevalence of mastitis decreased during the next 20 years as seen in the successive national mastitis surveys [8–11]. At the same time, consumption of antibiotic intramammary products has decreased, which indicates that combatting SCM has not relied on antibiotic treatments [12].

Surveys are not directly comparable because methods and definitions differ, as do sampling schemes, which here comprised four samples during 1 year while the previous studies were based on a single sampling at one time point. However, based on the present study, though effects established were rather small, the same downward trend in the prevalence of SCM previously noted in Finland seems to continue.

Another factor which has had an impact on the udder health of Finnish dairy cows is their decreasing parity. In 1990, the average age of a dairy cow removed from the herd was 5.3 years, but in 2010 it was only 5.1 years [13]. Average parity of the herd decreases because of culling of the older cows and increasing the number of heifers after enlargement of the herd. The most common reasons for culling dairy cows in Finland are mastitis and fertility problems [13]. Premature culling of cows causes economic losses and addressing this problem is one of the biggest challenges for Finnish dairy farms [14].

During the twenty first century, general management of dairy herds as well as barn design and milking technology, improved in Finland, which also has contributed to the improved udder health reported in this study. The positive development of udder health of dairy cows contributes to the low SCC of the bulk milk in Finland. The geometric mean of bulk milk SCC in Finland has been under 150,000 cells/ml for 20 years, and it is the lowest in the European Union. However, although bulk milk SCC is related to udder health of the herd, it is not an accurate indicator of mastitis prevalence [15]. Milk from cows with high SCC is often separated from bulk milk, to maintain milk SCC in the premium class.

Prevalence and incidence of clinical and subclinical mastitis have been studied widely, but most published surveys have been based on random or 'convenience' samples [16–20]. Definitions used for mastitis also greatly differ among studies. To our knowledge, national dairy cow databases, covering the majority of dairy cows in a country, are available in Norway, Sweden and Denmark [7]. Similar national registers and the same definition of mastitis have been agreed on by the Committee for Milk Quality of the Nordic Dairy Organizations (NMSM) (personal communication, Laura Kulkas, Valio Ltd., December 2015). Because of the rather similar structure of dairy industry and the common definitions for mastitis, the present results could be applicable and used as a reference at least in the Nordic countries. In Sweden, the estimated SCM prevalence in 2012 using the SCC threshold of ≥200,000 cells/ml was 25.7% (personal communication, Håkan Landin, Växa Sverige, 2013), in Norway approximately 21.0% (personal communication, Olav Østerås, TINE advisory service, Norway, 2013), and in Denmark 26.0% [21]. Prevalence of mastitis in large Estonian herds, using a similar definition, was reported to be as high as 52.7% [22]. In a study comprising a random sample of large herds represented equally from all regions of the Netherlands, mean herd prevalence of SCM using the same SCC threshold as here was 12.8% in primipara and 27.1% in multipara [16]. Compared with figures presented in some other studies, the Finnish SCM prevalence of 19.0% in 2010 seems relatively low. Comparing mastitis prevalence studies from different countries or regions is however difficult due to different data collection protocols and study design. In addition, for instance, parity distribution of the cows included in the study should be considered.

Prevalence of CSCM

This was the first Finnish study reporting the prevalence of CSCM, i.e. proportion of cows with milk SCC chronically ≥200,000 cells/ml. The prevalence of CSCM decreased over 20 years from 20.4% (1991) to 16.1% (2010). It should be kept in mind that only cows that had all four sample results available for the year were included. It is possible that a considerable proportion of cows with CSCM were lost due to culling during the study year, i.e. the prevalence reported here may be underestimated. The prevalences of CSCM were not very much lower than those of SCM, indicating that many cows with CSCM actually have long-term udder health problems.

No published data are available on the proportion of cows with CSCM from countries other than Finland. In Sweden in 2012 the estimated figure was comparable with ours, 16.0% (personal communication, Håkan Landin, Växa Sverige, 2013). In our study, the factors associated with CSCM were Holstein breed, increasing parity and free stalls. In large herds producing high daily milk volumes, usually in free stalls, bulk milk SCC may be maintained more easily in the premium class (in Finland bulk milk SCC <250,000 cells/ml) without treatment or discarding milk from cows with high SCC due to SCM. The slight increase in the proportion of cows with CSCM during the past 10 years may be related to the extensive enlargement of the herds with cows of unknown udder health status. The lower odds for CSCM in 2010, despite the higher prevalence, could be due to the better management and environment of the cows in the new free stalls.

Our definition of CSCM was novel and based on the results of four samples during each study year that were available for the study. The real udder health status of the CSCM cows remains unknown as cows can have truly persistent (chronic) infections or be re-infected. After all, the only reliable method for defining an intramammary infection as chronic would be repeated sampling of the mammary quarter over a long period and strain-typing of the isolated organisms to confirm the presence of the same infecting agent in the quarter. Here, the time between sampling of the cow was considered long enough for a possible cure from mastitis after the previous sampling, which would indicate SCM in this study. More than four samples during the study year would have provided more precise information on the udder health of the cows.

Cow related factors associated with SCC, SCM and CSCM

Parity increased milk SCC and was associated with a higher OR for both SCM and CSCM. Our result supports the results from many previous studies [23, 24]. Mechanisms underlying this phenomenon are not fully understood, but could be related to the impairment of leukocyte functions with increasing age of the cow [25]. In principle, no other factor has been defined as an explicit cause of elevated milk SCC than intramammary infection [15]. The stress of subsequent lactation periods on the udder tissue and changes in udder conformation and depth increase exposure to intramammary infections [26]. Callosity of the teat end has also been recognized as a risk factor, and tends to increase with increasing parity [27].

Breed was another major factor related to SCC: Holsteins had significantly higher average SCC and higher OR for SCM and CSCM than Ayrshires. This result agrees with previous studies in which the Holstein breed was shown to be more susceptible to mastitis [19, 28–30]. The proportion of Holstein cows has continuously increased in Finland: in 1991 Holsteins represented 17.8% and Ayrshires 80.9% of dairy cows, but in 2010 the figures were 34.3 and 64.4%. Udder health improved among both breeds during the study period: the prevalence of SCM decreased in Holsteins from 26.3% (1991) to 20.8% (2010) and in Ayrshires from 21.4 to 18.0%, respectively. However, milk SCC increased in every parity group from 1991 to 2010, which is a reason for some concern. Udder health has been included as one of the most important factors for dairy cow breeding in Finland. Indexes like SCC, milking speed, leakage and the structure of the udder in daughter evaluation of the AI bulls, have been used in Finland for several decades. Cases of veterinary treated mastitis are also recorded and included in the breeding indexes. A possible threat in the future may be represented by increased use of genetic material from global breeding companies, which have no similar health data available. We assumed that the increase in SCC could be related to the increased milk production, but at least the milk yield for first 305 days lactation of the cow did not affect the SCC of the same cow.

The positive association between mastitis and milk yield is well established [31, 32]. Our results agree with earlier studies, but the effect we established was just moderate, yet statistically significant. Every 100 kg increase in the annual milk yield of a herd increased the average SCC of the herd by approximately 1000 cells/ml. This indicates that if the annual milk yield of a herd would increase from 10,000 to 12,000 kg, milk SCC of the herd would increase by 20,000 cells/ml, despite the year. In our study, high milk yield for the first 305 days had no impact on the milk SCC of the cow. Association of the milk yield and prevalence of SCM and CSCM was also very low (Tables 5, 6). High production herds with are usually managed expertly and breeding of the animals is systematic, which should improve udder health. In well-managed herds also treatment of mastitis is diagnosis-based and more efficient, which supports control of mastitis [33]. The dilution effect of the high milk yield on milk SCC may also play a role [31]. The only moderate increase of milk SCC seen here could be partly due to that phenomenon.

Cow composite milk SCC was higher for organic herds than conventional herds. A cow in an organic herd had in average 4300 cells/ml higher milk SCC than a cow in a conventional herd. This difference decreased during the study period, and in 2010 it was 3400 cells/ml. The proportion of cows with SCM was higher in organic herds (22.3%) compared with conventional herds (18.9%), which is consistent with the results on cow composite milk SCC. Results from previous studies comparing organic vs. conventional herds have been controversial. In a recent Canadian study the incidence rate of clinical mastitis was lower on organic farms than on conventional farms, but bulk milk SCC tended to be higher [20]. In a study carried out in the United Kingdom, no major differences were recorded between organic and conventional production [34]. In Sweden, where the requirements for organic production are similar as in Finland, cow composite milk SCC did not differ between the two production types [35]. Some studies reported similar results as here [36, 37]. In all studies cited, farm enrollment has been voluntary, which may create selection bias, possibly explaining discrepancies between the results. Factors explaining the higher cow milk SCC in organic farms could be avoidance of antibiotic treatments for mastitis, and lower milk yield in general compared with conventionally kept dairy cows, in addition to differences in management practices.

Herd related factors associated with SCC, SCM and CSCM

Free-stalls with AMS were strongly associated with a higher milk SCC of individual cows and herds, as well as with a higher prevalence of SCM, while herd size had only a moderate effect in increasing milk SCC. In Finland, larger herds are mostly housed in free-stalls and often have AMS, and smaller herds are usually kept in tie-stalls. Good management and milking hygiene, as well as professionalism of the farmer, can decrease average milk SCC of the herd [5, 38, 39]. Lower milk SCC of cows in tie stalls may be due to individual care of the cows, including closer monitoring of udder health. Milking hygiene and mastitis detection have not been optimal with AMS milking, but improvements have been made to new models of AMS [40]. Recommended grouping of cows according to udder health status in free-stalls with AMS has not been feasible because the herds are relatively small in Finland [41]. The design and functionality of free-stalls built after 2010, as well as their management, differ substantially from those in free-stalls built in 2001. In a recent study from Finland, AMS was not a significant risk factor for pathogen-specific intramammary infection [33].

Season and location of the farm

As previously reported, season had an impact on milk SCC [5, 42, 43]. SCC increased during late summer and was lowest during the cold and dry period in winter. Heat stress is known to affect milk SCC and milk production [44, 45], but may not be the most important factor under Finnish conditions. The summer season challenges ventilation systems in stalls and increasing warmth and humidity predispose cows to mastitis. According to Finnish legislation, cows in tie-stalls must graze at least 60 days during summer, but also free-stalls without grazing had a similar influence on SCC during late summer months (Fig. 2). Preventive measures for pathogen transmission in the summer season may be less efficient than during other seasons [46]. Using monthly test results would have provided more accurate knowledge on the seasonal effect, but those data were available for a very limited number of farms.

Location of the farm affected the results such that on farms located in West or South Finland both cow composite milk SCC and average SCC of the herd were higher than on farms in East and North Finland (Fig. 2). Accordingly, the risk for SCM and CSCM was lower in East and North Finland (Fig. 3). These findings may be linked to cultural, economic and management differences among farms in different parts of the country. Each area also has their own advisory services, which may slightly differ from each other.

Quality of the study and possible bias

The Finnish dairy industry has undergone substantial structural changes during two decades. The total number of herds has decreased from 40,188 in 1991 to 11,256 in 2010, cows from 445,600 (1991) to 289,339 (2010) [2], and average herd sizes have increased. The proportion of herds included in the Finnish national health monitoring and milk recording system has also considerably increased during the three decades. The change from 1991 to 2001 is notable and may represent selection bias in the present study. The proportion of cows included in 1991 was much lower than in the other study years, which may also indicate selection bias. However, the number of cows remains sufficiently high that we considered it to be a representative sample of Finnish dairy cows belonging the national health monitoring and milk recording system. The number of cows in free-stalls associated with the Finnish national health monitoring and milk recording system was zero in 1991 and 2001, but we decided to include AMS stalls, and present the data as a supplementary file with separate models for 2001 and 2010 because we considered the information to be important. The databases used were large and could be used as a representative sample of Finnish dairy cows in each study year, which gives confidence for the study. This was enabled by the Finnish national health monitoring and milk recording system database. Including only cows for which there were four milk samples per year may have caused some selection bias, but on the other hand requiring more samples per year had caused a considerable loss of cows. Due to the excessive number of recordings, most of the tested variables were statistically significant and fitted in the final models, despite elimination of the cows with missing information. Associations between the tested variables and SCM and CSCM seemed moderate. Making blind selection from the dataset could have emphasized the effect of some of the tested variables, but considerable information would have been lost. As SCM is affected by a variety of factors, which we did not study here, we consider the moderate associations to be sufficiently accurate.

Conclusions

This mastitis survey in Finland was the first that included cow composite milk SCC. Prevalence of CSCM was assessed for the first time. Prevalence of SCM in Finland decreased over the past three decades, from 22.3% (1991) and 20.1% (2001) to 19% (2010), the greatest reduction taking place during the first decade. Factors that possibly impacted the decreased risk for SCM are better breeding, management and housing of the dairy cows. Moreover, during the first decade national campaigns to improve udder health have contributed. The most significant cow and herd factors associated with SCM were increasing parity, Holstein breed, and free stalls with AMS. Prevalence of CSCM also decreased from 20.4% in 1991 to 16.1% in 2010; it was not much lower than that of SCM which indicates that most cows with SCM in fact had chronic mastitis. The Holstein breed and increasing parity were associated with CSCM. Prevalence of SCM has decreased but all the factors associated here with an increased milk SCC will continue to exist in the future. The Holstein breed will become more popular, and AMS is replacing conventional milking. These ongoing changes represent a challenge for dairy farm management and control of animal diseases such as SCM in the future. Regular surveys of mastitis prevalence would be useful to follow up on the situation and enable interventions to be made when needed.

Additional files

Additional file 1. Effect of different factors on prevalence of subclinical mastitis (SCM) in Finland in years 2001 and 2010.

Additional file 2. Estimated effects of different factors on cow composite milk SCC (somatic cell count) in Finland in 2001 and 2010.

Additional file 3. Estimated effects of different factors on herd milk SCC (somatic cell count) in Finland in 2001 and 2010.

Authors' contributions

HH participated in the analysis of the data and was in main responsible for drafting the manuscript. JV participated in the interpretation of the results and drafting the manuscript. HS participated in the analysis of the data and drafting the manuscript. TA participated in designing the study and drafting the manuscript. JJ was mainly responsible for the statistical analyses and participated in drafting the manuscript. SPe participated in designing the study and in drafting the manuscript. SPy participated in designing the study, was responsible for its coordination, and participated in drafting the manuscript. All authors read and approved the final manuscript.

Author details

[1] Department of Production Animal Medicine, Faculty of Veterinary Medicine, University of Helsinki, Paroninkuja 20, 04920 Saarentaus, Finland. [2] Veterinary Bacteriology Research Unit, Finnish Food Safety Authority Evira, Neulaniementie 4, 70210 Kuopio, Finland. [3] Oy 4Pharma Ltd., Mannerheimintie 44 A, 00260 Helsinki, Finland.

Acknowledgements

This study was funded by the Ministry of Agriculture and Forestry of Finland, Walter Ehrström Foundation and the Finnish Foundation of Veterinary Research. The authors would also like to thank Vesa Rainio for participating in designing the study and docent Tuula Honkanen-Buzalski who initiated the project.

Competing interests

The authors declare that they have no competing interests.

References

1. Natural Resources Institute Finland (Luke). Structural Development of Agriculture. Forecast of Structural Development. http://www.luke.fi/en/services. Accessed Jan 2017.
2. Natural Resources Institute Finland (Luke). Statistics. Number of Livestock 1990–2016. http://stat.luke.fi/en/number-of-livestock. Accessed Jan 2017.
3. IFCN, Dairy report 2015. ISSN 1610-434X. http://www.ifcndairy.org/en/downloads/index.php?catid=14. Accessed Jan 2017.
4. Hogeveen H, Huijps K, Lam TJGM. Economic aspects of mastitis: new developments. N Z Vet J. 2011;59:16–23.
5. Lievaart JJ, Barkema HW, Kremer WDJ, van den Broek J, Verheijden JHM, Heesterbeek JAP. Effect of herd characteristics, management practices, and season on different categories of the herd somatic cell count. J Dairy Sci. 2007;90:4137–44.
6. Landin H, Mörk M, Petterson G. Udder health in herds with automatic milking. In: Hogeveen H, Lam T, editors. Udder health and communication. Wageningen: Wageningen Academic Publishers; 2011. p. 385–90.
7. Rintakoski S. Epidemiological evaluation of the Nordic health registers for dairy cows—data transfer, validation and human influence on disease

recordings. Doctoral dissertation. Helsinki: University of Helsinki, Unigrafia; 2013.
8. Koiranen L, Nurmi E. Incidence of bovine mastitis in Finland. Suomen eläinlääkärilehti (Finnish Vet J). 1976;82:185–9.
9. Saloniemi H, Roine K. Field observations on the incidence of bovine clinical mastitis and teat diseases. Nord Veterinærmedicin. 1981;33:297–305.
10. Myllys V, Asplund K, Brofeldt T, Hirvelä-Koski V, Honkanen-Buzalski T, Junttila J, et al. Bovine mastitis in Finland in 1988 and 1995—changes in prevalence and antimicrobial resistance. Acta Vet Scand. 1998;39:119–26.
11. Pitkälä A, Haveri M, Pyörälä S, Myllys V, Honkanen-Buzalski T. Bovine mastitis in Finland 2004—prevalence, distribution of bacteria, and antimicrobial resistance. J Dairy Sci. 2004;87:2433–41.
12. Pyörälä S, Kaartinen L, Simojoki H, Kivilahti-Mäntylä K. Use of intramammary antimicrobials in Finland—towards lower consumption and targeted treatment of mastitis. 2012, Lisbon, Portugal; XXVII World Buiatrics Congress, 85-Abstracts, OC 14.
13. Heikkilä A. Replacement decisions on Finnish dairy farms—toward better economic performance with novel technology and sustainable herds. University of Helsinki. MTT Science 22. Tampere: Juvenes print–Suomen yliopistopaino Oy; 2013.
14. Heikkilä A, Nousiainen JI, Jauhiainen L. Optimal replacement policy and economic value of dairy cows with diverse health status and production capacity. J Dairy Sci. 2008;91:2342–52.
15. International Dairy Federation. Guidelines for the use and interpretation of bovine milk somatic cell counts (SCC) in the dairy industry. Bulletin of the International Dairy Federation. Belgium: IDF; 2013. p. 466.
16. van den Borne BHP, van Schaik G, Lam TJGM, Nielen M. Variation in herd level mastitis indicators between primi- and multiparae in Dutch dairy herds. Prev Vet Med. 2010;96:49–55.
17. Schwarz D, Diesterbeck US, Failing K, König S, Brügemann K, Zschöck M, et al. Somatic cell counts and bacteriological status in quarter foremilk samples of cows in Hesse, Germany-A longitudinal study. J Dairy Sci. 2010;93:5716–28.
18. Wilson DJ, Gonzalez RN, Das HH. Bovine mastitis pathogens in New York and Pennsylvania: prevalence and effects on somatic cell count and milk production. J Dairy Sci. 1997;80:2592–8.
19. Persson Waller K, Bengtsson B, Lindberg A, Nyman A, Ericsson Unnerstad H. Incidence of mastitis and bacterial findings at clinical mastitis in Swedish primiparous cows—influence of breed and stage of lactation. Vet Microbiol. 2009;134:89–94.
20. Levison LJ, Miller-Cushon EK, Tucker AL, Bergeron R, Leslie KE, Barkema HW, et al. Incidence rate of pathogen-specific clinical mastitis on conventional and organic Canadian dairy farms. J Dairy Sci. 2016;99:1341–50.
21. Katholm J, Bennedsgaard TW. Yversundhed i Danmark 2013. Dansk Vet Tidsskr. 2013;96:28–35.
22. Haltia L, Honkanen-Buzalski T, Spiridonova I, Olkonen A, Myllys V. A study of bovine mastitis, milking procedures and management practices on 25 Estonian dairy herds. Acta Vet Scand. 2006;48:22.
23. Hagnestam-Nielsen C, Emanuelson U, Berglund B, Strandberg E. Relationship between somatic cell count and milk yield in different stages of lactation. J Dairy Sci. 2009;92:3124–33.
24. Reksen O. Relationships between milk culture results and composite milk somatic cell counts in Norwegian dairy cattle. J Dairy Sci. 2008;91:3102–13.
25. Rainard P, Riollet C. Innate immunity of the bovine mammary gland. Vet Res. 2006;37:369–400.
26. Rogers GW. Index selection using milk yield, somatic cell score, udder depth, teat placement, and foot angle. J Dairy Sci. 1993;76:664–70.
27. Neijenhuis F, Barkema HW, Hogeveen H, Noordhuizen JPTM. Relationship between teat-end callosity and occurrence of clinical mastitis. J Dairy Sci. 2001;84:2664–72.
28. Sewalem A. Analysis of the relationship between somatic cell score and functional longevity in Canadian dairy cattle. J Dairy Sci. 2006;89:3609–14.
29. Heikkilä A, Nousiainen JI, Pyörälä S. Costs of clinical mastitis with special reference to premature culling. J Dairy Sci. 2012;95:139–50.
30. Bludau MJ, Maeschli A, Leiber F, Steiner A, Klocke P. Mastitis in dairy heifers: prevalence and risk factors. Vet J. 2014;202:566–72.
31. Green LE, Schukken YH, Green MJ. On distinguishing cause and consequence: do high somatic cell counts lead to lower milk yield or does high milk yield lead to lower somatic cell count? Prev Vet Med. 2006;76:74–89.
32. Koivula M, Mäntysaari EA, Negussie E, Serenius T. Genetic and phenotypic relationships among milk yield and somatic cell count before and after clinical mastitis. J Dairy Sci. 2005;88:827–33.
33. Taponen S, Liski E, Heikkilä A-M, Pyörälä S. Factors associated with intramammary infection in dairy cows caused by coagulase-negative staphylococci, *Staphylococcus aureus*, *Streptococcus uberis*, *Streptococcus dysgalactiae*, *Corynebacterium bovis* and *Escherichia coli*. J Dairy Sci. 2017;100:493–503.
34. Haskell MJ, Langford FM, Jack MC, Sherwood L, Lawrence AB, Rutherford KMD. The effect of organic status and management practices on somatic cell counts on UK dairy farms. J Dairy Sci. 2009;92:3775–80.
35. Fall N, Emanuelson U. Milk yield, udder health and reproductive performance in Swedish organic and conventional dairy herds. J Dairy Res. 2009;76:402–10.
36. Roesch M, Doherr MG, Blum JW. Performance of dairy cows on Swiss farms with organic and integrated production. J Dairy Sci. 2005;88:2462–75.
37. Nauta WJ, Baars T, Bovenhuis H. Converting to organic dairy farming: consequences for production, somatic cell scores and calving interval of first parity Holstein cows. Livestock Sci. 2006;99:185–95.
38. Dufour S, Frechette A, Barkema HW, Mussell A, Scholl DT. Effect of udder health management practices on herd somatic cell count. J Dairy Sci. 2011;94:563–79.
39. Barkema HW, Van der Ploeg JD, Schukken YH, Lam TJGM, Benedictus G, Brand A. Management style and its association with bulk milk somatic cell count and incidence rate of clinical mastitis. J Dairy Sci. 1999;82:1655–63.
40. Hovinen M, Pyörälä S. Invited review: udder health of dairy cows in automatic milking. J Dairy Sci. 2011;94:547–62.
41. Kivinen T, Hovinen M, Norring M, Seppä-Lassila L, Sarjokari K, Lätti M, et al. Grouping of cows on a dairy farm—aiming for fluent work and animal welfare [in Finnish]. Maito ja Me. 2014;1 Appendix: 1–24.
42. Yang L, Yang Q, Yi M, Pang ZH, Xiong BH. Effects of seasonal change and parity on raw milk composition and related indices in Chinese Holstein cows in northern China. J Dairy Sci. 2013;96:6863–9.
43. Østerås O, Sølverød L, Reksen O. Milk culture results in a large Norwegian survey—effects of season, parity, days in milk, resistance, and clustering. J Dairy Sci. 2006;89:1010–23.
44. West JW. Effects of heat-stress on production in dairy cattle. J Dairy Sci. 2003;86:2131–44.
45. Smith DL, Smith T, Rude BJ, Ward SH. Comparison of the effects of heat stress on milk and component yields and somatic cell score in Holstein and Jersey cows. J Dairy Sci. 2013;96:3028–33.
46. Barkema HW, Schukken YH, Lam TJGM, Beiboer ML, Benedictus G, Brand A. Management practices associated with low, medium, and high somatic cell counts in bulk milk. J Dairy Sci. 1998;81:1917–27.

16

The response of mute swans (*Cygnus olor*, Gm. 1789) to vaccination against avian influenza with an inactivated H5N2 vaccine

Beata Dolka*, Artur Żbikowski, Izabella Dolka and Piotr Szeleszczuk

Abstract

Background: Recent epidemics of highly pathogenic avian influenza (HPAI) produced an unprecedented number of cases in mute swans (*Cygnus olor*) in European countries, which indicates that these birds are very sensitive to the H5N1 virus. The HPAI outbreaks stirred a debate on the controversial stamping-out policy in populations of protected bird species. After preventive vaccination had been approved in the European Union, several countries have introduced vaccination schemes to protect poultry, captive wild birds or exotic birds in zoos against HPAI. The aim of this study was to investigate the immune response of wild mute swans to immunization with an inactivated AI H5N2 vaccine approved for use in poultry. The serological responses of mute swans were assessed by comparison with racing pigeons (*Columba livia*), a species which is characterized by different susceptibility to infection with the H5N1 HPAI virus and plays a questionable role in the ecology of influenza (H5N1) viruses.

Results: Swans were vaccinated once or twice at an interval of 4 weeks. The humoral immune response was evaluated by hemagglutination inhibition (HI) and NP-ELISA. The lymphocyte blast transformation test was used to determine the cell-mediated immune response. Higher values of the geometric mean titer (GMT) and 100 % seroconversion (HI $\geq$32) were noted in double vaccinated swans (1448.2) than in single vaccinated swans (128.0) or in double vaccinated pigeons (215.3). Significant differences in HI titers were observed between swans and pigeons, but no variations in ELISA scores were noted after the booster dose. Immunization of swans had no effect on the proliferative activity of lymphocytes.

Conclusions: The inactivated H5N2 vaccine was safe and immunogenic for mute swans and pigeons. Vaccination may have practical implications for swans kept in zoos, wildlife parks or rehabilitation centers. However, challenge studies are needed to prove the efficacy of the H5N2 AI vaccine.

Keywords: Avian influenza, H5N1, Vaccination, Inactivated vaccine, Mute swans, Racing pigeons

Background

Mute swans (*Cygnus olor*, Gm. 1789) of the order *Anseriformes* and other wild birds of the orders *Anseriformes* and *Charadriiformes* are important natural reservoirs of low pathogenic avian influenza (LPAI) viruses. LPAI viruses of subtypes H5 and H7 can evolve into HPAI (highly pathogenic avian influenza) viruses once introduced into poultry. In contrast to LPAIV, HPAI viruses are rarely detected in wild birds [1–4]. The first known report discussing the possible role of swans in the epidemiology of avian influenza was dedicated to whistling swans in Japan [5]. Following a massive HPAI outbreak in wild geese in 2005, the Qinghai-like HPAI virus H5N1 (clade 2.2) continued to spread across three continents, resulting in devastating losses in the poultry industry. Mute swans were the most frequently affected species of wild birds, particularly in Europe [3, 6–8]. Subsequent investigations revealed the sensitivity of swans to infections and variations in the pathobiology of the HPAI H5N1 virus [3, 7, 9]. Several studies have demonstrated that mute swans could

*Correspondence: beata_dolka@sggw.pl
Department of Pathology and Veterinary Diagnostics, Faculty of Veterinary Medicine, Warsaw University of Life Sciences-SGGW, Nowoursynowska 159c St., 02-776 Warsaw, Poland

be vectors of HPAI H5N1 over short distances, and that they represent a new avian host in HPAI virus ecology [6, 7]. Mute swans were recognized as a source of infection in the first global cases of HPAI H5N1 infections passed by birds to humans [10]. Further studies demonstrated that the opportunities for swan-to-human transmission of H5N1 were extremely rare [11]. In AI surveillance programs, mute swans were an effective indicator species (sentinel birds) in the epidemiology of HPAI [3, 7]. Since 2010, HPAI H5N1 viruses have become enzootic and evolved dynamically to form multiple H5 HA clades [4, 12]. Between 2014 and 2015, various HPAIV H5 subtypes of several clades have spread rapidly and globally in poultry and wild birds [12, 13]. Furthermore, mute swans (Sweden 2015) and other swan species were affected by the novel reassortant H5N8 virus [8].

Unlike swans, pigeons were long regarded as a species that is highly resistant or minimally susceptible to infection with HPAIV [14–16]. However, according to the recent literature, pigeons' susceptibility to H5N1 virus and their role in AI epidemiology have been questioned [16, 17]. Avian influenza is still an unsolved problem for the racing pigeon industry, mainly due to a lack of detailed regulations. The restrictions put on poultry in connection to suspected and confirmed HPAI outbreaks also apply to domestic pigeons. Thus vaccination may be a solution to avian influenza problem in racing pigeon industry.

The global strategy for the control and eradication of HPAI involves strict administrative procedures, including confinement, stamping-out and pre-emptive culling [18, 19]. The application of radical solutions to healthy, valuable, endangered and protected species of birds (held in captivity) was met with high opposition for ethical, social, and environmental reasons [20]. Pursuant to the provisions of Council Directive 2005/94/EC, AI vaccination was approved in EU as an additional measure disease control and an alternative to pre-emptive culling. The vaccination strategy should be carried out only in combination with biosecurity measures [21–23]. In the EU, commercial inactivated AI vaccines were licensed for use only in chickens and Pekin ducks, but they were also shown to be effective in other bird species [24–26]. It should be noted that only individual species of wild birds kept in captivity can be considered for AI vaccination. Many studies demonstrated that vaccine-induced antibody responses in birds were determined by the species, vaccine type or dose [25, 27]. However, little is known about vaccination of swans and pigeons against HPAI H5N1 [26, 27, 42, 48].

In view of the above, the aim of this study was to evaluate the immune response of mute swans immunized against AI with an inactivated vaccine. The serological response of swans was compared with that of racing (domestic) pigeons (*Columba livia f. domestica*) immunized with the same vaccine. Pigeons were compared with mute swans based on differences in the susceptibility of the two species to H5N1 HPAIV.

Methods

Mute swans

Eleven free-living mute swans were captured in early spring in central Poland. Immature swans of both sexes (2-year-old males n = 4, 36.4 %; females n = 7, 63.6 %) were marked with ornithological rings and transported to the Agricultural Experiment Station of the Warsaw University of Life Sciences. They were placed in individual boxes and exposed to the natural light–dark cycle. Feed and water were provided ad libitum.

Vaccine

Birds were immunized with the Nobilis® Influenza H5N2 vaccine based on an inactivated, whole avian influenza virus (A/duck/Potsdam/1402/86, European strain) inducing an HI titer of $\geq 6.0 \log_2$ (MSD Animal Health, Boxmeer, Netherlands). The vaccine strain has 90 % nucleotide sequence homology to the HA gene of the H5N1 HPAI field strain A/turkey/Turkey/1/05; clade 2.2 (1530 base pairs, including basic cleavage site), and 92.4 % homology based on the amino acids sequence [30]. The vaccine was chosen based on its specific subtype, availability, licensing considerations, safety and efficacy data for poultry and other birds, and DIVA (Differentiating Infected from Vaccinated Animals) guidelines [18, 28–30]. The Nobilis® Influenza H5N2 vaccine is commercially available and has been approved by the European Commission and the European Medicines Agency [31].

Experimental design

Vaccination of mute swans

Mute swans were divided into two experimental groups (D1, D2, n = 8) and one control group (C, n = 3). Each group contained birds of both sexes: D1 (n = 4): 1 male and 3 females; D2 (n = 4): 2 males and 2 females; C (n = 3): 1 male and 2 females. Birds were manually restrained for vaccine administration. Group D1 swans were vaccinated once (day 0). Swans from group D2 were vaccinated twice: on day 0 and 4 weeks later (4-week interval). The dose was adjusted for body weight. Birds were given a dose of 1 ml. The vaccine was administered subcutaneously to the nape of the neck. The control group was not vaccinated.

Vaccination of racing pigeons for comparative analysis

Four young racing pigeons aged 3–12 months were vaccinated twice according to the schedule for D2 mute swans.

The vaccine was administered subcutaneously in the dorsal region of the neck. Each pigeon (body weight >400 g) received a dose of 0.5 ml. Pigeons were kept at the Small Animal Clinic of the Faculty of Veterinary Medicine at the Warsaw University of Life Sciences (SGGW). They were placed in individual cages (450 mm × 900 mm) with ad libitum access to water and feed, temperature of 22–25 °C and humidity of 50–70 %. The birds were exposed to 10 h of light per day.

Safety monitoring

During the study, swans and pigeons were observed twice daily and were weighed before the first vaccine administration and then every 7 days. After immunization, vaccine tolerance and any side effects, in particular localized reactions at the injection site, were recorded. Birds were also observed for adverse effects [25].

Serological tests

Blood samples from the medial metatarsal vein were collected 5 times: before the first vaccination (0) and in weeks 2, 4, 6, and 8. At these dates, the presence of H5 subtype-specific antibodies in serum samples was determined by the hemagglutination inhibition test (HI). The HI test was performed according to standard procedures using 4 HAU of commercially available H5 heterologous antigen (A/chicken/Belgium150/99soncke99/150v6, H5N2) (GD Animal Health, Deventer, the Netherlands). HI titers were expressed in $\log_2$, where 4 $\log_2$ (HI $\geq$16) was the minimum positive titer [15, 23]. The geometric mean titer (GMT), seroconversion (SR) and protection rates (PR) were determined with the use of methods described in previous studies [25, 27, 32]. According to Bertelsen et al. [32] the SR and PR were expressed as the percentage of birds with titers higher than or equal to 16 and 32, respectively. Similarly to other authors, we assumed for the purpose of this study a HI titer $\geq$32 could be considered protective [25, 32].

The presence of AI type-specific antibodies was determined by NP (nucleoprotein)–blocking ELISA (FlockChek AI MultiS-Screen Ab Test Kit, IDEXX Laboratories, Inc., Westbrook, Maine USA). ELISA results were analyzed using xChek® ver. 3.3 software (IDEXX Laboratories, Inc., Westbrook, Maine USA). The mean S/N ratio (sample to negative control ratio) and coefficient of variation (% CV, standard deviation divided by the mean) were presented. The S/N cut-off was set at <0.5 to identify antibody-positive samples.

Before vaccination (day 0), serum samples were examined for the presence of NDV antibodies in the HI test to reduce the risk of possible cross-reactions and false positive results. The NDV antigen, LaSota strain (GD Animal Health, Deventer, the Netherlands) was used in HI [23, 29].

Evaluation of cell-mediated immunity by the Lymphocyte Blast Transformation Test

Lymphocytes from heparinized peripheral blood sampled from swans were separated by the gradient centrifugation method using Gradisol L (Aqua-Med, Poland) and were washed in supplemented Eagle's medium (Biomed Lublin, Poland). Cells were adjusted to 2.0×10^6 cells/ml in Eagle's medium with fetal calf serum, and 100 μl from each well was transferred to 96-well plates. Lymphocyte cultures were stimulated by two non-specific T cell mitogens: phytohemagglutinin (PHA) and concanavalin A (ConA) (Sigma-Aldrich, USA), as well as a specific stimulator: inactivated AIV H5 antigen (A/Chicken/Belgium150/99, LPAI H5N2). Each mitogen (100 μl) was added in triplicate at a final concentration of 5.0, 2.5 and 1.25 μg/ml for PHA and ConA and with HA activity of 1/8 and 1/16 for Ag H5. The cultures were incubated for 72 h at 41 °C. Radiolabeled ^{3}H-thymidine (40 MBq/ml) (Lacomed, Czech Republic) was added for the final incubation of 24 h at 41 °C. Controls included unstimulated labeled and unlabeled cells. The general procedure was adopted based on the literature [33–35]. After incubation, the cells were deposited on glass fiber discs with a cell harvester (Skatron, Norway), and the amount of incorporated radioactivity was measured with the Wallac 1414 WinSpectral liquid scintillation counter (PerkinElmer Life Sciences, Wallac Oy, Turku, Finland). T-cell proliferative activity was expressed by the stimulation index (SI). Proliferation was regarded as significant at SI $\geq$2 [36].

Virus isolation

Before vaccination, cloacal swabs from swans and pigeons were collected in tubes containing a liquid medium: sterile phosphate buffered saline—PBS (BIOMED, Lublin, Poland) with an antibiotics (Antibiotic Antimycotic Solution 100× , Sigma, USA). Clarified supernatant fluids from swabs were inoculated (0.2 ml) in embryonated 11-day-old chicken eggs. The eggs were incubated at 37 °C for 72 h and candled daily. Amnio-allantoic fluid was harvested and tested in the hemagglutination assay (HA). HA-negative samples (derived from swans) were passaged three times using undiluted amnio-allantoic fluids as inoculum. One passage was performed for samples derived from pigeons. Three eggs per sample were used in every passage [23, 29].

Molecular tests

RNA was isolated from amnio-allantoic fluids and cloacal swabs using the QIAamp Viral RNA Mini Kit (Qiagen, Germany). The presence of AIV was tested by matrix (M) gene-based Real-Time RT-PCR using the OneStep RT-PCR Kit (Qiagen, Germany) [37]. For more specific detection of the H5 subtype (including Eurasian isolates), the H5 gene was amplified by Real-Time RT-PCR and RT-PCR [38, 39]. The presence of NDV was checked by RT-PCR [40]. Two inactivated H5N1 antigens (A/whooper swan/Germany/R65-2/06, A/turkey/England/250/07) and the NDV antigen were used as positive controls.

Statistical analysis

The results were processed in Statistica 10.0 software. Group means were compared by the t-test for variables with normal distribution and in the Mann–Whitney U test for other distributions. Three or more groups of variables were compared against normal distribution by one-way analysis of variance for completely randomized or repeated measures and Fisher's multiple comparison procedure. The Kruskal–Wallis test was used to compare non-normal distributions. The results were expressed as arithmetic means and standard deviation (SD). Geometric means were calculated for selected variables. The results were regarded as significant at $P < 0.05$ and highly significant at $P < 0.01$.

Results

Safety

Mute swans and pigeons showed no clinical signs of disease before vaccination. All swans were in good health, and their average body weight was determined at 8.3 ± 1.2 kg (8.8 ± 0.5 kg in males, 8.0 ± 1.4 kg in females).

No adverse effects were observed. The final body weight of the swans decreased by 1.1 kg during the study period, but the differences in the average body weight of experimental and control group birds were not statistically significant ($P > 0.05$). The behavior of vaccinated swans did not differ from that of control swans. Cases of mortality or injuries due to handling, catching and manual restraint were not observed.

Serological tests

Before vaccination (day 0), swans and pigeons tested seronegative for AIV/H5 in HI and NP-ELISA. The unvaccinated control remained seronegative throughout the entire 8-week experiment. Serum samples tested before the experiment, gave negative results for NDV in HI.

Post-vaccination HI titers in mute swans

Vaccine antibody responses in the HI test are shown in Fig. 1a. Statistically non-significant (NS) differences were found between groups in week 0. In weeks 2, 4, 6 and 8, the mean $\log_2$ HI titers in D1 and D2 birds were significantly higher ($P < 0.01$) than in the control group. Beginning from week 2, highly significant differences ($P < 0.01$) in HI titer values were observed in groups D1 and D2. However, 25 % of vaccinated swans were negative in the HI test two weeks after the administration of the first dose. Four weeks after the first vaccination the overall GMT was 152, and SR (HI ≥ 16), PR (HI ≥ 32) reached for the first time 100 %. After the administration of the booster dose, antibody titers in group D2 increased significantly by 2.5 $\log_2$ and were higher ($P < 0.01$) than in group D1. The highest antibody titers were noted in weeks 6 and 8 in groups D1 (7.0 $\log_2$) and D2 (10.5 $\log_2$). At the end of study (week 8), GMT was approximately 11-fold higher (GMT 1448.2) in swans administered a booster vaccine than in swans that were vaccinated only once (GMT 128.0). In week 8, SR and PR reached 100 % (HI ≥ 16 and ≥ 32) in D1 and D2 swans. No statistically significant differences were found in group C during the study.

Post-vaccination HI titers in racing pigeons

The results of the HI assays are shown in Fig. 1b. The titers were positive between week 2 (after the first vaccine dose) and the end of the experiment. In week 4, the overall GMT was determined at 45.3, and SR reached for the first time 100 %. The earliest sampling point when PR reached 100 % was two weeks after booster dose (week 6). The highest antibody titer in pigeons (8.0 $\log_2$), 100 % SR and PR were noted in week 8. Significant differences ($P < 0.05$) in $\log_2$ HI titer values between pigeons and swans were noted in weeks 2 and 6, whereas highly significant differences ($P < 0.01$) were observed in weeks 4 and 8. In general, antibody titers in D2 swans were higher ($P < 0.05$) than in pigeons after the first and second vaccination. No significant differences were found between groups at week 0.

ELISA results in mute swans

The results of the NP-ELISA are shown in Fig. 2a. No differences were found between the groups in week 0. After vaccination, highly significant differences ($P < 0.01$) were noted in S/N values in groups D1, D2 relative to the values noted before vaccination and the control group. In weeks 2, 4, 6 and 8, highly significant differences ($P < 0.01$) in the S/N ratio were noted between C, D1 and D2, whereas no significant differences were observed between D1 and D2. The mean S/N values after the first vaccination were determined at 0.106, CV 48.8 % (week 2) and 0.082, CV 24.2 % (week 4). The mean S/N values in group D1 reached 0.110 (CV 45.5 %) in week 6 and were somewhat higher in week 8 (S/N 0.126, CV 52.4 %). The booster dose induced a minor decrease in S/N to 0.066 (CV 13.4 %) in group D2 in week 6. In group D2, S/N values were determined at 0.070 (CV 10.9 %) in week 8. Statistically non-significant (NS) differences were found in group C during the study.

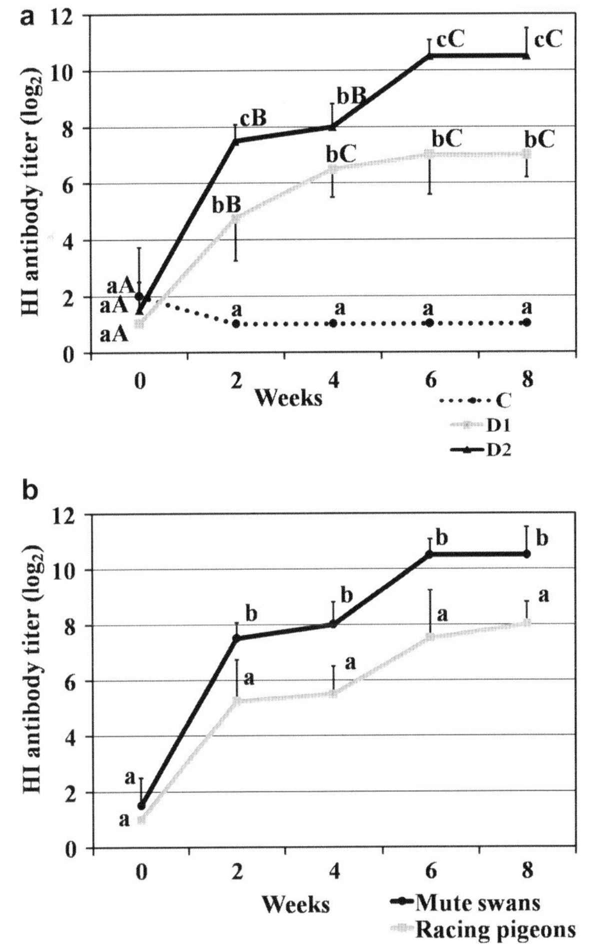

Fig. 1 **a** Mean $\log_2$ HI titers against the H5N2 antigen in control (C) and vaccinated mute swans (D1, D2). **b** Mean $\log_2$ HI titers against the H5N2 antigen in mute swans (group D2) and racing pigeons. Interpretation: HI $\geq$ 4 $\log_2$ (16) positive, HI < 4 $\log_2$ (16) negative. *Small letters* (*a, b, c*) denote significant differences in $\log_2$ HI titers between groups in successive weeks based on the results of the Kruskal–Wallis test. *Capital letters* (*A, B, C*) denote significant differences in $\log_2$ HI titers between weeks (*0, 2, 4, 6, 8*) within groups based the results of the on Kruskal–Wallis test

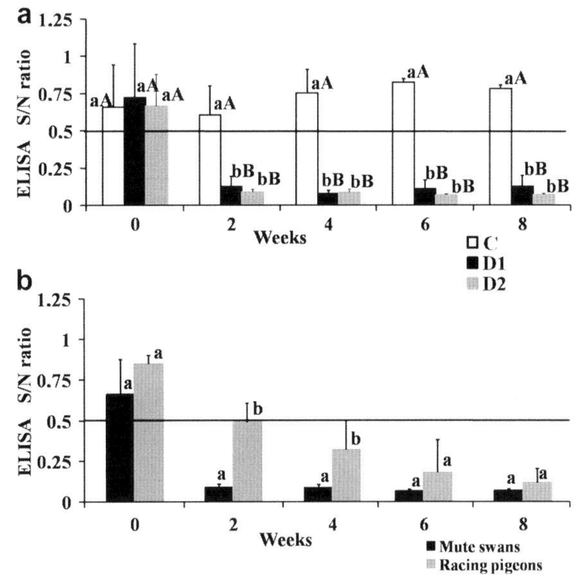

Fig. 2 **a** Mean values of the S/N ratio in ELISA for control and vaccinated mute swans (groups C, D1, D2). **b** Mean values of the S/N ratio in ELISA for mute swans (group D2) and racing pigeons. Interpretation: cut-off: S/N = 0.5, S/N < 0.5 positive, S/N $\geq$ 0.5 negative. *Small letters* (*a, b*) denote significant differences in the values of the S/N ratio between groups in successive weeks based on the results of Fisher's multiple comparison procedure. *Capital letters* (*A, B*) denote significant differences in the values of the S/N ratio between weeks (*0, 2, 4, 6, 8*) within groups

ELISA results in racing pigeons

Vaccinated pigeons tested positive for NP antibodies in ELISA (Fig. 2b). After the first vaccination, S/N values were determined at 0.488 (CV 20.8) in week 2, 0.321 (CV 48.6 %) in week 4, and they were significantly higher than in swans ($P < 0.01$ in week 2 and $P < 0.05$ in week 4). After the administration of the booster vaccine, the lowest S/N value (0.115, CV 53.9 %) was observed in week 8. A tendency towards higher S/N values was not observed in pigeons (in weeks 2, 4, 6 and 8). Statistically non-significant differences in S/N values were found between swans and pigeons (in weeks 6 and 8) after the second vaccine dose.

Lymphocyte blast transformation test

The results of the lymphocyte blast transformation test showed no difference between control and vaccinated animals (Table 1).

Virus isolation

Amnio-allantoic fluids from eggs inoculated with the medium from cloacal samples collected before vaccination, produced negative results in the HA test.

Molecular tests

All samples (cloacal swabs and amnio-allantoic fluids from eggs inoculated with the medium from cloacal samples) tested negative for AIV in Real-Time RT-PCR (M gene-based) and in the H5 subtype-specific PCR assays. NDV RNA was not detected by RT-PCR.

Discussion

Several schedules of AI vaccination for exotic birds have been proposed [41–44], but specific antibody titers with confirmed protective levels for mute swans and racing pigeons have not yet been identified. The present study was carried out to analyze the immune responses of wild mute swans vaccinated with an inactivated AI H5N2 vaccine licensed for use in chickens in the EU. To the best

Table 1 In vitro proliferative responses (SI ± SD) of peripheral blood lymphocytes after stimulation with PHA, ConA mitogens and H5 antigens in mute swans from control and experimental groups (C, D1, D2)

Mitogen concentrations [μg/ml] or antigen (HA titer)	Week[NS]	SI ± SD values in groups of mute swans[NS]		
		C	D1	D2
PHA 5.0 μg/ml	0	1.29 ± 0.13	0.68 ± 0.78	1.31 ± 1.10
	4	0.90 ± 0.06	1.26 ± 0.18	0.96 ± 0.13
	8	1.22 ± 0.06	1.20 ± 0.36	1.20 ± 0.09
PHA 2.5 μg/ml	0	1.14 ± 0.13	0.77 ± 1.02	1.43 ± 0.33
	4	1.16 ± 0.23	0.55 ± 0.14	0.90 ± 0.62
	8	1.41 ± 0.09	1.73 ± 0.38	1.53 ± 0.16
PHA 1.25 μg/ml	0	1.59 ± 0.44	1.5 ± 0.58	1.88 ± 0.28
	4	1.26 ± 0.36	1.01 ± 0.18	1.21 ± 0.74
	8	1.17 ± 0.86	2.41 ± 1.49	1.09 ± 0.34
ConA 5.0 μg/ml	0	1.27 ± 0.18	1.46 ± 0.06	1.74 ± 0.59
	4	0.92 ± 0.07	1.98 ± 1.02	1.21 ± 0.34
	8	1.14 ± 0.11	1.26 ± 0.45	1.84 ± 0.51
ConA 2.5 μg/ml	0	1.44 ± 0.33	1.85 ± 0.46	1.67 ± 0.51
	4	1.02 ± 0.16	2.18 ± 1.08	1.58 ± 0.91
	8	1.70 ± 0.37	1.86 ± 0.63	3.16 ± 1.46
ConA 1.25 μg/ml	0	1.82 ± 0.26	1.41 ± 0.14	1.15 ± 0.48
	4	1.06 ± 0.18	0.99 ± 0.64	1.29 ± 0.67
	8	1.93 ± 0.87	1.69 ± 0.00	3.17 ± 1.51
H5 (HA 1/8)	0	0.96 ± 0.05	1.29 ± 0.09	0.80 ± 0.58
	4	1.01 ± 0.07	0.56 ± 0.25	0.90 ± 0.00
	8	1.24 ± 0.22	1.18 ± 0.42	1.2 ± 0.15
H5 (HA 1/16)	0	1.04 ± 0.38	0.83 ± 0.43	1.03 ± 0.46
	4	0.77 ± 0.10	0.45 ± 0.20	0.79 ± 0.00
	8	1.27 ± 0.26	1.60 ± 0.81	1.31 ± 0.11

NS no statistically significant differences based on analysis of variance and Fisher's multiple comparisons in SI between weeks and groups for a given mitogen

of our knowledge, this is the first study to investigate the serological responses induced by AI vaccination in mute swans. The antibody response of swans was compared with that of racing pigeons.

According to the literature, inactivated H5N2 vaccines are well tolerated by domestic waterfowl and zoo birds [25, 41]. The vaccine used in the present study was safe for swans and pigeons. Our findings corroborate the results of studies which demonstrated that AI vaccines approved for use in poultry induced an immune response in non-target avian species [27, 30, 41]. Other authors noted 100 % SR in *Anseriformes* or in black swans after the first dose of an inactivated H5N2 vaccine [41, 44]. In this study, seroconversion was not observed in all swans after the first vaccination, which could point to variations in early response. Our results are in agreement with the findings of other authors who demonstrated differences in immune responses within the same bird species [32, 41, 45]. In our study, the overall GMT in mute swans after the first dose was higher than the known GMT values for black swans and other *Anseriformes* [26, 41, 44, 45], and it was lower than reported in *Accipitriformes, Phoenicopteriformes* [27, 44]. Based on the literature, the differences induced by vaccination are observed between and within taxonomic orders. It could be assumed that single dose of the vaccine may induce relatively high antibody titers in mute swans. However, the type of H5 vaccine strain may have impact on the antibody responses [25, 27, 30].

Similarly to other studies, the effect of a booster dose was clearly demonstrated in this study [22, 25, 42, 44]. High seroconversion (100 %) was induced by booster dose of an inactivated H5N2 vaccine in black swans and other *Anseriformes* [41, 44], whereas lower seroconversion was also reported [27]. We observed dissimilar kinetics of the anti-NP and anti-HA antibodies after vaccination. The differences in NP-ELISA scores between D1 and D2 were not statistically significant throughout the study (week 2, 4, 6, 8). The findings indicate, that booster dose of vaccine did not have a significant impact on the increase of anti-NP titers, in contrast to anti-HA titers. The results highlight the role of anti-HA antibodies in the immune response to AI vaccination.

Elevated GMT in mute swans supported the observations made in black-necked swans, coscoroba swans and trumpeter swans, but differed from the values reported in whistling swans where GMT was low [30]. The H5N2 vaccine used in this study and H5N9 vaccines induced lower overall GMT and seroconversion in different species of *Anseriformes* than in mute swans [26, 27, 30, 32]. However, the differences in HI titers can be attributed to species-specific factors, vaccination schedules or differences in HI assays.

A clear relationship between HI titers and protection against AIV of the same HA subtype [2, 22] was reported in chickens, but it was not noted in mute swans. Studies of ducks demonstrated that vaccines characterized by high protein homology of HA1 with the challenge strain (89–100 % of amino acid similarities) delivered the best protection results [46]. This study relied on the assumption that vaccination in mute swans would produce similar results. The strains of HPAI viruses subtype H5N1 circulating at that time in Poland belonged to clade 2.2 [15]. Based on the high percentage (90–92.4 %) of homology of the vaccine strain with strains H5N1 (clade 2.2), we suggested that both antigenic and genetic distance between vaccine strain and circulating field strains in Poland can be considered the same (or very similar). Antigenically drifted avian influenza viruses decreased the effectiveness of commercial poultry vaccines, but not all antigenic variants of HPAIV H5N1 evaded vaccine-induced immunity in birds [46, 47]. Some studies revealed that genetically more distant vaccines could protect ducks against infection with H5N1 viruses [46]. In our study, a potent antibody response was observed in mute swans, but its role in conferring immunity against heterologous viruses needs to be further investigated.

In this study, booster vaccination was needed for all racing pigeons to produce titers of ≥ 32. The overall GMT was similar to that of rock pigeons vaccinated with the H5N6 vaccine [48], but was lower than obtained by H7N1 vaccine [42]. Unlike in this experiment, the same H5N2 vaccine induced lower antibody titers and seroconversion in *Columbiformes* [27, 30]. In this study, species-specific differences in vaccine-induced antibody titers were noted between mute swans and racing pigeons. The overall GMT in pigeons was approximately sevenfold lower than in swans. Our findings are consistent with the results reported in *Anseriformes* which developed stronger immune responses to inactivated vaccines than *Columbiformes* [26, 30, 48]. Selected species-specific factors, such as the role played by a given species in avian influenza epidemiology, AIV ecology and its susceptibility to HPAIV infection, could influence on the vaccine-induced antibody titers.

In our study, the vaccine promoted the development of both subtype H5 and type A influenza specific antibodies (anti-NP antibodies) in swans and pigeons. The significance of the antibody response to NP-induced by vaccination has not been fully elucidated. Anti-NP antibodies are not neutralizing, but according to recent reports, they could play a role in the promotion of cellular immunity [49].

Immunization of mute swans had no effect on the proliferative activity of lymphocytes. Our results were in agreement with data demonstrating that immunization of ducks with an inactivated vaccine did not increase the cellular response [34, 36]. Higgins et al. [34] suggested that ducks could have detectable levels of serum antibodies when the cell-mediated immune response is not detected in the lymphocyte transformation test. Further research into cellular immune responses in *Anseriformes* is needed to validate this hypothesis.

Conclusions

The present study demonstrated that immunization of mute swans with an inactivated H5N2 vaccine is safe and induced a strong humoral immune response. Humoral responses in swans were higher than in pigeons, but the induced antibody titers exceeded the levels presumed to confer immunity in poultry [2, 25, 27, 32]. A booster dose is recommended to enhance and maintain antibody titers. Our results could have practical implications for vaccination strategies for captive swans in zoos, wildlife parks or rehabilitation centers. Under extraordinary circumstances, vaccination of racing pigeons may be a useful strategy to save these birds from indoor confinement and pre-emptive culling (especially valuable individuals) due to the potential risk of AI outbreak. It could allow to continue the long-term breeding work and thus avoid economic losses. The challenge studies are needed to prove the efficacy of the H5N2 AI vaccine, in particular against the new H5 virus variants, and to formulate conclusive recommendations for immunization.

Abbreviations

AI: avian influenza; AIV: avian influenza virus; APMV-1 (NDV): avian paramyxovirus serotype 1 (Newcastle Disease Virus); GMT: geometric mean titer; HAU: hemagglutinating units; HI: hemagglutination inhibition; HPAI: highly pathogenic avian influenza; SI: stimulation index; LBTT: lymphocyte blast transformation test; PR: protection rate; SR: seroconversion rate.

Authors' contributions

BD involved in the design of the study, coordinated the experiment, carried out the practical work, analyzed the data and wrote the paper. AŻ, ID, PS participated in collecting samples and vaccination. PS involved in the design of the study, contributed significantly to the study and critically revised the manuscript. All authors read and approved the final manuscript.

Acknowledgements

We thank MSD Animal Health for the vaccine used in this study. We thank Dr. M. Slomka (VLA-Weybridge, UK) and Prof. L. B. Brydak (Department of

Influenza Research, NIPH—NIH, Poland) for control strains, A. Budyta (ornithologist) for help in the fieldwork, Polish Association of Racing Pigeon Breeders (PZHGP) for racing pigeons.

Competing interests
The authors declare that they have no competing interests.

Funding
This scientific work was co-financed by the European Social Fund (ESF) and the national budget within Integrated Regional Operational Programme (IROP), Action 2.6 "Regional Strategy for Innovation and Transfer of Knowledge", own project Mazowieckie voivodeship "Punjab Doctoral Scholarship" 0547/3.

References
1. Alexander DJ. A review of avian influenza in different bird species. Vet Microbiol. 2000;74:3–13.
2. Tian G, Zhang S, Li Y, Bu Z, Liu P, Zhou J, et al. Protective efficacy in chickens, geese and ducks of an H5N1-inactivated vaccine developed by reverse genetics. Virology. 2005;341:153–62.
3. Teifke JP, Klopfleisch R, Globig A, Starick E, Hoffman E, Wolf PU, et al. Pathology of natural infections by H5N1 highly pathogenic avian influenza virus in mute (*Cygnus olor*) and whooper (*Cygnus cygnus*) swans. Vet Pathol. 2007;44:137–43.
4. Verhagen JH, van der Jeugd HP, Nolet BA, Slaterus R, Kharitonov SP, de Vries PP, et al. Wild bird surveillance around outbreaks of highly pathogenic avian influenza A(H5N8) virus in the Netherlands, 2014, within the context of global flyways. Euro Surveill. 2015;20:21–32.
5. Otsuki K, Kawaoka Y, Nakamura T, Tsubokura M. Pathogenicity for chickens of avian influenza viruses isolated from whistling swans and a black-tailed gull in Japan. Avian Dis. 1982;26:314–20.
6. Nagy A, Machova J, Hornickova J, Tomci M, Nagl I, Horyna B, et al. Highly pathogenic avian influenza virus subtype H5N1 in mute swans in the Czech Republic. Vet Microbiol. 2007;120:9–16.
7. Feare CJ. Role of wild birds in the spread of highly pathogenic avian influenza virus H5N1 and implications for global surveillance. Avian Dis. 2010;54:201–12.
8. OIE. Update on avian influenza in animals (type H5 and H7). 2016. http://www.oie.int/animal-health-in-the-world/update-on-avian-influenza/2016/. Accessed 19 Oct 2016.
9. Kalthoff D, Breithaupt A, Teifke JP, Globig A, Harder T, Mettenleiter TC, et al. Highly pathogenic avian influenza virus (H5N1) in experimentally infected adult mute swans. Emerg Infect Dis. 2008;14:1267–70.
10. Yamamoto Y, Nakamura K, Yamada M, Ito T. Zoonotic risk for influenza A (H5N1) infection in wild swan feathers. J Vet Med Sci. 2009;71:1549–51.
11. Wallensten A, Salter M, Bennett S, Brown I, Hoschler K, Oliver I. No evidence of transmission of H5N1 highly pathogenic avian influenza to humans after unprotected contact with infected wild swans. Epidemiol Infect. 2010;138:210–3.
12. Adlhoch C, Gossner C, Koch G, Brown I, Bouwstra R, Verdonck F, et al. Comparing introduction to Europe of highly pathogenic avian influenza viruses A (H5N8) in 2014 and A(H5N1) in 2005. Euro Surveill. 2014;19:20996.
13. Lee DH, Torchetti MK, Winker K, Ip HS, Song CS, Swayne DE. Intercontinental spread of Asian-origin H5N8 to North America through Beringia by migratory birds. J Virol. 2015;89:6521–4.
14. Liu Y, Zhou J, Yang H, Yao W, Bu W, Yang B, et al. Susceptibility and transmissibility of pigeons to Asian lineage highly pathogenic avian influenza virus subtype H5N1. Avian Pathol. 2007;36:461–5.
15. Śmietanka K, Minta Z, Wyrostek K, Jóźwiak M, Olszewska M, Domańska-Blicharz AK, et al. Susceptibility of pigeons to clade 1 and 2.2 high pathogenicity avian influenza H5N1 virus. Avian Dis. 2011;55:106–12.
16. Abolnik C. A current review of avian influenza in pigeons and doves (*Columbidae*). Vet Microbiol. 2014;170:181–96.
17. Mansour SM, ElBakrey RM, Ali H, Knudsen DE, Eid AA. Natural infection with highly pathogenic avian influenza virus H5N1 in domestic pigeons (*Columba livia*) in Egypt. Avian Pathol. 2014;43:319–24.
18. Swayne DE, Suarez DL, Sims LD. Influenza. In: Swayne DE, Glisson JR, McDougald LR, Nolan LK, Suarez DL, Nair V, editors. Diseases of poultry. Hoboken: Wiley; 2013. p. 181–218.
19. Terrestrial Animal Health Code, vol. 1–2. OIE, 2016. http://www.oie.int/international-standard-setting/terrestrial-code/access-online/. Accessed 19 Oct 2016.
20. Śmietanka K, Minta Z, Domańska-Blicharz K, Tomczyk G, Wijaszka T. Avian influenza H5N1 outbreak in a flock of mute swans in the city of Toruń, Poland, in 2006. Bull Vet Inst Pulawy. 2008;52:491–5.
21. CEC. Council Directive 2005, 94, EC of 20,on December 2005 Community measures for the control of avian influenza and repealing Directive 92/40/EEC. Off J Eur Comm. 2006;L10:16–65.
22. Van den Berg T, Lambrecht B, Marché S, Steensels M, Van Borm S, Bublot M. Influenza vaccines and vaccination strategies in birds. Comp Immunol Microbiol Infect Dis. 2008;31:121–65.
23. Manual of Diagnostic Tests and Vaccines for Terrestrial Animals, OIE (2016) Chapter 2.03.04. (Avian Influenza), Chapter 2.03.14. (Newcastle Disease), Section 3.7.0 Recommendations for the manufacture of vaccines. http://www.oie.int/manual-of-diagnostic-tests-and-vaccines-for-terrestrial-animals/. Accessed 19 Oct 2016.
24. Koch G, Steensels M, van den Berg T. Vaccination of birds other than chickens and turkeys against avian influenza. Rev Sci Tech. 2009;28:307–18.
25. Lécu A, De Langhe C, Petit T, Bernard F, Swam H. Serologic response and safety to vaccination against avian influenza using inactivated H5N2 vaccine in zoo birds. J Zoo Wildl Med. 2009;40:731–43.
26. Vergara-Alert J, Fernández-Bellon H, Busquets N, Alcántara G, Delclaux M, Pizarro B, et al. Comprehensive serological analysis of two successive heterologous vaccines against H5N1 avian influenza virus in exotic birds in zoos. Clin Vaccine Immunol. 2011;18:697–706.
27. European Food Safety Authority (EFSA). Scientific Opinion Scientific opinion on: vaccination against avian influenza of H5 and H7 subtypes as a preventive measure carried out in Member States in birds kept in zoos under Community approved programmes. EFSA-Q-2006-156. EFSA J. 2007;450:1–35.
28. Capua I, Cattoli G, Marangon S. DIVA-a vaccination strategy enabling the detection of field exposure to avian influenza. Dev Biol (Basel). 2004;119:229–33.
29. 2006/437/EC: Commission Decision of 4 August 2006 approving a diagnostic manual for avian influenza as provided for in Council Directive 2005/94/EC. Off J E Union. Vol. 49. 31.08.2006. L237, p. 1–27. http://eur-lex.europa.eu/legal-content/EN/ALL/?uri=CELEX:32006D0437. Accessed 4 Aug 2006.
30. Philippa J, Baas C, Beyer W, Bestebroer T, Fouchier R, Smith D, et al. Vaccination against highly pathogenic avian influenza H5N1 virus in zoos using an adjuvanted inactivated H5N2 vaccine. Vaccine. 2007;25:3800–8.
31. European medicines agency-EMA. Nobilis influenza H5N2: EPAR-product information. http://www.ema.europa.eu/ema/index.jsp?curl=pages/medicines/veterinary/medicines/000118/vet_med_000147.jsp&mid=WC0b01ac058001fa1c.
32. Bertelsen MF, Klausen J, Holm E, Grøndahl C, Jørgensen PH. Serological response to vaccination against avian influenza in zoo-birds using an inactivated H5N9 vaccine. Vaccine. 2007;25:4345–9. doi:10.1016/j.vaccine.2007.03.043.
33. Bertram EM, Jilbert AR, Kotlarski L. Optimization of an in vitro assay which measures the proliferation of duck T lymphocytes from peripheral blood in response to stimulation with PHA and ConA. Dev Comp Immunol. 1997;21:299–310.
34. Higgins DA, Henry RR, Kounev ZV. Duck immune responses to *Riemerella anatipestifer* vaccines. Dev Comp Immunol. 2000;24:153–67.
35. Kapczynski DR. Detection of cell-mediated immune response to avian influenza viruses. Methods Mol Biol. 2014;1161:199–215.

36. Lambrecht B, Gonze M, Meulemans G, van den Berg TP. Assessment of the cell mediated immune response in chickens by detection of chicken interferon-gamma in response to mitogen and recall Newcastle disease viral antigen stimulation. Avian Pathol. 2004;33:343–50.
37. Spackman E, Senne DA, Myers TJ, Bulaga LL, Garber LP, Perdue ML, et al. Development of a real time reverse transcriptase PCR assay for type A influenza virus and the avian H5 and H7 haemagglutination subtypes. J Clin Microbiol. 2002;40:3256–60.
38. Slomka MJ, Coward VJ, Banks J, Löndt BZ, Brown IH, Voermans J, et al. Identification of sensitive and specific avian influenza polymerase chain reaction methods through blind ring trials organized in the European Union. Avian Dis. 2007;51:227–34.
39. Slomka MJ, Pavlidis T, Banks J, Shell W, McNally A, Essen S, et al. Validated H5 Eurasian real–time reverse transcriptase-polymerase chain reaction and its application in H5N1 outbreaks in 2005–2006. Avian Dis. 2007;51:373–7.
40. Creelan JL, Graham DA, McCullough SJ. Detection and differentiation of pathogenicity of avian paramyxovirus serotype 1 from field cases using one-step reverse transcriptase–polymerase chain reaction. Avian Pathol. 2002;31:493–9.
41. Oh S, Martelli P, Hock OS, Luz S, Furley C, Chiek EJ, et al. Field study on the use of inactivated H5N2 vaccine in avian species. Vet Rec. 2005;157:299–300.
42. Philippa JD, Munster VJ, Hv Bolhuis, Bestebroer TM, Schaftenaar W, Beyer WE, et al. Highly pathogenic avian influenza (H7N7): vaccination of zoo birds and transmission to non-poultry species. Vaccine. 2005;23:5743–50.
43. Obon E, Bailey TA, O'Donovan D, McKeown S, Kent J, Joseph S, et al. Humoral response to H5N2 vaccination in exotic birds in the United Arab Emirates. Vet Rec. 2007;161:860–1.
44. Furger M, Hoop R, Steinmetz H, Eulenberger U, Hatt JM. Humoral immune response to avian influenza vaccination over a six-month period in different species of captive wild birds. Avian Dis. 2008;52:222–8.
45. Cagle C, To TL, Nguyen T, Wasilenko J, Adams SC, Cardona CJ, et al. Pekin and Muscovy ducks respond differently to vaccination with a H5N1 highly pathogenic avian influenza (HPAI) commercial inactivated vaccine. Vaccine. 2011;29:6549–57.
46. Van der Goot JA, van Boven M, Stegeman A, van de Water SG, de Jong MC, Koch G. Transmission of highly pathogenic avian influenza H5N1 virus in Pekin ducks is significantly reduced by a genetically distant H5N2 vaccine. Virology. 2008;382:91–7.
47. Swayne DE, Lee CW, Spackman E. Inactivated North American and European H5N2 avian influenza virus vaccines protect chickens from Asian H5N1 high pathogenicity avian influenza virus. Avian Pathol. 2006;35:141–6.
48. Philippa JD, Bestebroer TM, Baas C, van der Bildt MW, Fouchier RA, van Amerongen G, et al. Protection of rock pigeons (*Columba livia*) against highly pathogenic influenza (H5N1) by inactivated H5N6 vaccine. In: Vaccination of non-domestic animals against emerging virus infections. Thesis, Erasmus Medical Centre: Rotterdam, The Netherlands, 2008; 142–59.
49. LaMere MW, Lam HT, Moquin A, Haynes L, Lund FE, Randall TD, et al. Contributions of antinucleoprotein IgG to heterosubtypic immunity against influenza virus. J Immunol. 2011;186:4331–9.

Cross-sectional survey on the use and impact of the Danish national antibiotic use guidelines for companion animal practice

Lisbeth Rem Jessen[1*], Tina Møller Sørensen[1], Zenia Littau Lilja[1], Maja Kristensen[1], Tine Hald[2] and Peter Damborg[3]

Abstract

Background: The Danish antibiotic use guidelines for companion animal practice were published by the Danish Veterinary Association in 2012. Since then, national surveillance data indicate a 10% reduction in the total use of antibiotics for companion animals, particularly a marked reduction in the use of third generation cephalosporins. The aim of the study was to assess if and how the guidelines have impacted diagnostic and antibiotic prescription habits of the users, and to identify user perceived barriers to implementation.

Results: An online questionnaire was sent to all 882 members of the Danish Small Animal Veterinary Association in October 2015. The survey was completed by 151 veterinarians. Respondents most frequently consulted the recommendations on skin and urinary tract infections (UTI), and users generally reported a high degree of adherence to the recommendations. Sixty-five per cent indicated that the guidelines had influenced their habits in one or more of the areas being investigated, i.e. perioperative use of antibiotics, use of first line antibiotics for the treatment of pyoderma or UTI, and/or use of microbiological diagnostics. Perioperative use of antibiotics for clean surgeries was uncommon, irrespective of whether respondents had consulted the relevant recommendations or not. On the contrary, significant differences in the prescribing habits between guideline users and non-users were observed for pyoderma and UTI, suggesting an impact of the guidelines towards more prudent antimicrobial use. The diagnostic habits were examined in a subgroup of 63 guideline users. Of those, 19 and 39% reported frequent use of culture and susceptibility (C&S) testing prior to treating pyoderma and UTI respectively, whereas 68–84% reported C&S testing in the event of poor response to treatment or recurrence of infections. The main barriers for implementation of therapeutic recommendations were confidence in old prescribing practices and unavailability of recommended drugs. The main barriers for C&S testing were good experience with empiric treatment, and the owners' financial situation.

Conclusions: The findings suggest a positive influence of the national antibiotic guidelines on prescription patterns among companion animal practitioners in Denmark. Sustained campaign activity is encouraged and should include promotion of bacteriological testing.

Keywords: Bacteriological testing, Culture, Rational antimicrobial use, Prescription patterns, Pyoderma, Questionnaire, Sensitivity, Susceptibility, Urinary tract infections, UTI

Background

Antibiotic consumption is widely recognized as the main driver for the selection of antibiotic resistant bacteria, and rational antimicrobial use is therefore considered one of the most important strategies in combatting antimicrobial resistance [1]. Rational antimicrobial use may be defined as usage resulting in clinical resolution while selecting minimally for antimicrobial resistance. Several international and national guidelines for antimicrobial use have been developed over the last decade to help

*Correspondence: lrmj@sund.ku.dk
[1] Department of Veterinary Clinical Sciences, University of Copenhagen, Dyrlægevej 16, 1870 Frederiksberg C, Denmark
Full list of author information is available at the end of the article

companion animal veterinarians towards this goal [2–6]. Such guidelines are written as clinical practice guidelines indicating diagnostic criteria for—and recommended therapy (drug, dose, duration) of—the most common bacterial infectious diseases in companion animals.

When implemented at hospital or practice level, clinical practice guidelines hold a huge potential to impact prescribing habits of veterinary clinicians and promote prudent use of antibiotics [7].

In Sweden, national antibiotic use guidelines for companion animals [5] were first published in 2003 and later revised in 2009. Since then the use of antibiotics, in particular cephalosporins, fluoroquinolones and potentiated aminopenicillins, has dropped markedly [8]. In a survey conducted in 2012 on antibiotic use and prescribing habits among veterinary practitioners from seven European countries, Swedish practitioners reported a very low use of critically important antibiotics for companion animals [9] and, as the sole country, indicated antibiotic guidelines as the most important factor influencing their prescription habits [10].

In Denmark, national antibiotic use guidelines for companion animals were published in November 2012 [6] and distributed in a booklet format to all members of the Danish Small Animal Association (DSAVA). The guidelines are available also as PDF downloads (Danish and English) and as a smartphone/tablet application. All versions are free of charge. Between 2012 and 2016, national consumption data indicate a 10% reduction in the total use of antibiotics for companion animals, including an almost 40% reduction in the use of third generation cephalosporins [11]. However, it is unknown to what extent such changes may be attributable to the use of the guidelines.

The aim of this survey was to assess if and how the Danish national antibiotic use guidelines for companion animals have impacted diagnostic habits and antibiotic prescription patterns of users, and to identify user perceived barriers to implementation of recommendations.

Methods

A questionnaire (Additional file 1) was designed to investigate (1) if and to which extent the guidelines were consulted, (2) impact of the guidelines on prescriber habits within the following areas: perioperative use of antibiotics, prescription patterns for infections of the skin and urinary tract (UTI), and use of culture and susceptibility testing (C&S) and, (3) the practitioners attitude to the guidelines, and their perception of the utility and applicability in practice.

The questionnaire was tested in a small focus group of four practitioners before being launched as an electronic survey using TricTrac Student, (http://www.trictrac.com). The survey was accessible from October to November 2015, and during this period a link to the questionnaire was sent twice by e-mail to all 882 members of DSAVA. Participation in the survey was anonymous, and respondents could choose to participate in a draw for prizes (Additional file 2).

The Danish national guidelines consists of different chapters each providing infection-specific diagnostic and therapeutic recommendations. Respondents having consulted a specific set of recommendations (e.g. treatment of skin infections) were defined as "users" of those recommendations, regardless of whether they indicated adherence or not to the recommendations. Respondents who had not consulted the specific set of recommendations were defined as "non-users".

The questionnaire consisted of 86 questions, of which 73 where multiple choice and 13 were open. Open questions reported in this paper all relate to personal therapeutic habits. The majority of questions were open to all participants. However, questions regarding adherence to specific recommendations were only asked to *users*.

The questionnaire was divided in three parts. In the first part, participants were asked information on gender, age, graduation year, practice location, type of practice, and presence of any written antibiotic policy in their practice. In the second part, participants were asked questions related to their use of—and adherence to—the different recommendations of the guidelines. This included questions related to (i) their perioperative use of antibiotics and choice of treatment for pyoderma and UTI, and (ii) their diagnostic habits with regards to use of C&S. Finally, in the third part, participants were asked questions related to their perception of the guidelines and barriers for implementation. The questionnaire in original language (Danish) is available upon request. The criteria for evaluating adherence are listed in Table 1.

Descriptive statistics were performed using Excel 2013, Microsoft Office. Chi square tests were performed for comparison of habits between guideline users and non-users (SAS Enterprise Guide 2013). Study power and margin of error was calculated using EpiInfo v7.2.0.1. $P < 0.05$ was considered statistically significant.

Results

The questionnaire was completed by 151 companion animal practitioners, corresponding to 17% (151/882) of the DSAVA members. This resulted in a statistical power of approximately 85%, a confidence level of 95%, and a margin of error of 7.3% for the survey.

The distribution of age, gender and geographical location (Additional file 2) of the 151 respondents was similar to that of the entire group of 882 DSAVA members (Figs. 1, 2 and 3). Thirty per cent (46/151) of the clinics had a written antibiotic policy.

Table 1 Criteria for evaluating if specific therapeutic practices were in accordance with the national guideline recommendations

Indication	Assessment of accordance	
	In accordance	Not in accordance
Use of perioperative antibiotics	In 0–10% of clean surgeries	In > 10% of clean surgeries
Treatment of superficial pyoderma	Topical treatment alone Topical treatment in combination with a lincosamide	Topical treatment in combination with systemic antibiotics other than lincosamide Systemic treatment alone
Treatment of cystitis	Amoxicillin or potentiated sulfonamides	Systemic treatment other than amoxicillin or potentiated sulfonamides

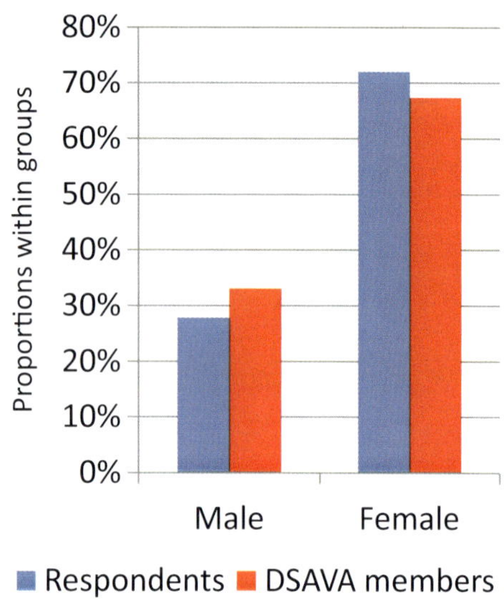

Fig. 1 Gender distribution of the 151 respondents and the 882 Danish Small Animal Association (DSAVA) members

Consultation of the guidelines

Of the 151 respondents, 145 (96%) reported they had consulted the guidelines. Twelve per cent (18/151) had never heard of the smartphone/tablet application, and among those that knew of the application, 59% (78/133) preferred the booklet or PDF format, whereas 38% (51/133) preferred the smartphone/tablet application. Three per cent (4/133) had never used the guidelines or did not know which version they had used.

Respondents most frequently consulted the recommendations on skin infections (78%, 118/151) and UTI (64%, 96/151). Between 73 and 92% (32/44 and 109/118) of users indicated adherence to the recommendations they had consulted (Fig. 4).

Prescribing habits and diagnostics

In total, 98 out of 151 respondents (65%) answered that the antibiotic guidelines had influenced their habits in one or more of the following areas: use of perioperative

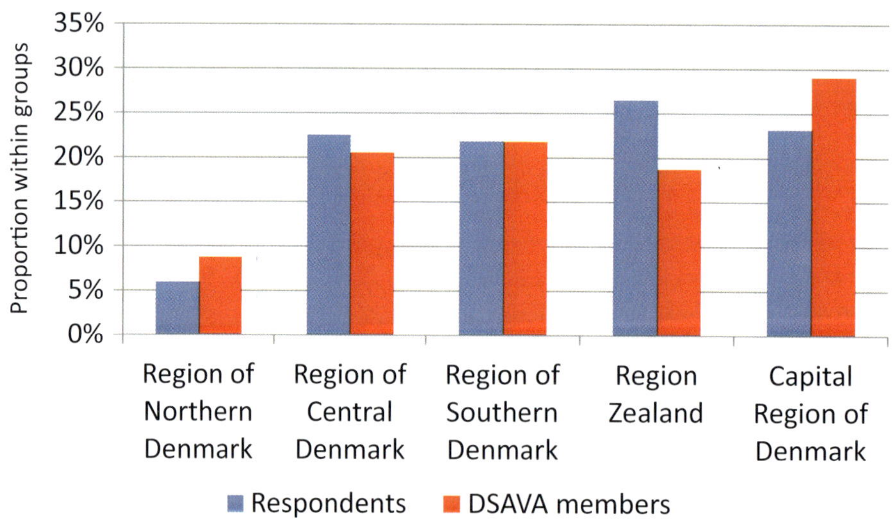

Fig. 2 Geographical location in Denmark of the 151 respondents and the 882 Danish Small Animal Association (DSAVA) members

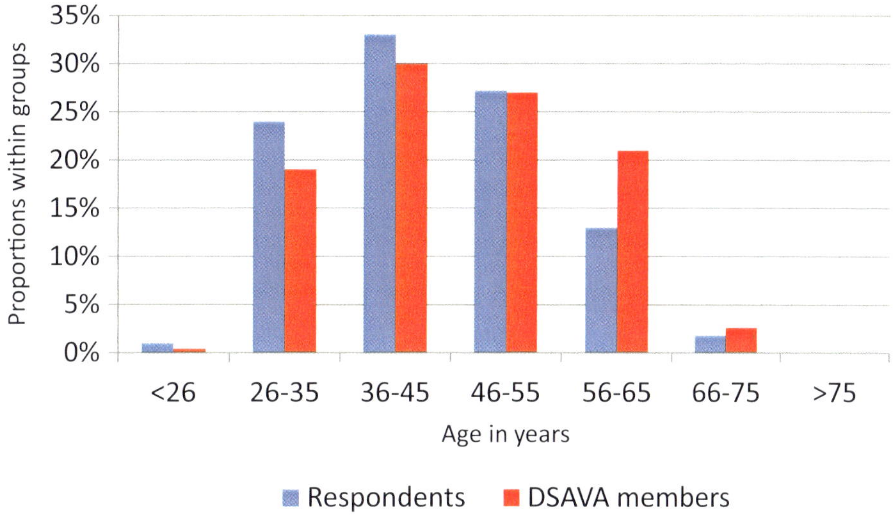

Fig. 3 Age distribution of the 151 respondents and the 882 Danish Small Animal Association (DSAVA) members

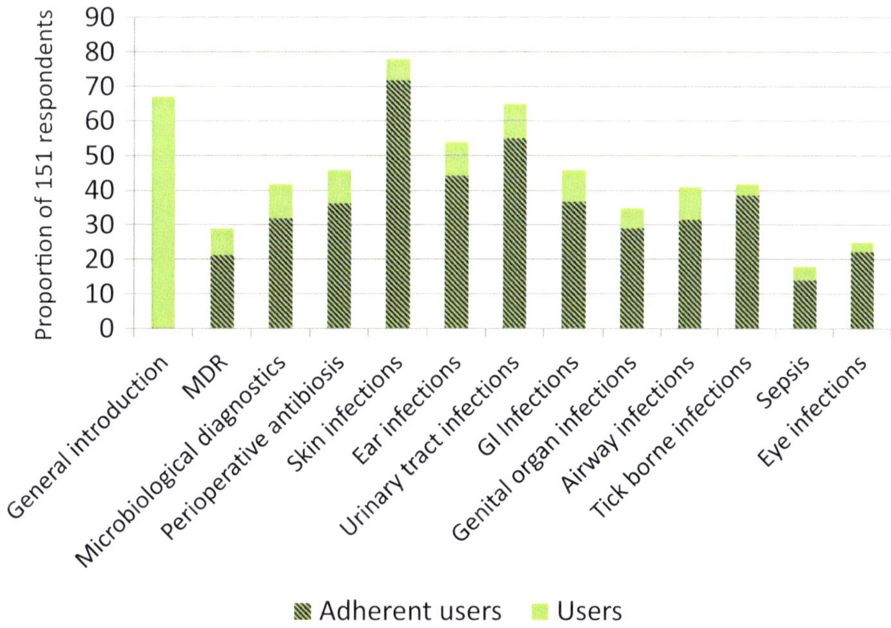

Fig. 4 The proportion of respondents consulting the different recommendations of the antibiotic use guidelines (users). Shaded area of the columns are the proportion of users answering yes to the following question: "Do you predominately adhere to the recommendations in this area?"

antibiotics, choice of treatment for pyoderma and/or UTI, and/or use of culture and susceptibility testing.

Perioperative antibiotics

In total, 66 out of 151 respondents (44%) indicated that the guidelines had led them to reduce their perioperative use of antibiotics. When asked specifically about their habits, 75% (113/151) reported peri- or postoperative use of antibiotics in less than 10% of clean surgeries, which was in accordance with the recommendations (Table 1). Among the 70 respondents who had consulted the guideline recommendations on perioperative antibiotics (users), this proportion was 81% (57/70), and among the 81 who had not consulted the recommendations (non-users), the proportion was 69% (56/81). There was no significant difference between users and non-users ($P = 0.083$).

Skin infections

In total, 68 out of 151 respondents (45%) indicated that the guidelines had influenced their choice of treatment for canine superficial pyoderma. When asked about their first line treatment for canine superficial pyoderma, 65% (96 out of 147 respondents replying to the question) reported use of topical treatment alone or in combination with systemic lincosamides. Both of these treatment regimens are in accordance with the recommendations (Table 1). Among the 116 respondents who had consulted the recommendations on skin infection (users), this proportion was 70% (81/116), and among the 31 who had not consulted the recommendations (non-users) the proportion was 48% (15/31) (Fig. 5). The difference between users and non-users was statistically significant (P = 0.026).

Urinary tract infections

In total, 36 out of 151 respondents (24%) indicated that the guidelines had influenced their choice of treatment

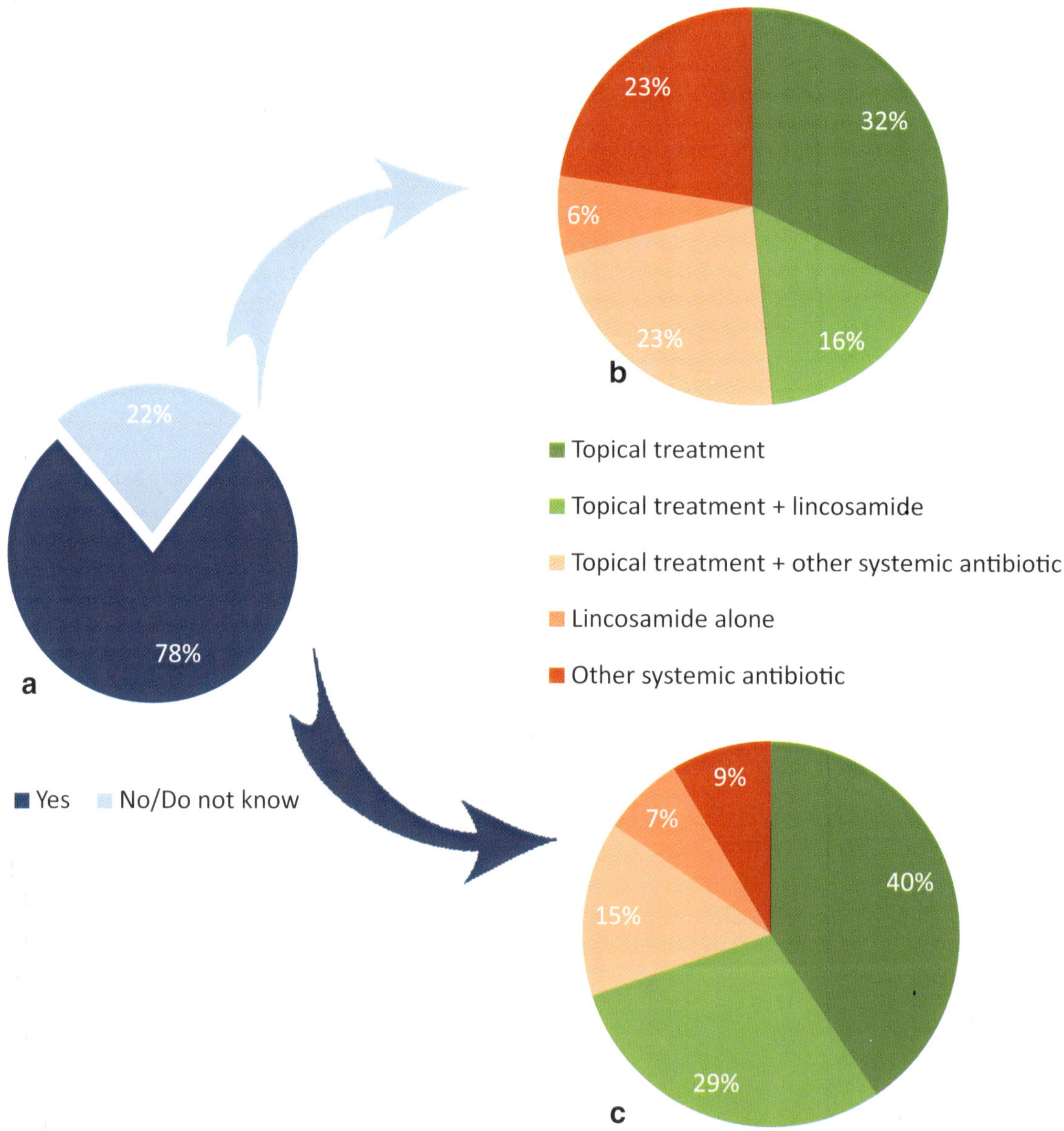

Fig. 5 Users and non-users choice of first line treatment for superficial pyoderma. **a** Proportion of the 151 respondents answering yes (users) or no (non-users) to the following question: "Have you consulted the recommendations on skin infections?". **b** Choice of first line treatment for superficial pyoderma among the 31 non-users. **c** Choice of first line treatment for superficial pyoderma among the 116 users

for UTI. When asked about their first line treatment for cystitis, 51% (74 out of 144 respondents replying to the question) reported use of amoxicillin or potentiated sulfonamides in accordance with the recommendations (Table 1). Among the 93 respondents who had consulted the recommendations on UTI (users) this proportion was 59% (55/93), and among the 51 who had not consulted the recommendations (non-users) the proportion was 37% (19/51) (Fig. 6). The difference between users and non-users was statistically significant ($P = 0.012$).

Culture and susceptibility testing

Questions regarding C&S testing were intended for all respondents, but by programming error only the 63 respondents who had consulted the recommendations on microbiological diagnostics (users) were asked. In total, 35 of those 63 users (56%) replied that consulting the guidelines had increased their use of C&S testing. The proportions of users performing C&S testing in different suggested clinical scenarios are listed in Table 2.

Users of the chapter on microbiological diagnostics answered to the question "In which of the following

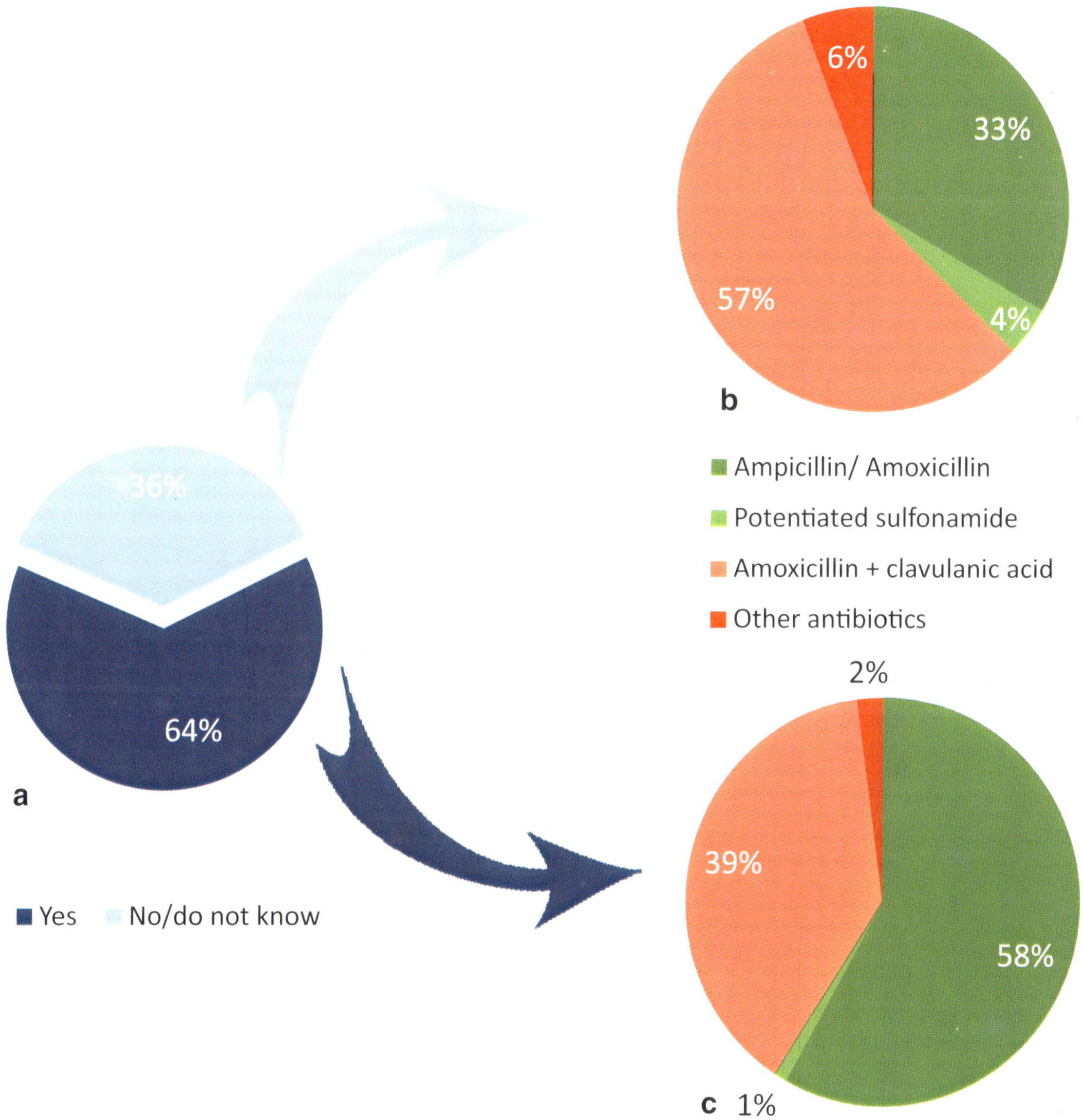

Fig. 6 Users and non-users choice of first line treatment for cystitis. **a** Proportion of the 151 respondents answering yes (users) or no (non-users) to the following question: "Have you consulted the recommendations on urinary tract infections?". **b** Choice of first line treatment for cystitis among the 51 non-users. **c** Choice of first line treatment for cystitis among the 93 users

Table 2 Proportion of users performing culture and susceptibility testing in different clinical scenarios

Scenarios	Number of users (%) n = 63
When I treat pyoderma (any type) with systemic antibiotics	12 (19)
When I treat UTI (any type) with antibiotics	25 (39)
When I treat recurrent pyoderma with systemic antibiotics	53 (84)
When I treat recurrent UTI with antibiotics	50 (79)
When I treat rare infections	35 (55)
When empiric treatment fails	43 (68)
I rarely perform C&S	1 (2)
Other	6 (10)

scenarios do you usually perform C&S?". Multiple answers were allowed.

User perception of barriers for implementation

The majority of respondents (95%, 144/151) fully agreed that the national Danish antibiotic use guidelines for companion animals is an important initiative, and 77% (116/151) fully agreed that guidelines can reduce the occurrence of antibiotic resistance in companion animals in Denmark.

The following main barriers for not adhering to the therapeutic recommendations of the guidelines were identified among the respondents: confidence in old prescribing practices (46%, 69/151), unavailability of products registered for dogs and cats (34%, 52/151), difficulties dosing the drug (e.g. due to odd tablet size) (31%, 47/151), costs (30%, 46/151), lack of time for consulting the guidelines (25%, 38/151), limited number of antibiotic drugs available on site (23%, 35/151), owners difficulties in administering drugs (18%, 27/151).

The main barriers for performing C&S among the 63 users were the owners' financial situation (70%, 44/63) and good experience with empiric treatment (60%, 38/63). Furthermore, 25% (16/63) of users noted that it is not necessary to perform C&S as often as the guideline recommends, and 21% (13/63) noted that they never or rarely encounter infections with antibiotic resistant bacteria.

Discussion

The survey indicates that the guidelines have been positively received among the respondents, of which the majority indicated adherence to the recommendations. To better investigate the direct and indirect impact of guidelines on prescription habits, a comparison of actual antibiotic prescriptions before and after guideline publication would be ideal. Since such data were not available, we compared the choice of treatment in specific scenarios for users vs. non-users of the guidelines. This comparison showed a significant difference between the two groups with regard to treatment of pyoderma and UTI (Figs. 5 and 6). Although the causal relationship cannot be established with certainty, the results suggest that the guidelines have influenced the habits of its readers towards more rational antimicrobial use. On the other hand, there was no apparent effect of the guidelines on perioperative use of antibiotics, since both users and non-users reported very limited use of antibiotics for this indication. This result likely reflects the restrictive use of antibiotics in surgery that is well established amongst veterinarians in Denmark, which could be due to many years of teaching aseptic surgical techniques to veterinary students. Accordingly, the guideline emphasizes what is generally known about perioperative antibiotic use, instead of changing a treatment paradigm.

When comparing the results for pyoderma and UTI, the survey shows that recommendations for skin infections were not only being consulted more frequently, they are also being converted into practice more successfully. Even among the practitioners not consulting the guidelines on pyoderma (non-users) their choices were nearly 50% in accordance with the recommendations. This result is probably explained by campaigning activity conducted by the Danish Veterinary Dermatological Network (DVEN) prior to and following the publication of the guidelines, and illustrates the great importance of active dissemination and campaigns.

The Danish guidelines recommend frequent use of C&S testing, including for all cases of suspected pyoderma and UTI. One rationale behind this recommendation is the relatively high consumption of antibiotics for these common indications [9, 12]. Furthermore, multidrug-resistant pathogens like methicillin-resistant *Staphylococcus pseudintermedius* (MRSP) and extended-spectrum beta-lactamase (ESBL)-producing *Enterobacteriaceae* have emerged in companion animals, and these pathogens occur primarily in the skin and the urinary tract, respectively [13]. Unfortunately, the habits for C&S testing were only examined among the respondents consulting the section on microbiological diagnostics, and the difference between guideline users and non-users could not be assessed. However, the survey clearly indicates that, even though 56% of users reported an increased use of C&S testing this is not routinely performed for pyoderma and UTI, except in recurrent cases (Table 2). The result is not surprising, as recommending broad use of C&S testing represents a major shift of paradigm, which takes time to implement. In a European survey from 2012 [10], 51% of companion animal practitioners reported using C&S

testing for complicated or non-responding cases only, and 16% reported to rarely or never use it. Interestingly, broad use of sensitivity testing was much more widespread among Swedish practitioners participating in that survey.

As anticipated from other studies of veterinary antibiotic prescription patterns [10, 14], financial costs were a commonly reported barrier in our study, and 70% of respondents reported the owners financial situation to be a limiting factor for performing bacteriological diagnostics. This is in line with surveys on veterinary prescription patterns in North America where 65% [14] and 84% [15] of participants reported costs as a barrier to recommending C&S testing. In that regard it should be noted that the costs of C&S testing are relatively modest, at least in Scandinavia, and in most instances lower than the costs associated with treatment failure (e.g. repeated veterinary consultations and antibiotic treatments). Regardless, as long as diagnostic testing relies on owner/client economy, test costs will remain a potential barrier to antibiotic stewardship. In light of this situation, companion animal veterinarians must educate owners on the importance and benefits of this practice prior to antimicrobial treatment.

The survey indicates that a variety of factors influence the adherence to therapeutic recommendations, and that practical barriers such as unavailability of recommended drugs for veterinary use, odd tablet size, and ease of administration play an important role. Similarly, ease of administration was identified as a factor influencing antibiotic prescription patterns in a cross sectional survey among companion animal veterinarians in the UK [16]. To exemplify the problems of availability, potentiated sulfonamides are recommended as first choice for several conditions in the guidelines, but unfortunately from March 2015 no oral product for companion animal use has been available on the Danish market. Other commonly recommended drugs, including amoxicillin have been in short supply on the Danish market periodically. Such barriers are difficult to foresee and to solve by the authors of the guidelines, who base recommendations on clinical effect and knowledge of selection pressure and critical importance of drugs. Recommending more than one drug for each condition may partly overcome this problem.

The response rate on this survey was 17%, which is low in a small and well defined population with a presumed interest in the topic. The reason for this is unknown but falls within a general trend of decreased response rates in epidemiological studies [17, 18]. The response rate might have improved by directly contacting the practitioners, or offering further incentives to participants. Irrespectively, a low response rate is not necessarily problematic if demographic representation and study power is adequate [19], which was the case in our study. Of importance, the investigation relied on voluntary participation. This could have biased the results (selection bias) towards a higher degree of adherence to the guidelines, as the respondents may have an increased interest in antibiotic use.

The criteria for evaluating if specific therapeutic practices were in accordance with the guideline recommendations were to some extent subjective (Table 1). To exemplify, we considered topical antiseptic treatment both with and without a lincosamide as appropriate for treatment of superficial pyoderma, even though the guidelines recommend topical treatment alone as the first line. The rationale behind the decision was the lack of distinction between first episode cases and recurring cases in the questionnaire. Many respondents therefore added comments that topical treatment was their first choice for superficial pyoderma with combination therapy being applied only for difficult, non-responsive, or recurrent cases.

Conclusions

The findings suggest a positive influence of the national antibiotic use guidelines on prescription pattern among companion animal practitioners in Denmark. This is supported by national consumption data, since the use of particularly some important broad-spectrum drugs like third generation cephalosporins has markedly dropped since the guidelines were published. The vast majority of respondents had consulted the guidelines and perceived them as useful despite issues such as limited availability of certain drugs. Future campaigns are strongly encouraged to promote implementation of the recommendations in practice. Campaigns should focus on infections for which antibiotics are commonly prescribed, and on the use of diagnostic testing.

Authors' contributions

LRJ conceived the study, supervised the master thesis project, participated in the data analyses and drafted the manuscript. TMS co-supervised the master thesis project, participated in the design of the study, conducted the data analyses and critically revised the manuscript. ZLL conducted the master thesis project, the data analyses, and critically revised the manuscript. MK conducted the master thesis project, the data analyses, and critically revised the manuscript. TH co-supervised the master thesis project, participated in the design of the study and critically revised the manuscript. PPD conceived the study, supervised the master thesis project, participated in the data analyses and critically revised the manuscript. All authors read and approved the final manuscript.

Author details

[1] Department of Veterinary Clinical Sciences, University of Copenhagen, Dyrlægevej 16, 1870 Frederiksberg C, Denmark. [2] National Food Institute,

Technical University of Denmark, Kemitorvet, Building 204, 2800 Kgs. Lyngby, Denmark. [3] Department of Veterinary and Animal Sciences, University of Copenhagen, Stigbøjlen 4, 1870 Frederiksberg C, Denmark.

Acknowledgements
We wish to acknowledge all the practitioners for participating in this study and Helle Elkjær Johansen from the DSAVA for mediating contact to the DSAVA members.

Competing interests
The authors declare that they have no competing interests. LRJ and PPD were involved as academic coordinators and editors in the first edition of the Danish National Guidelines for Antibiotic Use in Companion Animals.

Funding
The draw for prizes was funded by the Danish Small Animal Association (DSAVA). No other external funding was granted for this study.

References

1. World Health Organization. Draft global action plan on antimicrobial resistance. 2014. http://www.who.int/drugresistance/global_action_plan/en/. Accessed 30 June 2017.
2. Weese JS, Blondeau JM, Boothe D, Breitschwerdt EB, Guardabassi L, Hillier A, et al. Antimicrobial use guidelines for treatment of urinary tract disease in dogs and cats: antimicrobial guidelines working group of the international society for companion animal infectious diseases. Vet Med Int. 2011;2011:263768.
3. Lappin MR, Blondeau J, Boothe D, Breitschwerdt EB, Guardabassi L, Lloyd DH, et al. Antimicrobial use guidelines for treatment of respiratory tract disease in dogs and cats: antimicrobial guidelines working group of the International Society for Companion Animal Infectious Diseases. J Vet Intern Med. 2017;31:279–94.
4. Hillier A, Lloyd DH, Weese JS, Blondeau JM, Boothe D, Breitschwerdt E, et al. Guidelines for the diagnosis and antimicrobial therapy of canine superficial bacterial folliculitis (Antimicrobial Guidelines Working Group of the International Society for Companion Animal Infectious Diseases). Vet Dermatol. 2014;25(163–75):e42–63.
5. Swedish Veterinary Association. Guidelines for the clinical use of antibiotics in the treatment of dogs and cats (Antibiotikapolicy för Hund- och Kattsjukvård), vol. 2. Sweden: SVS; 2009. http://www.sva.se/upload/Redesign2011/Pdf/antibiotika/antibiotikapolicy_2009.pdf.
6. Jessen LR, Damborg P, Spohr A, Schjøth B, Wiinberg B, Houser G et al. Antibiotic use guidelines for companion animal practice (Antibiotikavejledning til familiedyr), vol. 1: Den Danske Dyrlægeforenings Sektion for Hund, Kat & Smådyr, SvHKS, Emdrupvej 28A, 2100 København Ø; 2012. https://www.ddd.dk/organisatorisk/sektionsmaadyr/Documents/Antibiotikavejledning_Interaktiv_HIGH.pdf.
7. Weese JS. Investigation of antimicrobial use and the impact of antimicrobial use guidelines in a small animal veterinary teaching hospital: 1995–2004. J Am Vet Med Assoc. 2006;228:553–8.
8. Greko C. Reduction of sales of antimicrobials for dogs—Swedish experiences. The FECAVA symposium, 2013. EJCAP. 2013;23:55–60.
9. De Briyne N, Atkinson J, Pokludova L, Borriello SP. Antibiotics used most commonly to treat animals in Europe. Vet Rec. 2014;175:325.
10. De Briyne N, Atkinson J, Pokludova L, Borriello SP, Price S. Factors influencing antibiotic prescribing habits and use of sensitivity testing amongst veterinarians in Europe. Vet Rec. 2013;173:475.
11. DANMAP 2016. Use of antimicrobial agents and occurrence of antimicrobial resistance in bacteria from food animals, food and humans in Denmark. Denmark: DTU-Food/SSI; 2016. https://www.danmap.org/~/media/Projekt%20sites/Danmap/DANMAP%20reports/DANMAP%202016/DANMAP_2016_web.ashx.
12. Rantala M, Holso K, Lillas A, Huovinen P, Kaartinen L. Survey of condition-based prescribing of antimicrobial drugs for dogs at a veterinary teaching hospital. Vet Rec. 2004;155:259–62.
13. Wieler LH, Ewers C, Guenther S, Walther B, Lubke-Becker A. Methicillin-resistant staphylococci (MRS) and extended-spectrum beta-lactamases (ESBL)-producing Enterobacteriaceae in companion animals: nosocomial infections as one reason for the rising prevalence of these potential zoonotic pathogens in clinical samples. Int J Med Microbiol. 2011;301:635–41.
14. Fowler H, Davis MA, Perkins A, Trufan S, Joy C, Buswell M, et al. A survey of veterinary antimicrobial prescribing practices, Washington State 2015. Vet Rec. 2016;179:651.
15. AVMA Task Force for Antimicrobial Stewardship in Companion Animal Practice. Understanding companion animal practitioners' attitudes toward antimicrobial stewardship. J Am Vet Med Assoc. 2015;247:883–4.
16. Hughes LA, Williams N, Clegg P, Callaby R, Nuttall T, Coyne K, et al. Cross-sectional survey of antimicrobial prescribing patterns in UK small animal veterinary practice. Prev Vet Med. 2012;104:309–16.
17. Galea S, Tracy M. Participation rates in epidemiologic studies. Ann Epidemiol. 2007;17:643–53.
18. Hohwu L, Lyshol H, Gissler M, Jonsson SH, Petzold M, Obel C. Web-based versus traditional paper questionnaires: a mixed-mode survey with a Nordic perspective. J Med Internet Res. 2013;15:e173.
19. McCrum-Gardner E. Sample size and power calculations made simple. Int J Ther Rehabil. 2010;17:10–4.

Cross-sectional study on risk factors for Porcine Reproductive and Respiratory Syndrome virus sow herd instability in German breeding herds

Christina Nathues[1,2], Eltje Janssen[3], Andrea Duengelhoef[3], Heiko Nathues[4†] and Elisabeth grosse Beilage[3*†]

Abstract

Background: Porcine Reproductive and Respiratory Syndrome virus (PRRSV) stability, besides meeting production targets, is also a requirement for several control options of PRRS in pig breeding farms. This study aimed to investigate the frequency of, and risk factors associated with, PRRSV instability in pig breeding farms in northern Germany. In 120 sow herds, a questionnaire on production and management parameters was filled, and blood samples from 30 suckling pigs from 10 different litters were taken and examined using real-time polymerase chain reaction (PCR).

Results: PRRSV was detected in 32 herds (27%), thus classified as PRRSV-unstable. According to multivariable logistic regression analysis, a suckling period ≤ 21 days, a low distance between the cadaver collection site and the actual sow barn, ≥ 2 pig herds in a 1000 m radius, presence of external employees, a time interval between purchase of gilts of ≤ 9 weeks and a 1- or 2-weekly farrowing rhythm were associated with a higher risk of PRRSV instability.

Conclusions: External and internal biosecurity as well as management factors were associated with PRRSV instability, which could be targeted by farmers and veterinarians to help them to achieve PRRSV PCR-negative status and in the control of PRRS.

Keywords: Herd management, Herd prevalence, PRRS control, Risk factors

Background

Pig herds infected with Porcine Reproductive and Respiratory Syndrome virus (PRRSV) often develop corresponding clinical diseases in sows, boars and/or their offspring. It has been shown that the frequency of disease outbreaks and the severity of clinical symptoms in a herd are driven by virulence of the particular PRRSV isolate and risk factors, such as co-infections or lack of gilt acclimatisation [1, 2]. Vaccination against the Porcine Reproductive and Respiratory Syndrome (PRRS) is possible and commonly applied [3], but does not always sufficiently prevent clinical diseases [4], neither does it offer the possibility of elimination of the virus at farm level [5].

Taking these limitations of PRRS control by vaccination into account, additional measures are necessary. In order to control PRRS in such herds, different options are available at farm level, including close and rollover and test and removal [6–9]. However, these two options require herd stability in terms of (non-existent) PRRSV transmission from dams to their offspring. They usually work sufficiently only if no further vertical transmission of PRRSV from sows to suckling pigs occurs and only PRRSV negative piglets are weaned. Therefore, appropriate evaluation of the breeding herd PRRSV status and assessment of potential risk factors influencing it are important. According to Holtkamp's definition, PRRSV stability [10] is the absence of virus circulation within the herd over

*Correspondence: Elisabeth.grosse.beilage@tiho-hannover.de
†Heiko Nathues and Elisabeth grosse Beilage contributed equally to the study
[3] Field Station for Epidemiology, University of Veterinary Medicine Hannover, Buescheler Strasse 9, 49456 Bakum, Germany
Full list of author information is available at the end of the article

a 90-day period, based on four consecutive negative polymerase chain reaction (PCR) herd testings every 30 days, or more frequently, of at least 30 suckling pigs at weaning age from 30 different litters. Moreover, there shall be no clinical signs consistent with PRRS observed in the particular breeding herd. Virus detection classifies a herd as unstable.

The aim of this study was to investigate the frequency of PRRSV instability among professional pig breeding farms in northern Germany and the associations between different farm and management characteristics, respectively, and PRRS PCR-status in these herds.

Methods

Study herds and data collection

A cross-sectional study was conducted in north-western Germany, the most pig-dense region in Germany. A total of 120 sow herds was included in the study. Inclusion and exclusion criteria were a size of the smallest farrowing group of minimum 12 sows, and the use of an electronic recording system for reproductive performance indicators. Overall, 201 herds were pre-selected. They were member of one out of five different advisory units and they were all contacted first by their (veterinary) advisor. Only herds, where the farmer agreed to participate in the study voluntarily, were included in the final sample. Between July 2011 and November 2012, the herds were examined once, evenly distributed over the whole study period. Herd examination consisted of (1) filling in a paper-based questionnaire on production and management parameters in personal interviews with the farmers (all parameters are listed in an additional file, separately for numerical variables (Additional file 1) and in categorical variables (Additional file 2); (2) taking blood samples from 30 suckling pigs from 10 different litters (3 piglets per litter/17–21 days of age/all randomly chosen) by puncture of the *vena jugularis externa*. Blood samples were taken to the laboratory (Field Station for Epidemiology) and examined for PRRSV with a commercially available real-time PCR kit (Tetracore Inc., Rockville, USA) in pools, each containing the 3 samples from the suckling pigs of the same litter. Due to limited time and financial resources, the sampling protocol of sampling all herds once was not strictly in line with Holtkamp's definition of PRRSV stability [10], requiring various consecutive herd testings. Thus, whereas a positive PCR result clearly classifies a herd as unstable, a lack of PRRSV detection at sampling does not proof that a herd is stable. For this reason, in the course of this manuscript we would like to use the term "PCR negative" to describe the absence of virus circulation in the herd at the time of sampling.

Data analysis

Data from questionnaires and laboratory results were stored in a spreadsheet program (Microsoft® Excel® 2016, Microsoft Corporation, Redmond, WA, USA); statistical analyses were conducted in R studio for R version 3.0.1 (R Core Team 2013, Vienna, Austria).

Descriptive statistics were calculated for all variables (indicated in Additional files 1 and 2). The herd status as result of PCR testing was defined as the main outcome variable. A herd was classified as PCR positive if at least one blood sample was tested positive by PCR; otherwise, it was classified as PCR negative. Univariable associations between all variables and PCR status were tested with χ^2 test or Fisher's Exact test for categorical variables and Mann/Whitney-U test for numerical variables. Categorical variables exhibiting very low numbers in certain categories were recoded (summing up two categories into one new one). An example is the production rhythm, where only few herds had a 2-weekly or 5-weekly rhythm, so that the different weekly rhythms were summarized in the two categories "1- or 2-weekly" and "3-, 4- or 5-weekly". Numerical variables were checked for linear relationship with the outcome variable by creating scatterplots and adding smoothed lines (function *lowess*). If this was not fulfilled, variables were categorized following biologically or otherwise plausible boundaries (e.g. suckling period up to vs. more than the legally required 21 days), or according to three equal quantiles (herd size, time interval between purchase of gilts). All variables showing a p-value of ≤ 0.1 in the univariable analysis were treated as candidate variables for a multivariable logistic regression model, and tested for associations among them (Spearman correlation coefficient for numerical variables and Cramer's V/Phi-coefficient (function *assocstats* from the R *vcd* package). In the case of two variables showing a correlation coefficient (R) of 0.5 or higher, the biologically more plausible variable was retained. Additionally, the full model containing the 86 complete observations for all candidate variables was checked for multi-collinearity by calculating the general variance inflation factor (function *vif* of the *car* package). Based on the full model, a step-wise backward selection process was conducted using R function *step (direction ="both")*, based on Akaike's as well as Bayesian Information Criterion (AIC and BIC). In addition, a manual backward selection based on Likelihood Ratio-Test (LRT, significance level: $p \leq 0.05$) was performed on the full model to check if this would result in the same final model. The LRT was used as well to compare the resulting two different final models. Two-way Interactions were tested between all variables of the final models.

Results

Of the 120 herds in this study, PRRSV was detected in 32 herds, whereas 88 herds were tested PCR negative. Positive results were distributed evenly over the study period; no influence of the season was seen. The median herd size over all herds was 240 sow places or 2091 pigs (excluding suckling pigs) in total. Most of the herds were farrow-to-finish herds (n = 86), the remaining herds were piglet producers selling nursery pigs (n = 29) or suckling pigs (n = 5). Further herd characteristics and univariable comparisons between PCR positive and PCR negative herds are displayed in Additional files 1 and 2.

The results of multivariable logistic regression analyses (full and final models) are presented in Table 1. Due to multi-collinearity with several other variables (e.g. farrowing rhythm or presence of external staff), herd size was not included in the full model, because it was deemed the less directly effect-related variable. Alternative full models including herd size alone and in conjunction with the highly correlated variables both led to the same final model after variable selection.

The final model after manual backward selection (final model 2; automated stepwise selection based on BIC resulted in the same final model) contained four variables significantly associated with herd status (based on LRT).

Herds working with a suckling period >21 days had an odds ratio (OR) of 0.23 for being PCR positive thus unstable, compared to herds with a suckling period of ≤21 days [95%-confidence interval (CI) 0.05–0.88]. Every additional meter distance between the cadaver collection site and the actual sow barn decreased the chance of being unstable (OR 0.99, CI 0.98–0.99). Herds with ≥2 pig herds in their vicinity (1000 m radius) had a 9.91-fold higher chance of being unstable than herds with maximum one other herd in their vicinity (CI 2.35–60.8). The OR of being unstable for herds with external employees (people employed for taking care of the pigs, i.e. not belonging to the herd owning family or household) compared to herds without external employees was 4.52 (CI 1.34–17.43).

The final model after automated step-wise backward selection based on AIC (final model 1) included the same variables as final model 2: the distance between sow barn and pick-up location for carcasses (OR 0.98, CI 0.97–0.99), the number of farms in their vicinity (OR 17.78, CI 3.52–138.06), presence of external employees (OR 5.46, CI 1.39–26.24) and the suckling period (OR 0.25, CI 0.05–1.16) remained significant. Two additional variables were the time interval between purchase of gilts—an interval of 9 weeks had an OR of 0.49 (CI 0.059–2.79), an interval of 10 or more weeks an OR of 0.16 (CI 0.03–0.75) compared with smaller intervals—and a 3- or more-weekly farrowing rhythm had an OR of 0.35 (CI 0.09–1.23). Although the latter three variables were not significant according to the set α-level, the LRT for comparison of the two final models gave a p-value of 0.04. This, together with the lower AIC, indicated a superiority of the larger final model 1 (automated step-wise backward selection) to explain the observed data. No significant interactions were found between any two variables of the final models.

Discussion

This study aimed to investigate the frequency of PRRSV instability among professional pig breeding farms and to assess risk factors for PRRSV instability in German sow herds. Knowledge about PRRSV status in terms of virus circulation is crucial for both, farmers and veterinary practitioners, when planning actions for controlling PRRSV infections in pig herds by different prevention measures [10]. Since the presence of risk factors can influence this status, and also the efficiency of various control measures, the assessment of these risk factors in individual herds needs appropriate attention. The presented investigation is the first cross-sectional study describing the prevalence of 'PRRSV unstable herds' and risk factors in professional pig farms in Germany, which are also typical for other North European countries with intensive production systems, e.g. Denmark and The Netherlands. Due to time and financial constraints, the applied sampling protocol to assess the herd status by testing it at one point in time differed from Holtkamp's proposed methodology of four repeated testings over 90 days [10]. Therefore, it cannot be stated for all herds tested negative in this study that they were actually PRRSV stable according to Holtkamp. However, with the high number of animals sampled per herd, we assume that an overall negative PCR result gives sufficient evidence of lack of virus circulation in weaning-age pigs in this herd, at least at the time of sampling. On the other hand, from this result, it cannot be concluded that a herd is truly PRRSV negative or provisionally negative as defined by Holtkamp categories IV and III, nor is a distinction between stable (category II) and (provisionally) negative possible. This would require a more intense sampling protocol and an evidenced outbreak history, which was not available for study herds, since PRRSV is endemic in the region for years and vaccine coverage against PRRSV is high. However, for our main purpose of the study, which was to assess virus circulation in the breeding herd, i.e. suckling pigs, this distinction is deemed to have limited relevance.

A sample of herds that have been selected from an institutional database was examined in this study. The total herd size was neither a primary selection nor inclusion criterion, but due to the minimum number of 12 sows per farrowing group that was requested for the

Table 1 Results of full model, final model 1 (automated step-wise backward selection based on akaike information criterion AIC) and 2 (manual backward selection): coefficients (Coeff.), standard error (SE) and p-value of the wald test (Wald) for each separate category of a variable as well as likelihood ratio-test (LRT) indicating the p-value of the overall variable (final models only)

Variable/category	Full model			Final model 1				Final model 2			
	Coeff.	SE	Wald	Coeff.	SE	Wald	LRT	Coeff.	SE	Wald	LRT
(Intercept)	−1.00	2.59	0.70	−1.10	1.00	0.27		−1.75	0.91	0.05	
Suckling period (days)											
≤21											
≥22	−1.53	1.02	0.13	−1.37	0.80	0.09	0.08	−1.49	0.71	0.04	0.03
Sows—genetic											
Danbred											
BHZP or Topigs	−1.27	1.02	0.22								
PIC, Hülsenberger, Hermitage, other	−1.97	1.08	0.07								
Time interval between purchase of gilts (weeks)											
<9											
9	−1.63	1.38	0.24	−0.72	0.95	0.45	0.06				
10–52	−2.55	1.10	0.02	−1.82	0.84	0.03					
Time interval in which sows are sent to slaughter (weeks)	0.08	0.29	0.79								
Time interval between pick-up of carcasses (days)	0.02	0.10	0.83								
Distance between sow barn and pick-up location for carcasses (m)	−0.02	0.01	0.09	−0.02	0.01	0.03	0.01	−0.01	0.01	0.06	0.03
Quarantine/acclimatization unit—number of gilts per compartment (n)	0.01	0.03	0.71								
Pig density in county											
Low											
High	1.48	0.89	0.10								
Number of other pig farms within 1000 m distance											
≤1											
≥2	3.94	1.33	<0.01	2.88	0.92	0.00	<0.001	2.29	0.81	0.01	<0.001
Boar semen—purchase from PRRSV unsuspicious boar stud											
No											
Yes	−0.83	0.81	0.31								
Hygiene lock											
No clear separation											
Clear separation	0.88	1.21	0.47								
Employment of external staff											
No											
Yes	1.29	0.86	0.13	1.70	0.74	0.02	0.01	1.51	0.65	0.02	0.01

Table 1 (continued)

Variable/category	Full model			Final model 1				Final model 2			
	Coeff.	SE	Wald	Coeff.	SE	Wald	LRT	Coeff.	SE	Wald	LRT
Farrowing rhythm											
1- or 2-weekly											
3-, 4- or 5-weekly	−0.90	0.85	0.29	−1.06	0.66	0.11	0.10				
Suckling pigs—age at ear tagging (day)											
1st											
≥ 2nd	−0.96	0.86	0.26								
Suckling pigs—2nd standard antibiotic treatment											
No											
Yes	−0.42	0.82	0.61								
Sows—vaccination against PRRSV											
No											
Yes	−0.09	1.32	0.94								
AIC	94.9			81.8				84.0			

BHZP "Bundes Hybrid Zucht Programm", German commercial provider of hybrid sows, *PIC* "Pig Improvement Company", North American commercial provider of hybrid sows purpose of obtaining all samples in 1 day (i.e. at least 10 l in the farrowing area expected), the average herd size of farms herein was considerably high (> 300 sows/herd). At the same time the average number of sows in German breeding farms was 211 (Source: http://www.destatis.de), in Dutch breeding farms 240 (Source: http://www.thepigsite.net) and in Danish breeding farms 422 (Source: http://www.lf.dk). Therefore, the study population examined here is size-wise considered as being representative for the target population, i.e. the intensive pig farming systems in northern Europe.

The sample size used in this study was derived from the 'within-herd' sampling protocol in order to assess the PRRSV status' according to Holtkamp et al. [10]. The protocol per sampling was slightly modified as well, taking samples from three piglets per litter instead of only one, and, thus, not perfectly matching the recommendation, but close to. However, this compromise was necessary considering the smaller herd size of European sow farms compared to those in the USA, where the sampling protocol according to Holtkamp et al. [10] had been developed. Farms accommodating approximately 300 sows (average in this study) usually maintain farrowing groups of 15 (1 week farrowing rhythm) to a maximum of 45 sows (3 week farrowing rhythm), which precludes the accessibility of 30 different litters every time in every farm.

Statistical analyses and the modelling approach used herein were conducted following a standard, i.e. well-established, protocol (variable selection, selection of final model, etc.). Two different approaches were used to obtain the final model after multivariable logistic regression, in order to check the robustness of the results. The fact that both final models contained the same set of statistically significant variables confirmed this. Nevertheless, the final model after automated step-wise backward selection based on AIC (final model 1) contained two additional variables. Although these did not exhibit p-values below the significance level of 0.05, they apparently help to explain parts of the overall variation in the data, as can be deducted from the better AIC value of this final model compared to the other one.

The variable 'number of sows' was not considered in the final multivariable models in spite of being known as a common confounder in herd level risk factor studies [11] due to the very strong association with other variables (particularly total herd size and staff). Alternative full models built in the modelling process that included this variable, yielded exactly the same final model as described above; herd size had always dropped out as non-significant. Concerning the possible causal pathway, we acknowledge that herd size itself can have a direct effect on virus circulation, given that in larger herds the possibility of having naïve subpopulations of, e.g. gilts is higher. Nevertheless, we think that the biggest proportion of its influence is rather indirect: in the study region, bigger herds tend to be run more professionally, with a higher chance for external employees, they have a different farrowing rhythm, often wean piglets earlier or have shorter intervals for the purchase of gilts; factors that are assumed to have a more direct influence on the herd status. Given the fact that the influence of herd size in risk factor studies has been described elsewhere, it was decided to focus on the other variables.

The significant protective effect of a longer suckling period is in contrast to the idea of reducing the risk of vertical pathogen transmission by keeping this period, i.e. time under risk, as short as possible. This principle of protecting piglets from sow's infection by early separation and thereby reducing the time under exposure has been successfully implemented with the 'segregated early weaning' to combat *Mycoplasma hyopneumoniae* transmission from sows to their offspring [2]. However, in the present study, results indicate that any risk of PRRSV transmission from the dam to their offspring is not increasing over time, but decreasing. Similar observations of a reduced risk of PRRSV infection with longer suckling periods have been made in another study [12], whereas elsewhere the length of this period was not linked in any way to PRRSV infection in pigs from these litters [13]. It can be hypothesized that no increased risk of infection is observed here, because sows (in stable herds) transfer neutralizing and non-neutralizing PRRSV specific antibodies to suckling pigs. The neutralizing PRRSV specific antibodies are protecting them from corresponding infection up to 5 weeks of life [14]. The non-neutralizing antibodies are suspected in potentially assisting viral clearance in already infected animals by Antibody-dependent cellular phagocytosis (ADCP), Antibody-dependent complement-mediated cytotoxicity (CDC) and other mechanisms, which have been described for immune reactions directed to human immunodeficiency virus [15]. Such a phenomenon would explain a decreased PRRSV positivity in piglets from herds with a longer suckling period. Piglets in the present study were aged 17–21 days at sampling, whereby it can be anticipated that piglets in herds with a longer suckling period tended to be a few days older than piglets in herds with only 3 weeks of suckling period, where the actual weaning age is often 20 days of age or even less. The transfer of neutralizing maternally derived antibodies and their protective effect in receiving pigs as assumed in this study is in contrast to the epidemiology of *M. hyopneumoniae* infection, where antibodies do not prevent from infection at all. Another hypothesis could be that piglets weaned after a shorter suckling period are less resistant, contract PRRSV infection more easily after weaning and shed higher amounts of virus. Since in the most predominant farming systems in the investigated region sows and weaned pigs are kept at the same location, these weaned pigs might destabilize the whole sow herd. Finally, the possibility that farms could have reduced the suckling period in an attempt to control PRRSV infection does not seem likely because herds mostly were not aware of any clinical impact of PRRSV.

The influence of the proximity of neighbouring herds, i.e. number of other pig herds within a 1000 m radius, and of the pig density on the likelihood of the sow herd PRRSV PCR status are indicating an airborne transmission of PRRSV, which has been suggested and described elsewhere [2, 12, 16]. The frequency of such an event is widely unknown and is obviously depending on environmental factors determining the stability of PRRSV outside the host [17]. All study herds were located in an area of Germany, where endemic PRRSV infection of nearly all pig herds has been observed earlier [18] and sampling was conducted during a period of 1 year, thus covering all seasons and various environmental conditions. Therefore, airborne transmissions of PRRSV isolates of different virulence, etc. between herds in this region must be assumed and their occurrence is high likely associated to the distance between the farms, i.e. pig density. Once a new (more pathogenic) PRRSV isolate is successfully transmitted into a pig herd, destabilization is depending on cross-protection induced by the previous PRRSV infection in the pigs [18].

The increasing distance between the barn and the storage bin for dead pigs was observed as being protective in terms of PRRSV instability. This might be related to the content of the bin itself, i.e. pigs that potentially died from PRRS and still harbor PRRSV [18], or the fact that emptying the bin requires a rendering truck coming close to the barn. This rendering truck is usually not clean, because it is used for collection of cadaver from several farms per day. It has been shown that both, the tires of a truck and the boots of the driver, can transmit PRRSV, when no sufficient hygienic precautions are in place [18].

A similar impact on the PRRSV status by a lack in the external biosecurity could be speculated with regards to external employees. There are numerous reports pointing out the importance of an adequate hygiene lock and further requirements for visitors and personnel before entering a pig farm [18, 19]. Considering a higher number of people having regular access to the barns, implies an increased risk of someone not totally fulfilling or even omitting hygiene procedures, thereby lowering both, internal and external biosecurity. Apart from the numerical increase of people entering the farm, it is well known that farm employees are less aware of the necessity and the correctness of best hygiene practice as compared to farm owners [20]. Taking these potential risks together it is conclusive that pig farms with external employees are more prone to the entry of new isolates of PRRSV and within-herd circulation of PRRSV, both leading to PRRSV instability.

The factor 'Time interval between purchase of gilts: 9 weeks' indicated a trend in the Final Model 1, but was not significantly associated with the PRRSV status. The same applies to the factor 'Farrowing rhythm: 3-, 4- or 5-weekly'. Regarding the latter one it can be hypothesized that farms operating with a 1- or 2-week farrowing rhythm have a less strict separation of piglets of different age and, therefore, a higher chance of within herd transmission of pathogens. In farms with a 3-, 4- or 5-week rhythm, the older group is already or nearly weaned, when new piglets are born, thereby preventing a transfer of pathogens by staff or other vectors between the different farrowing compartments for the corresponding farrowing group.

Conclusions

The PRRSV status could be determined with an adopted sampling and testing protocol that suits smaller pig herds as compared to the USA. In 27% of the study herds PRRSV was detected in suckling pigs indicating PRRSV instability. The PRRSV status in German sow herds of average size relies on external and internal biosecurity (pig density in the area, rendering management, external employees), as well as on farm specific management factors (suckling period). Before or while taking actions to control PRRS by known measures, farmers and veterinarians should also eliminate risk factors in the herd and select appropriate measures accordingly.

Additional files

Additional file 1. Descriptive statistics for numerical variables: mean, standard deviation (SD), median (Med), minimum (Min), Maximum (Max) and test result of the Mann/Whitney-U Test (p-value) between PRRSV-positive (pos), i.e. unstable, and PRRSV-negative (neg) herds.

Additional file 2. Categorical variables: number of herds in PRRSV positive (pos) and PRRSV negative (neg) herds per category and result of Chi square/Fisher's Exakt test (p-value).

Authors' contributions

CN collected the data, analysed the results and proposed the manuscript. EJ assisted with sample and data collection on farm, while AD assisted with analyses of the samples in the laboratory. HN and EgB jointly supervised the project and assisted in analysing the results and drafting the manuscript. All authors read and approved the final manuscript.

Author details

[1] Veterinary Public Health Institute, Department of Clinical Research & Veterinary Public Health, Vetsuisse Faculty, University of Bern, Schwarzenburgstrasse

155, 3097 Liebefeld, Switzerland. [2] Federal Food Safety and Veterinary Office, Schwarzenburgstrasse 155, 3003 Bern, Switzerland. [3] Field Station for Epidemiology, University of Veterinary Medicine Hannover, Buescheler Strasse 9, 49456 Bakum, Germany. [4] Clinic for Swine, Department of Clinical Veterinary Medicine, Vetsuisse Faculty, University of Bern, Bremgartenstrasse 109a, 3012 Bern, Switzerland.

Acknowledgements
The authors are grateful for the famers' attendance in this study. Moreover, the technical support of Mechthild Busemann in the laboratory is acknowledged.

Competing interests
The authors declare that they have no competing interests.

Funding
This study was funded intramurally by the Field Station for Epidemiology, University of Veterinary Medicine Hannover.

References

1. Baysinger AK, Dewey CE, Straw BE, Brumm MC, Schmitz J, Doster A, et al. Risk factors associated with endemic reproductive deficiencies caused by PRRSV infection. J Swine Heal Prod. 1997;5:179–87.
2. Rosendal T, Dewey C, Friendship R, Wootton S, Young B, Poljak Z. Association between PRRSV ORF5 genetic distance and differences in space, time, ownership and animal sources among commercial pig herds. Transbound Emerg Dis. 2016;63:e185–93.
3. Pileri E, Mateu E. Review on the transmission porcine reproductive and respiratory syndrome virus between pigs and farms and impact on vaccination. Vet Res. 2016;47:108.
4. Thanawongnuwech R, Suradhat S. Taming PRRSV: revisiting the control strategies and vaccine design. Virus Res. 2010;154:133–40.
5. Cano JP, Dee SA, Murtaugh MP, Pijoan C. Impact of a modified-live porcine reproductive and respiratory syndrome virus vaccine intervention on a population of pigs infected with a heterologous isolate. Vaccine. 2007;25:4382–91.
6. Dee SA, Molitor TW. Elimination of porcine reproductive and respiratory syndrome virus using a test and removal process. Vet Rec. 1998;143:474–6.
7. McCaw M, FitzSimmons M, Daniels C, Allison G, Gillespie T, Thacker E, et al. Field experiences with different methods of controlling PRRS virus. In: Zimmerman J, Yoon K-J, editors. 2003 PRRS Compend A Compr Ref Porc Reprod Respir Syndr Pork Prod Vet Pract Res. Producer E. National Pork Board; 2003. p. 90–115. http://proposal.pork.org/Resources/3152/2003PRRSCompendium.aspx#.V0aYsOR0dU4.
8. Yang JS, Moon HJ, Lee CS, Park SJ, Song DS, Kang BK, et al. Elimination of porcine reproductive and respiratory syndrome virus from a seedstock breeding farm and a supplying boar stud by a modified test and removal method. Vet Rec. 2008;162:333–7.
9. Corzo CA, Mondaca E, Wayne S, Torremorell M, Dee S, Davies P, et al. Control and elimination of porcine reproductive and respiratory syndrome virus. Virus Res. 2010;154:185–92.
10. Holtkamp DJ, Polson DD, Torremorell M, Morrison B, Classen DM, Becton L, et al. Terminology for classifying swine herds by porcine reproductive and respiratory syndrome virus status. Swine Heal Prod. 2011;19:44–56.
11. Dohoo I, Martin W, Stryhn H. Veterinary epidemiologic research. Charlottetown: VER Inc.; 2009.
12. Velasova M, Alarcon P, Williamson S, Wieland B. Risk factors for porcine reproductive and respiratory syndrome virus infection and resulting challenges for effective disease surveillance. BMC Vet Res. 2012;8:184.
13. Fablet C, Marois-Créhan C, Grasland B, Simon G, Rose N. Factors associated with herd-level PRRSV infection and age-time to seroconversion in farrow-to-finish herds. Vet Microbiol. 2016;192:10–20.
14. Geldhof MF, Van Breedam W, De Jong E, Lopez Rodriguez A, Karniychuk UU, Vanhee M, et al. Antibody response and maternal immunity upon boosting PRRSV-immune sows with experimental farm-specific and commercial PRRSV vaccines. Vet Microbiol. 2013;167:260–71.
15. Rahe MC, Murtaugh MP. Effector mechanisms of humoral immunity to porcine reproductive and respiratory syndrome virus. Vet Immunol Immunopathol. 2017;186:15–8.
16. Lambert M-È, Arsenault J, Poljak Z, D'Allaire S. Epidemiological investigations in regard to porcine reproductive and respiratory syndrome (PRRS) in Quebec, Canada. Part 2: prevalence and risk factors in breeding sites. Prev Vet Med. 2012;104:84–93.
17. Hermann J, Hoff S, Muñoz-Zanzi C, Yoon K-J, Roof M, Burkhardt A, et al. Effect of temperature and relative humidity on the stability of infectious porcine reproductive and respiratory syndrome virus in aerosols. Vet Res. 2007;38:81–93.
18. Grosse Beilage E, Rohde N, Krieter J. Seroprevalence and risk factors associated with seropositivity in sows from 67 herds in north-west Germany infected with *Mycoplasma hyopneumoniae*. Prev Vet Med. 2009;88:255–63.
19. Holtkamp DJ, Yeske PE, Polson DD, Melody JL, Philips RC. A prospective study evaluating duration of swine breeding herd PRRS virus-free status and its relationship with measured risk. Prev Vet Med. 2010;96:186–93.
20. Mardesen M. Assessment of knowledge, compliance and attitudes of english and Spanish speaking farm employees towards biosecurity practices. In: 48th Am Assoc Swine Vet Annu Meet. 2017. p. 57–8.

α-Tocopherol and β-carotene concentrations in feed, colostrum, cow and calf serum in Swedish dairy herds with high or low calf mortality

Maria Torsein[1,2*], Ann Lindberg[3], Catarina Svensson[4], Sören Krogh Jensen[5], Charlotte Berg[2] and Karin Persson Waller[4,6]

Abstract

Background: A study of herd-level risk factors for calf mortality in large Swedish dairy herds showed low serum concentrations of α-tocopherol and β-carotene in 1–7 day old calves to be more common in high mortality herds. Therefore, we aimed to investigate if calf mortality risk at herd level is associated with concentrations of α-tocopherol and/or β-carotene at individual level in feed, colostrum, cow and calf serum, while controlling for herd level covariates. Inclusion criteria were affiliation to the Swedish official milk recording scheme, herd size of ≥ 120 milking cows/year, calf mortality risk (day 1–90) of at least 6% (high mortality; HM) or less than 1% (low mortality; LM) and located within one of two regions in southern Sweden. This cross-sectional study was performed in 2010 in 19 ($n_{HM} = 9$; $n_{LM} = 10$) dairy herds. Questionnaires were used to collect information about feed and routines for colostrum feeding. Feed (n = 57), colostrum (n = 162), cow serum (n = 189) and calf serum samples (n = 187) were collected and analysed for α-tocopherol and β-carotene. Other analyses e.g. total serum protein, fat content, and total solids in colostrum were also performed. Linear regression models with vitamin concentrations in feed, colostrum, cow and calf serum as outcome were performed.

Results: Calves in HM herds had lower concentrations of α-tocopherol in serum than calves in LM herds, but the effect depended on total protein status in serum of the calf ($P = 0.036$). Calves from herds that fed transition milk for 3 days or more had higher α-tocopherol concentrations in serum than calves from herds feeding transition milk up to 2 days ($P = 0.013$). Fat percentage in colostrum was positively associated with α-tocopherol ($P < 0.001$) and β-carotene concentrations in colostrum ($P < 0.001$). A diet containing ≥ 20% (in kg dry matter) maize silage of the total ration was negatively associated with β-carotene concentration in cow serum ($P = 0.001$).

Conclusions: High calf mortality risks were associated with lower concentrations of α-tocopherol in calf serum for calves with failure of passive transfer. Feeding transition milk longer was associated with higher concentrations of α-tocopherol in calf serum. In HM herds, evaluation of the calves' α-tocopherol status is recommended.

Keywords: Calf mortality, Colostrum, Transition milk, Vitamin A, Vitamin E

Background

Calf mortality is complex and often multi-factorial in its nature, at the same time it is an economic and ethical burden for the cattle industry. For these reasons, it is important to determine factors influencing calf mortality. In a previous study of herd-level risk factors for calf mortality in large Swedish dairy herds [1], low serum concentrations of α-tocopherol (vitamin E) and β-carotene in 1–7 day old calves were found to be more common in

*Correspondence: maria.torsein@gardochdjurhalsan.se
[2] Department of Animal Environment and Health, Swedish University of Agricultural Sciences, P.O. Box 234, 532 23 Skara, Sweden
Full list of author information is available at the end of the article

high mortality (HM) herds than in low mortality (LM) herds.

Vitamin E comprises eight fat soluble compounds, tocopherols and tocotriols, of which α-tocopherol has the highest activity and is the major tocopherol found in blood and milk in cows [2]. Vitamin E is an antioxidant and thereby protects cells from oxidative damage. Several studies have reported that the serum α-tocopherol concentration in calves is important for their immune system [3–5]. Furthermore, Carter et al. [6] demonstrated that calves with respiratory tract disease supplemented with α-tocopherol had lower treatment costs compared to non-supplemented calves indicating a quicker recovery. Moreover, α-tocopherol has been shown to exert a protective effect on leukocytes participating in the defence against *Mannheimia haemolytica* [7].

Among carotenoids, β-carotene is the main dietary precursor of vitamin A (retinol) in cattle [8]. β-Carotene can be degraded to higher or lower extent in the rumen due to differences between the carotenoid supplement form. β-Carotenes in forage passes the rumen, i.e. have been shown to be degraded to a lower extent, whereas carotenoids supplemented as purified products have been shown to be degraded to a higher extent [8]. β-Carotenes can be converted into vitamin A in numerous cell types, but this occurs mainly in enterocytes and hepatocytes [8]. Absorbed β-carotene is transported with lipids to the liver [9, 10]. β-Carotene is an antioxidant and has immune regulatory properties [11]. A deficiency could lead to a higher risk of infections, exemplified by the increased risk of diarrhoea in calves seen during the first week after birth when the dam has inadequate β-carotene concentration in colostrum, or if the serum concentrations of the calves are low [12–14].

Only negligible amounts of α-tocopherol and β-carotene are transferred from cow to calf via the placenta [15–17], and hence colostrum is the major vitamin source for the newborn calf. Adequate colostrum intake from cows fed adequate amounts of vitamins is therefore essential for supplying calves with fat-soluble vitamins. Roughage is the cows major natural source for α-tocopherol and β-carotene, but it is difficult to predict vitamin concentrations in the roughage, as it is highly variable depending on plant species, maturity of the plant, and harvest conditions [18]. Moreover, the vitamin concentration in silage often decreases during storage [19]. Vitamins can also be supplemented in the cow's diet, which can impact the vitamin status of the cow. Biological and genetic factors of the cow, and the cow's dry matter intake at the time around calving are other factors that affect the concentration of vitamins in colostrum [20, 21]. Hence, the vitamin concentration in colostrum, as well as the vitamin status of the calves, is often unknown.

To evaluate if vitamin status is associated with calf mortality, more knowledge on associations between feed vitamin status, cow vitamin status, colostrum feeding and calf vitamin status is needed. Therefore, we aimed to evaluate concentrations of α-tocopherol and β-carotene in feed, colostrum and cow and calf serum at individual/sample level to test the hypothesis that calf mortality risk at herd level is associated with low average serum concentrations of α-tocopherol and/or β-carotene at individual/sample level, while controlling for other individual/sample and herd level covariates.

Methods

Study design

This cross-sectional study was performed in 19 dairy herds from the south of Sweden from January 14th to April 1st, 2010. As previously mentioned, we aimed to evaluate concentrations of α-tocopherol and β-carotene in HM and LM herds. Therefore, for each of the two vitamins, α-tocopherol and β-carotene, we investigated four different outcomes in the chain of events: vitamin concentrations in feed, colostrum and cow and calf serum at the individual or sample level.

Selection of herds

The Swedish official milk recording scheme (SOMRS) produces its annual statistics based on periods ranging from September 1st up to and including August 31st the following year. This time period is used hereafter and referred to as 2008/09, 2009/10, etc. Since SOMRS data on herd size and calf mortality risks were intended to be used for the selection of the herds, the primary inclusion criteria were consequently set to be affiliation to SOMRS. Secondly the herds were selected based on geographic region, their herd size between 2006/2007 and 2008/2009 ($\geq$ 120 cows), and their calf mortality risk in 1–90 days old calves 2008/2009. For logistic reasons herds from two regions in southern Sweden were selected, the former county of Skaraborg and south of Älvsborg (hereafter referred to as Skaraborg), and the county of Halland together with the eastern part of the county Skåne (Additional file 1). With the hypothesis that low vitamin concentrations contribute to calf mortality, we selected herds that were highly different in calf mortality to generate a study population where risk factors contributing to the variation in vitamin status would be more easily identified. Therefore, we included herds with a calf mortality risk (2008/09) of at least 6% (High Mortality, HM) or less than 1% (Low Mortality, LM).

Herds conforming to the inclusion criteria were contacted by mail and by phone, until five HM herds and five LM herds from each of the two regions had agreed to participate. One HM herd from Skaraborg was excluded from the study due to the diagnosis of Q-fever in the herd. A replacement herd was not included because the study had already started. Hence, 19 herds participated in the study, 10 LM herds and nine HM herds.

Collection of data

As previously mentioned, data on herd size, calf mortality, and milk production were obtained from the SOMRS. During the study period January 14th, 2010 to April 1st, 2010 each herd was visited by the same veterinarian (the first author) three to five times for collection of questionnaires, information on feeding routines for individual calves and samples.

Questionnaire

Upon the first visit, a questionnaire was used to collect information about the feeding of cows and heifers close to calving and about routines for feeding colostrum to calves. The questionnaire had been reviewed by two veterinarians being specialists in ruminant medicine prior to the study. It comprised eight semi-closed or open questions (Additional file 2), and took approximately 15 min to complete. The farmers completed the questionnaire independently. It included questions about feeding routines and the rations of the roughage of dry cows and heifers near calving, including how minerals and vitamins were given to heifers and cows 1 month before calving and around the time of calving. This information was used to create three variables; "percentage grass silage of total diet (DM)", "percentage maize silage of total diet (DM)", way of feeding supplements". Information about the general herd-level strategies for colostrum management, for example way of feeding colostrum, was also collected from the questionnaire and used to create the variable "herd-level percentage calves given colostrum manually" (i.e. fed by the farmer).

Data regarding feeding routines for individual calves

The farmers were instructed to fill in individual forms (Additional file 3) for up to ten calves per herd concerning the feeding routines during the calves' first 7 days of life, i.e. what type of milk source that was fed and how long the calf stayed with their mother. For practical reasons information was not recorded specifically for calves subsequently blood sampled by the veterinarian. The information from the forms was used to create two herd-level variables: "herd-level median volume of the first colostrum meal given manually to each calf" and "herd-level median total volume of colostrum given manually the first day postpartum to each calf".

Sampling and analyses of samples

Handling of collected samples

Samples collected at the herd visits by the veterinarian (feed, blood and bulk milk) were kept cool in a cooler box, whereas colostrum samples collected by the farmers were kept cool in a refrigerator until the samples were sent by mail to the National Veterinary Institute (SVA) in Uppsala, Sweden, on the day of collection. If collected on a Friday or a Saturday the samples were refrigerated at 4 °C until sent, to reach the laboratory on a weekday.

Feed samples

At each visit, one pooled sample per herd of the roughage in the diet of dry cows and heifers near calving, i.e. grass silage or total mixed ration (TMR), was collected, resulting in a total of maximum three samples per herd ($n = 57$ samples; 27 from HM herds and 30 from LM herds). For each sample, information about when the roughage had been harvested and how it had been stored until feeding was included. This information was used to form eight variables: "first-harvest grass in feed sample" (0/1), "second-harvest grass in feed sample" (0/1), "third-harvest grass in feed sample" (0/1), "TMR" (0/1) "Region" (Halland/former Skaraborg), "Grass stored as round bales" 0/1), "Grass stored in bunker silos" (0/1), "Grass stored in tower silos" (0/1). To get a representative pooled sample, ten subsamples were collected from different parts of the feed bunk, of the dry cows or heifers near calving. The subsamples were pooled in a big plastic bag and mixed thoroughly, and approximately 1.5 L of the pooled feed sample was transferred into a new clean plastic bag. Then, air was evacuated and the bag was closed. At SVA, feed samples were stored at − 20 °C, until they later were sent to Aarhus University, Department of Animal Science, Research Center Foulum, Tjele, Denmark (RCF) and analysed for concentrations of α-tocopherol and β-carotene as described by Müller et al. [22].

Colostrum samples

Upon the first visit by the veterinarian, the farmers were provided with materials and written instructions for sampling colostrum from up to 10 cows per herd. All colostrum samples (178 samples from 19 herds; 83 HM herds and 95 LM herds) were collected by the farmers. The farmers were instructed to hand-milk equal amounts from each udder quarter into a clean cup (containing 40 mL), stir the sample with a disposable spoon and then pour the mixed sample into two sterile 10 mL tubes without additives and also into one 50 mL tube containing 50 μL of 20% bronopol and 0.2% methylene blue. Samples were to be collected by the farmers within 6 h post-partum and to be kept cool in a refrigerator until they were sent by mail to SVA, as described above. They were also asked to fill in a form about sampling date, time after calving when the sample was taken, parity and breed of the sampled cows and information on whether milk leakage had occurred (definition: milk puddle more than 15 cm in diameter) during the last 14 days pre-partum. For practical reasons, it was not possible to take colostrum samples from the same cows that were blood sampled.

Colostrum samples that were older than 7 days on their arrival at SVA were excluded from analysis. Of the 178 colostrum samples, 11 samples (3 HM and 8 LM) were later omitted due to blood content in colostrum. At SVA, fresh colostrum samples were analysed for contents of total solids using the Brix scale, as an indicator of immunoglobulin contents [23], with a digital refractometer (PAL-1, Atago Co., Ltd., Tokyo, Japan). Furthermore, 162 of the 167 fresh colostrum samples (78 HM and 84 LM samples) were analysed for fat, protein and lactose contents by mid-infrared spectroscopy (Fourier Transform Instrument, FT 120, Foss Electric) at the Swedish University of Agricultural Sciences (SLU), Department of Animal Nutrition and Management, Uppsala, Sweden. Consequently, five samples of fresh colostrum could not be analysed for fat, protein and lactose due to too high viscosity. Aliquots of colostrum samples were stored at SVA at − 20 °C, until they later were sent to RCF and analysed for concentrations of α-tocopherol and β-carotene as described by Jensen and Nielsen [24].

Blood samples of cows and calves

At each visit, the veterinarian collected blood samples from cows at 2–7 days post calving and calves at 2–7 days of age, up to a maximum total number of 10 samples from cows and 10 samples from calves per herd. When possible, mother–offspring pairs were sampled. Blood samples were collected from the coccygeal vessels of selected cows (189 samples from 19 herds; 90 HM and 99 LM), and from the jugular vein of selected calves (187 samples from 19 herds; 89 HM and 98 LM) in vacuumed tubes without additives. Altogether, 164 mother–offspring pairs were sampled from the herds (79 HM and 85 LM pairs), i.e. 87 and 88% of the collected samples from cows and calves, respectively, were paired samples. Information on parity number and breed of the sampled animals was also collected.

Upon arrival, blood samples were centrifuged and serum was collected. Serum samples were analysed for concentrations of total protein by adding 40 μL fresh sera to an optical refractometer (Leica Microsystems Inc., Buffalo, NY, US). Aliquots of serum were stored at − 20 °C, until they later were sent to RCF analysed for concentrations of α-tocopherol and β-carotene as described by Jensen and Nielsen [24].

Bulk milk samples

As a result of a legislated control program, salmonellosis is very rare in Swedish cattle [25]. Salmonella status was therefore only determined using one bulk milk sample per herd (n = 39; 19 from HM herds and 20 from LM herds). Bulk milk samples were collected in 10 mL sterile plastic tubes for later analysis of antibodies to *S. dublin* and *S. typhimurium* as described by Nyman et al. [25], using commercial ELISAs (PrioCheck® Salmonella Ab bovine Dublin and PrioCheck® Salmonella Ab bovine (O-antigens: 1, 4, 5, 9, 12), Prionics AG, Schlieren-Zurich, Switzerland).

Data editing and statistical analyses

Data editing, descriptive statistics and multivariable analyses were performed using Stata®version 11 (Stata Corporation, College Station, TX, USA).

As stated previously, our outcome variables were concentrations of α-tocopherol and β-carotene in feed, colostrum, cow serum and calf serum, and analysed at sample level. Thus, eight statistical models were built. To approximate the normal distribution, the outcome variables "α-tocopherol concentration in feed", "α-tocopherol concentration in colostrum", "α-tocopherol concentration in calf serum", "β-carotene concentration in feed", "β-carotene concentration in colostrum" and "β-carotene concentration in calf serum" were transformed using the natural logarithm (ln). Linear multivariable regression, controlling for clustering within herds, was used to investigate associations between the concentration of vitamins, at individual (i.e. sample level), and the predictor variables, using Stata's "cluster" option. Predictor variables used in the different models are given in Tables 1 and 2.

The hypothesized causal relationships between the outcomes and the predictor variables were outlined using causal diagrams to identify potential confounding effects and intervening variables. In the models: "α-tocopherol concentration in calf serum" and "β-carotene concentration in calf serum", variables regarding colostrum management were not entered since they all were regarded as interveners with the variable "total protein", measured in calf serum. Variables not considered to have intervening effects were entered in the multivariable regression models after correlations between variables were assessed. Correlations between variables qualifying for inclusion in the multivariable analyses were assessed using Spearman's rank correlation coefficients. For the models: "α-tocopherol concentration in feed" and "β-carotene concentration in feed", strong and significant correlations were present between three variables; first-, second- and third harvest grass in feed sample, respectively. The variables with the highest explanatory power (based on

Table 1 Results of univariable analyses (continuous variables), tested for associations with type of herd (high mortality/low mortality)

Model/variable	High mortality			Low mortality			*P* value[a]
	25 pct.	Median	75 pct.	25 pct.	Median	75 pct.	
Model feed[b] (n = 57)							
Herd size 2008/09	154	175	222	141	151	170	0.28
% Grass silage of total diet	27	37	42	29	41	60	0.45
Model colostrum[b] (n = 162)							
Fat[c] (%)	3.44	4.95	7.30	2.65	3.82	6.56	0.10
Herd size 2008/09	154	175	222	141	151	170	0.34
Total solids (Brix%)	21.2	23.4	26.1	19.9	22.4	25.1	0.20
Model cow (n = 189)							
Herd size 2008/09	154	175	222	141	151	170	0.28
% Grass silage of total diet	27	37	42	29	41	60	0.45
Model calf[b]							
Herd size 2008/09	154	175	222	141	151	170	0.28
Median herd level concentration of vitamin (α-tocopherol/β-carotene) in colostrum (μg/mL)	0.59/0.07	0.90/0.11	1.19/0.17	0.72/0.08	1.07/0.15	1.44/0.20	0.030/0.18

[a] Tested with univariable logistic regression, with cluster on herd, of its association with type of herd (high mortality/low mortality)

[b] Outcome transformed with a natural logarithm (ln) to approximate normal distribution

[c] Five missing values

pseudo R^2) were chosen, i.e. with α-tocopherol as outcome the variable "third-harvest grass in feed sample" (pseudo-R^2: 0.009) and for β-carotene "first-harvest grass in feed sample" (pseudo-R^2: 0.014), and these variables were consequently used in their respective model.

For the models "α-tocopherol concentration in colostrum" and "β-carotene concentration in colostrum" the samples containing blood were omitted due to potential bias since they had significantly higher Brix% and protein concentration compared to colostrum samples not containing blood.

Before running the multivariable models, all candidate predictor variables were evaluated with univariable regression models (with vitamin concentrations as outcomes), controlling for clustering within herd, in order to detect possible bias and to explore the variables. Hence, the univariable regression models were not used to qualify variables to the multivariable models; rather, the predictors were included in the multivariable models according to our a priori constructed causal diagram, regardless of P value. The predictor variables and some data from the variables of the collected samples were also evaluated with univariable regression with type of herd (HM/LM) as outcome, as presented in Tables 1, 2, 3, and further explored with Wilcoxon rank sum test or χ^2 test (Chi square test) to further analyse possible associations between the variables.

The multivariable models were run using a manual stepwise backward procedure, where variables associated with the outcome at $P \leq 0.05$ were retained in the model until all variables in the model were significant. All variables excluded during the reduction were then re-entered and kept if the P value was ≤ 0.05 or if the parameter estimate of another variable changed more than 20%, indicating confounding [26].

Two-way interactions (considered biologically plausible by the investigator) between variables in the reduced model were tested one by one and kept if the P value was ≤ 0.05. To control for potential bias due to a skewed distribution of breed between groups (the distribution of Swedish Red, Swedish Holstein and Mixed breed in HM herds was 16, 74 and 10%, respectively; and 55, 39 and 6%, respectively, in LM herds), we forced the variables "group (HM/LM)" and "breed" into all models, except for the two models with vitamin concentration in feed as outcomes, where "breed" was not considered to be a biologically plausible predictor. Additionally, for the two models with vitamin concentration in feed as outcomes, the variable "TMR (feeding total mixed rations/not feeding total mixed rations)" was also forced into the models to control for the fact that feed samples from TMR herds are accounting for the total ration, but only for the grass silage in non-TMR herds.

To identify potentially influential observations, plots of Pearson's residuals (r) versus the predicted values as well as univariable kernel density estimation curves were constructed. Observations with divergent values, i.e. $-3 \leq r \geq 3$, were considered outliers and their

Table 2 Results of univariable analyses (categorical variables), tested for associations with type of herd: high mortality (HM) or low mortality (LM)

Model/variable	Class	HM	LM	*P* value[a]
Model feed[b] (n = 57)				
Feeding TMR	Yes	18	21	
	No	9	9	0.88
First harvest grass in feed sample[c]	Yes	12	15	
	No	15	12	0.64
Percentage maize silage of total diet (%)	< 20	18	24	
	≥ 20	9	6	0.26
Third harvest grass in feed sample[d]	Yes	18	16	
	No	9	11	0.74
Type of herd (HM/LM)		27	30	
Model colostrum[b] (n = 162)				
Breed	SR	15	46	
	SH/MB	65	41	0.063
Hours post-partum sample was collected	< 1	19	28	
	> 1 ≤ 3	37	30	
	> 3–6	24	29	0.15
Milk leakage occurred pre-partum	Yes	6	13	
	No	64	74	0.25
	Missing	10	0	
Parity	1	20	22	
	2	24	34	
	3	16	13	
	4–8	20	18	0.68
Type of herd (HM/LM)		80	87	
Model cow (n = 189)				
Breed	SR	14	54	
	SH	67	39	
	MB	9	6	0.12
Day post partum cow was sampled	2–3	33	40	
	4–5	31	36	
	6–7	26	23	0.80
Feeding TMR	Yes	18	21	
	No	9	9	0.88
Parity	1	37	39	
	2	21	31	
	3–8	32	29	0.55
Percentage maize silage of total diet (DM)	Tested in model feed, see above			
Type of herd (HM/LM)		90	99	
Model calf[b] (n = 187)				
Age of calf when sampled (days)	2–3	30	42	
	4–5	30	33	
	6–7	29	23	0.53
Breed	SR	15	52	
	SH/MB	74	46	0.052
Total protein (g/L)	≥ 55	59	58	
	< 55	30	40	0.52

Table 2 continued

Model/variable	Class	HM	LM	*P* value[a]
Transition milk is given (days)	≥ 3	59	88	
	< 3	20	10	0.42
Type of herd (HM/LM)		89	98	

SR Swedish Red, *SH* Swedish Holstein, *MB* mixed breed

[a] Tested with univariable logistic regression, with cluster on herd, of its association with type of herd (HM: high mortality; LM: low mortality)

[b] Outcome transformed with a natural logarithm (*ln*) to approximate normal distribution

[c] Variable used only for the model "β-carotene concentration in feed"

[d] Variable used only for the model "α-tocopherol concentration in feed"

influence on the models were further evaluated. In the model "β-carotene concentration in cow serum" three observations showed slightly high residuals. One outlier was excluded since the concentration of vitamin was questionably high (β-carotene: 9.39 μg/mL serum) and because this observation alone made the variable "days post-partum" significant. The two other observations were kept in the model since they did not influence the model and their β-carotene concentrations were reasonable.

For each significant continuous variable in each model, we calculated the predicted effect on the concentration of fat soluble vitamins of moving from the first quartile of the predictor to the third quartile. These predicted effects are provided as examples to visualise the magnitude of the associations found in our material.

Results

Descriptive statistics on data collected at the individual level

Predictor variables used in the different models are, as previously mentioned, given in Tables 1 and 2. The distributions of the variables generated from the collected material (feed, colostrum, cow serum and calf serum) are given in Table 3, for HM and LM herds, respectively.

From the forms regarding feeding routines of individual calves, the following herd-level data was obtained; the median of the variable "Percentage of calves given colostrum manually" was 92% (range 22–100%) in HM herds and 100% (range 15–100%) in LM groups; the median for all herds (n = 18; 1 HM herd missing) was 100%. The volume of the first colostrum feeding given manually to individual calves varied from 0.5 to 4 L with a median value of 2.5 L for both HM and LM calves. The median total volume of colostrum given manually to individual calves the first day postpartum was 3.25 L for HM herds (range 1–8 L) and 4 L in LM herds (range 0.5–8 L). The median number of days (at herd level) that the calves were fed

Table 3 Distribution of variables analysed in collected samples and results of univariable analyses

Model/variable	High mortality (HM)			Low mortality (LM)			*P* value[a]
	25 pct.	Median	75 pct.	25 pct.	Median	75 pct.	
Model feed (nHM = 27; nLM = 30)							
α-Tocopherol (mg/kg DM)	30.30	46.41	70.95	44.98	63.81	75.18	0.50
β-Carotene (mg/kg DM)	15.3	28.3	35.1	20.6	36.6	42.2	0.33
Number of days from collection of sample until arrival at lab	1	1	2	1	2	3	0.75
Model colostrum (nHM = 80[b]; nLM = 87[b])							
α-Tocopherol (μg/mL colostrum)	1.58	2.62	5.68	0.91	2.25	4.37	0.085
β-Carotene (μg/mL colostrum)	0.47	0.75	1.74	0.29	0.74	1.45	0.14
Total solids (Brix%)	21.20	23.35	26.05	19.90	22.40	25.10	0.20
Fat[c] (%)	3.44	4.95	7.30	2.65	3.82	6.56	0.10
Lactose[c] (%)	2.82	3.10	3.31	3.01	3.21	3.50	0.003
Protein[c] (%)	12.39	13.65	15.48	11.07	13.02	14.77	0.21
Number of days from collection of sample until arrival at lab	1	3	5	1	3	4	0.61
Model cow (nHM = 90; nLM = 99)							
α-Tocopherol (μg/mL serum)	1.75	2.34	2.75	1.98	2.59	3.00	0.17
β-Carotene (μg/mL serum)	2.17	2.95	4.09	2.40	3.37	4.46	0.39
Number of days from collection of sample until arrival at lab	1	1	2	1	2	3	0.74
Model calf (nHM = 89; nLM = 98)							
α-Tocopherol (μg/mL serum)	0.59	0.90	1.19	0.72	1.07	1.44	0.030
β-Carotene (μg/mL serum)	0.07	0.11	0.17	0.08	0.15	0.20	0.18
Total protein (g/L)	53	57	61	53	57	62	0.77
Age (days) of the calf at sampling	3	4	6	3	4	5	0.32
Number of days from collection of sample until arrival at lab	1	1	2	1	2	4	0.77

[a] Tested with univariable logistic regression with cluster on herd of its association with type of herd (HM/LM)

[b] Samples with blood in colostrum omitted ($n_{HM} = 3$; $n_{LM} = 8$)

[c] Five missing values

with transition milk were 3 days (range 2–7 days) for HM herds and 4 days (range 1.5–7 days) for LM herds.

Descriptive statistics on data collected at the herd level

From SOMRS, herd data were collected to do the selection of herds for enrolment in the study. The median calf mortality risk (2008/09) in calves 1–90 days of age in HM herds was 9% (range 6–15%) and in LM herds 0% (range 0–0%). For herd size (2006/07; 2008/09) and annual herd milk production (in kg ECM 2008/09), see Table 4.

One HM herd stored their grass silage as round bales; one LM herd stored their grass silage mainly in a bunker silo, but also as round bales, while the rest of the herds stored all their grass silage in bunker silos. Most of the herds fed a total mixed ration to the cows (70% of HM herds and 67% of LM herds), 8 of 10 herds in Halland/Skåne and 5 of 9 herds in Skaraborg. The median percentage grass in DM of the full ration was 36.3% (range 20–68.9%) and 42.1% (range 18–60%) in Halland/Skåne and Skaraborg, respectively. Herds feeding TMR had significantly (P = 0.024) higher percentage of maize silage DM of full ration (Additional file 4). The median percentage maize silage DM of the full ration was significantly higher in Halland/Skåne (P = 0.005) with 17.2% (range 0–28.7%) and 0% (range 0–29.5%) in Halland/Skåne and Skaraborg, respectively (Additional file 5). All herds fed vitamin and mineral supplements to cows and heifers before calving. All bulk milk samples analysed were negative for antibodies against *S. typhimurium* and *S. dubli*n.

Multivariable analyses

α-Tocopherol

The results of the four multivariable analyses for α-tocopherol are presented in Table 5.

Feed model No effect of type of herd, i.e. HM/LM herd, was identified. A higher percentage of grass silage (DM) of total diet was associated with higher concentrations of α-tocopherol in the analysed feed samples (P = 0.008), corresponding to a difference of 1.30 mg/kg DM when comparing the 25th percentile [27.2% grass silage (DM) of full ration] to the 75th percentile [57.5% grass silage (DM) of full ration] (95% confidence interval 1.081–1.55).

Table 4 Descriptive herd data from 19 Swedish dairy herds with high or low calf mortality risk

Variable	High mortality (n = 9)			Low mortality (n = 10)			*P* value[a]
	25 pct.	Median	75 pct.	25 pct.	Median	75 pct.	
ECM (kg)/year 2008/09	8475	9516	10,207	9265	10,234	10,409	0.24
Herd size[b] 2006/07	153	184	226	129	134	169	0.071
Herd size[b] 2008/09	154	175	222	141	151	170	0.28
% Herd expansion[c]	– 0.058	– 0.013	0.11	– 0.040	0.074	0.10	0.80

[a] Tested with univariable logistic regression, of associations with type of herd

[b] Cows/year

[c] Calculated as [(herd size 2008/09 – herd size 2006/07)/Herd size 2008/09]

Feed samples containing grass from the third harvest of the season had lower concentrations of α-tocopherol than feed samples not containing grass from the third harvest ($P = 0.006$). Lower concentrations of α-tocopherol were seen in feed samples coming from herds using TMR, compared to herds not using TMR ($P < 0.001$). However, an interaction was observed between region and TMR ($P = 0.006$), implying that the difference in concentration of α-tocopherol in feed samples was only significant for herds in region Halland/Skåne. Baseline herds (herds not feeding TMR in region Halland/Skåne) had a higher concentration of α-tocopherol corresponding to a difference of 0.45 mg/kg DM in feed compared to herds feeding TMR, in the same region.

Colostrum model No effect of type of herd was found. Breed was significantly associated with the concentration of α-tocopherol in colostrum ($P = 0.001$), with higher concentrations in Swedish Holstein and mixed breed than in Swedish Red. Colostrum with a higher content of total solids (Brix%) was associated with a higher concentration of α-tocopherol ($P = 0.005$), corresponding to a difference of 1.25 μg/mL colostrum (95% confidence interval 1.09–1.44), when comparing the 25th percentile (Brix 20.4%) to the 75th percentile (Brix 25.4%). A higher content of fat in colostrum was also associated with a higher concentration of α-tocopherol ($P < 0.001$), corresponding to a difference of 3.11 μg/mL colostrum (95% confidence interval 2.48–3.91), when comparing the 25th percentile (2.91% fat) to the 75th percentile (7.1% fat).

Cow model No effect of type of herd was seen. Parity was significantly associated with α-tocopherol in serum ($P = 0.005$), with lower concentrations in cows in third to eight parities, as compared to first parity cows.

Calf model Calves in HM herds had lower α-tocopherol serum concentrations than calves in LM herds. An interaction between total protein and type of herd (HM/LM) was observed, but was only significant for HM herds ($P = 0.036$). For those herds, calves with total protein < 55 g/L, i.e. failure of passive transfer (FPT), had significantly lower α-tocopherol serum concentrations, compared to baseline herds (LM and total protein ≥ 55 g/L). Swedish Holstein calves or calves of mixed breed had significantly higher α-tocopherol serum concentrations compared to Swedish Red calves ($P = 0.043$). Calves from herds that fed transition milk for 3 days or more had significantly higher serum concentrations of α-tocopherol ($P = 0.13$).

β-Carotene

The results of the four multivariable analyses for β-carotene are presented in Table 6.

Feed model No effect of type of herd was identified. The concentration of β-carotene in feed was lower in herds using TMR ($P < 0.001$), and in region Halland/Skåne ($P = 0.034$), compared to herds not using TMR and region Skaraborg, respectively. Feed samples containing grass from the first harvest of the season had higher concentration of β-carotene compared to feed samples without grass from the first harvest of the season ($P = 0.001$).

Colostrum model No effect of type of herd was shown. A higher content of fat in colostrum was associated with a higher concentration of β-carotene ($P < 0.001$). However, an interaction between fat and breed was observed. That means that the effect of fat is different for the different breeds. When comparing a difference in fat content in colostrum, and taking breed into account; corresponding to the 25th and 75th percentiles; i.e. 2.91 and 7.1% fat, respectively, it was shown that Swedish Red had higher concentration (1.61 μg/mL; $P = 0.038$) of β-carotene in colostrum compared to Swedish Holstein or mixed breed (95% confidence interval 1.17–2.20), Although Swedish Holstein cows had higher fat content in colostrum, the interaction means that Swedish Red cows had higher β-carotene concentration per unit of fat, given the other variables in the model. Total solids (Brix%) in

Table 5 Results from multivariable linear regression models of the associations between predictors and concentration of α-tocopherol

Model/variable	Class	α-Tocopherol concentration			
		Estimate	Robust std. err.	*P* value	95% CI
Model feed α-tocopherol[a] (mg/kg DM; n = 57)					
Constant		3.59	0.14	< 0.001	3.29–3.90
Herd size		0.0023	0.00053	< 0.001	0.0012–0.034
Region	Halland/Skåne	Baseline	–	–	–
	Skaraborg	0.28	0.14	0.065	− 0.19 to 0.58
Third harvest in feed sample	No	Baseline	–	–	–
	Yes	− 0.36	0.12	0.006	− 0.60 to − 0.12
TMR[b]	No	Baseline	–	–	–
	Yes	− 0.80	0.12	< 0.001	− 1.07 to − 0.54
Interaction: TMR × region				0.006	
	TMR: no × Halland/Skåne	Baseline	–	–	–
	TMR: yes × Halland/Skåne	− 0.80	0.13	< 0.001	− 1.07 to − 0.53
	TMR: no × Skaraborg	0.28	0.14	0.065	− 0.19 to 0.58
	TMR: yes × Skaraborg	0.08	0.11	0.48	− 0.15 to 0.32
Type of herd[b]	LM	Baseline	–	–	–
	HM	0.054	0.11	0.615	− 0.17 to 0.28
% Grass silage of total diet		0.86	0.28	0.008	0.26–1.45
Model colostrum α-tocopherol (μg/mL)[a] (n = 162)					
Constant		− 1.68	0.32	< 0.001	− 2.34 to − 1.02
Breed[b]	SR	Baseline	–	–	–
	SH/MB	0.45	0.12	0.001	0.21–0.69
Fat[c] (%)		0.20	0.023	< 0.001	0.15–0.25
Herd size		0.0014	0.00046	0.006	0.0004/–0.0024
Type of herd[b]	LM	Baseline	–	–	–
	HM	− 0.11	0.11	0.34	− 0.35 to 0.13
Total solids (Brix%)		0.042	0.013	0.005	0.015–0.069
Model cow α-tocopherol (μg/mL) (n = 189)					
Constant		2.77	0.18	< 0.001	2.40–3.14
Breed[b]				0.10	
	SR	Baseline	–	–	–
	SH	− 0.33	0.14	0.027	− 0.62 to − 0.04
	MB	− 0.30	0.19	0.13	− 0.70 to 0.10
Parity				0.0053	
	1	Baseline	–	–	–
	2	0.26	0.15	0.10	− 0.057 to 0.57
	3–8	− 0.32	0.13	0.028	− 0.60 to − 0.040
Type of herd[b]	LM	Baseline	–	–	–
	HM	− 0.099	0.15	0.53	− 0.42 to 0.23
Model calf serum α-tocopherol[a] (μg/mL) (n = 187)					
Constant		0.026	0.11	0.82	− 0.20 to 0.25
Breed[b]	SR	Baseline	–	–	–
	SH/MB	0.24	0.11	0.043	− 0.0081 to 0.48
Days transition milk is fed (days)	≥ 3	Baseline	–	–	–
	< 3	− 0.21	0.076	0.013	− 0.37 to − 0.052
Total protein (g/L)	≥ 55	Baseline	–	–	–
	< 55	− 0.16	0.11	0.16	− 0.40 to 0.073

Table 5 continued

Model/variable	Class	α-Tocopherol concentration			
		Estimate	Robust std. err.	*P* value	95% CI
Type of herd[b]	LM	Baseline	–	–	–
	HM	− 0.17	0.14	0.219	− 0.47 to 0.12
Interaction: type of herd × total protein (g/L)				0.036	
	LM × total protein ≥ 55	Baseline	–	–	–
	LM × total protein < 55	− 0.16	0.11	0.16	− 0.40 to 0.072
	HM × total protein ≥ 55	− 0.17	0.14	0.22	− 0.47 to 0.11
	HM × total protein < 55	− 0.68	0.14	< 0.001	− 0.97 to − 0.40

SR Swedish Red, *SH* Swedish Holstein, MB mixed breed

[a] Outcome transformed with a natural logarithm (ln) to approximate normal distribution

[b] Forced into model

[c] Five missing values

colostrum was positively associated with the concentration of β-carotene in colostrum (P = 0.007). A comparison between the 25th percentile (Brix 20.4%) and the 75th percentile (Brix 25.4%) showed higher β-carotene concentration corresponding to a difference of 1.27 μg/mL colostrum (95% confidence interval 1.08–1.59).

Cow model No effect of type of herd was identified. Having a total ration containing more or equal to 20% maize silage DM was associated with significantly lower concentration of β-carotene in cow serum (P = 0.001). Swedish Holstein cows had significantly lower concentrations of β-carotene in serum than Swedish Red cows (P < 0.001).

Calf model No effect of type of herd was found. A significant negative association between FPT and concentrations of β-carotene in calf serum was found (i.e. lower concentrations in calves with FPT). However, an interaction between breed and FPT was observed (P = 0.002). This interaction means that the effect of FPT on the concentration of β-carotene in calf serum is different for the different breeds with significantly lower concentrations of β-carotene in calves of Swedish Holstein or mixed breed calves, compared to calves of Swedish Red.

Discussion

The evaluation of α-tocopherol and β-carotene in feed, colostrum, cow and calf serum revealed that only low α-tocopherol status at the calf level was associated with high calf mortality risk at herd level. However, the low α-tocopherol status of the calf was related to the total protein status of the calf, which is a proxy for adequate colostrum intake. Still, no differences between HM and LM herds were found regarding colostrum routines in the univariable analyses. Different routines regarding the feeding of transition milk were identified, with significant higher concentrations of α-tocopherol in calf serum from herds feeding transition milk for 3 days or more.

Vitamins in feed

Roughage is the major natural source of α-tocopherol and β-carotene for the cow, but it is difficult to predict vitamin concentrations in the feed, as these are highly variable depending on plant species, maturity of the plant, harvest and storage conditions [18]. Influence of harvest number was shown in the feed models in our study with lower concentrations of α-tocopherol in feed samples containing grass from third harvest and higher concentrations of β-carotene in feed samples containing grass from first harvest. The results of season is in contrast to findings by Jensen et al. [27], who reported higher concentrations of α-tocopherol and β-carotene in a grass-clover mixture in late season (Aug–Oct) and lower in June as compared to the average concentration for the whole season. The reason for the difference is unknown but the vitamin concentration in grass is also highly dependent on when in the vegetative phase the grass is harvested, which might have affected the result. Such data were, however, not collected in this study. Having a high proportion of grass silage of the total ration was positively associated with α-tocopherol concentrations in the feed samples. The importance of grass silage for cow vitamin status was shown in a Danish study in which milk from cows fed grass silage had a higher concentration of α-tocopherol and β-carotene than milk from cows fed maize silage [28]. Mogensen et al. [29] also reported that increasing the proportion of maize silage at the expense of grass-clover silage decreased the milk content of β-carotene.

Table 6 Results from multivariable linear regression models of the associations between predictors and concentration of β-carotene

Model/variable	Class	β-Carotene concentration			
		Estimate	Robust std. err.	*P* value	95% CI
Model feed β-carotene (mg/kg DM)[a] (n = 57)					
Constant		3.50	0.10	< 0.001	3.28–3.72
First harvest in feed sample	No	Baseline	–	–	–
	Yes	0.64	0.17	0.001	0.29–1.00
Region	Halland/Skåne	Baseline	–	–	–
	Skaraborg	0.38	0.17	0.034	0.032–0.73
TMR[b]	No	Baseline	–	–	–
	Yes	− 0.99	0.14	< 0.001	− 1.28 to − 0.70
Type of herd[b]	LM	Baseline	–	–	–
	HM	− 0.15	0.17	0.38	− 0.51 to 0.20
Model colostrum β-carotene (μg/mL)[a] (n = 162)					
Constant		− 2.81	0.38	< 0.001	− 3.6 to − 2.02
Breed	SR	Baseline	–	–	–
	SH/MB	0.69	0.25	0.013	0.16 to 1.21
Fat[c] (%)		0.26	0.27	< 0.001	0.20 to 0.32
Interaction: fat (%) × breed	Fat[c] (%) × breed SR	Baseline	–	–	–
	Fat[c] (%) × breed SH/MB	− 0.11	0.036	0.005	− 0.19 to − 0.038
Total solids (Brix%)		0.048	0.016	0.007	0.015 to 0.081
Type of herd[b]	LM	Baseline	–	–	–
	HM	− 0. 62	0.16	0.69	− 0.39 to 0.26
Model cow serum β-carotene (μg/mL) (n = 189)					
Constant		4.28	0.21	< 0.001	3.85–4.71
Breed[b]				0.0003	
	SR	Baseline	–	–	–
	SH	− 1.27	0.25	< 0.001	− 1.78 to − 0.75
	MB	− 0.55	0.32	0.10	− 1.23 to 0.12
Percentage maize silage (DM) of total ration	< 20%	Baseline	–	–	–
	≥ 20%	− 1.08	0.27	0.001	− 1.66 to − 0.50
Type of herd[b]	LM	Baseline	–	–	–
	HM	0.16	0.27	0.56	− 0.41 to 0.73
Model calf serum β-carotene[a] (μg/mL; n = 187)					
Constant		− 1.84	0.08	< 0.001	− 2.01 to − 1.67
Breed[b]	SR	Baseline	–	–	–
	SH/MB	− 0.06	0.12	0.61	− 0.31 to 0.018
Interaction: breed × total protein (g/L)			0.036		
	SR × total protein ≥ 55	Baseline	–	–	–
	SR × total protein < 55	− 0.21	0.11	0.078	− 0.44 to 0.026
	SH/MB × total protein ≥ 55	− 0.062	0.12	0.61	− 0.31 to 0.18
	SH/MB × total protein < 55	− 0.78	0.15	< 0.001	− 1.08 to − 0.047
Total protein (g/L)	≥ 55	Baseline	–	–	–
	< 55	− 0.21	0.11	0.078	− 0.44 to 0.026
Type of herd[b]	LM	Baseline	–	–	–
	HM	− 0.18	0.15	0.23	− 0.49 to 0.12

SR Swedish Red, *SH* Swedish Holstein, *MB* mixed breed

[a] Outcome transformed with a natural logarithm (ln) to approximate normal distribution

[b] Forced into model

[c] Five missing values

For both α-tocopherol and β-carotene, feed samples taken in herds feeding TMR had lower vitamin concentrations than in herds not feeding TMR, although for α-tocopherol the association was dependent on region. This was expected as grain and other protein sources are fairly low in vitamin concentration. Another possible explanation for the lower concentrations in TMR might be related to the percentage grass or maize silage (DM) used in the TMR.

As vitamins may be lost during storage, differences in vitamin concentrations could be due to different methods for storing silage. In a Swedish study, it was concluded that there is a greater risk of α-tocopherol losses in silage stored as round-bales compared to in silage stored in bunker silos [19]. However, with only two herds in the study storing their silage in round-bales, the overall effect of storage in round bales is considered negligible.

Vitamins in colostrum

Breed was also associated with vitamin concentrations in colostrum as Swedish Holstein cows, and cows of mixed breeds had higher concentrations of α-tocopherol and β-carotene than Swedish Red cows. This indicates a role of genetics in vitamin secretion into milk as observed previously [30]. In a study by Jensen et al. [20], significant effects of sire on concentrations of both α-tocopherol and β-carotene in milk, milk fat and also for the total secretion of fat-soluble vitamins into milk were shown. In the present study, we did not instruct the farmers to empty the udder completely at milking. Hence, the first colostrum milk yield is unknown and hence, differences in vitamin concentration in colostrum between the breeds could also be an effect of dilution. However, Swedish Holstein is a breed with higher milk production and should therefore be expected to have lower vitamin concentrations due to dilution. This is not supported by our data, which actually showed the opposite situation. We believe that the risk of bias is small and that the samples taken reflect the actual vitamin concentration that the farmers give to the calves when practising their usual colostrum management routines.

The content of fat in colostrum was positively associated with the concentrations of the two vitamins in colostrum, i.e. colostrum with higher fat content also had higher vitamin concentrations. This was expected, and a logical finding, since the vitamins are fat-soluble. The content of total solids was also positively associated with the concentrations of the two vitamins in colostrum. However, the variable total solids only explained a small proportion of the variation in vitamins in colostrum (data not shown). Therefore, estimation of total solids using the method applied here (a Brix refractometer) to predict the content of vitamins is questionable. To the authors' knowledge there is, however, no reliable cow-side test for fat content in colostrum. Hence, this could be an area for future development.

Vitamins in cow serum

The concentrations of α-tocopherol and β-carotene measured in cow serum reflects the total ration consumed by the cow. Having a total ration containing more or equal to 20% maize silage (DM) was associated with significantly lower concentration of β-carotene in cow serum. This is in line with other studies, which have shown maize silage to be very low in vitamin content [18]. As previously mentioned, several studies have found a positive association between vitamin-rich feed and/or vitamin supplements given, and vitamin concentrations in milk, and some of these studies conclude that a vitamin-rich feed also is associated with vitamin concentrations in plasma [31, 32].

Breed was associated with β-carotene concentration in cow serum; cows of Swedish Holstein and mixed breed had lower β-carotene concentrations in cow serum than Swedish Red cows, but the opposite was found for these vitamins in colostrum. For α-tocopherol in cow serum there was only a tendency for an effect of breed with lower concentrations in Swedish Holstein cows than in Swedish Red cows. The differences between breeds are probably due to genetic factors of importance for the ability to absorb vitamins in the digestive tract, or to secrete vitamins into the udder [20]. There may also have been differences between dietary fat content in the diets, but unfortunately, we have no information on dietary fat in diets for these herds. According to Goff and Stabel [21] secretion of α-tocopherol into the udder around calving is a major reason for the decreased plasma concentration observed in cows at this point in time. In both colostrum models, Swedish Holstein was associated with higher concentrations of the fat-soluble vitamins compared to Swedish Red. As above mentioned, with significant lower or a tendency for lower concentrations of β-carotene and α-tocopherol in cow serum, respectively, it seems reasonable to hypothesise that it could be an effect of colostrogenesis. However, as the blood and colostrum samples came from different cows we cannot draw any firm conclusions regarding causality. The concentrations of α-tocopherol in cows' serum in the present study are comparable with other Scandinavian studies [20, 33].

Vitamins in calf serum

The bulk milk samples from all herds were free from antibodies to *Salmonella*, which means that it is unlikely that salmonellosis contributed to calf mortality in this study. We found that calves in HM herds had lower concentrations of α-tocopherol in serum during the first week after birth than calves in LM herds. This association depended, however, on the total protein content of the calf serum. This is partly in line with Torsein et al. [1], who reported that the proportion of calves with inadequate concentration of α-tocopherol and β-carotene in serum was significantly higher in herds with high calf mortality risks day 1–90. In that study, which was conducted at the herd level, correlations between inadequate levels of α-tocopherol or β-carotene and failure of passive transfer could not be identified. In the present study, however, we found that calves with FPT were associated with lower concentrations of β-carotene concentration in calf serum. However, the association depended on the breed of the calves, i.e. only in calves of Swedish Holstein or mixed breed FPT was associated with lower concentrations of β-carotene in calf serum. For α-tocopherol, however, the association depended on type of herd, i.e. calves from HM herds and with failure of passive transfer were associated with lower concentrations of α-tocopherol in calf serum. Nevertheless, in this study we were not able to find any associations between colostrum management and type of herd (HM/LM), nor detect any significant difference in total protein content in serum between HM and LM herds. The lower concentrations of α-tocopherol in calves in HM herds can therefore not be fully explained by different colostrum routines and is also likely related to the quality of the feed and feeding management. We did find that calves from herds that fed transition milk for 3 days or more had higher α-tocopherol serum concentrations than calves from herds feeding transition milk up to 2 days only. The median (herd level) number of days the calves were fed with transition milk was 3 days for HM herds and 4 days for LM herds. Transition milk is sometimes mixed with colostrum and if so, the calves are offered a milk source with presumably high vitamin content.

Study design

Our aim was to investigate if calf mortality risk at herd level is associated with concentrations of α-tocopherol and/or β-carotene at individual level in feed, colostrum, cow and calf serum. A benefit of modelling the concentrations in separate models is that intervening between variables that lie along the same causal pathway is avoided. Since this study did not aim to follow how the vitamin uptake from the feed correlates to vitamin concentration in the cow and, then to the vitamin concentration in colostrum and later concentration in the calf at individual level, we did not focus on getting samples from that chain since the evaluation of the previous step in the causal chain were at herd level in the models. Still, a high percentage of the samples from cows and calves were indeed mother/offspring pairs. However, our primary aim was to look at vitamin concentrations at different steps and evaluate them as an indicator for the herds' vitamin status. Because of this, some associations may have remained undetected.

Conclusions

Our hypothesis that inadequate α-tocopherol and β-carotene concentrations in calf serum were associated with high calf mortality risks could only be confirmed for α-tocopherol, but the effect depended on total protein status of the calf. In herds with high calf mortality, evaluation of the calves' α-tocopherol status is recommended. Feeding transition milk for 3 days or more was associated with higher α-tocopherol concentrations in calf serum. High proportions of maize silage (DM) in the total diet were associated with lower concentrations of β-carotene in cow serum. Breed was associated with vitamin concentrations in colostrum.

Additional files

Additional file 1. Map of Sweden showing the 19 herds in the study; 9 herds with high calf mortality (HM) and 10 herds with low calf mortality (LM). Black: county of Skaraborg and south of Älvsborg. Grey: County of Halland. Blue: County of Skåne. Red: High mortality herds. Green: Low mortality herds.

Additional file 2. Vitamin E and beta carotene in cow/calf/colostrum. Questionnaire.

Additional file 3. Forms for individual calves regarding feeding routines.

Additional file 4. Differences of proportion of maize in 19 Swedish dairy herds with high (n = 9) or low (n = 10) calf mortality risk, day 1–90, feeding total mixed ration (TMR) or not.

Additional file 5. Regional differences concerning proportion of maize of total diet in 19 Swedish dairy herds with high (n = 9) or low (n = 10) calf mortality risk, day 1–90.

Abbreviations

DM: dry matter; FPT: failure of passive transfer, total protein < 55 g/L; HM: herd with high calf mortality risk; LM: herd with low calf mortality risk; SOMRS: Swedish Official Milk Recording Scheme; SVA: National Veterinary Institute, Uppsala, Sweden; RCF: Aarhus University, Department of Animal Science, Research Center Foulum, Tjele, Denmark.

Authors' contributions

KPW was project coordinator and designed the study together with MT, AL, CS, SKJ. MT coordinated the study; performed all herd visits, collected the samples in the study, performed the data analysis and drafted the manuscript. MT, KPW, AL, CS, SKJ and CB revised the manuscript. All authors read and approved the final manuscript.

Author details

[1] Farm & Animal Health, Uddetorp Röda huset, 532 96 Skara, Sweden. [2] Department of Animal Environment and Health, Swedish University of Agricultural Sciences, P.O. Box 234, 532 23 Skara, Sweden. [3] Department of Disease Control and Epidemiology, National Veterinary Institute, 751 89 Uppsala, Sweden. [4] Department of Clinical Sciences, Swedish University of Agricultural Sciences, P.O. Box 7054, 75007 Uppsala, Sweden. [5] Department of Animal Science, Aarhus University, Research Centre Foulum, P.O. Box 50, 8830 Tjele, Denmark. [6] Department of Animal Health and Antimicrobial Strategies, National Veterinary Institute, 751 89 Uppsala, Sweden.

Acknowledgements
The authors thank the participating farmers for their interest and support. The authors would also like to thank Hanna Lindqvist, Swedish University of Agricultural Sciences, Skara, Sweden, and Carin Clason, Växa Sverige, Falkenberg, Sweden, for valuable cooperation, and all technical staff analysing the samples, with special thanks to Maria Persson, National Veterinary Institute, Uppsala, Sweden.

Competing interests
The authors declare that they have no competing interests.

Availability of data and materials
The datasets generated during and/or analysed during the current study are not publicly available due to certain restrictions concerning confidentiality. Some data were used under license for the current study, and are therefore not publicly available. The datasets are available from the corresponding author on reasonable request and with permission from Farm & Animal Health and Växa Sverige.

Funding
The study was supported financially by the Swedish Farmers' Foundation for Agricultural Research, Award Number V0930002.

References

1. Torsein M, Lindberg A, Sandgren CH, Waller KP, Törnquist M, Svensson C. Risk factors for calf mortality in large Swedish dairy herds. Prev Vet Med. 2011;99:136–47.
2. Pehrson B, Hakkarainen J. Vitamin E status of healthy Swedish cattle. Acta Vet Scand. 1986;27:351–60.
3. Reddy PG, Morrill JL, Minocha HC, Morrill MB, Dayton AD, Frey RA. Effect of supplemental vitamin E on the immune system of calves. J Dairy Sci. 1986;69:164–71.
4. Rajaraman V, Nonnecke BJ, Franklin ST, Hammell DC, Horst RL. Effect of vitamins A and E on nitric oxide production by blood mononuclear leukocytes from neonatal calves fed milk replacer. J Dairy Sci. 1998;81:3278–85.
5. Higuchi H, Nagahata H. Effects of vitamins A and E on superoxide production and intracellular signalling of neutrophils in Holstein calves. Can Vet J. 2000;64:69–75.
6. Carter JN, Gill DR, Krehbiel CR, Confer AW, Smith RA, Lalman DL, et al. Vitamin E supplementation of newly arrived feedlot calves. J Anim Sci. 2005;83:1924–32.
7. Urban-Chmiel R, Hola P, Lisiecka U, Wernicki A, Puchalski A, Dec M, et al. An evaluation of the effects of α-tocopherol and ascorbic acid in bovine respiratory disease complex occurring in feedlot calves after transport. Livest Sci. 2011;141:53–8.
8. Nozière P, Graulet B, Lucas A, Martin B, Grolier P, Doreau M. Carotenoids for ruminants: from forages to dairy products. Anim Feed Sci Technol. 2006;131:418–50.
9. Chew BP. Vitamin A and β-carotene on host defense. J Dairy Sci. 1987;70:2732–43.
10. Rizzo A, Ceci E, Pantaleo M, Mutinati M, Spedicato M, Minoia G, et al. Evaluation of blood and milk oxidative status during early postpartum of dairy cows. Animal. 2013;7:118–23.
11. Chew BP. Role of carotenoids in the immune response. J Dairy Sci. 1993;76:2804–11.
12. Lotthammer KH. Importance of β-carotene for the fertility of dairy cattle. Feedstuffs. 1979;52:36–8.
13. Puls R. Vitamin levels in animal health. Diagnostic data and bibliographies. Clearbrook: Sherpa Int.; 1994.
14. Kume S, Toharmat T. Effect of colostral β-carotene and vitamin A on vitamin and health status of newborn calves. Livest Prod Sci. 2001;68:61–5.
15. Van Saun RJ, Herdt TH, Stowe HD. Maternal and fetal vitamin E concentrations and selenium–vitamin E interrelationships in dairy cattle. J Nutr. 1989;119:1156–64.
16. Nonnecke BJ, Horst RL, Waters WR, Dubeski P, Harp JA. Modulation of fat-soluble vitamin concentrations and blood mononuclear leukocyte populations in milk replacer-fed calves by dietary vitamin A and β-carotene. J Dairy Sci. 1999;82:2632–41.
17. Zanker IA, Hammon HM, Blum JW. β-Carotene, retinol and α-tocopherol status in calves fed the first colostrum at 0–2, 6–7, 12–13 or 24–25 hours after birth. Int J Vitam Res. 2000;70:305–10.
18. Mogensen L, Kristensen T, Søegaard K, Jensen SK, Sehested J. Alfa-tocopherol and beta-carotene in roughages and milk in organic dairy herds. Livest Sci. 2012;145:44–54.
19. Nadeau E, Johansson B, Jensen SK, Olsson G. Vitamin content of forages as influenced by harvest and ensiling techniques. In: Grassland science in Europe, vol. 9. Zürich: vdf Hochschulverlag AG an der ETH Zurich; 2004. p. 891–3.
20. Jensen SK, Johannsen AKB, Hermansen JE. Quantitative secretion and maximal secretion capacity of retinol, β-carotene and α-tocopherol into cows' milk. J Dairy Res. 1999;66:511–22.
21. Goff J, Stabel J. Decreased plasma retinol, α-tocopherol, and zinc concentration during the periparturient period: effect of milk fever. J Dairy Sci. 1990;73:3195–9.
22. Muller CE, Moller J, Jensen SK, Uden P. Tocopherol and carotenoid levels in baled silage and haylage in relation to horse requirements. Anim Feed Sci Technol. 2007;137:182–97.
23. Bielmann V, Gillan J, Perkins NR, Skidmore AL, Godden S, Leslie KE. An evaluation of Brix refractometry instruments for measurement of colostrum quality in dairy cattle. J Dairy Sci. 2010;93:3713–21.
24. Jensen SK, Nielsen KN. Tocopherols, retinol, β-carotene and fatty acids in fat globule membrane and fat globule core in cows' milk. J Dairy Res. 1996;63:565–74.
25. Nyman A-K, Agren E, Bergstrom K, Wahlstrom H. Evaluation of the specificity of three enzyme-linked immunosorbent assays for detection of antibodies against Salmonella in bovine bulk milk. Acta Vet Scand. 2013;55:5.
26. Dohoo IR, Wayne M, Stryhn H. Veterinary epidemiologic research. 2nd ed. Charlottetown: AVC Inc; 2009. p. 864.
27. Jensen SK, Søegaard K, Sehested J, Lindqvist H, Nadeau E. Indflydelse af høstmetode og konservering på vitamin-og fedtsyreindhold. Intern Rep Husb. 2010;27:15–20.
28. Havemose MS, Weisbjerg MR, Bredie WLP, Nielsen JH. Influence of feeding different types of roughage on the oxidative stability of milk. Int Dairy J. 2004;14:563–70.
29. Mogensen L, Vestergaard JS, Fretté X, Lund P, Weisbjerg MR, Kristensen T. Effect of toasting field beans and of grass-clover: maize silage ratio on milk production, milk composition and sensory quality of milk. Livest Sci. 2010;128:123–32.
30. Ramalho HMM, Santos J, Casal S, Alves MR, Oliveira MBPP. Fat-soluble vitamin (A, D, E, and β-carotene) contents from a Portuguese autochthonous cow breed—Minhota. J Dairy Sci. 2012;95:5476–84.
31. Kaewlamun W, Okouyi M, Humblot P, Remy D, Techakumphu M, Duvaux-Ponter C, et al. The influence of a supplement of β-carotene given during the dry period to dairy cows on colostrum quality, and β-carotene status, metabolites and hormones in newborn calves. Anim Feed Sci Technol. 2011;165:31–7.
32. Weiss WP, Hogan JS, Wyatt DJ. Relative bioavailability of all-rac and RRR vitamin E based on neutrophil function and total α-tocopherol and isomer concentrations in periparturient dairy cows and their calves. J Dairy Sci. 2009;92:720–31.
33. Meglia GE, Jensen SK, Lauridsen C, Waller KP. α-Tocopherol concentration and stereoisomer composition in plasma and milk from dairy cows fed natural or synthetic vitamin E around calving. J Dairy Res. 2006;73:227–34.

20

Clinical evaluation of constant rate infusion of alfaxalone–medetomidine combined with sevoflurane anesthesia in Thoroughbred racehorses undergoing arthroscopic surgery

Hirotaka Tokushige[1*], Asuka Kushiro[1], Atsushi Okano[1], Tatsuya Maeda[1], Hideki Ito[1], Ai Wakuno[2], Shun-ichi Nagata[3] and Minoru Ohta[4]

Abstract

Background: Alfaxalone has a number of pharmacological properties which are desirable for constant rate infusion (CRI). Previously, the co-administration of alfaxalone and medetomidine is shown to be suitable for short-term anesthesia in horses. However, the use of alfaxalone–medetomidine CRI with inhalational anesthesia under surgical procedures have not been investigated in clinical cases. The aim of the present study was to evaluate the clinical efficacy of alfaxalone–medetomidine CRI in sevoflurane-anesthetized Thoroughbred racehorses undergoing arthroscopic surgery. Sevoflurane requirement, cardiovascular function, and induction/recovery quality were compared between horses maintained with sevoflurane in combination with medetomidine CRI (3 μg/kg/h) (Group M; n = 25) and those maintained with sevoflurane in combination with alfaxalone–medetomidine CRI (0.5 mg/kg/h and 3 μg/kg/h, respectively) (Group AM; n = 25).

Results: The mean end-tidal sevoflurane concentrations were significantly lower in Group AM (1.8 ± 0.2%) than in Group M (2.4 ± 0.1%). The mean dobutamine infusion rate required for maintaining mean arterial blood pressure within the target values (60–80 mmHg) was significantly lower in Group AM (0.53 ± 0.20 μg/kg/min) than in Group M (0.85 ± 0.32 μg/kg/min). Induction and recovery scores were not significantly different between two groups. However, excitatory response during recovery were observed in five horses in Group AM. The mean plasma alfaxalone concentrations were stable throughout the maintenance period (0.77 ± 0.12 to 0.85 ± 0.13 μg/mL), and decreased significantly immediately after standing (0.32 ± 0.07 μg/mL).

Conclusions: Alfaxalone–medetomidine CRI reduced sevoflurane requirement by approximately 26% with good maintenance of cardiopulmonary function in Thoroughbred racehorses undergoing arthroscopic surgery. Sevoflurane in combination with alfaxalone–medetomidine CRI may be a clinically effective anesthetic technique for Thoroughbred racehorses. However, 20% of horses administered alfaxalone showed remarkable excitatory response during recovery. Greater attention to excitatory response may be advisable if alfaxalone is used for induction or maintenance of anesthesia. A larger study is needed to explore the clinical relevance of these findings.

Keywords: Alfaxalone–medetomidine, Constant rate infusion, Equine anesthesia, Racehorse, Recovery, Sevoflurane

*Correspondence: Hirotaka_Tokushige@jra.go.jp
[1] Racehorse Clinic, Miho Training Center, Japan Racing Association (JRA), 2500-2 Mikoma, Miho-mura, Inashiki-gun, Ibaraki 300-0493, Japan
Full list of author information is available at the end of the article

Background

Among the volatile anesthetic agents commonly used in equine anesthesia, sevoflurane has the advantages of rapid induction of anesthesia, easy control of anesthetic depth and rapid recovery due to its low blood solubility [1–3]. However, sevoflurane is known to cause dose-dependent cardiopulmonary depression, which increases the risk of peri-anesthetic mortality and death [4–7]. Therefore, balanced anesthesia is often used to reduce the requirements of inhalation anesthetics and to thereby minimize their cardiovascular depressant effects in equine practice [8].

Most balanced anesthetic protocols include the use of an α2-adrenoceptor agonist because of their potent sedative and analgesic effects [8]. One such α2-adrenoceptor agonist is medetomidine, whose short half-life, selectivity, and potency make it suitable for use as a constant rate infusion (CRI) for balanced anesthesia in horses [9–12]. In a previous study, we found that medetomidine CRI (3.0 μg/kg/h) reduced the sevoflurane requirement for arthroscopic surgery by approximately 10% in Thoroughbred racehorses, resulting in good maintenance of cardiopulmonary function, and an improvement in the quality of recovery from anesthesia [13]. However, the anesthetic sparing effect of medetomidine CRI on sevoflurane was insufficient to minimize the negative cardiovascular effects of sevoflurane, and cardiovascular depression during the maintenance period still remained a concern.

Alfaxalone is a synthetic neuroactive steroid that acts on the gamma aminobutyric acid $(GABA)_A$ receptors in the central nervous system and produces unconsciousness and muscle relaxation. Several experimental trials of alfaxalone in horses have been reported [14–18]. It is reported that the effects of alfaxalone in relation to induction of anesthesia, recovery quality, and cardiopulmonary response in Thoroughbred horses are similar to the effects of ketamine and thiopental [18], and that alfaxalone has a number of pharmacological properties which are desirable for CRI in horses [14, 19]. It is also reported that the co-administration of alfaxalone and medetomidine as CRI after induction of anesthesia with alfaxalone is suitable for short-term anesthesia in horses undergoing field castration [20]. Therefore, a further reduction in sevoflurane requirement would be expected if alfaxalone–medetomidine CRI was combined with sevoflurane anesthesia.

The purpose of this study was to assess the clinical efficacy of alfaxalone–medetomidine CRI in sevoflurane-anesthetized Thoroughbred racehorses undergoing arthroscopic surgery. In this study, sevoflurane requirement, cardiopulmonary function, and induction/recovery quality were compared between horses maintained with sevoflurane in combination with medetomidine CRI (Group M) and those maintained with sevoflurane in combination with alfaxalone–medetomidine CRI (Group AM).

Methods

Animals

Our study included 50 Thoroughbred racehorses with chip fractures of the carpal bones undergoing arthroscopic surgery. The surgery was performed on a single leg or both legs by randomly assigned experienced surgeons. The horses were assigned randomly to Group M or Group AM (25 horses in each group). In Group M, anesthesia was maintained with sevoflurane in combination with medetomidine CRI; in Group AM, anesthesia was maintained with sevoflurane in combination with alfaxalone plus medetomidine CRI. The mean ± standard deviation (SD) age and body weight were, respectively, 3.3 ± 0.5 years old and 470 ± 21 kg in Group M and 3.1 ± 0.7 years old and 465 ± 28 kg in Group AM. All horses were subjected to preanesthetic blood testing and electrocardiography. Food, but not water, was withheld for 12 h prior to anesthesia.

Experimental protocol

All horses were premedicated with medetomidine (Dorbene; Vetcare Oy, Salo, Finland) (5.0 μg/kg, IV) and midazolam (Dormicum; Astellas Pharma Inc., Tokyo, Japan) (20 μg/kg, IV) together. Anesthesia was induced in the horses in Group M by a rapid injection of 5% guaifenesin (5% Guaifenesin; Shinyo Pure Chemicals Co., Ltd., Osaka, Japan) (100 mg/kg, IV) with thiopental sodium (Ravonal; Mitsubishi Tanabe Pharma Co., Osaka, Japan) (4.0 mg/kg, IV); anesthesia in Group AM was induced by guaifenesin (the same volume as in Group M) with alfaxalone (Alfaxan; Jurox Pty Ltd., Rutherford, Australia) (1.0 mg/kg, IV). A scoring scale of 1–5 (G1: poor, G2: marginal, G3: fair, G4: good, G5: excellent) was used for the subjective assessment of induction of anesthesia [21]. After induction of anesthesia, horses were intubated endotracheally and positioned in dorsal recumbency. Anesthesia was maintained with sevoflurane (Sevofrane; Maruishi Pharmaceutical Co., Ltd., Osaka, Japan) and oxygen (approximately 5 L/min) using an intermittent positive pressure ventilator (MOK 94; Silver Medical Co., Tokyo, Japan) with a peak airway pressure of 25 cmH_2O to maintain the arterial carbon dioxide tension $(PaCO_2)$ between 45 and 55 mmHg.

A base-apex lead electrocardiogram was used to monitor heart rate (HR) and rhythm. A 20-G catheter was placed in the facial artery for arterial blood pressure measurements and arterial blood sample collections. Arterial blood pressures were measured directly through the catheter by a transducer system. Respiratory gas was collected continuously, and the end-tidal sevoflurane concentrations (ET_{SEVO}) was determined by infrared absorption. The ET_{SEVO} was recorded throughout anesthesia, and HR, systolic arterial blood pressure (SAP), diastolic arterial blood pressure (DAP) and mean arterial blood pressure (MAP) were recorded every 5 min by an anesthesia monitoring system (BP608; Omron Colin Co., Ltd., Tokyo, Japan). Arterial blood samples were collected every 15 min and $PaCO_2$, arterial oxygen partial pressure (PaO_2) and pH were immediately analyzed by a blood-gas analyzer (ABL800 FLEX; Radiometer Co., Ltd., Tokyo, Japan).

Throughout the maintenance period, horses in Group M received medetomidine CRI at a constant rate of 3.0 μg/kg/h and horses in Group AM received medetomidine CRI at a constant rate of 3.0 μg/kg/h and alfaxalone CRI at a constant rate of 0.5 mg/kg/h. The vaporizer setting of sevoflurane was based on observation of standard clinical signs to achieve a surgical plane of anesthesia. Anesthetic depth was judged to be light if movement, brisk palpebral response, spontaneous nystagmus, or sudden changes in arterial blood pressure and HR were observed. Lactated Ringer's solution was administered intravenously at a rate of approximately 10 mL/kg/h throughout anesthesia. Dobutamine (Dobutrex; Shionogi & Co., Ltd., Osaka, Japan) was infused to maintain MAP between 60 and 80 mmHg.

Horses in the two groups were allowed to recover without assistance and were given no additional sedatives. Oxygen was supplied until adequate spontaneous respiration appeared, and then the endotracheal tube was removed. The behavior and clinical response course of recovery were scored according to Mama's report [21] as follows: G5 (excellent, single coordinated effort to stand with minimal to no ataxia), G4 (fair, single attempt to stand with some ataxia), G3 (good, quiet recovery with more than one attempt to stand), G2 (marginal, uncoordinated attempts to stand with or without minor injury) and G1 (poor, multiple, uncoordinated attempts resulting in major or life-threatening injury). The number of attempts to stand and the times from the end of anesthesia to the appearance of spontaneous respiration, extubation, first movement, sternal recumbency, first attempt to stand, and standing were recorded.

Plasma alfaxalone analysis

Blood samples were collected from 10 out of 25 horses in Group AM after induction of anesthesia; at 15, 30, and 45 min after connection to the breathing circuit; and immediately after standing. All blood samples were immediately placed on ice, and then the plasma was separated from the blood and frozen at −20 °C. Alfaxalone in plasma was extracted by liquid–liquid extraction using methyl tert-butyl ether. The extracted substance was analyzed using liquid chromatography–tandem mass spectrometry consisted of Shimadzu prominence HPLC system (Shimadzu Co., Tokyo, Japan) and AB Sciex QTRAP 4000 mass spectrometer (AB Sciex, Framingham, MA, USA).

Statistical analysis

Age, body weight, mean ET_{SEVO}, mean dobutamine infusion rate, blood gas data, duration of anesthesia, recovery time, induction score, and recovery score were compared between the two groups by using the Mann–Whitney's U-test. Two-way repeated-measures ANOVA tests were applied to compare cardiovascular data between the two groups. One-way repeated-measures ANOVA tests were applied to compare plasma alfaxalone concentrations in Group AM. The Tukey's Kramer-test for multiple comparisons was applied when significant differences were identified. Values are given as mean ± SD, and statistical significance was set at $P < 0.05$.

Results

No abnormality was found in any of the horses based on the results of the preanesthetic blood examination and electrocardiography. There was no significant difference in age or in body weight between the two groups. Duration of the anesthesia was 55 ± 12 min in Group M and 60 ± 11 min in Group AM, and these were not significantly different. The mean ET_{SEVO} values during the maintenance period (Fig. 1) were significantly lower ($P < 0.001$) in Group AM (1.8 ± 0.2%) than in Group M (2.4 ± 0.1%). The cardiovascular parameters HR, SAP, DAP, and MAP did not change significantly throughout the maintenance, and there were no significant differences between the two groups (Table 1). The mean dobutamine infusion rate required to maintain mean arterial blood pressure within the target values (60–80 mmHg) was significantly lower ($P < 0.001$) in Group AM (0.53 ± 0.20 μg/kg/min) than in Group M (0.85 ± 0.32 μg/kg/min). The mean values of $PaCO_2$ and PaO_2 in Group AM (48 ± 3 mmHg and 461 ± 49 mmHg, respectively) were not significantly different from those in Group M (51 ± 3 mmHg and 474 ± 46 mmHg, respectively).

Induction and recovery scores were not significantly different between the two groups (Fig. 2). The scores for recovery in Group AM were G5 for 6 horses, G4 for 10 horses, G3 for 4 horses and G2 for 5 horses. Remarkable excitatory response at attempts to stand were observed in 5 horses classified as G2. The mean times from the end of anesthesia until the appearance of spontaneous respiration, extubation, first movement, sternal recumbency, first attempt to stand, and standing in Group AM (9 ± 5 min, 17 ± 6 min, 44 ± 12 min, 62 ± 14 min,

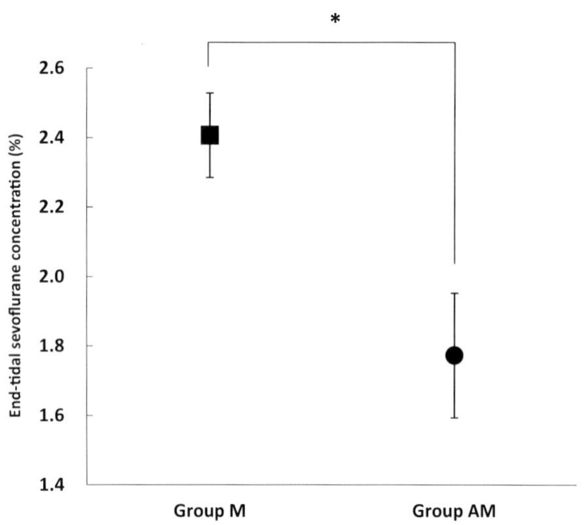

Fig. 1 Mean end-tidal sevoflurane concentration during the maintenance of anesthesia. Horses in Group M (n = 25) (black square) were maintained with sevoflurane in combination with medetomidine CRI; horses in Group AM (n = 25) (black circle) were maintained with sevoflurane in combination with alfaxalone–medetomidine CRI. *Significant difference between the two groups ($P < 0.001$), *P*: probability

68 ± 13 min, and 72 ± 14 min, respectively) were not significantly different from those in Group M (10 ± 8 min, 18 ± 8 min, 46 ± 12 min, 61 ± 10 min, 64 ± 10 min and 65 ± 9 min, respectively).

The plasma alfaxalone concentrations immediately after induction of anesthesia, during the maintenance of anesthesia, and after standing in Group AM are shown in Fig. 3. The mean plasma alfaxalone concentration immediately after induction (1.12 ± 0.20 μg/mL) was significantly higher than the concentrations during the maintenance and after standing ($P < 0.01$, $P < 0.01$, respectively). The mean plasma alfaxalone concentrations during the maintenance (0.77 ± 0.12 to 0.85 ± 0.13 μg/mL) were stable and did not change significantly throughout the maintenance. The mean plasma alfaxalone concentration significantly decreased immediately after standing (0.32 ± 0.07 μg/mL) ($P < 0.01$).

Discussion

The ET_{SEVO} providing a surgical plane of anesthesia for horses anesthetized with sevoflurane is reported to be 2.5–2.8% for orthopedic surgery [22]. We have reported that medetomidine CRI reduced the mean ET_{SEVO} concentrations during surgery for arthroscopic surgery by approximately 10% [13]. In the present study, the mean ET_{SEVO} in Group AM necessary to maintain the surgical plane of anesthesia during arthroscopic surgery was 1.8%, which was equivalent to approximately 80% of the minimum alveolar concentration (MAC) of sevoflurane in horses (2.31 ± 0.11%) [23]. The balanced anesthesia used in Group AM resulted in an approximately 26% reduction in ET_{SEVO} compared to that in Group M. All horses used in this study had the same fracture characteristics, and so the surgical stimuli were considered to be of a similar extent in both groups. Therefore, the potent anesthetic effect of alfaxalone is suggested to have compensated for the reduction in sevoflurane concentration.

There is currently limited information regarding the effects that alfaxalone CRI has on the doses of inhalation anesthetics required. In sheep, infusion of alfaxalone at 0.42 mg/kg/h resulted in a 22% reduction in the desflurane expiratory fraction required for maintenance of anesthesia [24]. In the current study, CRI of alfaxalone (0.5 mg/kg/h) resulted in mean ET_{SEVO} values of 1.8% over the duration of the surgical procedure. However,

Table 1 Cardiovascular parameters during the maintenance of anesthesia in the horses of Group M and Group AM

Variable	Group	Time after connection to breathing circuit (min)				
		0	15	30	45	60
HR (beats/min)	M	30 ± 3	27 ± 3	26 ± 3	27 ± 3	27 ± 3
	AM	31 ± 4	28 ± 4	27 ± 3	27 ± 3	28 ± 3
SAP (mmHg)	M	n/a	93 ± 8	97 ± 8	101 ± 9	104 ± 9
	AM	n/a	94 ± 6	102 ± 10	104 ± 9	101 ± 4
DAP (mmHg)	M	n/a	51 ± 8	54 ± 7	55 ± 7	56 ± 7
	AM	n/a	51 ± 7	59 ± 6	60 ± 7	57 ± 6
MAP (mmHg)	M	n/a	63 ± 8	68 ± 7	70 ± 7	71 ± 7
	AM	n/a	64 ± 7	73 ± 5	74 ± 4	72 ± 5

Data are presented as mean ± standard deviation (SD)

Horses in Group M (n = 25) were maintained with sevoflurane in combination with medetomidine CRI; horses in Group AM (n = 25) were maintained with sevoflurane in combination with alfaxalone–medetomidine CRI

HR heart rate, *SAP* systolic arterial blood pressure, *DAP* diastolic arterial blood pressure, *MAP* mean arterial blood pressure, *n/a* not applicable

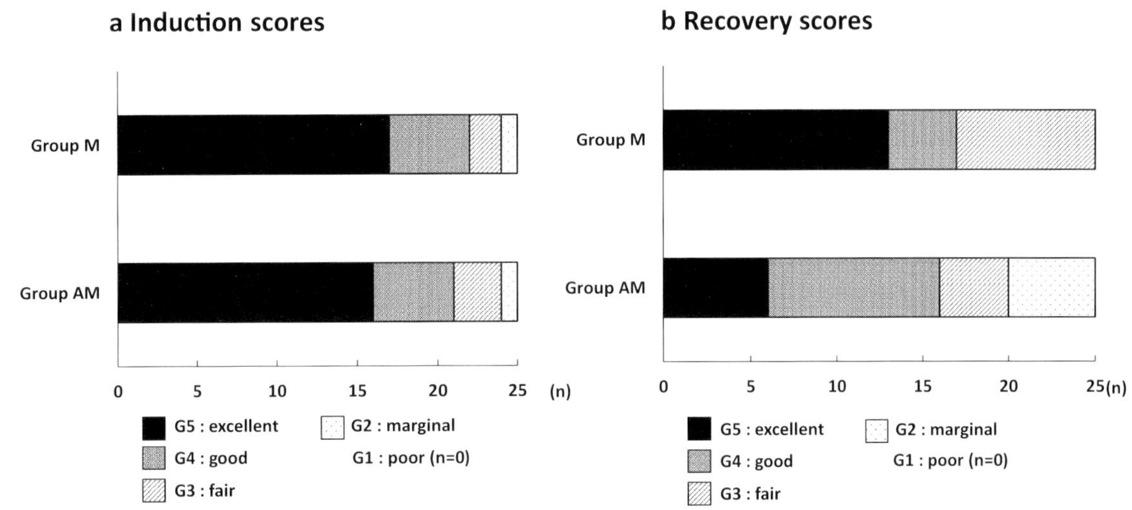

Fig. 2 Induction scores (**a**) and recovery scores (**b**). Horses in Group M (n = 25) were maintained with sevoflurane in combination with medetomidine CRI; horses in Group AM (n = 25) were maintained with sevoflurane in combination with alfaxalone–medetomidine CRI

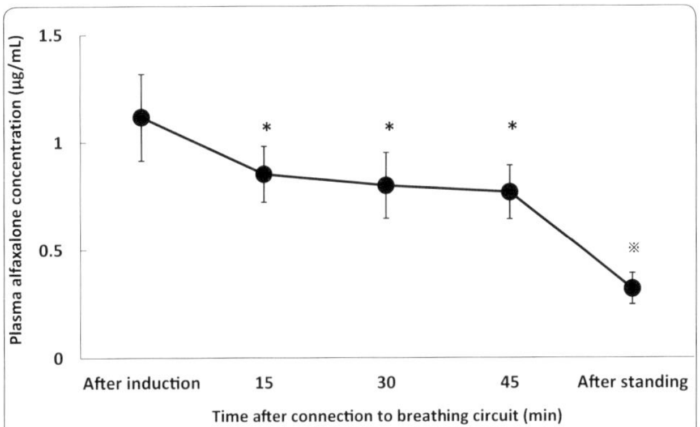

Fig. 3 Plasma alfaxalone concentration immediately after induction, during maintenance, and after standing in Group AM. Horses in Group AM (n = 25) were maintained with sevoflurane in combination with alfaxalone–medetomidine CRI. *Significantly different from the values immediately after induction of anesthesia ($P < 0.01$), ※significantly different from the values immediately after induction of anesthesia and during sevoflurane maintenance ($P < 0.01$), *P*: probability

crucially, the design of the present study had limitations with respect to detecting the sevoflurane-sparing effects of alfaxalone CRI because the induction agent used in each group was different (thiopental versus alfaxalone). Nevertheless, Wakuno et al. [18] reported that thiopental and alfaxalone showed similar effects in relation to induction of anesthesia and cardiopulmonary responses. In this study, in anticipation of the clinical applicability of alfaxalone, anesthesia in Group AM was induced by a loading dose of alfaxalone followed by CRI at a dose sufficient to maintain a stable plasma concentration of alfaxalone during the surgical procedure. Although it was difficult to make accurate comparisons owing to the different induction agents and the absence of an experimental MAC reduction study, we considered that alfaxalone CRI had a moderate degree of sevoflurane-sparing effect in horses.

In the present study, the mean ET_{SEVO} values in Group AM were 1.8%; the infusion rates of alfaxalone and medetomidine used were selected on the basis of preliminary studies and experimental work involving these drugs determined in the references of previous reports [13, 24, 25]. Granados et al. [24] reported that a loading dose of alfaxalone of 1.0 mg/kg followed by a maintenance dose of 0.42 mg/kg/h reduced the desflurane requirement in sheep by 22%. Ambros et al. [25] reported that a maintenance dose of 0.42 mg/kg/h produced clinically acceptable anesthetic quality and hemodynamic values ideal for use as a CRI in dogs. When medetomidine CRI (3.0 µg/kg/h) was applied during sevoflurane anesthesia, the sevoflurane dose required for maintenance of anesthesia was significantly lower than when sevoflurane was used alone [13]. In this study, a loading alfaxalone dose of 1.0 mg/kg followed by a maintenance dose of 0.5 mg/kg/h was considered to contribute to the ET_{SEVO} value of 1.8% of in Group AM. In addition, the infusion rate of alfaxalone effectively maintained stable plasma alfaxalone concentrations and there were no observations of light anesthesia with surgical stimulation. Although meaningful comparisons between previous studies and the present study are difficult, the infusion of alfaxalone and medetomidine would be expected to provide an effective balanced anesthesia in horses similar to that in other species because of the adequate anesthetic depth throughout the maintenance period.

It is essential that any anesthetic technique used in horses maintains adequate cardiopulmonary function. In our study, there was no significant difference between Group M and Group AM in terms of heart rate and arterial blood pressure. HR was stable and was maintained at an adequate value during anesthesia. MAP in Group AM was maintained within the target values (60–80 mmHg) throughout the operation. Sevoflurane induces a dose-dependent decrease in hemodynamic variables in horses, so reducing the dose of sevoflurane may promote cardiovascular stability and improve perianesthetic care [1, 6, 26]. Hence, the reduction in dobutamine requirement is suggested to be a result of the better cardiovascular function. On the other hand, the difference in the induction agents used might also have influenced the dobutamine infusion rates in the present study. There is limited information regarding the cardiopulmonary effects of alfaxalone in horses, but in dogs, a 2-h infusion of alfaxalone resulted in only mild hemodynamic changes, with cardiac variables (cardiac index, heart rate, systemic vascular resistance, arterial blood pressure) remaining stable and not differing significantly from baseline values [25].A previous study in horses showed no significant difference between thiopental and alfaxalone in terms of their effects on arterial blood pressure [18]. From those results it is suggested that the combination alfaxalone–medetomidine CRI minimized cardiovascular depression as a result of reducing the sevoflurane requirement, and that alfaxalone–medetomidine CRI contributed to the significant decrease in the requirement of dobutamine for maintenance of MAP within the target values. However, the level of improvement of cardiovascular depression was moderate. Therefore, we consider that small to moderate amounts of inotropic agents will still be necessary.

With respect to effects in the induction phase, there was no significant difference in induction score between the two groups. The induction dose of alfaxalone used in the current study was chosen based on the results of a previous study that reported there was no statistically significant difference in the quality of anesthetic induction between alfaxalone (1.0 mg/kg, IV) and thiopental (4.0 mg/kg, IV), and that all inductions were of an acceptable quality [18]. Therefore, no difference in induction grade between alfaxalone and thiopental was recognized in the present study.

In the recovery phase, the qualities were clinically acceptable in Group AM; however, remarkable excitatory response at attempts to stand were observed in 5 out of 25 horses. Recovery quality depends on many factors including the horse's physical status, duration of anesthesia, and the anesthetic drugs used [27, 28]. It was considered that sevoflurane would have been washed out from the body more quickly in Group AM than in Group M because the mean ET_{SEVO} values in Group AM were significantly lower than those in Group M. However, there was no significant difference in recovery quality between the two groups. A major concern when using alfaxalone infusion to maintain anesthesia is that accumulation of the drug or its active metabolites may occur, resulting in prolonged and potentially ataxic and uncontrolled recoveries [20]. Goodwin et al. [29] reported unacceptable recoveries in horses recovering from 3-h general anesthesia with an infusion of alfaxalone of 3 mg/kg/h. Others reported that alfaxalone induced central nervous system excitation and that induction of anesthesia with alfaxalone was associated with poor recovery [30, 31]. In the current study, the adverse effects of alfaxalone might remain in the attempt to stand because the plasma alfaxalone concentration after standing in Group AM was 0.32 ± 0.07 µg/mL. The excitation of 20% of horses during recovery has potential for an increased risk of major or life-threatening injury when using alfaxalone. We consider that horses administered alfaxalone should be given additional sedatives and be assisted, and so recovery quality might be improved. Anyway, the present results indicate that further investigation is required to explore the clinical relevance of excitatory response induced by alfaxalone because 25 horses are not many with regards to more severe consequences.

Conclusions

Alfaxalone–medetomidine CRI reduced sevoflurane requirement by approximately 26% with good maintenance of cardiopulmonary function in Thoroughbred racehorses undergoing arthroscopic surgery. Sevoflurane in combination with alfaxalone–medetomidine CRI may be a clinically effective anesthetic technique for Thoroughbred racehorses. However, 20% of horses administered alfaxalone showed remarkable excitatory response during recovery. Greater attention to excitatory response may be advisable if alfaxalone is used for induction or maintenance of anesthesia. A larger study is needed to explore the clinical relevance of these findings.

Abbreviations

ANOVA: analysis of variance; CRI: constant rate infusion; DAP: diastolic arterial blood pressure; ET_{SEVO}: end-tidal sevoflurane concentrations; HR: heart rate; IV: intravenous; MAP: mean arterial blood pressure; *p*: probability; $PaCO_2$: arterial carbon dioxide tension; PaO_2: arterial oxygen partial tension; SAP: systolic arterial blood pressure; SD: standard deviation.

Authors' contributions

HT, AW, and MO designed the study. HT, AK, AO, TM, and HI performed the anesthesia. HT and SN participated in the acquisition of data, interpreting and analyzing the results. All authors participated in writing and editing of the manuscript. All authors read and approved the final manuscript.

Author details
[1] Racehorse Clinic, Miho Training Center, Japan Racing Association (JRA), 2500-2 Mikoma, Miho-mura, Inashiki-gun, Ibaraki 300-0493, Japan. [2] Racehorse Clinic, Ritto Training Center, JRA, 1028 Misono, Ritto-shi, Shiga 520-3085, Japan. [3] Analytical Chemistry Section, Laboratory of Racing Chemistry, 1731-2 Tokami-cyo, Utsunomiya-shi, Tochigi 320-0851, Japan. [4] Equine Research Institute, JRA, 1400-4 Shiba, Shimotsuke-shi, Tochigi 329-0412, Japan.

Competing interests
The authors declare that they have no competing interests.

Acknowledgements
Not applicable.

References

1. Aida H, Steffey EP, Pascoe JR, Yarbrough TB, Takahashi T, Hiraga A, Hobo S, Smith BL, Steffey MA, Jones JH. Use of sevoflurane for anesthetic management of horses during thoracotomy. Am J Vet Res. 2000;61:1430–7.
2. Carroll GL, Hooper RN, Rains CB, Martinez EA, Matthews NS, Hartsfield SM, Beleau MH. Maintenance of anaesthesia with sevoflurane and oxygen in mechanically-ventilated horses subjected to exploratory laparotomy treated with intra- and post operative anaesthetic adjuncts. Eq Vet J. 1998;30:402–7.
3. Wallin RF, Regan BM, Napoli MD, Stern IJ. Sevoflurane: a new inhalational anesthetic agent. Anesth Analg. 1975;54:758–66.
4. Aida H, Mizuno Y, Hobo S, Yoshida K, Fujinaga T. Cardiovascular and pulmonary effects of sevoflurane anesthesia in horses. Vet Surg. 1996;25:164–70.
5. Driessen B, Nann L, Benton R, Boston R. Differences in need for hemodynamic support in horses anesthetized with sevoflurane as compared to isoflurane. Vet Anaesth Analg. 2006;33:356–67.
6. Grosenbaugh DA, Muir WW. Cardiorespiratory effects of sevoflurane, isoflurane, and halothane anesthesia in horses. Am J Vet Res. 1998;59:101–6.
7. Steffey EP. Pharmacology. Inhalation anesthetics. In: Thurmon JC, Tranquilli WJ, Benson GJ, editors. Lumb and jones' veterinary anesthesia. 3rd ed. Baltimore: The Williams and Wilkins; 1996. p. 297–329.
8. Valverde A. Balanced anesthesia and constant-rate infusions in horses. Vet Clin Eq. 2013;29:89–122.
9. Bettschart-Wolfensberger R, Clarke KW, Vainio O, Aliabadi F, Demuth D. Pharmacokinetics of medetomidine in ponies and elaboration of a medetomidine infusion regime which provides a constant level of sedation. Res Vet Sci. 1999;67:41–6.
10. Creighton CM, Lemke KA, Lamont LA, Horney BS, Riley CB. Comparison of the effects of xylazine bolus versus medetomidine constant rate infusion on cardiopulmonary function and depth of anesthesia in horses anesthetized with isoflurane. J Am Vet Med Assoc. 2012;240:991–7.
11. Grimsrud KN, Mama KR, Steffey EP, Stanley SD. Pharmacokinetics and pharmacodynamics of intravenous medetomidine in the horse. Vet Anaesth Analg. 2012;39:38–48.
12. Ringer SK, Kalchofner K, Boller J, Fürst A, Bettschart-Wolfensberger R. A clinical comparison of two anesthetic protocols using lidocaine or medetomidine in horses. Vet Anaesth Analg. 2007;34:257–68.
13. Tokushige H, Ohta M, Okano A, Kuroda T, Kakizaki M, Ode H, Aoki M, Wakuno A, Kawasaki K. Effects of medetomidine constant rate infusion on sevoflurane requirement, cardiopulmonary function, and recovery quality in Thoroughbred racehorses undergoing arthroscopic surgery. J Eq Vet Sci. 2015;35:83–7.
14. Goodwin WA, Keates HL, Pasloske K, Pearson M, Sauer B, Ranasinghe MG. The pharmacokinetics and pharmacodynamics of the injectable anaesthetic alfaxalone in the horse. Vet Anaesth Analg. 2011;38:431–8.
15. Keates HL, van Eps AW, Pearson MR. Alfaxalone compared with ketamine for induction of anaesthesia in horses following xylazine and guaifenesin. Vet Anaesth Analg. 2012;39:591–8.
16. Klöppel H, Leece EA. Comparison of ketamine and alfaxalone for induction and maintenance of anaesthesia in ponies undergoing castration. Vet Anaesth Analg. 2011;38:37–43.
17. Leece EA, Girard NM, Maddern K. Alfaxalone in cyclodextrin for induction and maintenance of anaesthesia in ponies undergoing field castration. Vet Anaesth Analg. 2009;36:480–4.
18. Wakuno A, Aoki M, Kushiro A, Mae N, Kodaira K, Maeda T, Yamazaki Y, Ohta M. Comparison of alfaxalone, ketamine and thiopental for anaesthetic induction and recovery in Thoroughbred horses premedicated with medetomidine and midazolam. Eq Vet J. 2017;49:94–8.
19. Goodwin WA, Keates HL, Pasloske K, Pearson M, Sauer B, Ranasinghe MG. Plasma pharmacokinetics and pharmacodynamics of alfaxalone in neonatal foals after an intravenous bolus of alfaxalone following premedication with butorphanol tartrate. Vet Anaesth Analg. 2012;39:503–10.
20. Goodwin WA, Keates HL, Pearson M, Pasloske K. Alfaxalone and medetomidine intravenous infusion to maintain anaesthesia in colts undergoing field castration. Eq Vet J. 2013;45:315–9.
21. Mama KR, Steffey EP, Pascoe PJ. Evaluation of propofol for general anesthesia in premedicated horses. Am J Vet Res. 1996;57:512–6.
22. Ohta M, Oku K, Yamanaka T, Mizuno Y. Anesthetic management with sevoflurane and oxygen for orthopedic surgeries in racehorses. J Vet Med Sci. 2000;62:1017–20.
23. Aida H, Mizuno Y, Hobo S, Yoshida K, Fujinaga T. Determination of the minimum alveolar concentration (MAC) and physical response to sevoflurane inhalation in horses. J Vet Med Sci. 1994;56:1161–5.
24. Granados MM, Domínguez JM, Fernández-Sarmiento A, Funes FJ, Morgaz J, Navarrete R, Carrillo JM, Rubio M, Muñoz-Rascón P, Gómez IA, Gómez-Villamandos R. Anaesthetic and cardiorespiratory effects of a constant-rate infusion of alfaxalone in desflurane-anaesthetised sheep. Vet Rec. 2012;171:125.
25. Ambros B, Duke-Novakovski T, Pasloske KS. Comparison of the anesthetic efficacy and cardiopulmonary effects of continuous rate infusions of alfaxalone-2-hydroxypropyl-beta-cyclodextrin and propofol in dogs. Am J Vet Res. 2008;69:1391–8.
26. Steffey EP, Mama KR, Galey FD, Puschner B, Woliner MJ. Effects of sevoflurane dose and mode of ventilation on cardiopulmonary function and blood biochemical variables in horses. Am J Vet Res. 2005;66:606–14.
27. Hubbell JA. Recovery from anaesthesia in horses. Eq Vet Educ. 1999;11:160–7.
28. Young SS, Taylor PM. Factors influencing the outcome of equine anaesthesia: a review of 1314 cases. Eq Vet J. 1993;25:147–51.
29. Goodwin WA, Keates HL, Pasloske K, Pearson M, Shiels I, Sauer B. Total intravenous anesthesia (TIVA) in the horse with alfaxalone. In: Clutton ER and W Communications, editors. Proceedings of 10th world congress of veterinary anesthesia. Glasgow; 2009. p. 87.
30. Jiménez CP, Mathis A, Mora SS, Brodbelt D, Alibhai H. Evaluation of the quality of the recovery after administration of propofol or alfaxalone for induction of anaesthesia in dogs anaesthetized for magnetic resonance imaging. Vet Anaesth Analg. 2012;39:151–9.
31. Mathis A, Pinelas R, Brodbelt DC, Alibhai HI. Comparison of quality of recovery from anaesthesia in cats induced with propofol or alfaxalone. Vet Anaesth Analg. 2012;39:282–90.

Development of the Finnish neurological function testing battery for dogs and its intra- and inter-rater reliability

Anna Fredrika Boström[1*], Heli Katariina Hyytiäinen[1], Petteri Koho[2], Sigitas Cizinauskas[3] and Anna Katrina Hielm-Björkman[1]

Abstract

Background: The Finnish neurological function testing battery for dogs (FINFUN) was developed to meet the increasing demand for objective outcome measures in veterinary physiotherapy. The testing battery should provide consistent, reproducible results and have established face and content validity. Internal consistency and intra- and inter-rater reliability of the FINFUN were also investigated.

Results: The FINFUN comprised 11 tasks: lying, standing up from lying, sitting, standing up from sitting, standing, proprioceptive positioning, starting to walk, walking, trotting, walking turns and walking stairs. A score from 0 to 4, (0: unable to perform task, 4: performing task with normal motor function) was given for each task, the maximum score being 44. Twenty-six dogs were filmed when performing the FINFUN. Seven observers scored the performances from the video recordings. The FINFUN was considered to have appropriate face and content validity based on a pilot study, clinical experience and critical reflection of the development process. Its internal consistency was excellent, with no Cronbach's alpha values below 0.922. The intra-rater reliability for total score of experienced observers was almost perfect: 0.999 (observer 1) and 0.994 (observer 2). The inter-rater reliability for both experienced and novice observers' total scores was also almost perfect (0.919–0.993). Analysis of each individual task showed substantial intra-rater and inter-rater agreement for the tasks "lying" and "sitting".

Conclusions: The FINFUN is an objective, valid and reliable tool with standardized scoring criteria for evaluation of motor function in dogs recovering from spinal cord injury.

Keywords: Inter-rater reliability, Intra-rater reliability, Motor function, Neurology, Outcome measure, Physiotherapy, Testing battery, Validity

Background

Dogs recovering from different grades of paralysis caused by disease or trauma to the nervous system are seen daily in veterinary hospitals and rehabilitation practices [1, 2]. Veterinary physiotherapy is an important part of the modern treatment regime for these neurological patients [3]. Maintenance and enhancement of functional ability in affected dogs is important to ensure rapid recovery and a good quality of life, and physiotherapy has been shown to be beneficial for dogs recovering from intervertebral disc disease [3–5], fibrocartilaginous embolism [6] and degenerative myelopathy [7].

In human neurology, the physiotherapist evaluates and trains everyday motor function with the aim of the individual being able to continue with work and activities of daily living [8]. Objective evaluation of motor function and change over time is important and requires accurate and repeatable measurements and reliable instruments [8]. Human neurological physiotherapy has several established, validated and reliable functional outcome measures for patients with spinal cord injury and stroke that are used in both clinical practice and research [8–12].

*Correspondence: anna.bostrom@helsinki.fi
[1] Department of Equine and Small Animal Medicine, Faculty of Veterinary Medicine, University of Helsinki, P.O. Box 57, 00014 Helsinki, Finland
Full list of author information is available at the end of the article

The demand for efficient, safe and evidence-based physiotherapy strategies is increasing also in veterinary medicine, creating a need for sensitive validity and reliability testing instruments to assess the recovery from and effects of different interventions [13]. To the authors' knowledge, there are no functional testing batteries that evaluate overall motor function of dogs with neurological disease. Overall motor function comprises functional everyday tasks like sitting and standing, transitions from lying or sitting to standing, from standing to walking and ambulation at different speeds. No testing battery so far include voluntary motor functions progressing towards more advanced locomotion and activities of daily living, and is as well convenient to use in both clinical practice and research. Objective outcome measures should be validated and evaluated for internal consistency and intra-and inter-rater reliability [12, 14]. Face validity considers whether users or experts agree that the instrument is measuring what it is intended to measure, and content validity is the degree to which all tasks in the measure assess the same domain of interest [12]. Internal consistency means that all tasks in the instrument measure the same attribute [12, 14]. Intra-rater reliability is the degree to which scores on the instrument obtained by one trained observer agree with the scores obtained when the same observer administers the measure on another occasion [12]. Inter-rater reliability is the degree to which scores on the instrument obtained by one trained observer agree with the scores obtained by another trained observer [12, 14].

Validated outcome measures are consistently used in the experimental setting to quantify the progress in the animal's locomotor function [15, 16], but implementing them in clinical practice is not straightforward [17]. In small animal clinical practice, the veterinary modifications of the human Frankel score for spinal cord injury are frequently used for injury classification and outcome determination, but it does not quantify walking [18–21]. The Texas Spinal Cord Injury Score (TSCIS) was created to provide reliable measurements for location and degree of injury as well as to determine outcome in dogs with spinal cord injury [21], but it is limited by the functional evaluation of the ability to walk [21]. Previous studies present useful validated methods to quantify both the ability to walk and the quality of walking [17, 22–24], but these scales do not include any other components of the dog's functional ability.

The aim of this study was to develop a neurological function testing battery that would measure overall motor function in canine patients. The testing battery would provide consistent, reproducible results independent of neurological disease (i.e. intervertebral disc disease or fibrocartilaginous embolism). The testing battery would need to be cost-effective and convenient to use by veterinary physiotherapists in both clinical and research settings. Further aims were to establish the face and content validity of the testing battery and to investigate its internal consistency and intra- and inter-rater reliability.

We hypothesized that the Finnish neurological function testing battery for dogs (FINFUN) would be valid for assessment of motor function in dogs with neurological disease and that it would display high internal consistency and intra- and inter-rater reliability.

Methods

Development of the test

The FINFUN was designed based on a human functional outcome measure, the Motor Assessment Scale [11], the Basso, Beattie, Bresnahan (BBB) Scale for spinal cord injured rats [15], the five recovery stages in dogs with acute spinal cord injuries [22] and the clinical experience of the research team. The general instructions and scoring criteria of the FINFUN can be found in Additional file 1. The FINFUN consists of 11 tasks of progressive difficulty; 'lying', 'standing up from lying', 'sitting', 'standing up from sitting', 'standing', 'proprioceptive positioning in affected limbs', 'start to walk from standing', 'walking', 'running', 'walking turns' and 'walking stairs'.

In each task, the dog´s performance is given a numeric score from 0 to 4, where 0 indicates that the dog is unable to perform the task at all and 4 indicates that the dog is able to perform the complete task with normal motor function or with motor function at the level prior to disease/injury. Two animal physiotherapists (AB and HH) and an ECVN Diplomate (SC) developed the scoring criteria. To ensure consistency in the scoring process, each task is described thoroughly and the criteria for each score in the tasks are specified (Additional file 1).

The testing battery includes a section for comments, where information relevant to the assessment (method of support, method of motivation, medication) can be recorded. This section makes it possible to distinguish between the dog not being able to perform a task physically or just being restricted by support, motivation or the surgeon's restrictions. To ensure standardized scoring, the FINFUN criteria are additionally accompanied by general instructions for use, specifying equipment and environment requirements as well as providing instructions regarding assistance and motivation of the tested dogs. The scoring time is approximately 15 min.

The FINFUN was validated in both the English and Finnish languages. The general instructions and scoring criteria were created in English and translated to Finnish by a native speaker for the Finnish-speaking observers. The text was then translated back to English and checked by a native speaker from the English language editing services.

A pilot study on intra- and inter-rater reliability was undertaken on 10 dogs with different grades of paralysis. The results showed the FINFUN to have excellent intra- and inter-rater reliability [25]. After the pilot study, one author (AB) used the FINFUN in clinical practice and the scoring criteria were further adjusted according to clinical experience and critical reflections with the observers in the pilot study.

Observer training

Seven observers volunteered for this study. They were all trained human physiotherapists, specialized in animal physiotherapy. They had all been involved in the pilot study and were thus familiar with the testing battery. Two of the observers were considered experienced, i.e. had worked with neurological patients daily during the last 2 years, and the remaining five were considered novices, i.e. had worked with neurological cases only occasionally. The observers received training in the use of the testing battery, and they practiced the evaluation process both live and from video recordings. The observers were instructed to familiarize themselves with the test criteria thoroughly beforehand. The observers scored the performances from the video recordings of at least eight dogs on their own to establish a routine in the scoring process. The scoring process was revised on the test date, and the observers had the opportunity to ask questions about the testing battery itself or the scoring process before the actual study started. The performances used in the training were not included in the study.

Study protocol

Twenty-six dogs of different breeds recovering from spinal cord injury caused by intervertebral disc disease, fibrocartilaginous embolism, arachnoidal cyst or neoplasia, were referred to physiotherapy (AB) by the treating veterinary surgeon, where they were evaluated using the FINFUN. The evaluation was part of their agreed routine physiotherapy assessment carried out by an animal physiotherapist (AB). Ethical approval was not required as the evaluation was carried out during standard clinical practice. The dogs were filmed (with owner consent) from the front, behind and both sides while performing the different tasks using a digital video camera. The video recordings were stored on a computer. All observers, except AB, were blinded to the diagnosis and background data of the dogs, as the included dogs had been her patients. All observers consented to patient confidentiality by signing the FINFUN scoring sheet once the scoring was completed. The video recordings were shown to the observers twice and the seven observers evaluated the dogs' performances from the video recordings according to the FINFUN scoring criteria.

Inter- and intra-rater reliability

The five novice and two experienced observers scored the dogs from the video recordings according to the test criteria on the same occasion, blinded to each others′ scores. Inter-rater reliability was evaluated for each individual task as well as for the FINFUN sum score for novice and experienced observers separately.

The two experienced observers scored the dogs from the video recordings according to the test criteria on two different occasions with a 3-week interval. The observers were blinded to each others' and the previous scores. Intra-rater reliability was evaluated for each individual task as well as for the FINFUN sum score.

Statistical analysis

Mean and standard deviation were used to summarize the descriptive data of the studied dogs. The internal consistency was tested using Cronbach's alpha. The intra- and inter-rater reliability was analyzed using Intra-class correlation coefficient (ICC), two-way mixed model and absolute agreement, with a confidence interval of 95%. The reliability was reported as follows: slight agreement: 0.01–0.20, fair agreement: 0.21–0.40, moderate agreement: 0.41–0.60, substantial agreement: 0.61–0.80, almost perfect agreement: 0.81–1.00 [26]. SPSS, version 19 (IBM, New York, NY, USA) was used in the analysis.

Results

Animals

Of the 26 evaluated dogs, 10 were female and 16 male. Their mean age was 5.0 ± 2.2 years and their mean weight 13.5 ± 9.9 kg. The breed, sex, age, weight, diagnosis and mean, standard deviation (SD) and range of scores for each dog are displayed in Table 1. Magnetic resonance imaging or myelography confirmed the diagnosis in all dogs, and 22 dogs had surgical hemilaminectomy and 2 dogs dorsal laminectomy prior to the physiotherapy referral.

Face and content validity

The FINFUN was considered to meet the criteria for good face and content validity. The novice observers agreed with the test developers that the testing battery covered the most essential components for evaluation of functional ability in dogs with neurological disease hence the criterion for good face validity was met. The criteria for the content validity was met, as there was consensus amongst all participants in this study, that each item measured motor function relevant for dogs with neurological disease. This was confirmed by clinical

Table 1 Descriptive information on the studied dogs

Dog	Breed	Sex	Age (years)	Weight (kg)	Diagnosis/treatment	Mean score (SD)	Range score
1	Mixed	F	8	25.1	T12-L1 disc extrusion, hemilaminectomy	20.3 (2.0)	18–23
2	Dachshund, short-haired	M	5	12.0	T12-13 disc extrusion, hemilaminectomy	9.7 (1.6)	7–12
3	Mixed	M	1	8.0	L1-2 disc extrusion, hemilaminectomy	8.6 (1.7)	5–10
4	Welsh corgi cardigan	F	6	16.5	T12-13 disc extrusion, hemilaminectomy	24.6 (1.6)	22–26
5	Bernese mountain dog	M	7	49.3	L7-S1 disc protrusion, dorsal laminectomy	36.4 (1.7)	34–38
6	Pinscher	F	4	15.0	T11-13 disc extrusion, hemilaminectomy	34.0 (1.6)	32–36
7	Miniature poodle	M	3	7.5	L4-5 disc extrusion, hemilaminectomy	24.1 (2.0)	21–27*
8	Coton de tulear	F	4	5.0	L1-2 disc extrusion, hemilaminectomy	28.9 (1.2)	27–31
9	Dachshund, short-haired	M	9	11.0	T13-L1 disc extrusion, hemilaminectomy	33.6 (1.5)	32–36
10	Tibetan terrier	M	7	12.6	T12-13 disc extrusion, hemilaminectomy	35.6 (2.4)	33–40*
11	Cocker spaniel	F	6	15.8	T12-13 disc extrusion, hemilaminectomy	15.9 (2.1)	14–19
12	French bulldog	M	4	13.8	L1-2 disc extrusion, hemilaminectomy	23.1 (0.9)	22–24
13	Dachshund, wire-haired	M	3	10	T13-L1 disc extrusion, hemilaminectomy	28.3 (1.7)	27–31
14	Dachshund, wire-haired	F	4	5.6	T12-13 disc extrusion, hemilaminectomy	31.9 (0.9)	31–33
15	Mix	F	9	6.2	T12-13 disc extrusion, hemilaminectomy	27.1 (1.6)	24–29
16	Dachshund long haired	M	8	7.5	T12-13 disc extrusion, hemilaminectomy	13.7 (1.0)	12–15
17	Coton de tulear	M	7	8.0	L1-2 disc extrusion, hemilaminectomy	31.0 (1.6)	29–34
18	Dachshund, wire-haired	M	4	5.9	T12-13 disc extrusion, hemilaminectomy	30.9 (2.5)	27–35*
19	Dachshund, short-haired	F	4	8.0	L4-5 disc extrusion, hemilaminectomy	28.7 (0.8)	28–30
20	French bulldog	M	5	16.5	T5-7 arachnoidal cyst, dorsal hemilaminectomy	31.7 (1.6)	30–34
21	Saluki	M	6	28.0	Fibrocartilaginous embolism, conservative treatment	6.4 (1.4)	4–8
22	Dachshund, wire-haired	M	3	12.0	T12-13 disc extrusion, hemilaminectomy	29.4 (1.0)	28–31
23	Doberman	F	5	29.3	T12-L1 osteochondromatosis, hemilaminectomy	25.3 (1.8)	23–27
24	Mixed	F	2	4.4	L1-2 disc extrusion, hemilaminectomy	10.3 (2.6)	7–14*
25	Dachshund, wire-haired	M	3	9.6	T12-13 disc extrusion, hemilaminectomy	37.0 (2.3)	33–40*
26	Löwchen	M	2	7.5	T12-13 disc extrusion, conservative treatment	15.1 (0.9)	14–16

The breed, age, weight and mean ± standard deviation (SD) and range for the given scores for each dog with all observers' scores considered. Dogs with a wide range in the scores (> 5 points) are indicated with an asterisk (*)

F female, *M* male

observations showing that dogs with higher functional ability (walking or running for longer distances or requiring less support) got higher scores.

Internal consistency

All of the observers showed excellent internal consistency, with none below 0.922. Excluding one task at a time from the analysis showed that exclusion of 'lying' (task 1), 'sitting' (task 3) and 'proprioceptive positioning' (task 6) would increase Cronbach's alpha for all observers, albeit not enough to alter the internal consistency significantly.

Inter-rater reliability

The results for the inter-rater reliability are shown in detail in Table 3. The inter-rater reliability between the experienced observers' total score was almost perfect (ICC 0.993, 95% CI (0.984–0.997)). The agreement ranged from substantial to almost perfect for the separate tasks (0.705–0.993), with 'lying' and 'sitting' being the tasks with low ICC values and large standard error measures (Table 3). Inter-rater reliability between novice observers' total scores was almost perfect (ICC (3.5) 95% CI 0.993 (0.988–0.997)) and substantial for 'sitting' (95% CI 0.697 (0.465–0.848)). Inter-rater reliability for all observers' total scores was almost perfect (ICC (3.7) 95% CI 0.996 (0.993–0.998)) and was almost perfect for all tasks, except '*sitting*', for which it was substantial (0.793).

Intra-rater reliability

Intra-rater reliability for observer 1 total score was almost perfect ICC 0.996, 95% CI (0.991–0.998), ranging from substantial to almost perfect for the separate tasks 0.668–0.957. The observer 2 intra-rater reliability was almost perfect ICC (3.2) 0.994, 95% CI (0.981–0.998) for the total score and for all separate tasks, except 'sitting', for which it was moderate 0.464 (− 089 to 0.748) (Table 2).

Table 2 Intra-rater reliability for individual tasks and sum score of the testing battery

Task	Intra-rater correlation observer 1 (95% CI)	Intra-rater correlation observer 2 (95% CI)
Lying	0.943 (0.873–0.974)	1.000
Standing up from lying	0.957 (0.904–0.981)	0.979 (0.952–0.991)
Sitting	0.668 (0.224–0.855)	0.464 (−089 to 0.748)
Standing up from sitting	0.938 (0.861–0.972)	0.917 (0.770–0.966)
Standing	0.976 (0.946–0.989)	0.933 (0.844–0.971)
Proprioceptive positioning	0.988 (0.974–0.995)	0.961 (0.915–0.983)
Start to walk from standing	0.986 (0.970–0.994	0.986 (0.970–0.994)
Walking	0.989 (0.975–0.995)	0.990 (0.977–0.995)
Running	0.984 (0.966–0.993)	0.994 (0.987–0.997)
Walking turns	0.983 (0.961–0.993)	0.978 (0.952–0.990)
Walking stairs	0.976 (0.948–0.989)	0.984 (0.964–0.993)
Total score	0.996 (0.991–0.998)	0.994 (0.981–0.998)

The intra-class correlation coefficient and confidence intervals for the two experienced observers (observer 1 and observer 2). Data are shown for each individual task and for the FINFUN total score

Discussion

The FINFUN was designed to meet the demand for an objective, validated and reliable functional outcome measure in veterinary physiotherapy. This study shows the FINFUN to be valid and reliable between observers and to provide reproducible results when dogs with different grades of paralysis are assessed from video recordings.

Development of the test

The development of functional testing batteries must be transparent and well described [13]. This report includes detailed information regarding the development of the testing battery and the educational level, experience and training of the observers. Both human and veterinary outcome measures were used in the development process of the FINFUN [11, 15, 22]. The MAS evaluates task-related interventions in human patients with acute stroke using simple scoring criteria and the tasks are separate actions, which enable them to be used as separate entities based on the information required [11]. These features were desirable in the FINFUN. The ordinal scale used in the FINFUN was chosen according to Olby et al. [22], and the test criteria regarding movement quality were determined based on the in the BBB Locomotor Rating Scale [15].

The FINFUN consists of activities of daily living that are applicable to any pet dog and that progress from easier tasks to more challenging ones. 'Start to walk from standing' (task 7) was included as a separate task from walking, as dogs with upper motor neuron lesion may succeed in standing due to normal or increased extensor tone in the hind limbs [27], but they cannot initiate movement or take weight-bearing steps. During activities of daily living the dogs need to move safely and independently through turns, hence walking turns were included. It was challenging to motivate dogs to walk a figure of eight, resulting in a risk for the handler interfering with a dog's performance. This task showed, however, good reliability and was easily assessed by the observers.

'Running' (task 9) and 'walking stairs' (task 11) require strength, causing some physical stress to the patient. Dogs recovering from trauma or spinal surgery may not be permitted to run or walk stairs for several weeks post-operatively. Including such tasks in the FINFUN could therefore be questioned, although many households require running and walking stairs for independent locomotion [28]. The FINFUN scoring criteria takes this into account and allows a dog to receive some points for stair climbing and running if it is able to perform the tasks with strong support. Additionally, the assessor may use the comments section to record whether the dog is not yet permitted to perform these tasks due to postsurgical restrictions. The dogs in this study were considered fit enough by their veterinary surgeon to perform all of the tasks. The owners were informed that these activities are not permitted in the home environment at this point of recovery, and they were allowed to withdraw their dog from the running or stair-climbing tasks.

Face and content validity

The thorough development process, including the translation, the pilot study and the clinical experience with critical reflection of the FINFUN in relation to already reported functional tests, contributed to sufficient face and content validity. The FINFUN users and the small animal neurologist in this study considered the FINFUN to measure overall motor function. Further investigation is needed to determine whether the FINFUN provides results consistent with those of another validated measure (criterion validity) [12, 14].

Internal consistency

The results show appropriate internal consistency, indicating that the FINFUN measures what it is intended to measure. A high Cronbach's alpha is considered to increase the reliability of a measure [29]. On the other hand, a high alpha is not always desired because closely correlated tasks may suggest redundancy, and tasks very similar to each other could be considered for exclusion from the testing battery [30]. However, all of the original tasks were maintained in the FINFUN because an extensive measure is more reliable than a more compact one as

Table 3 Inter-rater reliability for individual tasks and the sum score of the testing battery

Task	Inter-rater experienced (n = 2) (95% CI)	Inter-rater novice (n = 5) (95% CI)	Inter-rater all (n = 7) (95% CI)
Lying	0.705 (0.341–0.868)	0.919 (0.857–0.959)	0.932 (0.881–0.966)
Standing up from lying	0.954 (0.896–0.980)	0.970 (0.947–0.985)	0.982 (0.969–0.991)
Sitting	0.758 (0.457–0.892)	0.697 (0.465–0.848)	0.793 (0.646–0.894)
Standing up from sitting	0.911 (0.638–0.968)	0.939 (0.885–0.970)	0.978 (0.962–0.989)
Standing	0.953 (0.881–0.980)	0.966 (0.940–0.983)	0.975 (0.958–0.987)
Proprioceptive positioning	0.988 (0.974–0.995)	0.968 (0.944–0.984)	0.983 (0.971–0.991)
Start to walk from standing	0.973 (0.941–0.988)	0.988 (0.978–0.994)	0.992 (0.985–0.996)
Walking	0.978 (0.951–0.990)	0.975 (0.956–0.987)	0.986 (0.976–0.993)
Running	0.977 (0.950–0.990)	0.962 (0.931–0.981)	0.978 (0.962–0.989)
Walking turns	0.968 (0.910–0.987)	0.967 (0.941–0.983)	0.981 (0.967–0.990)
Walking stairs	0.971 (0.936–0.987)	0.975 (0.956–0.988)	0.984 (0.972–0.992)
Sum score	0.993 (0.984–0.997)	0.993 (0.988–0.997)	0.996 (0.993–0.998)

The intra-class correlation coefficient and confidence intervals for the experienced and novice observers as well as for all observers combined. Data are shown for each individual task and for the FINFUN total score

it increases variance, and thus, reliability [30]. Additionally, each task was considered clinically relevant, justifying that all tasks in the testing battery be retained [31].

Intra-rater reliability

The high intra-rater agreement for observer 1 can be explained by the fact that the studied dogs had been her patients. On the other hand, high intra-rater reliability has also been found in expert observers evaluating motor function in human stroke patients [11] and forelimb locomotion in rats with experimental unilateral cervical spinal cord injury [32]. Observer 2 showed moderate agreement for 'sitting' (task 3), but almost perfect agreement for the other tasks. A re-check of the scoring sheets showed this observer to be consistently stricter in the second scoring for 'sitting' in most dogs. This could be explained by the video assessment and interpretation of the scoring criteria. In general, the observers found it challenging to, from the videos, distinguish between motivating the dog to maintain a desired position and providing support. The handler was stroking the dog on several occasions to calm it down. This could be interpreted as motivation to maintain position for the required time, but it could also be considered support because light support is defined as touching the dog < 5 times during the performance (Additional file 1). Evaluation of motor function from video recordings has the disadvantage, that the observer is able to evaluate only that exact performance, possibly missing details that would have been detectable in the live situation.

Inter-rater reliability

Previous validated functional outcome measures have shown high inter-rater agreement [21, 22, 33]. The inter-rater reliability in this study was very promising, with little variance in the confidence intervals (Table 3) between observers, regardless of whether or not they were experienced. Relative to the FINFUN, the more brief TSCIS, a functional scale evaluating gait, proprioceptive positioning and nociception, showed substantial agreement in weighted kappa scores (0.72–01.00) and confidence intervals between moderate (0.42) and perfect (1.0). However, in their study the observers were of different educational levels and had received no training [21].

Previous studies emphasize the importance of observer training when developing numerical scales to assess motor function since training reduces observer-related errors [11, 15, 34]. Novice observers may adapt quickly to scoring routines [17], and the observers volunteering for this study were involved also in the pilot study. Thus, they were familiar with the scoring process before undertaking the training, and this has certainly influenced the results positively. In accordance with previous reports, a learning curve was noted in this study [22]. The experiences from the pilot study and the training revealed that observers needed to practice the FINFUN at least eight times in order to feel comfortable in the scoring process. A similar amount of practice in the development of functional scoring in dogs with spinal cord injury has been reported [22]. Considering this, to achieve such high level of agreement as is presented here, the required practice scoring should be approximately 15 times.

Interestingly, the agreement is higher for the FINFUN sum score than for the separate tasks (Tables 2 and 3), indicating that observers agreed very well on the dogs' overall function. However, there is variation >5 points in the scores given for dogs 7, 10, 18, 24 and 25 (Table 1, dogs marked with an asterisk). These were dogs with good motor function (dogs 7, 10, 18 and 25) or very poor motor function (dog 24). Novice observers may not detect small details or mistakes in dogs' motor function, therefore giving the dogs with good function a score of 4 (normal), whereas an experienced observer may be stricter, giving the same dog only a score of 3 (independent performance, mistakes occurring). This is in concordance with a previous study in which observers evaluating forelimb function in rats found that rating individuals with higher function was more difficult [32]. Increased observation time for specific periods and details may reduce the risk of missing important signs in the evaluation of locomotion [15]. Therefore, the FINFUN should be used so that the dog is allowed to perform the task more than once if needed and the best performance recorded. This gives the observer more time to decide on the score in the live situation, and this would correspond to the situation in clinical practice.

When validating a testing battery, it is of outmost importance that it is done under standardized conditions [12]. The frequently used video assessment ensures standardization in the evaluation of motor function [15, 23]. A recent study aiming to create a scoring system to detect the worse limb in dogs with thoracolumbar myelopathy found evaluations from video recordings to give higher inter-rater agreement than live evaluations [35]. In the current study, video assessment was chosen to reduce bias by enabling observers to assess the same performance of the dogs at the same time, excluding possible interfering factors from the environment, and thus, contributing to high reliability. This procedure also saved the patients the unnecessary stress of having several observers attending the therapy sessions. The dogs were filmed at the clinic in a standardized manner and the same person handled all the dogs during the video recordings. This was done to ensure that the handler would be as consistent as possible with amount of support or motivation for all the included dogs.

Although FINFUN showed high intra- and inter-rater reliability, it also has to be able to provide the practitioner with clinically relevant information. Based on the face and content validity we can argue that the FINFUN measures functional ability in the dog, providing scores that appear clinically relevant to the users in this study. The testing battery generated scores corresponding to the different grades of paralysis and no obvious floor or ceiling effect was noted. However, estimating the clinical relevance numerically with statistical tests was not within the scope of this study. This study focused on developing the testing battery itself and reliable scoring criteria. Still, the determination of the clinical relevance is a very important study that should follow the current one and further include determination of the sensitivity, specificity and responsiveness of the testing battery.

Limitations

This study included only dogs with paraparesis or paraplegia, so this sample will not give variation in scoring of 'lying' (task 1), as perhaps would patients with tetraparesis. Most observers have scored 'lying' high (3 or 4), which may have influenced the overall results. Although different severities of paralysis were represented in the studied sample, no normal dogs were included. Therefore the sensitivity or specificity of the testing battery could not be evaluated. One of the observers (AB) was not blinded to the studied dogs, as they were her patients. By the time of the study, several months had passed since the video recordings. However, it cannot be excluded that not being blinded to the patients might have increased the reliability in the scoring for AB. The FINFUN does not distinguish between affected limbs, as does, for example, the TSCIS [21]. However the FINFUN allows possible discrepancy between limbs to be noted subjectively in the comments section. Considering the discussion above, the FINFUN scoring system may not be sensitive enough to evaluate the quality of near-normal movement. Therefore, the authors suggest the use of another validated scale focusing on assessment of walking quality [23, 24] simultaneously with the FINFUN, particularly when assessing already ambulatory patients.

The FINFUN is a tool designed to assess the overall function and quality of movement of canine patients to provide adequate information on the performance level of activities of daily living. It is to be used by veterinary physiotherapists working in the hospital setting, in both clinical practice and research. Further comparison with other, already validated, outcome measures should be carried out in future studies. Research regarding the construct validity of the FINFUN and its responsiveness to change in live dogs is underway.

Conclusions

The FINFUN meets the demands of the growing field of physiotherapy and rehabilitation in veterinary medicine as an objective, valid and reliable tool with standardized scoring criteria for evaluation of motor function in dogs recovering from spinal cord injury.

Authors' contributions

AB designed the FINFUN and the study, collected and analyzed the data and edited the manuscript. HH edited the FINFUN scoring criteria, collected the data and edited the manuscript. PK performed the statistical analysis and interpretation of results and edited the manuscript. AH-B planned the validation, assisted in the statistical analysis and edited the manuscript. SC designed the FINFUN and the study and edited the manuscript. All authors read and approved the final manuscript.

Author details

[1] Department of Equine and Small Animal Medicine, Faculty of Veterinary Medicine, University of Helsinki, P.O. Box 57, 00014 Helsinki, Finland. [2] Rehabilitation Orton, Tenholantie 10, 00280 Helsinki, Finland. [3] Small Animal Hospital Aisti, Virtatie 9, 01600 Vantaa, Finland.

Acknowledgements

The authors thank the volunteer observers, animal physiotherapists Anu Rautakallio, Heidi Koskinen, Hanne Kalliomäki, Pirkko Lindfors and Minna Roukka.

Competing interests

The authors declare that they have no competing interests.

Funding

Not applicable.

References

1. Brisson BA. Intervertebral disc diease in dogs. Vet Clin North Am Small Anim Pract. 2010;40:829–58.
2. Sims C, Waldron R, Marcellin-Little DJ. Rehabilitation and physical therapy for the neurologic veterinary patient. Vet Clin North Am Small Anim Pract. 2015;45(1):123–43.
3. Hodgson MM, Bevan JM, Evans RB, Johnson TI. Influence of in-house rehabilitation on the postoperative outcome of dogs with intervertebral disk herniation. Vet Surg. 2017;46:566–73.
4. Ruddle TL, Allen DA, Schertel ER, Barnhart MD, Wilson ER, Lineberger JA, et al. Outcome and prognostic factors in non-ambulatory Hansen type I intervertebral disc extrusions: 308 cases. Vet Comp Orthop Traumatol. 2006;19:29–34.
5. Gallucci A, Dragone M, Menchetti T, Gagliardo T, Pietra M, Cardinali M, et al. Acquisition of involuntary spinal cord locomotion (spinal walking) in dogs with irreversible thoracolumbar spinal cord lesion. 81 dogs. J Vet Intern Med. 2017;31:492–7.
6. Gandini G, Cizinauskas S, Lang J, Fatzer R, Jaggy A. Fibrocartilaginous embolism in 75 dogs: clinical findings and factors influencing the recovery rate. J Small Anim Pract. 2003;44(2):76–80.
7. Kathmann I, Cizinauskas S, Doherr MG, Steffen F, Jaggy A. Daily controlled physiotherapy increases survival time in dogs with suspected degenerative myelopathy. J Vet Intern Med. 2006;20(4):927–32.
8. Carr JH, Shepherd RB. Measurement. Neurological rehabilitation: optimizing motor performance. 2nd ed. Edinburgh: Churchill Livingstone; 2010. p. 57–74.
9. Yavuz N, Tezyürek M, Akyüz M. A comparison of two functional tests in quadriplegia: the quadriplegia index of function and the functional independence measure. Spinal Cord. 1998;36:832–7.
10. Keith RA, Granger CV, Hamilton BB, Sherwin FS. The functional independence measure: a new tool for rehabilitation. Adv Clin Rehabil. 1987;1:6–18.
11. Carr Jh, Shepherd RB, Nordholm L, Lynne D. Investigation of a new motor assessment scale for stroke patients. Phys Ther. 1985;65(2):175–80.
12. Finch E, Brooks D, Stratford P, Mayo N. Why measurement properties are important. Physical rehabilitation outcome measures: a guide to enhanced clinical decision-making. 2nd ed. Ontario: Canadian Physiotherapy Association; 2002. p. 26–41.
13. Hyytiäinen H. Developing a physiotherapeutic testing battery for dogs with stifle dysfunction. Doctoral Thesis, University of Helsinki. 2015.
14. Berg A. Outcome measures in animal physiotherapy. In: McGowan C, Goff L, editors. Animal physiotherapy, assessment, treatment and rehabilitation of animals. 2nd ed. Singapore: Wiley Blackwell; 2016. p. 347–63.
15. Basso M, Beattie M, Bresnahan J. A sensitive and reliable locomotor scale for open field-testing in rats. J Neurotrauma. 1994;12(1):1–21.
16. Ward PJ, Herrity AN, Harkema SJ, Hubscher CH. Training-induced functional gains following spinal cord injury. Neural Plast. 2016. https://doi.org/10.1155/2016/4307694.
17. Song RB, Basso MD, da Costa RC, Fisher LC, Mo XM, Moore SA. Adaptation of the Basso–Beattie–Bresnahan locomotor rating scale for use in a clinical model of spinal cord injury in dogs. J Neurosci Methods. 2016;1(268):117–24.
18. Frankel HL, Hancock DO, Hyslop G, Melzack J, Michaaelis LS, Ungar GH, et al. The value of postural reduction in the initial management of closed injuries of the spine with paraplegia and tetraplegia. Paraplegia. 1969;7:179–92.
19. Ingram EA, Kale DC, Balfour RJ. Hemilaminectomy for thoracolumbar Hansen type I intervertebral disk disease in ambulatory dogs with or without neurologic deficits: 39 cases (2008–2010). Vet Surg. 2013;42(8):925–31.
20. Van Wie EY, Fosgate GT, Mankin JM, Jeffrey ND, Kerwin SC, Levine GJ, et al. Prospectively recorded versus medical record-derived spinal cord injury scores in dogs with intervertebral disc herniation. J Vet Intern Med. 2013;27:1273–7.
21. Levine G, Levine J, Budke C, Kerwin S, Au J, Vinayak A, et al. Description of a newly developed spinal cord injury scale for dogs. Prev Vet Med. 2009;89:121–7.
22. Olby N, De Risio L, Munana K, Wosar M, Skeen T, Sharp N, et al. Development of a functional scoring system in dogs with acute spinal cord injuries. Am J Vet Res. 2001;62(10):1624–8.
23. Olby NJ, Lim JH, Babb K, Back K, Domaracki C, Williams K, et al. Gait scoring in dogs with thoracolumbar spinal cord injuries when walking on a treadmill. BMC Vet Res. 2014. https://doi.org/10.1186/1746-6148-10-58.
24. Song RB, Oldach MS, Basso MD, da Costa RC, Fisher LC, Mo XM, et al. A simplified method of walking track analysis to assess short-term locomotor recovery after acute spinal cord injury caused by thoracolumbar intervertebral disc extrusion in dogs. Vet J. 2016;210:61–7.
25. Boström A, Hyytiäinen H, Koho P, Cizinauskas S. Development of a functional test for neurologically impaired dogs. Pilot testing for reliability. Poster presentation. In: Proceedings of the 9th international symposium on rehabilitation and physical therapy in veterinary medicine, Minneapolis, USA. 2008.
26. Landis JR, Koch GG. The measurement of observer agreement for categorical data. Biometrics. 1977;33(1):159–74.
27. Lorentz MD, Coates JR, Kent M. Neurologic history, neuroanatomy and neurologic examination. Handbook of veterinary neurology. 5th ed. St. Louis: Elsevier Saunders; 2011. p. 2–36.
28. Millard RP, Headrick JF, Millis DL. Kinematic analysis of the pelvic limbs of healthy dogs during stair and decline slope walking. J Small Anim Pract. 2010;51(8):419–22.
29. Metsämuuronen J. Internal reliability of the measurement (validity) [Mittauksen sisäinen luotettavuus (validiteetti)]. Basics of research in human sciences [Tutkimuksen tekemisen perusteet ihmistieteessä]. Jyväskylä: Gummerus Kirjapaino Oy; 2009. p. 145–8.
30. Wadhwa G, Aikat R. Development, validity and reliability of the 'Sitting Balance Measure' (SBM) in spinal cord injury. Spinal Cord. 2016;54:319–23.
31. Streiner DL. Starting at the beginning: an introduction to coefficient alpha and internal consistency. J Pers Assess. 2003;80(1):99–103.
32. Singh A, Krisa L, Frederick KL, Sandrow-Feinberg H, Stackhouse SK, Murray M, et al. Forelimb locmotor rating scale for behavioral assessment of recovery after unilateral cervical spinal cord injury in rats. J Neurosci Methods. 2016;15(226):124–31.
33. Phoole JL, Whitney SL. Motor assessment scale for stroke patients: concurrent validity and interrater reliability. Arch Med Rehabil. 1988;69(3):195–7.

A veterinary perspective on One Health in the Arctic

Christian Sonne[1*], Robert James Letcher[2], Bjørn Munro Jenssen[1,3,4], Jean-Pierre Desforges[1], Igor Eulaers[1], Emilie Andersen-Ranberg[1], Kim Gustavson[1], Bjarne Styrishave[5] and Rune Dietz[1]

Abstract

Exposure to long-range transported industrial chemicals, climate change and diseases is posing a risk to the overall health and populations of Arctic wildlife. Since local communities are relying on the same marine food web as marine mammals in the Arctic, it requires a One Health approach to understand the holistic ecosystem health including that of humans. Here we collect and identify gaps in the current knowledge of health in the Arctic and present the veterinary perspective of One Health and ecosystem dynamics. The review shows that exposure to persistent organic pollutants (POPs) is having multiple organ-system effects across taxa, including impacts on neuroendocrine disruption, immune suppression and decreased bone density among others. Furthermore, the warming Arctic climate is suspected to influence abiotic and biotic long-range transport and exposure pathways of contaminants to the Arctic resulting in increases in POP exposure of both wildlife and human populations. Exposure to vector-borne diseases and zoonoses may increase as well through range expansion and introduction of invasive species. It will be important in the future to investigate the effects of these multiple stressors on wildlife and local people to better predict the individual-level health risks. It is within this framework that One Health approaches offer promising opportunities to survey and pinpoint environmental changes that have effects on wildlife and human health.

Keywords: Contaminants, Greenland, Hg, Humans, Inuits, Mercury, Persistent organic pollutants, Polar bears, POPs, Seals, Sled dogs, Whales

Background

One Health aims to improve health and well-being through the prevention of risks and the mitigation of effects of crises that originate at the interface between humans, animals and their various environments (http://www.onehealthglobal.net). Given the close relationship between wildlife, sled dogs and humans in the North Atlantic, in combination with long-term biomonitoring programs using multiple veterinary tools over the last three decades, an Arctic One Health approach requires focus on few key species and study areas that interlink wildlife, human and ecosystem health. The present review will therefore discuss clinical and veterinary studies on polar bears (*Ursus maritimus*), ringed seals (*Pusa hispida*), narwhals (*Monodon monoceros*), killer whales (*Orcinus orca*), domestic sled dogs (*Canis familiaris*), and humans (*Homo sapiens*), and how shared information on these provide a base from which One Health can be operated. The focus will be on exposure of Arctic wildlife and Inuit populations to long-range transported contaminants and its interactions with climate change and infectious diseases (zoonoses).

Search strategy

We conducted this literature review to give a systematic overview of the current knowledge on environmental contaminants and zoonosis in the Arctic and how it links to climate change in a multiple stressors framework. From our own working knowledge in the field, we identified "persistent organic pollutants (POPs)", "mercury (Hg)" and "zoonoses" relevant for the Arctic and the link to "climate change" as overall themes/keywords. We used ScienceDirect, PubMed, Google, Google Scholar, ISI

*Correspondence: cs@bios.au.dk
[1] Department of Bioscience, Arctic Research Centre (ARC), Aarhus University, Faculty of Science and Technology, Frederiksborgvej 399, PO Box 358, 4000 Roskilde, Denmark
Full list of author information is available at the end of the article

Web of Knowledge/Web of Science and Springer Link to locate peer-reviewed scientific articles and reports, using the thematic keywords "immune", "endocrine", "neuro", "bone", "diseases" and "multiple stressors" either alone or in combination. We also used dissertations and AMAP reports to obtain information from the grey literature. Although we attempted to be systematic within the scope of the review, we acknowledge that this is not an exhaustive representation of all the material that may exist in the scientific literature.

The arctic environment as a sink for pollutants

Hunting and fishing have always been an important part of Arctic human existence in this harsh northern environment [1–6], and their intensity has increased with a growing Arctic human population bringing along more effective hunting methods, including larger and faster boats and fishing vessels, riffles and gillnets. Adding to these local stressors on Arctic ecosystems, anthropogenic pollution has become a ubiquitous problem that is particularly relevant in the Arctic environment [6–8]. In addition to elevated mercury (Hg), an array of anthropogenic chlorinated, brominated, and fluorinated persistent organic pollutants (POPs), all alien substances, have been introduced to the Arctic [1, 7, 9–14]. More specifically, the 1850s marked the period of early industrialization and was associated with elevated Hg emissions [10], whereas the onset of the 1940s marked the onset of large-volume worldwide use of industrial chemicals and pesticides. POPs and Hg typically originate from industrial and household emissions at temperate regions and are transported via global atmospheric and oceanic pathways that result in deposition in the Arctic environment [6, 7, 9, 11, 12, 15].

Arctic fish and wildlife rely on energy-rich fatty tissues as their main energy source in the harsh Arctic environment [16, 17]. Fatty tissues typically host various natural lipophilic compounds, such as specific vitamins (A and D) and endogenous steroid hormones transported by portal and periphery blood supply among others [8, 18–23]. However, most POPs and methyl-Hg, the bioavailable chemical from of Hg, are highly lipophilic as well and are therefore readily stored in lipid-rich tissues. Additional low excretion of these compounds results in a net intake of POPs and Hg over time, referred to as bioaccumulation, and is moreover transferred from prey to predator along the food chain resulting in biomagnification. As a result, apex predators such as polar bears, Arctic fox (*Vulpes lagopus*), seal spp., whale spp. and seabird spp., are exposed to the highest concentrations occurring the Arctic environment, already a major sink for POPs and Hg as described above. Finally, indigenous northerners and their dogs are ultimate sinks due to their traditional consumption of the aforementioned wildlife [7, 13, 14, 24, 25]. Newer perfluorinated compounds [poly- and perfluoralkyl substances (PFASs)], in particular perfluorooctane sulfonate (PFOS) and other long-chained poly- and perfluorocarboxylic acid (PFCAs) are proteinophilic and also biomagnify due to high resistance to biological degradation [7].

Long-range transported pollutants have been extensively monitored in the Arctic due to the high exposure of Inuit populations, resulting from their consumption of a marine diet consisting especially of apex marine predators high in contaminants [2, 3, 6]. Such biomonitoring activities have shown that, among these POPs, polychlorinated biphenyls (PCBs) continue to dominate and are of the greatest exposure concern, despite their ban decades ago [7]. However, other high-concentration POPs, amongst which organochlorine pesticides (OCPs), brominated flame retardants (BFRs), PFASs, and Hg can also be found at concentrations that raise concerns for the health of top predators and humans [7, 11, 26–28].

Arctic wildlife and human health

POPs and Hg pose a health threat to Arctic top predators and humans because the compounds and their biotransformation metabolites have structural similarities to endogenous compounds. These anthropogenic compounds have been classified as endocrine disruptors or cellular toxicants acting via non-endocrine pathways, and thus negatively affect immune and neuro-endocrine functioning, growth and development, reproduction and general fitness [7, 8, 29]. Since the compounds potentially target different organ-tissues, the dietary exposure causes chronic and combined stress manifested through several health effects at the organism level [8, 30, 31].

There is evidence that high exposure poses a great risk to neonatal individuals during critical periods of development. Seasonal cycles of energy requirements for fasting, breeding, lactation, and migration lead to increased intake or catabolism of adipose tissue causing pulsed exposure to bioavailable contaminants circulating in the blood [32, 33]. In polar bears, for example, up to 70% of the total organochlorine body burden is transported from mother to offspring during lactation, resulting in cub adipose tissue concentrations that are approximately three times higher than those in their mothers [32, 34–37]. A female polar bears' very first cubs are believed to be especially vulnerable since high contaminant exposure can affect normal development and growth [7, 8, 31]. In a meta-study, it has recently been modelled that chlorinated and brominated POPs, singularly or collectively, were far better predictors of declines in population densities in 14 polar bear subpopulations than were human population density, harvest rate and sea ice extention

[38]. Indeed, circumarctic polar bear subpopulations are under influence of immunological, reproductive and carcinogenic consequences from POP exposure [27]. From a population conservation point of view, contaminants that reduce pregnancy, fecundity and survival in both males and females are among the most important to monitor in different Arctic subpopulations of polar bears, as well as other top predators and northerners relying on the same food web [39, 40].

East Greenland polar bears, killer whales, narwhals and ringed, harp (*Pagophilus groenlandicus*) and hooded seals (*Cystophora cristata*) carry very high concentrations of POPs and Hg [7, 11, 12, 15, 41]. Since Greenlanders in this region traditionally ingest significant quantities of adipose tissue from these species, they are among the Arctic people carrying the highest POP burdens [5, 6, 43, 44]. Such high exposure is likely to pose a health risk based on available literature on dioxin toxic equivalency factor (TEQ) and tolerable daily intake (TDI) guidelines [44, 45]. Human exposure to contaminants in Greenland has been evaluated from chemical analyses of prey species and food intake [5, 46, 47], showing that the TDI was exceeded for chlordane (CHL) by a factor of 3–6, while PCB exposure did not. However, none of these studies reported on polar bear and ringed seal blubber important to people's exposure in East Greenland, where POP loads are known to be four times larger than in west Greenland. According to Nielsen et al. [48] it is recommended that Greenlanders reduce their exposure to PCBs and CHL by reducing their blubber intake. The Arctic Monitoring and Assessment Programme (AMAP) is therefore concerned about Arctic human health within a contaminant exposure context and their studies do support observations that Greenland hunters are particularly exposed to high PCB concentrations due to frequent ingestion of polar bear, killer whale, narwhal and seal tissues [6, 44, 49–51]. Studies from the Russian Arctic have shown that dioxin, furans and PCB exposure of neo- and prenatal children exceeded TEQ TDI levels by up to 33 times in the year 2000 [5, 52]. It has been shown that blood concentrations of PFASs including PFOS in male Inuits from East Greenland can be two to three times higher as compared to the Faroese population where local exposure has already been attributed with effects on the immune system [53–55].

Although certain PFASs have been associated with developmental and hormonal effects, immunotoxicity, and tumour growth in rodents [56], the impact of these compounds on human health appear to be inconclusive [56, 57]. Of the PCBs found in Greenlanders, the congeners CB-77, CB-126 and CB-169 attain a coplanar configuration similar to the very toxic dioxins and furans, and are in fact commonly found in Arctic wildlife [3, 5, 58]. These coplanar PCB congeners are characteristically highly potent inducers of aryl hydrocarbon hydroxylase activity [3, 5]. Furthermore, for Greenlanders, significant correlations were found between blood contaminant concentrations and calculated daily intake of POPs [51]. Hg exposure of Inuit people is also of great health concern and has been recognised as a neuro-endocrine and immune health problem in the societies of Faroe Islands, West Greenland (Avanersuaq, Thule) and Canada [6, 11, 59].

Biomonitoring of wildlife health

Several of the environmental contaminants, such as PCBs and Hg are regulated by international agreements over the last 15 years through international treaties and conventions including the Stockholm Convention on POPs (http://chm.pops.int) and Minamata Convention on Hg (http://www.mercuryconvention.org). However, over the last two decades, the concentrations of the highly toxic PCBs, chlordane pesticides and Hg have remained essentially unchanged or even increased in polar bears inhabiting contaminant hot spots, such as Greenland and Hudson Bay [10, 12–14, 60, 61]. This is likely due to climate change effects on food web interactions, generational transfer, and continued secondary and unintentional emissions [12, 13, 17, 62]. For Hg, body burdens even appear to be continuously increasing in most top predators in the central Arctic reaching up to 20-fold baseline levels of pre-industrialisation [10, 11, 60, 63].

For three decades the AMAP program and associated subprograms have therefore monitored the health of Arctic wildlife and humans [1, 3, 5–7, 41, 60]. For the purpose of studying contaminant concentrations, spatial and temporal trends, and human exposure, these programs have used ringed seals and polar bears as key monitoring species [7, 64]. From the East Greenland region, a large number of organ–tissue samples from polar bears have been obtained since the 1980s as part of the traditional hunt [12, 42]. Likewise, from Svalbard, Canada and Alaska, adipose tissue and blood has been archived, facilitating the spatial and temporal trends which are further supported by similar samples from ringed seals [7]. With respect to East Greenland polar bears, histopathological, gross morphological and bone composition and morphological investigations have been carried out since 1999 [8, 31, 65, 66]. These studies have provided a unique opportunity to investigate the potential organ-specific effects of POP exposure [8]. Similar to polar bears, analyses of bone density and histopathology have been carried out on West Greenland ringed seal populations [67, 68] and on Alaska polar bears, ringed seals and whale spp. [69–72].

Interpretations and conclusions in wildlife health studies linked to contaminant exposure are typically based on correlational and descriptive interpretations, unavoidably confounded by a plethora of factors affecting the physiological state of a free-ranging animal. To improve the understanding of the effects of exposure to real-world contaminant cocktails experimental exposure studies have been performed on sled dogs and domesticated Arctic foxes, being possible surrogate model species for *Canidae* spp. In captive sled dogs and Arctic fox studies, which both included a cohort fed a naturally POP contaminated diet of minke whale (*Balaenoptera acutorostrata*) blubber, it has been possible to define and compare POP exposed and unexposed reference groups in direct relation to an array of effects such as on reproductive organs and other internal organs, the skeletal system, immune and endocrine systems, and POP dietary accumulation, biotransformation and toxicokinetics [7, 8, 31].

Biological effects

In the following sections we review the available literature of One Health in the Arctic (Fig. 1). We present and discuss the results from empirical studies of wildlife and compare these with controlled studies of sledge dogs and arctic foxes in the context of One Health and health effects in humans. The following sections are divided into first specific organ-systems and after that the relatively sparse information on multiple effects health effects are presented and discussed.

Chronic diseases

Chronic diseases, including diabetes, upper respiratory and recurrent middle ear infections, cancer, and osteoporosis, are becoming an epidemic in the Arctic and may be partially caused by chronic POP exposure and associated endocrine disruption [3, 5, 73]. It is apparent that subsistence hunters in East Greenland are exposed to mixtures of POPs that include both toxic parent compounds and also their derived metabolites [74]. Some POPs can induce (hepatic) cytochrome (CYP) 450 enzymes in Arctic people that may interfere with normal metabolic processes and homeostasis of various intrinsic hormones and vitamins influencing immunity and reproduction [1, 3, 5, 75, 76]. Likewise, Sandau et al. [77] found that metabolism of PCBs was significantly negatively correlated with thyroid hormones, namely free thyroxine, in northern peoples in the Ungava region in northern Quebec, Canada. These findings of associations between POP exposure, induction of CYP-450 enzymes, and changes in thyroid hormone concentrations, may play a role in the development of chronic diseases [5].

Bone mineral density

Studies of polar bears suggest that osteoporosis may be a problem for especially the male bears that do not have the evolutionary physiological mechanisms that females have, putting them at high risk of POP related bone

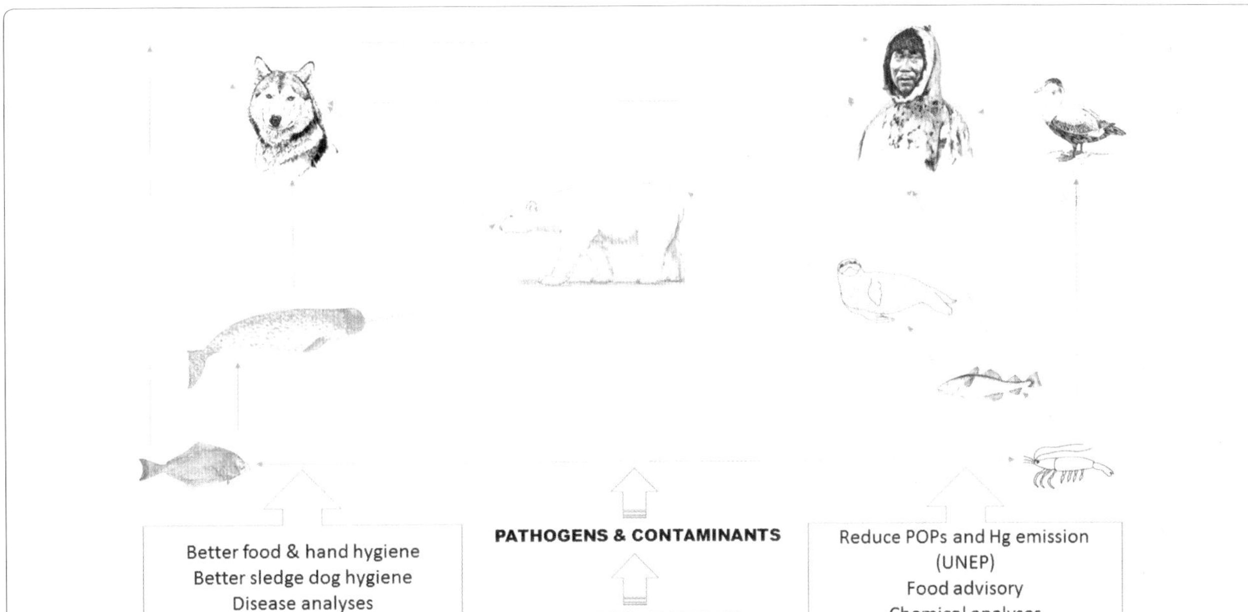

Fig. 1 A simplification of the marine food web and One Health in the Arctic. Climate change affect the presence of pathogens and composition of contaminants in Arctic wildlife that is handled and eaten by Inuits and sled dogs transferring contaminants and pathogens into the local societies. Inuits and sled dogs share microbiomes which increases the risk of zoonotic infections. Actions to be taken is given in callouts

mineral density declines [8, 66, 78]. The studies of polar bears have shown reductions in bone mineral density due to PCB exposure all supported by studies on seals in the Baltic Sea and alligators in Florida, USA [79–81].

A single study has been published on osteoporosis in relation to POP exposure in Greenlanders [82]. The study focused on quantitative ultrasound parameters (QUS) at the right calcaneus of 153 people from Southwest Greenland and found blood plasma CB-153 concentrations strongly and negatively associated with the three QUS parameters. While the relationship was no longer significant when normalizing for age and weight, people in Southwest Greenland belong to some of the lowest POP exposed Greenlanders and effects on bone composition are therefore not likely to occur [5, 6]. Another study of Cree women from Eastern James Bay in Canada showed that bone stiffness index was negatively associated to blood concentrations of CB-105 and CB-118 [83].

Endocrine disruption

Endocrine disruption from POP exposure is likely to be a challenge in Arctic wildlife [30, 84]. Polar bears have been in focus over the last decades and both steroid hormones and thyroid hormones seem to be impacted by POP parent compounds and their metabolites, mimicking hormone activity in both the transport pathways and receptor mechanisms and affecting overall health and survival [8, 30]. These investigations have been backed up by controlled experiments on sled dogs and Arctic foxes [8, 84]. Likewise, in Inuit peoples, disruption by POPs of the thyroid and steroid hormone endocrine axis is influencing physiological endpoints with effects on reproduction, cancer, and immunity [6, 85].

Studies on polar bears from Svalbard indicate that plasma steroid levels may be affected by POP exposure, particularly PCBs and their hydroxylated metabolites (OH-PCBs). In females, pregnenolone and androstenedione in the blood appeared to be significantly negatively correlated to several hydroxylated PCBs [86], indicating that these POPs may affect early or perhaps rate-limiting steps in steroidogenesis. The data also indicated that CYP-17 may be a target for OH-PCBs and consequently the reproductive potential of female polar bears. PCBs also appear to affect male plasma steroids, in particular androgen levels in Svalbard polar bears [87]. Concentrations of the most masculinizing steroids, dihydrotestosterone and testosterone, were negatively correlated to levels of a large number of PCB congeners.

Reproductive organs

Studying reproductive organs in wildlife is often based on necropsy samples as clinical investigations are rather difficult. Necropsy of human reproductive organs from Arctic populations has for ethical reasons not been studied, though the investigation of endocrinology and reproductive organs in wildlife and domesticated species (sled dogs and Arctic fox) can give some important information. For example, the presence of orchitis in polar bear testes [88] may be of importance while studying testicular dysgenesis syndrome in Inuits. Seasonal hormone and semen production in Arctic fox was found to be affected by POPs [89, 90]. Similarly, there are indications that the size of polar bear penis bone, testicles and ovaries may be inversely correlated to PCB concentrations [66, 88]. Such information may be of use in human medicine when autopsies are not an option and when POPs are suspected of having endocrine disruptive effects in humans.

Immune effects

Environmental contaminants have been shown to modulate all measurable aspects of cellular and humoral immunity in marine mammals [89]. Resistance against acute and chronic diseases also depends on the optimal function of the immune system [91, 92]. For years, POPs have been known to modulate immunity, and while the mechanisms of immune suppression are not fully understood, it includes both humoral cell-mediated systems [3, 92–95]. Several studies have reported immune effects in Arctic wildlife, including polar bears, ringed seals, sled dogs and Arctic foxes [8], demonstrating that contaminants are reaching levels that can cause significant changes in physiology and immune fitness, with important consequences for resistance to disease.

Polar bear immunity was assessed in a comprehensive study in Svalbard and Hudson Bay, and negative associations were found between PCB exposure and serum immunoglobulin G (IgG) levels, antibody titres against influenza virus and reovirus following immunizations, and lymphocyte proliferation [96, 97]. In a controlled study on Greenland sled dogs, exposed pups, but not adults, showed reduced and delayed IgG antibody production with circulating levels of IgG in all pups correlating to blood concentrations of several POPs [8]. Hepatic mRNA expression of interleukin-1β (IL-1β), an important pro-inflammatory cytokine, in ringed seals from Svalbard were positively correlated with hepatic POP levels [98]. Similarly, hepatic IL-1 mRNA expression was positively correlated with blubber PCB burdens in 41 ringed seals in northern Labrador, Canada [99]. These studies illustrate that in vivo real life exposure to contaminants cause measurable changes in immune function in Arctic wildlife, and thus likely humans.

In vitro experiments, where immune cells are exposed to contaminants under laboratory conditions in order to characterise effect levels, have also been carried-out in Arctic wildlife species. East Greenland ringed seal leukocytes were exposed to four PCB congeners (CB-138, -153, -169, and -180) and two PFASs, i.e. PFOS and perfluorooctanoic acid (PFOA), and it was found that PCBs but not PFASs cause significant suppression of lymphocyte proliferation at relevant environmental concentrations for seals [100]. Beluga whale (*Delphinapterus leucas*) leukocytes were also used to show that low levels of Hg exposure can cause significant reductions in lymphocyte proliferation and intracellular thiol production, and significant induction of metallothionein [101]. Altogether, studies of free-ranging animals and in vitro experiments suggest high contaminant loads in the Arctic can induce immune suppression which affect the ability to respond to intruding infectious pathogens as previously suggested for marine mammals [7, 8, 31, 89] and Inuit and other northern peoples [6]. For example, prenatal exposure to PCBs has been suspected to play a role in the relatively high incidence of acute respiratory infections and middle ear inflammation in Inuit children [6, 102–106].

Neurological effects

Multiple environmental contaminants can cross the blood–brain barrier and exert effects on the brain functioning thus causing neurobehavioral effects. Through various mechanisms, contaminants can influence mating and other reproductive behaviours, motivation, communication, aggression, dominance and other social behaviours, as well as learning and other cognitive abilities [29, 107]. Field studies of behavioural effects of POPs in polar bears are difficult to conduct due to logistical and ethical constraints. However, several POPs reported in brain tissue of polar bears [74, 108–112] are confirmed or suspected developmental neurotoxicants in humans and experimental animals [29, 107, 113, 114]. POPs might affect brain function or development through many mechanisms, for instance by interacting with brain neurotransmitter systems [113]. Also, the ability of some POPs to induce epigenetic changes could present a mechanistic pathway of neurodevelopmental perturbations [115–117]. Associations between neurochemical and epigenetic biomarkers and Hg levels in brain tissue have been reported for polar bears [11, 118, 119]. Despite relatively low concentrations of Hg, significant negative correlations were found between both Hg concentrations and *N*-methyl-D-aspartic acid (NMDA) glutamate receptors. NMDA glutamate and genomic methylation is important for animal health, behaviour, reproduction, and survival, and their reduction may have population-level effects for polar bears [120].

Another proposed mechanism of developmental neurotoxicity is through thyroid hormone disruption; thyroid hormones are essential for proper neurodevelopment of the foetus and early neonate [121, 122]. Thus, the high levels of POPs reported in 4-month old polar bear cubs [34] and their associated thyroid disrupting properties in cubs [123, 124] raises concern for neurodevelopmental effects in polar bears. The relatively high concentrations of several POPs reported in polar bear brains may cause adverse effects, with a possible heightened susceptibility during the more sensitive foetal and neonatal stages of brain development [29, 125]. Similarly to humans, this could alter behavioural traits and reduce cognitive abilities related to memory and learning in offspring. For polar bears, this could functionally reduce hunting skills or alter mating behaviour, and thus ultimately affect reproduction and survival.

Multiple stressors

In the previous section we discussed the important risk posed by environmental contaminants in Arctic wildlife and human populations for a wide range of physiological health endpoints. Arctic ecosystems, however, are being stressed by more than contaminants, resulting in a situation of multiple cumulative stress for wildlife and humans. Two major additional aspects to consider in the study of Arctic health is climate change and infectious diseases. Climate change has a duel impact, acting through alteration of food web pathways for contaminants [61, 126] and spreading and virulence of zoonotic diseases associated to sea ice conditions [127–129]. A pollution induced increase in disease rates due to immunotoxic effects of POPs and Hg can increase the likelihood and risk of disease transfer from animals to humans (zoonoses) as the proportion of infected Arctic wildlife increases [30, 89, 130–132]. A large volume of marine and terrestrial wildlife is consumed by humans in the Arctic, often raw and inadequately frozen, and this likely increases the risk of zoonotic diseases [8].

Climate change and contaminant exposure

Arctic wildlife have received considerable focus as they, depending on the regional subpopulation, are threatened most dramatically by climate change due to observed and projected loss of sea ice, which has important implications for ice-associated hunters like polar bears [133–135]. Modeling has shown that southernmost polar bear subpopulations in the Hudson Bay are at greatest risk, and will struggle to persist throughout this century [136]. In fact, models have also predicted two-thirds of the world's polar bears could disappear if greenhouse gas emissions continue to increase as predicted [134, 137]. This has been linked to the occupation of large home range sizes and the requirement of higher energetic costs and thus higher feeding rates, which can lead to increasing blood PCB concentrations [138, 139]. In some regions, the decline of sea ice extent has resulted in changes in the presence of seal species that polar bears prey upon, and this has been shown to cause increased bioaccumulation of certain POPs as more contaminated prey are being consumed [61, 140]. Dietary shift towards feeding on plants, berries and caribou (*Rangifer tarandus*) and seabird eggs [141–143] will most likely decrease and increase, respectively, the exposure to POPs. Furthermore, climate warming induced migration of warm water adapted fish species [144, 145] may act as biovectors increasing contaminant levels in marine Arctic ecosystems [146, 147], ultimately causing increased bioaccumulation and biomagnification of these compounds to humans and other high trophic marine wildlife [30, 126]. McDonald et al. [147] conducted a review on ecological impacts of global climate change on POP and Hg pathways and exposures in arctic marine ecosystems, and documented that lower sea ice extent mediated dietary changes were associated with higher contaminant levels in some populations of polar bears, ringed seals, and thick-billed murres (*Uria lomvia*), but the influence of changing trophic interactions on POP levels and trends varied widely in both magnitude and direction.

Climate change and infectious diseases

Climate change not only threatens to alter contaminant dynamics by changing Arctic ecosystems, but these same factors influencing the presence and extent of different species in the Arctic will have implications for the introduction of novel infectious diseases to the region. Climate change has been deemed the most important factor in the emergence of infectious diseases, and nowhere else in the world is climate change occurring as fast as in the polar regions [148, 149]. A warming climate may profoundly affect disease dynamics in the Arctic by changing the species composition and northward invasion of disease vectors and transport of pathogens [149, 150]. In addition, increased survival of infected animals during milder winters may further increase the risk of pathogen reservoir in marine mammals including that of zoonosis [149, 150]. Moreover and as discussed above immunotoxic contaminants may increase disease-related mortality and morbidity of Arctic marine mammals [129].

Perspectives and recommendations

Further efforts are required to understand the toxicokinetics and toxicodynamics of POPs and Hg in Greenland wildlife and peoples in this changing Arctic in order to better predict the individual-level health risks associated with contaminant exposure. Arctic top predators are sentinels for humans as they consume the same diet and act as potential vectors for zoonotic transfer to humans due to harvesting. Combining correlational studies on wildlife health with experimental work on surrogate species, such as the sled dog, will allow better understanding of the proximate toxic pathways behind exposure to contaminants and infectious diseases, their interactions, and the driving role of a rapidly changing climate. Doing this offers a promising One Health approach to survey and pinpoint environmental change and multiple stressors that may have effects on wildlife and human health [7, 8, 31, 151–153]. The warming Arctic climate is suspected to influence abiotic and biotic long-range transport and exposure pathways of contaminants to the Arctic. As a result there will be likely increases in POP exposure of Arctic wildlife and human populations, while exposure to vector-borne diseases and zoonoses may increase as well through range expansion and introduction from invasive species. Broad, and nevertheless in-depth studies on the occurrence and human health risk of Arctic zoonoses, and their interactive effects with climate change and contaminant exposure are pending, as well as an increased effort to educate the relevant groups of the public regarding safe handling of wildlife.

Abbreviations

AMAP: arctic monitoring and assessment program; BFRs: brominated flame retardants; BMD: bone mineral density; CHL: chlordane; Hg: mercury; IL: interleukin; IgG: immunoglobulin G; NMDA: *N*-methyl-D-aspartic acid; OH-PCBs: hydroxylated PCBs; OCPs: organochlorine pesticides; PCBs: polychlorinated biphenyls; PFASs: poly- and perfluoralkyl substances; PFOS: perfluorooctane sulfonate; PFCAs: poly- and perfluorocarboxylic acid; POPs: persistent organic pollutants; QUS: quantitative ultrasound parameters; TEQ: dioxin toxic equivalency factor; TDI: tolerable daily intake.

Authors' contributions

CS designed the review and produced the 1st draft and further revisions and submission of manuscript. RJL dealt with the precision of environmental contaminants, BMJ with the multiple stressors' framework, JPD with the immune sections, IE with the ecological framework, EAR with zoonosis, KG with PBPK modelling, BS with steroid hormones and RD with modelling and ecosystem effects. All authors read and approved the final manuscript.

Authors' information

CS is a wildlife veterinarian focusing on industrial chemicals and health effects in the Arctic. RJL is an environmental chemist focusing on legacy and emergent environmental chemicals in the Arctic and North America. BMJ is a wildlife biologist working on birds and marine mammals in the Arctic with a special focus on the thyroid hormone system. JPD is working on immune toxicology in North Atlantic predators. IE is ecologist focusing on food web dynamics and energy and nutrient flow. EAR is DVM with insights to infectious diseases in the Arctic. KG is specialised in applying PBPK modelling to contaminants in Arctic ecosystem wildlife. BS is specialised in analyses and interpretation of steroid hormones in Arctic predators. RD is wildlife biologist with insights to marine mammal biology and contaminant exposure.

Author details

[1] Department of Bioscience, Arctic Research Centre (ARC), Aarhus University, Faculty of Science and Technology, Frederiksborgvej 399, PO Box 358, 4000 Roskilde, Denmark. [2] Ecotoxicology and Wildlife Health Division, Environment and Climate Change Canada, National Wildlife Research Centre, Carleton University, Ottawa, ON K1A 0H3, Canada. [3] Department of Biology, Norwegian University of Science and Technology, 7491 Trondheim, Norway. [4] Department of Arctic Technology, The University Centre in Svalbard, PO Box 156, 9171 Longyearbyen, Norway. [5] Toxicology Laboratory, Department

of Pharmacy, Faculty of Health and Medical Sciences, University of Copenhagen, Universitetsparken 2, 2100 Copenhagen, Denmark.

Competing interests
The authors declare that they have no competing interests.

Funding
Nordic Council of Ministers (NMR NORDEN) is acknowledged for financial support to the project entitled Infectious Zoonotic Diseases Transmissible from harvested Wildlife to humans in the European Arctic (ZORRO). We also acknowledge BONUS BALTHEALTH that has received funding from BONUS (Art. 185), funded jointly by the EU, Innovation Fund Denmark (Grants 6180-00001B and 6180-00002B), Forschungszentrum Jülich GmbH, German Federal Ministry of Education and Research (Grant FKZ 03F0767A), Academy of Finland (Grant 311966) and Swedish Foundation for Strategic Environmental Research (MISTRA).

References
1. AMAP. Arctic Monitoring and Assessment Programme: AMAP assessment report—arctic pollution issues 1998; Oslo 1998. http://www.amap.no.
2. AMAP. Arctic Monitoring and Assessment Programme: AMAP assessment 2002—human health in the Arctic 2003; Oslo 2003. http://www.amap.no.
3. AMAP. Arctic Monitoring and Assessment Programme: AMAP assessment 2002—persistent organic pollutants in the Arctic 2004; Oslo 2004. http://www.amap.no.
4. AMAP. Arctic Monitoring and Assessment Programme: AMAP assessment 2002—heavy metals in the Arctic 2005; Oslo 2005. http://www.amap.no.
5. AMAP. Arctic Monitoring and Assessment Programme: AMAP assessment 2009—human health in the Arctic 2009; Oslo 2009. http://www.amap.no.
6. AMAP. Arctic Monitoring and Assessment Programme: AMAP assessment 2013—human health in the Arctic 2013; Oslo 2015. http://www.amap.no.
7. Letcher RJ, Bustnes JO, Dietz R, Jenssen BM, Jørgensen EH, Sonne C, et al. Effects assessment of persistent organohalogen contaminants in Arctic wildlife and fish. Sci Total Environ. 2010;408:2995–3043.
8. Sonne C. Health effects from long-range transported contaminants in Arctic top predators: an integrated review based on studies of polar bears and relevant model species. Environ Int. 2010;36:461–91.
9. Muir DCG, de Wit CA. Trends of legacy and new persistent organic pollutants in the circumpolar Arctic: overview, conclusions, and recommendations. Sci Total Environ. 2010;408:3044–51.
10. Dietz R, Outridge PM, Hobson KA. Anthropogenic contribution to mercury levels in present-day Arctic animals—a review. Sci Total Environ. 2009;407:6120–31.
11. Dietz R, Basu N, Braune B, O'Hara T, Letcher R, Scheuhammer T, et al. What are the toxicological effects of mercury in Arctic biota? Sci Total Environ. 2013;443:775–90.
12. Dietz R, Rigét FF, Sonne C, Born EW, Bechshøft T, McKinney MA, et al. Part 2: three decades (1984–2010) of flame retardant trends in East Greenland polar bears (*Ursus maritimus*). Environ Int. 2013;59:494–500.
13. Letcher RJ, Morris AD, Dyck M, Sverko E, Reiner E, Blair DAD, et al. Legacy and (re)emerging halogenated persistent organic pollutants in polar bears from a contamination hotspot in the Arctic, Hudson Bay Canada. Sci Total Environ. 2018;610–611:121–36.
14. Rigét F, Vorkamp K, Bossi R, Sonne C, Letcher RJ, Dietz R. Twenty years of monitoring of persistent organic pollutants in Greenland biota. A review. Environ Pollut. 2016;217:114–23.
15. Pedro S, Boba C, Dietz R, Sonne C, Rosing-Asvid A, Hansen M, et al. Blubber-depth distribution and bioaccumulation of PCBs and organochlorine pesticides in Arctic-invading killer whales. Sci Total Environ. 2017;601–602:237–46.
16. Butt CM, Berger U, Bossi R, Tomy GT. Levels and trends of poly- and perfluorinated compounds in the Arctic environment. Sci Total Environ. 2010;408:2936–65.
17. Houde M, De Silva AO, Muir DCG, Letcher RJ. Monitoring of perfluorinated compounds in aquatic biota: an updated review. Environ Sci Technol. 2011;45:7962–73.
18. Bechshøft TØ, Jakobsen J, Sonne C, Dietz R. Distribution of vitamin A (retinol) and E (α-tocopherol) in polar bear kidney: implications for biomarker studies. Sci Total Environ. 2011;409:3508–11.
19. Bechshøft TØ, Sonne C, Jakobsen J, Rigét FF, Born EW, Letcher RJ, et al. Vitamins A and E in liver, kidney, and whole blood from organohalogen exposed East Greenland polar bears sampled 1994–2008: reference values and temporal trends. Polar Biol. 2016;39:743–54.
20. Kirkegaard M, Sonne C, Dietz R, Jenssen BM, Letcher RJ. Organohalogens in a whale blubber supplemented diet reduce hepatic retinol and renal tocopherol concentrations in Greenland sled dogs. J Toxicol Environ Health Part A. 2010;73:773–86.
21. Kirkegaard M, Sonne C, Dietz R, Jenssen BM, Leifsson PS, Jensen JEB, et al. Testosterone concentrations and male genital organ morphology in Greenland sled dogs (*Canis familiaris*) dietary exposed to organohalogen contaminants. Toxicol Environ Chem. 2010;92:955–67.
22. Sonne C, Kirkegaard M, Jacobsen J, Jenssen BM, Letcher RJ, Dietz R. Altered 25-hydroxyvitamin D3 in liver tissue from Greenland sledge dogs (*Canis familiaris*) dietary exposed to organohalogen polluted minke whale (*Balaenoptera acuterostrata*) blubber. Ecotoxicol Environ Saf. 2014;104:403–8.
23. Sonne C, Dietz R, Rigét FF, Letcher RJ, Munk Pedersen K, Styrishave B. Steroid hormones in blood plasma from Greenland sledge dogs (*Canis familiaris*) dietary exposed to organohalogen polluted minke whale (*Balaenoptera acuterostrata*) blubber. Toxicol Environ Chem. 2014;96:273–86.
24. Sonne C, Andersen-Ranberg E, Rajala EL, Agerholm JS, Bonefeld-Jørgensen E, Desforges JP, et al. Prevalence of antibodies against *Brucella* spp. in West Greenland polar bears (*Ursus maritimus*) and East Greenland muskoxen (*Ovibos moschatus*). Polar Biol **(In review)**.
25. Sonne C, Andersen-Ranberg E, Rajala EL, Agerholm JS, Bonefeld-Jørgensen E, Desforges JP, et al. Seroprevalence for *Brucella* spp. in Baltic ringed seals (*Phoca hispida*) and East Greenland harp (*Pagophilus groenlandicus*) and hooded (*Cystophora cristata*) seals. Vet Immunol ImmunoPathol **(In review)**.
26. Brown TM, Macdonald RW, Muir DCG, Letcher RJ. The distribution and trends of persistent organic pollutants and mercury in marine mammals from Canada's Eastern Arctic. Sci Total Environ. 2017;618:500–17. https://doi.org/10.1016/j.scitotenv.2017.11.052.
27. Dietz R, Gustavson K, Sonne C, Desforges JP, Rigét FF, McKinney MA, et al. Physiologically-based pharmacokinetic modelling of immune, reproductive and carcinogenic effects from contaminant exposure in polar bears (*Ursus maritimus*). Environ Res. 2015;140:45–55.
28. Landrigan PJ, Fuller R, Acosta NJR, Adeyi O, Arnold R, Basu N, et al. The lancet commission on pollution and health. 2017.
29. Grandjean P, Landrigan PJ. Developmental neurotoxicity of industrial chemicals. Lancet. 2006;368(9553):2167–78.
30. Jenssen BM, Dehli Villanger G, Gabrielsen KM, Bytingsvik J, Ciesielski TM, Sonne C, et al. Anthropogenic flank attack on polar bears: interacting consequences of climate warming and pollutant exposure. Front Ecol. 2015;3:1–7.
31.. Sonne C, Letcher RJ, Bechshøft TØ, Rigét FF, Muir DCG, Leifsson PS, et al. Two decades of biomonitoring polar bear health in Greenland: a review. Acta Vet Scan. 2012;54:S15.
32. Polischuk SC, Norstrom RJ, Ramsay MA. Body burdens and tissue concentrations of organochlorines in polar bears (*Ursus maritimus*) vary during seasonal fasts. Environ Pollut. 2002;118:29–39.
33. Tartu S, Bourgeon S, Aars J, Andersen M, Polder A, Thiemann GW, Welker JM, Routti H. Sea ice-associated decline in body condition leads to increased concentrations of lipophilic pollutants in polar bears (*Ursus maritimus*) from Svalbard, Norway. Sci Total Environ. 2017;576:409–19.
34. Bytingsvik J, Lie E, Aars J, Derocher AE, Wiig Ø, Jenssen BM. PCBs and OH-PCBs in polar bear mother-cub pairs: a comparative plasma levels in 1998 and 2008. Sci Total Environ. 2012;417:117–28.
35. Dietz R, Rigét FF, Sonne C, Letcher RJ, Born EW, Muir DCG. Seasonal and temporal trends in polychlorinated biphenyls and organochlorine pesticides in East Greenland polar bears (*Ursus maritimus*), 1990–2001. Sci Total Environ. 2004;331:107–24.

36. Dietz R, Rigét FF, Sonne C, Muir DCG, Backus S, Born EW, et al. Age and seasonal variability of polybrominated diphenyl ethers in free-ranging East Greenland polar bears (*Ursus maritimus*). Environ Pollut. 2007;146:177–84.
37. Muir DCG, Backus S, Derocher AE, Dietz R, Evans TJ, Gabrielsen GW, et al. Brominated flame retardants in polar bears (*Ursus maritimus*) from Alaska, the Canadian Arctic, East Greenland, and Svalbard. Environ Sci Technol. 2006;40:449–55.
38. Nuijten RJM, Hendriks AJ, Jenssen BM, Schipper AM. Circumpolar contaminant concentrations in polar bears (*Ursus maritimus*) and potential population-level effects. Environ Res. 2016;151:50–7.
39. Pavlova V, Grimm V, Dietz R, Sonne C, Vorkamp K, Rigét FF, et al. Modelling population level effects of PCB contamination in East Greenland polar bears. Arch Environ Contam Toxicol. 2016;70:143–54.
40. Pavlova V, Nabe-Nielsen J, Dietz R, Sonne C, Grimm V. PCB contamination as a potential driver of mate—finding associated Allee effect in Svalbard polar bears: the implications from an individual based model. Proc Biol Sci. 2016;283:1843.
41. AMAP. Arctic Monitoring and Assessment Programme: AMAP assessment 2018—persistent organic pollutants in the Arctic 2018; Oslo 2018. http://www.amap.no.
42. Dietz R, Rigét FF, Sonne C, Born EW, Bechshøft T, McKinney MA, Letcher RJ. Part 1: three decades (1984–2010) of legacy contaminant trends in East Greenland polar bears (*Ursus maritimus*). Environ Int. 2013;59:485–93.
43. Lindh CH, Rylander L, Toft G, Axmon A, Rignell-Hydbom A, Giwercman A, et al. Blood serum concentrations of perfluorinated compounds in men from Greenlandic Inuit and European populations. Chemosphere. 2012;88:1269–75.
44. Sonne C, Dietz R, Letcher RJ. Chemical cocktail party in East Greenland: a first time evaluation of human organohalogen exposure from consumption of ringed seal and polar bear tissues and possible health implications. Toxicol Environ Chem. 2013;95:853–9.
45. Wielsoe M, Kern P, Bonefeld-Jorgensen EC. Serum levels of environmental pollutants is a risk factor for breast cancer in Inuit: a case control study. Environ Health. 2017;16:16.
46. Deutch B, Dyerberg J, Pedersen HS, Asmund G, Møller P, Hansen JC. Dietary composition and contaminants in north Greenland, in the 1970s and 2004. Sci Total Environ. 2006;370:372–81.
47. Johansen P, Muir DCG, Asmund G, Rigét FF. Human exposure to contaminants in the traditional Greenland diet. Sci Total Environ. 2004;331:189–206.
48. Nielsen E, Larsen JC, Ladefoged O. Risk assessment of contaminant intake from traditional Greenland food items. Danish Veterinary and Food Administration; 2006. p. 180. http://www.dfvf.dk.
49. AMAP. Arctic Monitoring and Assessment Programme: AMAP assessment 2011—mercury in the Arctic 2011; Oslo 2011. http://www.amap.no.
50. Bonefeld-Jørgensen E. Biomonitoring in Greenland: human biomarkers of exposure and effects—a short review. Rural Remote Health. 2010;10:1362.
51. Sonne C, Gustavson K, Rigét FF, Krüger T, Dietz R, Bonefeld-Jørgensen E. Physiologically based pharmacokinetic modeling of contaminants in Greenlanders: a new tool for monitoring levels and possible health effects? Environ Int. 2014;64:91–7.
52. Polder A, Gabrielsen GW, Odland JØ, Savinova TN, Tkachev A, Løken KB, Skaare JU. Spatial and temporal changes of chlorinated pesticides, PCBs, dioxins (PCDDs/PCDFs) and brominated flame retardants in human breast milk from northern Russia. Sci Total Environ. 2008;391:41–54.
53. Bonefeld-Jørgensen E, Long M, Bossi R, Ayotte P, Asmund G, Krüger T, et al. Perfluorinated compounds are related to breast cancer risk in Greenlandic Inuit: a case control study. Environ Health. 2011;10:88.
54. Grandjean P, Andersen EW, Budtz-Jørgensen E, Nielsen F, Mølbak K, Weihe P, et al. Serum vaccine antibody concentrations in children exposed to perfluorinated compounds. JAMA. 2012;307:391–7.
55. Long M, Bossi R, Bonefeld-Jørgensen EC. Levels and temporal trends of perfluoroalkyl acids in human serum from Greenland Inuit. Int J Circumpolar Health. 2012;71:17998.
56. Rand AA, Mabury SA. Is there a human health risk associated with indirect exposure to perfluoroalkyl carboxylates (PFCAs)? Toxicology. 2017;375:28–36.
57. Wilkinson JL, Hooda PS, Barker J, Barton S, Swinden J. Ecotoxic pharmaceuticals, personal care products, and other emerging contaminants: a review of environmental, receptor-mediated, developmental, and epigenetic toxicity with discussion of proposed toxicity to humans. Crit Rev Environ Sci Technol. 2016;46:336–81.
58. Sonne C, Leifsson PS, Dietz R, Born EW, Letcher RJ, Kirkegaard M, et al. Enlarged clitoris in wild polar bears (*Ursus maritimus*) can be misdiagnosed as pseudohermaphroditism. Sci Total Environ. 2005;337:45–58.
59. Grandjean P, Satoh H, Murata K, Eto K. Adverse effects of methylmercury: environmental health research implications. Environ Health Perspect. 2010;118:1137–45.
60. Dietz R, Born EW, Rigét FF, Aubail A, Sonne C, Drimmei RC, et al. Temporal trends and future predictions of mercury concentrations in Northwest Greenland polar bear (*Ursus maritimus*) hair. Environ Sci Technol. 2011;45:1458–65.
61. McKinney MA, Iverson SJ, Fisk AT, Sonne C, Rigét FF, Letcher RJ, et al. Global change effects on the long-term feeding ecology and contaminant exposures of East Greenland polar bears. Glob Change Biol. 2013;19:2360–72.
62. Letcher RJ, Boisvert G, Dyck M, Sonne C, Dietz R. Polar bears from two Arctic pollution hot spots: Comparison of recent levels of established and new perfluorinated sulfonic and carboxylic acids and precursors. Sci Total Environ. 2017 **(In review)**.
63. Rigét FF, Braune B, Bignert A, Wilson S, Aars J, Andersen M, et al. Temporal trends of Hg in Arctic biota, an update. Sci Total Environ. 2011;409:3520–6.
64. Rigét FF, Bossi R, Sonne C, Vorkamp K, Dietz R. Trends of perfluorochemicals in Greenland ringed seals and polar bears: indications of decreasing trends. Chemosphere. 2013;93:1607–14.
65. Pertoldi C, Sonne C, Wiig Ø, Baagøe HJ, Loeschcke V, Bechshøft TØ. East Greenland and Barents Sea polar bears (*Ursus maritimus*): adaptive variation between two populations using skull morphometrics as an indicator of gene flow. Hereditas. 2012;149:99–107.
66. Sonne C, Dyck M, Rigét FF, Bech-Jensen JE, Hyldstrup L, Letcher RJ, et al. Penile density and globally used chemicals in Canadian and Greenland polar bears. Environ Res. 2015;137:287–91.
67. Andersen-Ranberg. Metals and flukes in West Greenland ringed seals (*Pusa hispida*)—a histopathological, toxicological, parasitological and molecular study. M.Sc. thesis 2014, University of Copenhagen; p. 109.
68. Sonne-Hansen C, Dietz R, Leifsson PS, Hyldstrup L, Rigét FF. Cadmium toxicity to ringed seals (*Phoca hispida*)—an epidemiological study of possible cadmium induced nephropathy and osteodystrophy in ringed seals (*Phoca hispida*) from Qaanaaq in Northwest Greenland. Sci Total Environ. 2002;295:167–81.
69. Woshner VM. Concentrations and interactions of selected elements in tissues of four marine mammal species harvested by Inuit hunters in arctic Alaska, with an intensive histologic assessment, emphasizing the beluga whale. University of Illinois at Urbana—Champaign 2000; Urbana, Illinois 2000, Ph.D. Dissertation.
70. Woshner VM, O'Hara TM, Bratton GR, Suydam RS, Beasley VR. Concentrations and interactions of selected essential and non-essential elements in bowhead and beluga whales of Arctic Alaska. J Wildl Dis. 2001;37:693–710.
71. Woshner VM, O'Hara TM, Bratton GR, Beasley VR. Concentrations and interactions of selected essential and non-essential elements in ringed seals and polar bears of Arctic Alaska. J Wildl Dis. 2001;37:711–21.
72. Woshner VM, Knott K, Wells R, Willetto C, Swor R, O'Hara T. Mercury and selenium in blood and epidermis of bottlenose dolphins (*Tursiops truncatus*) from Sarasota Bay, FL: interaction and relevance to life history and hematologic parameters. EcoHealth. 2008;5:1–11.
73. Donaldson SG, Van Oostdam J, Tikhonov C, Feeley M, Armstrong B, Ayotte P, et al. Environmental contaminants and human health in the Canadian Arctic. Sci Total Environ. 2010;408:5165–234.
74. Gebbink WA, Sonne C, Dietz R, Kirkegaard M, Rigét FF, Born EW, et al. Tissue-specific congener composition of organohalogen and metabolite contaminants in East Greenland polar bears (*Ursus maritimus*). Environ Pollut. 2008;152:621–9.

75. Lagueux J, Pereg D, Ayotte P, Dewailly E, Poirier GG. Cytochrome P450 CYP1A1 enzyme activity and DNA adducts in placenta of women environmentally exposed to organochlorines. Environ Res. 1999;80:369–82.
76. Medehouenou TC, Larochelle C, Dumas P, Dewailly E, Ayotte P. Determinants of AhR-mediated transcriptional activity induced by plasma extracts from Nunavik Inuit adults. Chemosphere. 2010;80:75–82.
77. Sandau CD, Ayotte P, Dewailly E, Duffe J, Norstrom RJ. Pentachlorophenol and hydroxylated polychlorinated biphenyl metabolites in umbilical cord plasma of neonates from coastal populations in Québec. Environ Health Perspect. 2002;110:411–7.
78. Sonne C, Dietz R, Born EW, Rigét FF, Kirkegaard M, Hyldstrup L, et al. Is bone mineral composition disrupted by organochlorines in East Greenland polar bears (*Ursus maritimus*)? Environ Health Perspect. 2004;112:1711–6.
79. Herlin M, Kalantari F, Stern N, Sand S, Larsson S, Viluksela M, et al. Quantitative characterization of changes in bone geometry, mineral density and bio-mechanical properties in two rat strains with different Ah-receptor structures after long-term exposure to 2,3,7,8-tetrachlorodibenzo-*p*-dioxin. Toxicology. 2010;29:1–11.
80. Lind PM, Bergman A, Olsson M, Orberg J. Bone mineral density in male Baltic grey seal (*Halichoerus grypus*). Ambio. 2003;32:385–8.
81. Lind PM, Milnes MR, Lundberg R, Bermudez D, Örberg J, Guillette LJ. Abnormal bone composition in female juvenile American alligators from a pesticide-polluted lake (Lake Apopka, Florida). Environ Health Perspect. 2004;112:359–62.
82. Côté S, Ayotte P, Dodin S, Blanchet C, Mulvad G, Petersen HS, et al. Plasma organochlorine concentrations and bone ultrasound measurements: a cross-sectional study in peri-and postmenopausal Inuit women from Greenland. Environ Health. 2006;5:33.
83. Paunescu AC, Dewailly E, Dodin S, Nieboer E, Ayotte P. Dioxin-like compounds and bone quality in Cree women of Eastern James Bay (Canada): a cross-sectional study. Environ Health. 2013;12:54.
84. Sonne C, Letcher RJ, Jenssen BM, Desforges JP, Eulaers I, Andersen-Ranberg E, et al. Use of dogs to monitor remote locations: sledge dogs and the Artic environment. Springer Book **(In review)**.
85. Dallaire R, Dewailly E, Ayotte P, Muckle G, Laliberte C, Bruneau S. Effects of prenatal exposure to organochlorines on thyroid hormone status in newborns from two remote coastal regions in Quebec, Canada. Environ Res. 2008;108:387–92.
86. Gustavson L, Ciesielski TM, Bytingsvik J, Styrishave B, Hansen M, Lie E, et al. Hydroxylated polychlorinated biphenyls decrease circulating steroids in female polar bears (*Ursus maritimus*). Environ Res. 2015;138:191–201.
87. Ciesielski TM, Hansen IT, Bytingsvik J, Hansen M, Lie E, Aars J, et al. Relationships between POPs, biometrics and circulating steroids in male polar bears (*Ursus maritimus*) from Svalbard. Environ Pollut. 2017;230:598–608.
88. Sonne C, Leifsson PS, Dietz R, Born EW, Letcher RJ, Hyldstrup L, et al. Xenoendocrine pollutants may reduce size of sexual organs in East Greenland polar bears (*Ursus maritimus*). Environ Sci Technol. 2006;40:5668–74.
89. Desforges JPW, Sonne C, Levin M, Siebert U, De Guise S, Dietz R. Immunotoxic effects of environmental pollutants in marine mammals. Environ Int. 2016;86:126–39.
90. Sonne C, Torjesen PA, Berg KA, Fuglei E, Muir DCG, Jenssen BM, et al. Exposure to persistent organic pollutants reduces testosterone concentrations and affects sperm viability and morphology during the mating peak-period in a controlled experiment on farmed Arctic foxes (*Vulpes lagopus*). Environ Sci Technol. 2017;51:4673–80.
91. Janeway CA, Travers P, Walport M, Shlomchik M. Immune biology—the immune system in health and disease. 5th ed. New York: Garland Publishing, Taylor and Francis; 2001. p. 732.
92. Vos JG, Luster MI. Immune alterations. In: Kimbrough RD, Jensen AD, editors. Halogenated biphenyls, terphenyls, naphthalenes, dibenzodioxins, and related products. Amsterdam: Elsevier; 1989.
93. Hertz-Picciotto I, Park HY, Dostal M, Kocan A, Trnovec T, Sram R. Prenatal exposures to persistent and non-persistent organic compounds and effects on immune system development. Basic Clin Pharmacol Toxicol. 2008;102:146–54.
94. Klecha AJ, Barreiro Arcos ML, Frick L, Genaro AM, Cremaschi G. Immune-endocrine interactions in autoimmune thyroid diseases. Neuroimmunomodulation. 2008;15:68–75.
95. Tryphonas H. Immunotoxicity of polychlorinated-biphenyls—present status and future considerations. Exp Clin Immunogenet. 1994;11:149–62.
96. Lie E, Larsen HJS, Larsen S, Johansen GM, Derocher AE, Lunn NJ, et al. Does high organochlorine (OC) exposure impair the resistance to infection in polar bears (*Ursus maritimus*)? Part I: effect of OCs on the humoral immunity. J Toxicol Environ Health A. 2004;67:555–82.
97. Lie E, Larsen HJS, Larsen S, Johansen GM, Derocher AE, Lunn NJ, et al. Does high organochlorine (OC) exposure impair the resistance to infection in polar bears (*Ursus maritimus*)? Part II: possible effect of OCs on mitogen- and antigen-induced lymphocyte proliferation. J Toxicol Environ Health A. 2005;68:457–84.
98. Routti H, Arukwe A, Jenssen BM, Letcher RJ, Nyman M, Bäckman C, et al. Comparative endocrine disruptive effects of contaminants in ringed seals (*Phoca hispida*) from Svalbard and the Baltic Sea. Comp Biochem Physiol C Toxicol Pharmacol. 2010;152:306–12.
99. Brown TM, Ross PS, Reimer KJ, Veldhoen N, Danger NJ, Fisk AT, et al. PCB related effects thresholds as derived through gene transcript profiles in locally contaminated ringed seals (*Pusa hispida*). Environ Sci Technol. 2014;48:12952–61.
100. Levin M, Gebhard E, Jasperse L, Desforges JP, Dietz R, Sonne C, et al. Immunomodulatory effects of exposure to polychlorinated biphenyls and perfluoroalkyl acids in East Greenland ringed seals (*Pusa hispida*). Environ Res. 2016;151:244–50.
101. Frouin H, Loseto LL, Stern G, Haulena M, Ross PS. Mercury toxicity in beluga whale lymphocytes: limited effects of selenium protection. Aquat Toxicol. 2012;109:185–93.
102. Parkinson AJ. The Arctic human health initiative: a legacy of the international polar year 2007–2009. Int J Circumpolar Health. 2013;72:10.
103. Dallaire F, Dewailly E, Vézina C, Ayotte P, Muckle G, Bruneau S. Effect of prenatal exposure to polychlorinated biphenyls on incidence of acute respiratory infections in preschool Inuit children. Environ Health Perspect. 2006;114:1301–5.
104. Dewailly É, Ayotte P, Bruneau S, Laliberté C, Gingras S, Belles-Isles M, et al. Susceptibility to infections and immune status in Inuit infants exposed to organochlorines. Environ Health Perspect. 2000;108:205–11.
105. Dallaire R, Dewailly E, Ayotte P, Forget-Dubois N, Jacobson SW, Jacobson JL, et al. Growth in Inuit children exposed to polychlorinated biphenyls and lead during fetal development and childhood. Environ Res. 2014;134:17–23.
106. Weisglas-Kuperus N. Neurodevelopmental, immunological and endocrinological indices of perinatal human exposure to PCBs and dioxins. Chemosphere. 1998;37:1845–53.
107. Grandjean P, Landrigan PJ. Neurobehavioural effects of developmental toxicity. Lancet. 2014;13:330–8.
108. Greaves AK, Letcher RJ, Sonne C, Dietz R, Born EW. Tissue-specific concentrations and patterns of perfluoroalkyl carboxylates and sulfonates in East Greenland polar bears. Environ Sci Technol. 2012;46:11575–83.
109. Greaves AK, Letcher RJ, Sonne C, Dietz R. Brain region distribution and patterns of bioaccumulative perfluoroalkyl carboxylates and sulfonates in East Greenland polar bears (*Ursus maritimus*). Environ Toxicol Chem. 2013;32:713–22.
110. Krey A, Kwan M, Chan HM. Mercury speciation in brain tissue of polar bears (*Ursus maritimus*) from the Canadian Arctic. Environ Res. 2012;114:24–30.
111. Pedersen KE, Basu N, Letcher RJ, Greaves AK, Sonne C, Dietz R, et al. Brain region-specific perfluoroalkylated sulfonate (PFSA) and carboxylic acid (PFCA) accumulation and neurochemical biomarker responses in East Greenland polar bears (*Ursus maritimus*). Environ Res. 2015;138:22–31.
112. Pedersen KE, Basu N, Letcher RJ, Sonne C, Dietz R, Styrishave B. Per- and polyfluoroalkyl substances (PFASs)—new endocrine disruptors in polar bears (*Ursus maritimus*)? Environ Int. 2016;138:22–31.
113. Fonnum F, Mariussen E. Mechanisms involved in the neurotoxic effects of environmental toxicants such as polychlorinated biphenyls and brominated flame retardants. J Neurochem. 2009;111:1327–47.

114. Mariussen E. Neurotoxic effects of perfluoroalkylated compounds: mechanisms of action and environmental relevance. Arch Toxicol. 2012;86:1349–67.
115. Bollati V, Baccarelli A. Environmental epigenetics. Heredity. 2010;105:105–12.
116. Crews D. Epigenetic modifications of brain and behavior: theory and practice. Horm Behav. 2011;59:393–8.
117. Mill J, Petronis A. Pre- and peri-natal environmental risks for attention-deficit hyperactivity disorder (ADHD): the potential role of epigenetic processes in mediating susceptibility. J Child Psychol Psychiatry. 2008;49:1020–30.
118. Basu N, Scheuhammer AM, Sonne C, Dietz R, Letcher RJ. Is mercury in the environment of neurotoxic concern to polar bears? Environ Toxicol Chem. 2009;28:133–40.
119. Pilsner JR, Lazarus AL, Nam D, Letcher RJ, Scheuhammer T, Sonne C, et al. Mercury-associated DNA hypomethylation in polar bear brains via the LUminometric Methylation Assay (LUMA): a sensitive method to study epigenetics in wildlife. Mol Ecol. 2010;19:307–14.
120. Siegel GJ, Albers RW, Brady ST, Price DL. Basic neurochemistry. Molecular, cellular and medical aspects. 7th ed. Burlington: Elsevier Academic; 2006.
121. Ahmed EI, Zehr JL, Schulz KM, Lorenz BH, Don Carlos LL, Sisk CL. Pubertal hormones modulate the addition of new cells to sexually dimorphic brain regions. Nat Neurosci. 2008;11:995–7.
122. Zoeller RT, Crofton KM. Mode of action: developmental thyroid hormone insufficiency—neurological abnormalities resulting from exposure to propylthiouracil. Crit Rev Toxicol. 2005;35:771–81.
123. Bytingsvik J, Simon E, Leonards PEG, Lamoree M, Lie E, Aars J, et al. Transthyretin-binding activity of contaminants in blood from polar bear (*Ursus maritimus*) cubs. Environ Sci Technol. 2013;47:4778–86.
124. Simon E, van Velzen M, Brandsma SH, Lie E, Løken K, de Boer J, et al. Effect-directed analysis to explore the polar bear exposome: identification of thyroid hormone disrupting compounds in plasma. Environ Sci Technol. 2013;47:8902–12.
125. Rodier PM. Developing brain as a target of toxicity. Environ Health Perspect. 1995;103:73–6.
126. McKinney MA, Pedro S, Dietz R, Sonne C, Fisk AT, Roy D, et al. A review of ecological impacts of global climate change on persistent organic pollutant and mercury pathways and exposures in arctic marine ecosystems. Curr Zool. 2015;61:617–28.
127. Burek KA, Gulland FMD, O'Hara TM. Effects of climate change on Arctic marine mammal health. Ecol Appl. 2008;18:S126–34.
128. Harvell CD, Mitchell CE, Ward JR, Altizer S, Dobson AP, Ostfeld RS, et al. Climate warming and disease risks for terrestrial and marine biota. Science. 2002;296:2158–62.
129. Dudley JP, Hoberg EP, Jenkins EJ, Parkinson AJ. Climate change in the North American Arctic: a One Health perspective. EcoHealth. 2015;12:713–25.
130. Bradley M, Kutz SJ, Jenkins E, O'Hara TM. The potential impact of climate change on infectious diseases of Arctic fauna. Int J Circumpolar Health. 2005;64:468–77.
131. Greer A, Ng V, Fisman D. Climate change and infectious diseases in North America: the road ahead. CMAJ. 2008;178:715–22.
132. Jenkins EJ, Castrodale LJ, de Rosemond SJ, Dixon BR, Elmore SA, Gesy KM, et al. Tradition and transition: parasitic zoonoses of people and animals in Alaska, northern Canada, and Greenland. Adv Parasitol. 2013;82:33–204.
133. Derocher AE, Aars J, Amstrup SC, Cutting A, Lunn NJ, Molnár PK, et al. Rapid ecosystem change and polar bear conservation. Conserv Lett. 2013;6:368–75.
134. Durner GM, Douglas DC, Nielson RM, Amstrup SC, McDonald TL, Stirling I, et al. Predicting 21st-century polar bear habitat distribution from global climate models. Ecol Monogr. 2009;79:25–58.
135. Molnár PK, Derocher AE, Klanjscek T, Lewis MA. Predicting climate change impacts on polar bear litter size. Nat Commun. 2011;2:186.
136. Hamilton SG, de la Guardia LC, Derocher AE, Sahanatien V, Tremblay B, Huard D. Projected polar bear sea ice habitat in the Canadian Arctic Archipelago. PLoS ONE. 2014;9:e113746.
137. Amstrup SC, Marcot BG, Douglas DC. A Bayesian network modeling approach to forecasting the 21st century worldwide status of polar bears. In: DeWeaver ET, Bitz CM, Tremblay L-B, editors. Arctic sea ice decline: observations, projections, mechanisms, and implications, vol. 180. Washington, DC: American Geophysical Union; 2018. p. 213–68.
138. Olsen GH, Mauritzen M, Derocher AE, Sørmo EG, Skaare JU, Wiig O, et al. Space-use strategy is an important determinant of PCB concentrations in female polar bears in the Barents Sea. Environ Sci Technol. 2003;37:4919–24.
139. van Beest FM, Aars J, Routti H, Lie E, Andersen M, Pavlova V, Sonne C, et al. Spatiotemporal variation in home range size of female polar bears and correlations with individual contaminant load. Polar Biol. 2016;39:1479–89.
140. McKinney MA, Peacock E, Letcher RJ. Sea ice-associated diet change increases the levels of chlorinated and brominated contaminants in polar bears. Environ Sci Technol. 2009;43:4334–9.
141. Gormezano LJ, Rockwell RF. What to eat now? Shifts in polar bear diet during the ice-free season in western Hudson Bay. Ecol Evol. 2013;3:3509–23.
142. Iles DT, Petersen SL, Gormezano LJ, Koons DN, Rockwell RF. Terrestrial predation by polar bears: not just a wild goose chase. Polar Biol. 2013;36:1373–9.
143. Iverson SA, Gilchrist HG, Smith PA, Gaston AJ, Forbes MR. Longer ice-free seasons increase the risk of nest depredation by polar bears for colonial breeding birds in the Canadian Arctic. Proc R Soc B. 2014;281:20133128.
144. MacKenzie BR, Payne MR, Boje J, Hoyer JL, Siegstad H. A cascade of warming impacts brings bluefin tuna to Greenland waters. Glob Chang Biol. 2014;20:2484–91.
145. Valdimarsson H, Astthorsson OS, Palsson J. Hydrographic variability in Icelandic waters during recent decades and related changes in distribution of some fish species. ICES J Mar Sci. 2012;69:816–25.
146. Carrie J, Wang F, Sanei H, Macdonald RW, Outridge PM, Stern GA. Increasing contaminant burdens in an arctic fish, burbot (*Lota lota*), in a warming climate. Environ Sci Technol. 2010;44:316–22.
147. Macdonald RW, Harner T, Fyfe J. Recent climate change in the Arctic and its impact on contaminant pathways and interpretation of temporal trend data. Sci Total Environ. 2005;342:5–86.
148. IOM. Global climate change and extreme weather events: understanding the contributions to infectious disease emergency. Washington, DC: The National Academic Press, Institute of Medicine; 2008. p. 280.
149. Parkinson AJ, Butler JC. Potential impacts of climate change on infectious diseases in the Arctic. Int J Circumpolar Health. 2005;64:478–86.
150. Tryland M, Nesbakken T, Robertson L, Grahek-Ogden D, Lunestad BT. Human pathogens in marine mammal meat—a northern perspective. Zoonoses Publ Health. 2013;61:377–94.
151. Jenssen BM. Marine pollution: the future challenge is to link human and wildlife studies. Environ Health Perspect. 2003;111:A198–9.
152. Jenssen BM. Endocrine-disrupting chemicals and climate change: a worst-case combination for Arctic marine mammals and seabirds? Environ Health Perspect. 2006;114:76–80.
153. Weihe P, Debes F, Halling J, Petersen MS, Muckle G, Odland JØ, et al. Health effects associated with measured levels of contaminants in the Arctic. Int J Circumpolar Health. 2016;75:33805.

Protective role of the vulture facial skin and gut microbiomes aid adaptation to scavenging

Marie Lisandra Zepeda Mendoza[1], Michael Roggenbuck[2], Karla Manzano Vargas[1,3], Lars Hestbjerg Hansen[4], Søren Brunak[5,6], M. Thomas P. Gilbert[1,7] and Thomas Sicheritz-Pontén[1,5,8*]

Abstract

Background: Vultures have adapted the remarkable ability to feed on carcasses that may contain microorganisms that would be pathogenic to most other animals. The holobiont concept suggests that the genetic basis of such adaptation may not only lie within their genomes, but additionally in their associated microbes. To explore this, we generated shotgun DNA sequencing datasets of the facial skin and large intestine microbiomes of the black vulture (*Coragyps atratus*) and the turkey vulture (*Cathartes aura*). We characterized the functional potential and taxonomic diversity of their microbiomes, the potential pathogenic challenges confronted by vultures, and the microbial taxa and genes that could play a protective role on the facial skin and in the gut.

Results: We found microbial taxa and genes involved in diseases, such as dermatitis and pneumonia (more abundant on the facial skin), and gas gangrene and food poisoning (more abundant in the gut). Interestingly, we found taxa and functions with potential for playing beneficial roles, such as antilisterial bacteria in the gut, and genes for the production of antiparasitics and insecticides on the facial skin. Based on the identified phages, we suggest that phages aid in the control and possibly elimination, as in phage therapy, of microbes reported as pathogenic to a variety of species. Interestingly, we identified *Adineta vaga* in the gut, an invertebrate that feeds on dead bacteria and protozoans, suggesting a defensive predatory mechanism. Finally, we suggest a colonization resistance role through biofilm formation played by Fusobacteria and Clostridia in the gut.

Conclusions: Our results highlight the importance of complementing genomic analyses with metagenomics in order to obtain a clearer understanding of the host-microbial alliance and show the importance of microbiome-mediated health protection for adaptation to extreme diets, such as scavenging.

Keywords: Colonization resistance, Diet specialization, Metagenomics, Microbiome, Pathogens, Scavenging, Vulture

Background

Vultures are composed of two clades of carrion-scavenging birds that diverged more than 60 million years ago [1], the New World vultures (Cathartidae) and Old World vultures (Accipitridae). Vultures global populations are under serious threats due to e.g. collisions with wind-energy turbines [2], their use for traditional medicine [3], or ingestion of lead bullets from deer carcasses [4]. Vultures are known as "nature's clean-up crew", as they feed on tissues of animals that have died mainly from malnutrition, accidents, predation, and diseases [5–7]. Vultures are thus exposed to a variety of pathogens, including those that cause anthrax, tuberculosis, and brucellosis. A better understanding of various aspects for their biology are necessary, such as their susceptibility to the pathogens in their diet and their role in the transmission of infectious diseases [8, 9].

Vertebrate carcasses are very nutrient-rich resources. It has been speculated that the release of toxins and pathogenicity genes in the carcass microbiome are part of a

*Correspondence: thomassp@snm.ku.dk
[1] Centre for GeoGenetics, Natural History Museum of Denmark, University of Copenhagen, Øster Voldgade 5-7, 1350 Copenhagen K, Denmark
Full list of author information is available at the end of the article

microbial strategy for outcompeting other microbes [10, 11]. The main colonizers of a carcass are microbes originating from the microbiome of the animal when alive, some of which might become pathogenic in the carcass environment [12]. Other components of the post-mortem microbiome include soil-dwelling bacteria, nematodes, fungi, and insects [13]. In spite of the potentially serious health implications posed by their consumption, the pathogenic repertoire of the gut of these birds has not been fully characterized in relation to their possible implications in the environment. Thus, one of the most intriguing aspects of vulture biology is how they protect themselves against the health challenges posed by their dietary source. Physiologic, genetic and genomic analyses of different species of vultures have explored this aspect and identified genes associated with respiration, immunity, and gastric secretion as possible adaptations to its scavenging diet [14, 15]. For example, due to the previously reported very low stomach pH of a small sample of Old World vulture species [16], it has been suggested that the vulture stomach acidity serves as a filter of potential pathogens [14, 17].

With the genomic revolution, it has become apparent that besides genomic changes, host-associated microbiota plays an important role in diet specialization across vertebrates [18] and that the gut microbiome may play a highly relevant yet unexplored role in diet-driven speciation [19]. The gut microbiome is intimately related to digestion functions, such as energy harvest, nutrient acquisition, and intestinal homeostasis [20]. It has also been shown that the microbiome plays a health protective role to the host by interacting with the host's immune system and mediating colonization-resistance against pathogens [21, 22]. Furthermore, disorders in the microbiome can lead to diseases such as irritable bowel syndrome, inflammatory bowel disease, obesity, and diabetes [23–25]. In light of the key roles that host-microbiome relationships can play in adaptation, it has been acknowledged that vulture genomic adaptations alone may not provide the full answer to the vulture adaptation to scavenging [14]. However, neither the complete microbial taxonomic diversity (including non-bacterial microbes) nor the gene catalogue of the microbiome of any vulture species has been examined for their protective role against microbes that would normally pose serious health risks for other non-scavenging vertebrate species.

In order to evaluate the protective role of the vulture's facial skin and gut microbiome, we generated metagenomic datasets from facial skin swabs and gut samples for two species of New World vultures, the black vulture (*Coragyps atratus*) and the turkey vulture (*Cathartes aura*), and performed taxonomic and functional metagenomic analyses.

Methods

Sampling method and DNA sequencing

We generated DNA shotgun metagenome datasets from a subset of the samples used by Roggenbuck et al. [17]. Samples were collected over a period of several days in Tennessee, USA. Black vultures were live-trapped at deer carcasses and then transported to a central facility within a couple of hours of trapping. They were then euthanized with CO_2, necropsied, and sampled within 30–45 min of death. Turkey vultures were shot at roosts, bagged individually, and transported to the processing facility where they were refrigerated 2–6 h before necropsy and sampling. To collect the gut samples, carcasses were opened to expose the entire gastrointestinal tract. A section of around 3–4 cm of the large intestine (hereafter called gut) located 2–3 cm above the cloaca was isolated with a pair of medical haemostats. Afterwards, 2–3 mL of sterile water was injected through the wall of the intestine with a sterile single-use syringe. The haemostat-blocked section of the intestine was gently massaged with the needle still inserted, and then the wash liquid was aspirated with the syringe. The aspirant was injected into a sterile vial containing RNAlater. Facial skin samples were taken by using sterile polyester swabs saturated with sterile water and wiped across the facial skin of the vultures. Swab tips were cut off and immersed in sterile vials filled with RNAlater. DNA was extracted and the shotgun libraries for HiSeq PE 100 were prepared using the Nextera library building kit following the manufacturer's instructions, as in Roggenbuck et al. [17]. From the total of 48 different sampled individuals (25 black vultures, and 23 turkey vultures), we used 33 facial skin samples (17 black vultures; 16 turkey vultures) and 47 intestinal samples (25 black vultures; 22 turkey vultures).

Data processing

Two pipelines were used to process the raw reads. In the first approach, we removed adapter sequences and bases with quality <15 using Trimmomatic v0.32 [26]. Afterwards, in order to filter out non-bacterial reads derived from the vulture, human, and *Phi* phage (used as control required to increase library complexity on the Illumina HiSeq), the datasets were mapped against the bird genomes dataset of the avian phylogenomic project [27] (which includes the turkey vulture genome), the human (hg19), and the *Phi* phage genomes. Only the non-mapping reads were retained. The second approach was developed to take into account possible *k*-mer bias in the first bases of the reads that could have implications in the subsequent de novo assembly and gene prediction. To this end, we trimmed the first 16 bases of the reads with Trimmomatic v0.32. We then processed those reads with a Metagenomics Assembly and Gene Prediction

Toolkit (MOCAT) [28] to clean them of low quality bases and adaptors and screen them versus the turkey vulture, human, and *Phi* phage genomes.

Taxonomic profiling

We used MGmapper [29] to map with bwa v0.7.10 [30] the filtered cleaned reads against the next databases in full mode: MetaHitAssembly [31], HumanMicrobiome [32], ResFinder [33], Plasmid, Virulence, GreenGenes [34], and Silva [35]. We also mapped in chain mode to the next whole genome databases downloaded from GenBank in the given order: human, plants, vertebrates, invertebrates, protozoa, fungi, and viruses. The remaining non-mapping reads were mapped to the whole genome databases of bacteria. Using the unique mapping reads, we calculated the coverage (percentage of reference sequence covered by reads) of the identified species. The coverage was then used to filter the identifications as follows.

1. Relaxed filtering: In order to ensure the identification of low abundant taxa, we removed identifications with 90% of the abundance signal coming from only three samples.
2. Strict filtering: On top of the relaxed filtering, we removed the species with a coverage lower than the 1st quartile (Qu) value from the coverage distribution of the corresponding database.

With the filtered taxa, we classified the species as present in at least 90% and 50% of all the samples, thus defining a strict and a relaxed, respectively, taxonomic microbiome core.

For each database, we compared the taxa present only in the facial skin or gut datasets, those present in both, and those in significant differential abundance (P value < 0.05). To identify the differentially abundant species, we performed Wilcoxon and t-tests on the normalized abundance distribution of the identified species in the facial skin dataset versus the gut dataset. We also evaluated the taxonomic intra and inter sample variation between the facial skin and gut samples by calculating the Euclidean distances of their normalized abundances using the Ward.D method in R [36].

We then used the identifications of the relaxed filtering to test for microbial abundance correlations by calculating the Spearman correlation for each pairwise comparison of the microbes and calculated the P with a Bonferroni correction on those with a correlation value > 0.8 and < -0.7. We also examined the enrichment and depletion of taxa within the facial skin and gut microbiome. To this end, we calculated their mean abundance ($\bar{x}$) across the samples and compared them to the total distribution to calculate the Bonferroni corrected P. From these assignations, we also obtained a specific facial skin and gut core. As before, we defined two types of microbial cores: a strict one that retains those taxonomic identifications at the species level present in at least 80% of the samples of each sample type (facial skin or gut), and a relaxed one that retains those species present in at least 50% of the samples of each sample type.

We also identified the taxa of the top most abundant identified genes, which we defined as those genes with > 2000 mapping reads in the facial skin dataset and > 5000 in the gut dataset. We analysed the principal components (PCs) and rotation matrix of these taxa to identify the ones driving the variation within the facial skin and gut microbiomes. We defined "variation drivers" as those with an absolute rotation matrix value larger than the 3rd Qu value of the distributions from PC1, PC2 and PC3, and as "non-variation drivers" those with less than the 3rd Qu value of the distributions.

Besides the MGmapper identification, we used MOCAT as a complementary taxonomic identification method. For this approach, we used the taxonomic annotation given to the genes from the MOCAT strict nonredundant (NR) gene catalogue. This catalogue contains genes coding for proteins with a minimum length of 80 amino acids, not identified in low abundance, present only bacteria, fungi and virus, and that have an assigned Uniprot annotation (see "Methods"—"Functional profiling"). We analysed these identifications with MEGAN [37] having as input the search of the NR gene set catalogue against Uniprot using Ultra-Fast Sequence Search (USEARCH) [38].

Pathogenic characterization

We identified potential pathogens in the filtered bacterial and plasmid identifications. To this end, we obtained a list of the bacteria annotated with a disease from the database Pathosystems Resource Integration Center (PATRIC) [39]. In PATRIC, bacteria are annotated as pathogenic if they have been reported with experimental data as causative of a disease. We further added the pathogenicity classification level of bacterial strain using the list from van Belkum [40], which was developed by the Commissie Genetische Modificatie (COGEM). Pathogenicity classes are defined as follows. Class 1 represents species that are commonly non-pathogenic, although there may be differences in virulence among the bacterial strains that should be taken into account. Class 2 contains species that can cause diseases in humans or animals but are unlikely to spread in the human population. Class 3 encompasses species that cause serious human diseases and can disseminate in the human population. We used the metadata of the pathogenic strains obtained from PATRIC to identify whether or not the identified bacteria are capable of sporulation and of antimicrobial resistance, together with the reported disease and host. For the identification of pathogenic plasmids, we used the list from Ho-Sui et al. [41] on the association of virulence factors with genomic islands of pathogenic bacteria.

We then used R v3.1.1 [36] to examine the distribution of the total number of identified pathogenic bacteria. We grouped the samples by (i) vulture species (turkey and black vulture), and (ii) body sampling place (facial skin and gut). We then tested if the $\bar{x}$ of the distributions were significantly different with a two-tailed and one-tailed (alternate greater) t-test. Next, we examined the number of samples in which each pathogenic bacterial strain, plasmid, resistance gene, and virulence factor was present. In order to get a potentially pathogenic core, we identified those taxa present in 50% (relaxed core) and 90% (strict core) of the samples. We also identified the taxa present only in the facial skin or the gut microbiome.

Abundance analyses of potential pathogens

In order to analyse the abundance of the potentially pathogenic microbes across the samples, we first rescaled the number of unique mapping reads by their percentage in the sample. We then removed taxa present in low abundance (those with 90% of their signal coming from <4 samples). To determine if the identified potential pathogenic bacteria of facial skin and gut differed, we used the rescaled counts to build a dendrogram using a hierarchical clustering on the Euclidean distance. Afterwards, we examined which of the retained potentially pathogenic bacteria were present only on the facial skin or in the gut, and which ones were present in both. We then used a t-test to evaluate if the pathogenic bacterial abundance was statistically different by sample type and by vulture species.

16S bacterial taxonomic comparison

We compared the taxonomic bacterial identifications from both gut and facial datasets obtained with 16S analyses by Roggenbuck et al. [17] against the bacterial identifications from our metagenomics datasets using MGmapper, the taxonomic annotation of the de novo assembled genes with Uniprot, and the taxonomic identifications from the unmapped reads obtained with Double Index Alignment of Next-Generation Sequencing Data (DIAMOND) [42].

Functional profiling

We performed de novo assembly with the De Bruijn Graph De Novo Assembler with Uneven Depth sequencing data (IDBA-UD) [43] and predicted genes with Prodigal [44]. Afterwards, we generated a NR gene catalogue with USEARCH [38] by clustering the predicted genes with 90% identity and keeping the centroid sequences. We then searched the NR gene catalogue against Uniprot [45] with Ublast [38]. The resulting identifications were functionally and taxonomically annotated with the use of a customized python script. Finally, we used DIAMOND v0.6.4 [42] blastx to search the unmapped reads against Uniprot, keeping only the best hits for subsequent functional and taxonomic annotation.

For further functional assessment of the genes at the metabolic pathway level, we converted the Uniprot identifiers to the Kyoto Encyclopedia of Genes and Genomes (KEGG) [46] Enzyme Commission (EC) numbers and linked them to their corresponding metabolic pathway. Using the pathway classification information and the gene presence in each sample, we built a matrix for performing principal component analyses (PCA). Using the rotation matrix from the PCA we identified those pathways with an absolute rotation value within the minimum and 1st Qu values of the distributions of the PC1, PC2, and PC3. In order to distinguish the pathways driving most of the variation between the facial skin and gut microbiomes, we identified those pathways for which the absolute rotation value of their PC1, PC2, and PC3 was larger or equal to the 3rd Qu value of their corresponding distributions. We also obtained the Euclidean distances on the rescaled values of the matrices used for the PCAs.

As a second method, we used MOCAT with the Short Oligonucleotide Analysis Package for short-read de novo assembly (SOAPdenovo) v1.05 [47] for assembling the reads cleaned with the approach that removed their first 16 bases. Subsequently, we corrected the assembly for indels and chimeric regions with SOAPdenovo. Using Prodigal, we then predicted the genes from all the samples, pooled them, and built an NR gene catalogue with Uclust [38] using a 90% identity threshold. Facial skin and gut datasets were treated separately. In the MGmapper core definition approach, the NR gene catalogue was obtained for each sample, then the catalogues were pooled and the unique genes were kept to compare their presence or absence across the samples. In contrast, in this approach using MOCAT, we built the cores based on the abundance of the reads mapping to the NR gene catalogue. To this end, we first mapped the reads of each sample against the NR gene catalogue and rescaled the counts values. Then, we removed those genes in low abundance (<200 mapped reads), without a Uniprot annotation, and not derived from bacteria, archaea, virus, or fungi. We also removed genes coding for proteins with <80 amino acids aligned to a hit from the Uniprot database. From these proteins, we also obtained a strict core (at least 80% of the samples) and a relaxed core (at least 50% of the samples). We also identified the top most abundant proteins (those with >2000 mapping reads in the facial skin and >5000 in the gut samples). On the relaxed functional core, we performed pathway functional analyses of their EC numbers with KEGG.

Antibiotic resistance

In order to search for antibiotic resistance genes, besides searching the ResFinder database with MGmapper, we used the Resfams v1.2 database [48] and the associated profile hidden Markov models. We searched the de novo assembled NR gene set of each sample against the Resfams profiles with a software for multiple alignment using hidden Markov models (HMMER v3.0) [49].

Results

Metagenomic dataset

We produced a total of 342,279,763 raw read pairs from the facial skin samples and 512,803,778 from the gut samples. After cleaning and removing endogenous DNA by mapping against the bird genomes of the avian phylogenomic project [27], we obtained 79,938,910 read pairs from the facial skin samples (with a median of 1,378,000 read pairs per sample) and 144,877,366 from the gut samples (with a median of 1,118,000 per sample) (Additional file 1).

To prove the consistency of the taxonomic profiling between the two vulture species, we compared the number of identified microbial taxa in each species. We filtered the MGmapper [29] identifications of each whole-genome database by depth and breadth (percentage of covered reference sequence) of coverage and identified taxa differentially abundant in the facial skin and gut samples (Additional file 2). The number of identified bacteria was not significantly different between vulture species in the pooled datasets of facial skin and gut samples ($P=0.52$, $\bar{x}_{\text{black vulture}}=366.97$, $\bar{x}_{\text{turkey vulture}}=334.65$). There were no significant differences between vulture species in the number of identified species of fungi ($P=0.43$, $\bar{x}_{\text{black vulture}}=9$, $\bar{x}_{\text{turkey vulture}}=7.5$), viruses ($P=0.33$, $\bar{x}_{\text{black vulture}}=21$, $\bar{x}_{\text{turkey vulture}}=28.2$), plasmids ($P=0.68$, $\bar{x}_{\text{black vulture}}=186.85$, $\bar{x}_{\text{turkey vulture}}=173.65$), and protozoa ($P=0.21$, $\bar{x}_{\text{black vulture}}=12$, $\bar{x}_{\text{turkey vulture}}=9.62$). Also, the number of identified proteins with resistance to antibiotics did not differ between vulture species ($P=0.64$, $\bar{x}_{\text{black vulture}}=107.5$, $\bar{x}_{\text{turkey vulture}}=100.78$).

We compared our metagenomic bacterial identifications to those of Roggenbuck et al. [17]. A total of 735 bacterial operational taxonomic units were identified analysing the 16S sequences, of which 93 were not found among our metagenomics identifications with strict filtering. When using the pre-filtering identifications from the whole-genome bacterial database and those identifications from the GreenGenes [34] and Silva [35] databases, only 14 genera were not identified in our analysis (Additional file 1).

Taxonomic characterization

Compared to the gut, the facial skin microbiome had higher microbial richness in terms of number of taxa and variation between individuals ($P_{\text{protozoa}}=0.021$, $P_{\text{fungi}}=0.029$, $P_{\text{bacteria}}=0.0002$). However, there was no significant difference in abundance ($P_{\text{protozoa}}=0.514$, $P_{\text{fungi}}=0.47$, $P_{\text{bacteria}}=0.71$). Although the number of identified virus was not significantly different between facial skin and gut ($P=0.58$), viruses were statistically less abundant and variable in the facial skin than in the gut samples ($P=0.0002$, Euclidean distance$_{\text{facial skin}}=9.04$, Euclidean distance$_{\text{gut}}=13.14$). The most abundant bacterial genera in the facial skin microbiome were *Pseudomonas, Bacteroides,* and *Prevotella,* while the most abundant in the gut microbiome belonged to *Escherichia, Campylobacter,* and *Clostridium* (Additional file 3).

A total of 143 bacterial strains were significantly more abundant within the facial skin microbiome, 46 after the breadth filtering (mostly *Pseudomonas*). Within the gut microbiome, we identified 56 bacterial strains as the highest abundant, 33 after the breadth filtering (mostly *Escherichia* and *Campylobacter*). Bacterial strains most abundant in the facial skin dataset fell into three broad categories: (i) reported as potential human pathogens, (ii) associated with bioremediation (ionizing resistant, reducers of heavy metals, or oil degraders), and (iii) potentially beneficial (producers of antibiotics, insecticides and antifungals), usually intestinal bacteria, and related to water, plants, or soil. Those significantly more abundant in the gut dataset could be classified as: (i) reported as potential human pathogens, (ii) potentially beneficial, mostly intestinal or faecal bacteria from chicken, and (iii) fermenters and producers of intestinal metabolites.

From the mapping of the reads to the NR gene set catalogues obtained from MOCAT, the taxa of the top most abundant proteins in the facial skin microbiome were from *Sporidiobolales* (fungi), *Orthoretrovirinae* (virus), *Pleosporaceae* (fungi), *Bacillus cereus, Streptococcus* spp., and *Clostridiales.* While in the gut microbiome they were species from the genera *Bordetella, Mycobacterium, Chlamydia, Clostridium, Blautia* (a genus identified in the mammalian gut [50, 51]), and *Carnobacterium* (certain species inhibit the growth of *Listeria monocytogenes* in cured meats [52, 53]). The results from the search against Uniprot analysed with MEGAN (Figs. 1, 2) showed that in the facial skin microbiome the dominant population was *Proteobacteria,* followed by *Bacteroidetes, Firmicutes,* and *Actinobacteria,* with *Fusobacteria* in 12th place. Deeper examination of the *Proteobacteria* from the facial skin microbiome showed that the most

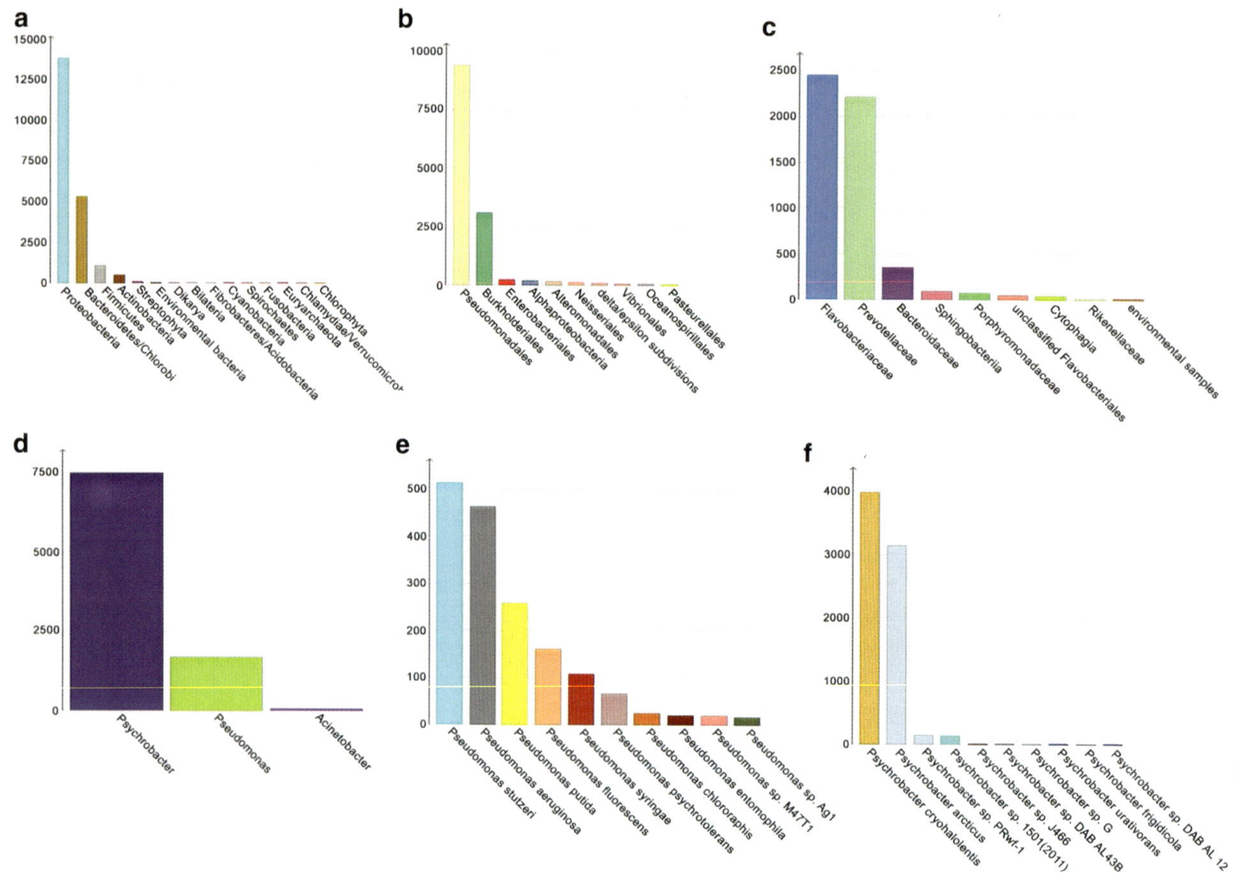

Fig. 1 Taxonomic profile of the most abundant facial skin microbiota with MEGAN filtered NR gene catalogue. **a** Phylum level, **b** Proteobacteria, **c** Bacteroidetes, **d** Pseudomonadales, **e** *Pseudomonas*, and **f** *Psychrobacter*

abundant taxa were *Burkholderiales* from the *Betaproteobacteria*, and *Pseudomonadales* from the *Gammaproteobacteria* (Fig. 1b). From the *Pseudomonadales*, the most abundant taxon was *Psychrobacter* (mainly *P. cryohalolentis*, and *P. articus*), followed by *Pseudomonas* (mainly *P. stutzeri*, *P. aeruginosa*, and *P. putida*) (Fig. 1d–f). From the *Bacteroidetes*, the most abundant taxa were *Prevotellaceae* (mainly *P. ruminicola*) and *Flavobacteriaceae* (mainly from unclassified *Flavobacteriaceae* followed by *Flavobacterium*) (Fig. 1c).

Firmicutes was the most abundant phylum in the gut microbiome, followed by *Proteobacteria*, *Fusobacteria* in the third place, and *Bacteroidetes* in much less abundant in the fourth place. The most abundant class within *Firmicutes* was *Clostridia* (Fig. 2b). Among the *Clostridiales*, the most abundant families were *Clostridiaceae*, *Peptostreptococcaceae* and *Lachnospiraceae* (Fig. 2d). The most abundant taxa in the genus *Clostridium* were the potentially pathogenic *C. perfringens* and *C. botulinum*, followed by the beneficial *C. carboxidovorans*, *C. sporogenes*, and *C. butyricum* (Fig. 2e). The most abundant taxa from the *Proteobacteria* were *Burkholderiales* (from the *Betaproteobacteria*), *Epsilonproteobacteria* (from the delta/epsilon subdivision), and *Enterobacteriales* (mainly from *Escherichia* from the *Gammaproteobacteria*) (Fig. 2c). The most abundant taxa in the *Fusobacteria* were the potentially pathogenic *Fusobacterium mortiferum*, *F. varium*, and *F. ulcerans* (Fig. 2f).

Many *Clostridia* that are part of the normal human gut microbiome were also found in the vulture gut, likely playing roles in digestion. For instance, *C. saccharolyticum* was significantly more abundant in the gut. This bacterium, which is present in sewage sludge, ferments various carbohydrates into acetic acid, hydrogen, carbon dioxide, and ethanol [54], functions for which we identified related genes in the vulture gut microbiome. We also identified genes for cellulose degradation in the gut, along with the cellulose degraders *C. cellulovorans* and *C. lentocellum* [55], which were significantly more abundant in the gut microbiome. The gut microbiome also contained *Bacteroides xylanisolvens*, which breaks down xylan [56] and for which we identified a gene related to

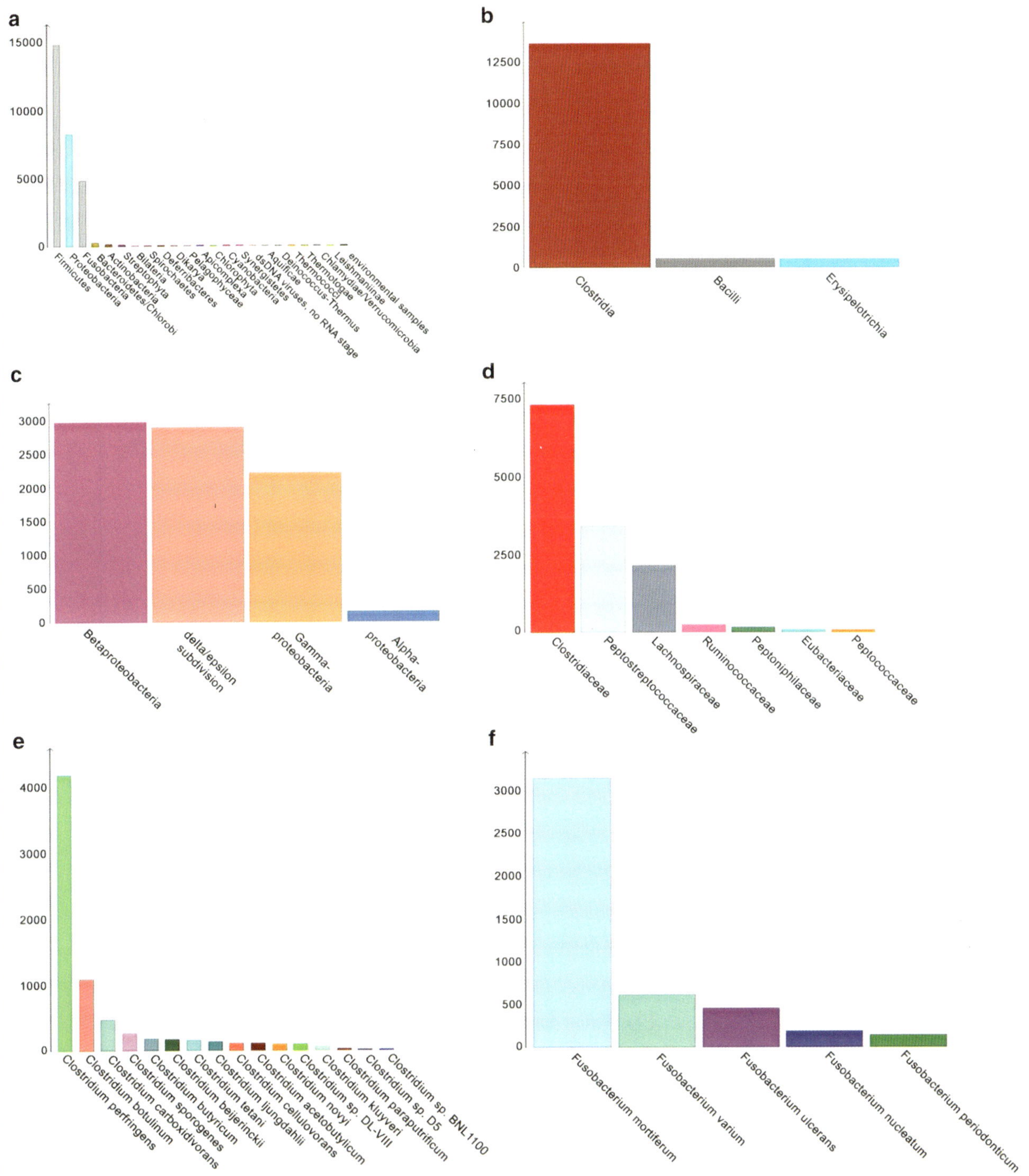

Fig. 2 Taxonomic profile of the most abundant gut microbiota with MEGAN filtered NR gene catalogue. **a** Phylum level, **b** Firmicutes, **c** Proteobacteria, **d** Clostridiales, **e** *Clostridium*, and **f** *Fusobacterium*

this function. Also, significantly more abundant in the gut microbiome than in the facial skin were the butanol producers *C. beijerinckii* [57] and *C. saccharobutylicum* [58].

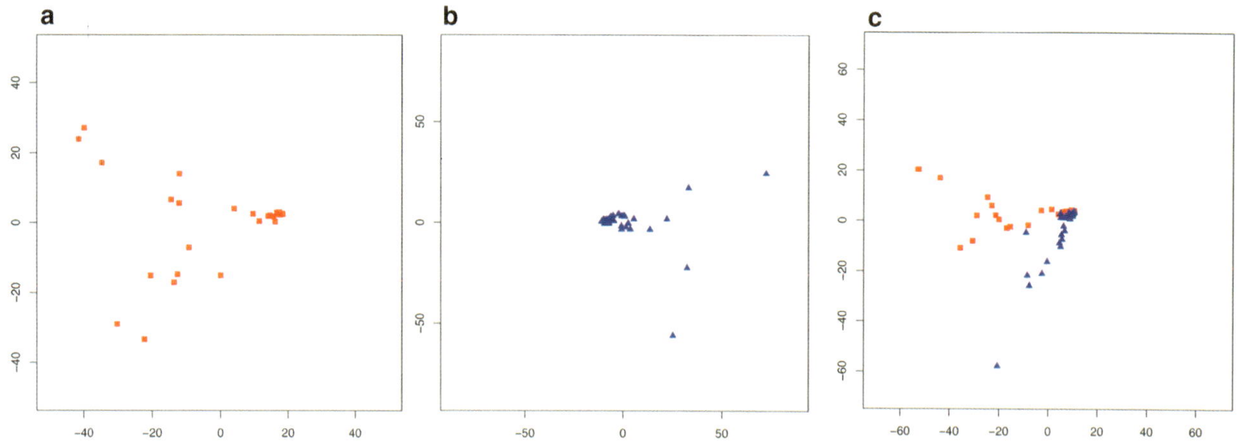

Fig. 3 PC1 vs PC2 of the taxonomic species level abundance. **a** Facial skin microbiome, **b** gut microbiome, and **c** species present in both facial skin (red squares) and gut (blue triangles)

We also identified protein coding genes involved in vitamin biosynthesis in the gut strict MOCAT NR functional core. For example, from the genera *Hydrogenophaga*, *Herbaspirillum*, and *Gordonia*, we identified the genes for D-threo-aldose 1-dehydrogenase, involved in ascorbate and aldarate metabolism, cobalamin biosynthesis, riboflavin biosynthesis, and vitamin B_1 biosynthesis; and 2-ketopantoate reductase, involved in vitamin B_5 production [59]. Using the MGmapper gene core, which does not take taxa into account, we identified a larger abundance of genes in the gut than in the facial skin microbiome that belong to the metabolism of cofactors and vitamins (e.g. folate biosynthesis, vitamin B_6 metabolism, riboflavin metabolism, and retinol metabolism). We also identified genes for the biosynthesis of various essential amino acids.

Comparison of the facial skin and gut microbiome variation

Based on the PCA of the abundance of the identified species in the facial skin and gut datasets (Fig. 3a, b), we found that the 803 species identified as driving the variation in the facial skin microbiome can be broadly grouped as: (i) pathogenic bacteria to a mammalian host (e.g. species from the genera *Bordetella*, *Gordonia*, *Shigella*, *Yersinia*, *Brucella*, *Prevotella*, and *Treponema*); (ii) soil or plant related; and (iii) related to mucosal surfaces and normal oral microbiome (*Neisseria* and *Nocardia*). Phages of *Salmonella*, *Aeromonas*, and *Erwinia* were also among the identifications driving variation. The 406 species not driving most of the variation included genera related to bioremediation (e.g. *Acinetobacter*), as well as other pathogens (species from the genera *Arcobacter* and *Brucella*), and phages of *Clostridium*, *Pseudomonas*, *Shigella*, and *Staphylococcus*.

In the gut samples, we identified 604 species that showed significant variation in abundance among the samples and 348 that were relatively uniformly distributed. The variation drivers included 112 potentially pathogenic bacteria, such as species from the genera *Listeria*, *Shigella*, *Yersinia*, *Bordetella*, *Shewanella*, *Erwinia*, and *Vibrio*. Bacteria that were non-drivers included species from the genera *Escherichia*, *Bacillus*, *Brucella*, and *Clostridium*, among others. Non-variation driver phages included phages for *Escherichia*, *Enterobacteria*, and *Shigella*. Phages driving variation included phages for *Clostridium*, *Yersinia*, and *Pseudomonas*.

Of the 879 microbial species shared by the facial skin and gut samples (Fig. 3c), we identified 553 species as driving variation (62.9%), and 326 as non-variation drivers (37.1%). Among the most important variation drivers were *Yersinia*, *Ralstonia*, *Rhizobium*, *Bifidobacterium*, *Bordetella*, *Listeria*, and *Burkholderia*. The non-variation drivers included *Brucella*, *Treponema*, *Clostridium*, and *Campylobacter*. Looking at the phages, only *Pseudomonas* phages were variation drivers, while non-variation drivers included phages for *Clostridium*, *Enterobacteria*, *Erwinia*, and *Shigella*.

Functional potential characterization

The PCA of gene abundance from the MOCAT NR gene set catalogue of the pooled facial skin and gut microbiomes annotated with KEGG showed less variation than the taxonomic profile in most of the pathway classes (Fig. 4).

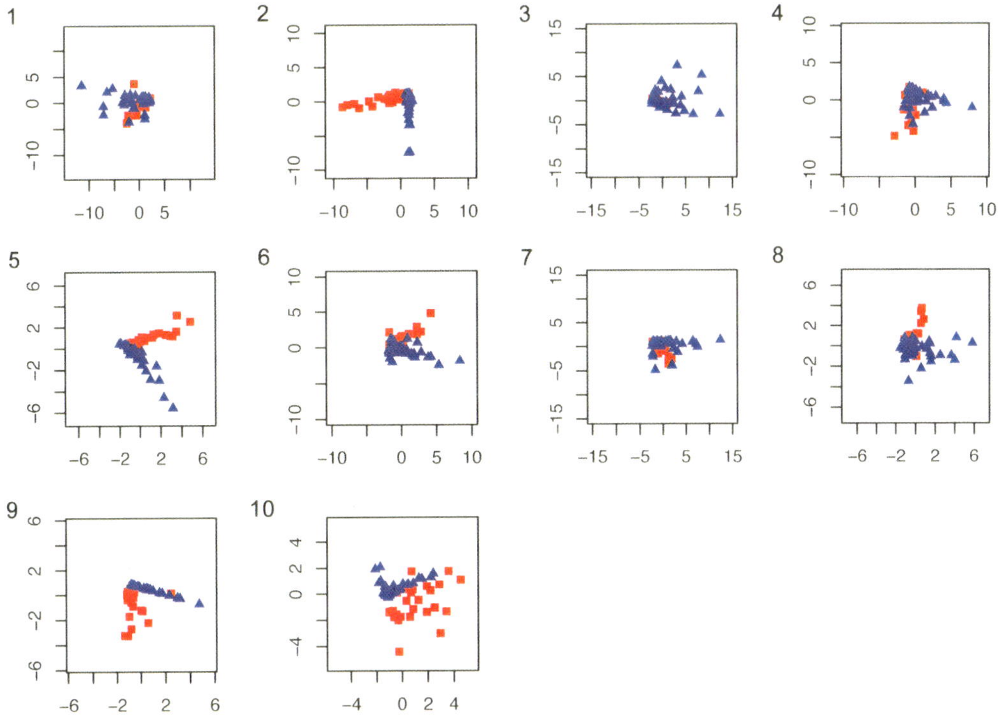

Fig. 4 PC1 vs PC2 of the gene abundance from each pathway class. Red squares represent facial skin samples, blue triangles represent gut samples. The examined pathway classes were: **1**—Amino acid metabolism. **2**—Metabolism of other secondary metabolites. **3**—Carbohydrate metabolism. **4**—Energy metabolism. **5**—Glycan biosynthesis and metabolism. **6**—Lipid metabolism. **7**—Metabolism of co-factors and vitamins. **8**—Metabolism of other amino acids. **9**—Metabolism of terpenoids and polyketides. **10**—Biodegradation and metabolism of xenobiotics

We also examined the number of proteins identified from each pathway class in the MGmapper NR protein set. PC1 of each pathway class explained 78–99% of the variance and clearly separated the pathway classes by their functional composition (Fig. 5). Examination of the rotation matrix showed that 60.4% (87) of the sub-pathways were responsible for the observed variation between the facial skin and gut microbiomes. Analysing variation by sample type, 57% of the sub-pathways in the facial skin (81 sub-pathways) and 56% (80 sub-pathways) in the gut datasets drive intra sample variation. We identified 59 variation driver genes with the largest (top 5%) mean abundance difference between facial skin and gut. Of those genes, 18 corresponded to amino acid metabolism (17 only present in gut samples and one in a single facial skin sample), 15 genes from carbohydrate metabolism (all in gut samples), and 7 genes corresponding to metabolism of cofactors and vitamins (all in gut samples). We found that 44% of the genes (921 out of the KEGG annotated 2093 pooled facial skin and gut relaxed gene cores) did not drive variation. The 46 genes with the smallest (bottom 5%) mean abundance difference between facial skin and gut were associated to the metabolism of amino acids, carbohydrates, cofactors and vitamins, glycan biosynthesis and metabolism, lipid metabolism, energy metabolism, chlorocyclohexane and chlorobenzene degradation, metabolism of terpenoids and polyketides, and metabolism of other amino acids.

Euclidean distance measures among the gut samples showed less intra sample type variation than the facial skin samples (Table 1, $P = 0.002$). The facial skin microbiome distances ranged from 3.2 to 6.2, while those in the gut microbiome ranged from 2.2 to 3.7. Analysis of all the functions together instead of per pathway class showed that the facial skin and gut microbiomes clearly separated into two different clusters. The MOCAT functional characterization yielded a total of 38,403 NR genes from the facial skin dataset and 50,106 NR genes from the gut dataset. Based on the normalized abundance of the mapping reads, we identified 1507 genes in the facial skin strict core and 7215 in the relaxed core, and 157 top abundant genes. We found 2512 genes in the gut strict core, 14,028 in the relaxed core, and 151 top abundant genes.

Core microbiome identification and attributes comparison

In the filtered MGmapper taxonomic profiling, we identified 1483 species in the facial skin samples, 638 of which

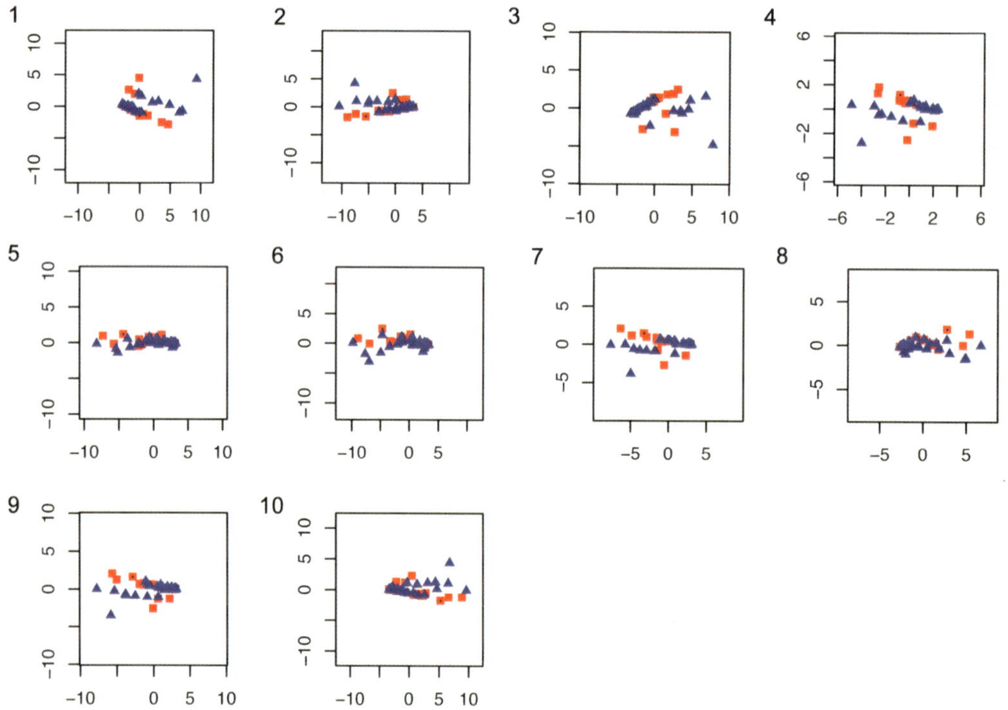

Fig. 5 PC1 vs PC2 of each pathway class protein counts. Red squares represent facial skin samples, blue triangles represent gut samples. The examined pathway classes were: **1**—Amino acid metabolism. **2**—Metabolism of other secondary metabolites. **3**—Carbohydrate metabolism. **4**—Energy metabolism. **5**—Glycan biosynthesis and metabolism. **6**—Lipid metabolism. **7**—Metabolism of co-factors and vitamins. **8**—Metabolism of other amino acids. **9**—Metabolism of terpenoids and polyketides. **10**—Biodegradation and metabolism of xenobiotics

Table 1 Distances between and within the facial skin and gut samples

Pathway	Facial skin vs facial skin	Gut vs facial skin	Gut vs gut
Amino acid metabolism	4.87	4.66	2.86
Biosynthesis of other secondary metabolites	5.97	5.97	3.68
Carbohydrate metabolism	4.1	4.48	3.58
Energy metabolism	3.33	3.27	2.17
Glycan biosynthesis and metabolism	3.24	3.67	3.22
Lipid metabolism	5.6	5.66	3.03
Metabolism of cofactors and vitamins	4.27	4.41	2.99
Metabolism of other amino acids	3.48	3.77	2.75
Metabolism of terpenoids and polyketides	4.57	4.94	3.18
Nucleotide metabolism	1.50	1.56	1.34
Xenobiotic biodegradation and metabolism	6.22	5.98	3.61

occurred in the relaxed core, and only 184 species that occurred in the strict core. In the gut microbiome, we found 1419 microbial species, with 322 present in the relaxed core, and 129 in the strict core. In the functional characterization, we identified a total of 238,065 NR unique bacterial genes in the facial skin microbiome and 387,951 NR unique bacterial genes in the gut microbiome (Additional file 3).

We compared the taxonomic and functional composition of the facial skin and gut microbiomes and examined the microbial attributes of the taxa identified from the annotations of the assembled genes (Additional file 3). We found ~26× more habitat-specialized microbes in the facial skin than in the gut microbiome (facial skin = 8373, gut = 320). Consistent with the anaerobic gut environment, the gut microbiome had ~5× more anaerobic or microaerophilic bacteria than the facial microbiome (gut = 34,749, facial skin = 6699). The functional pathways clearly separated by sample type were the metabolism of other secondary metabolites, the glycan biosynthesis and metabolism, and the lipid metabolism, followed to a lesser extent by the metabolism of xenobiotics and the metabolism of other amino acids (Fig. 4). From the energy metabolism class, the methane metabolism was among the most abundant functions in the facial skin and gut microbiomes.

Pathogenic characterization

There was no significant difference ($P = 0.44$) in the number of identified potentially pathogenic plasmids between the facial skin ($\bar{x} = 11.3$) and gut ($\bar{x} = 9.82$) microbiomes. Likewise, there was no statistical difference in their abundance between the facial skin and gut samples ($P = 0.78$). Furthermore, no potentially pathogenic plasmid was present in 90% of the samples. Among those present in at least 50% of the samples were plasmids from *Burkholderia vietnamiensis*, *Escherichia coli*, and *Ochrobactrum anthropic*. Potentially pathogenic plasmids present only in the facial skin microbiome were from opportunistic pathogens such as *Acinetobacter baumannii* and *Staphylococcus epidermidis*, which is usually part of the normal skin microbiome [60]. For example, the *O. anthropi* ATCC 49188 plasmid pOANT04 was present in 63 of the samples. *O. anthropi* is being increasingly recognized as a potentially problematic opportunistic and nosocomial human pathogen [61].

The Shiga toxin 1-converting phage BP-4795, which transmits virulence genes to its infected bacteria [62], was found in only five facial skin samples, and in 23 of the gut samples at various levels of abundance (max. coverage = 17.9%, max. mapping reads = 372). We also found the *Shigella* phage SfIV, which aids the virulence of *Shigella flexneri* [63], in 25 of the gut samples and 8 of the facial skin samples. We found that 75.2% of the identified pathogens are classified as level 2 pathogens in the facial skin samples (level 1 = 26 species, level 2 = 79 species), while 95.8% of those more abundant in the gut were classified as level 2 (level 1 = 2 species, level 2 = 46 species).

From the MGmapper strict core, the only protein identified in most of the facial skin samples (20 samples) and gut samples (36 samples) was an uncharacterized protein from *Chlamydophila psittaci*, an avian pathogen that causes avian chlamydiosis and epizootic outbreaks in mammals [64]. Among the viruses from this functional strict core, we found the avian endogenous retrovirus EAV-HP and the avian leucosis virus. We also identified in higher abundance in the gut dataset *Trichuris trichiura*, causative of trichuriasis in humans [65, 66] (max. mapping $\text{reads}_{\text{facial skin}} = 942$, max. mapping $\text{reads}_{\text{gut}} = 565{,}870$), and *Eimeria brunetti*, causative of haemorrhagic intestinal coccidiosis in poultry [67] (max. mapping $\text{reads}_{\text{facial skin}} = 30$, max. mapping $\text{reads}_{\text{gut}} = 1706$). More abundant in the facial skin dataset we identified the fly *Lucila cuprina* ($\bar{x}_{\text{gut}} = 11{,}910$, $\bar{x}_{\text{facial skin}} = 49{,}210$), which causes sheep strike [68].

We identified only 49 bacteria in the gut dataset with potential for sporulation, including *Fusobacterium necrophorum*, *Campylobacter jejuni*, and *L. monocytogenes* (Additional file 4). Regarding the bacteria reported as zoonotic pathogens, we could only identify *Streptococcus suis*, a pathogen capable of transmission from swine to humans [69]. Other identified bacteria with reported zoonotic capacity had very low abundance and were present in only one or two samples, so that they likely represent non-viable bacteria already dealt with by the vulture.

Discussion

Microbiome composition and variability

The comparison of our metagenomic bacterial identifications to those by Roggenbuck et al. [17] confirm the consistency of the taxonomic identifications. Given that we aim at characterizing the vulture scavenging-related microbiome, in light of previous observations that the facial skin and gut microbiota of turkey and black vultures largely overlap [17], we combined the datasets of both vulture species into one. The results from comparing the number and relative abundance of identified taxa in the two vulture species prove that their microbiomes are not statistically different ($P = 0.68$), and validate their joint use. We identified a strikingly large taxonomic and functional variation within the gut and facial skin datasets (Figs. 3, 4 and 6a). The observation that the functional profiles showed less variation than the taxonomic profiles could suggest a large amount of functional redundancy in the microbiota, or that there is a need for a common set of functions in order to thrive on the vulture's facial skin and gut. Examination of the PCA from the functional potential characterization suggests that the functional profile of the facial skin and gut microbiomes are very similar in most of the pathway classes, despite large within-sample type variation (Fig. 4). This suggestion is supported by the PCA of the number of identified proteins belonging to each pathway class (Fig. 5). This analysis further suggests that the relative abundance of the proteins rather than the presence/absence of them is one of the main factors distinguishing the facial skin from the gut microbiome functional profile. In comparison to the facial skin microbiome, the gut had less variation in the functional profile (Table 1, $P = 0.002$). This is consistent with the fact that the facial skin is the first part of the vulture's body to make contact with the carcass, thus potentially becoming contaminated by the carcass, which

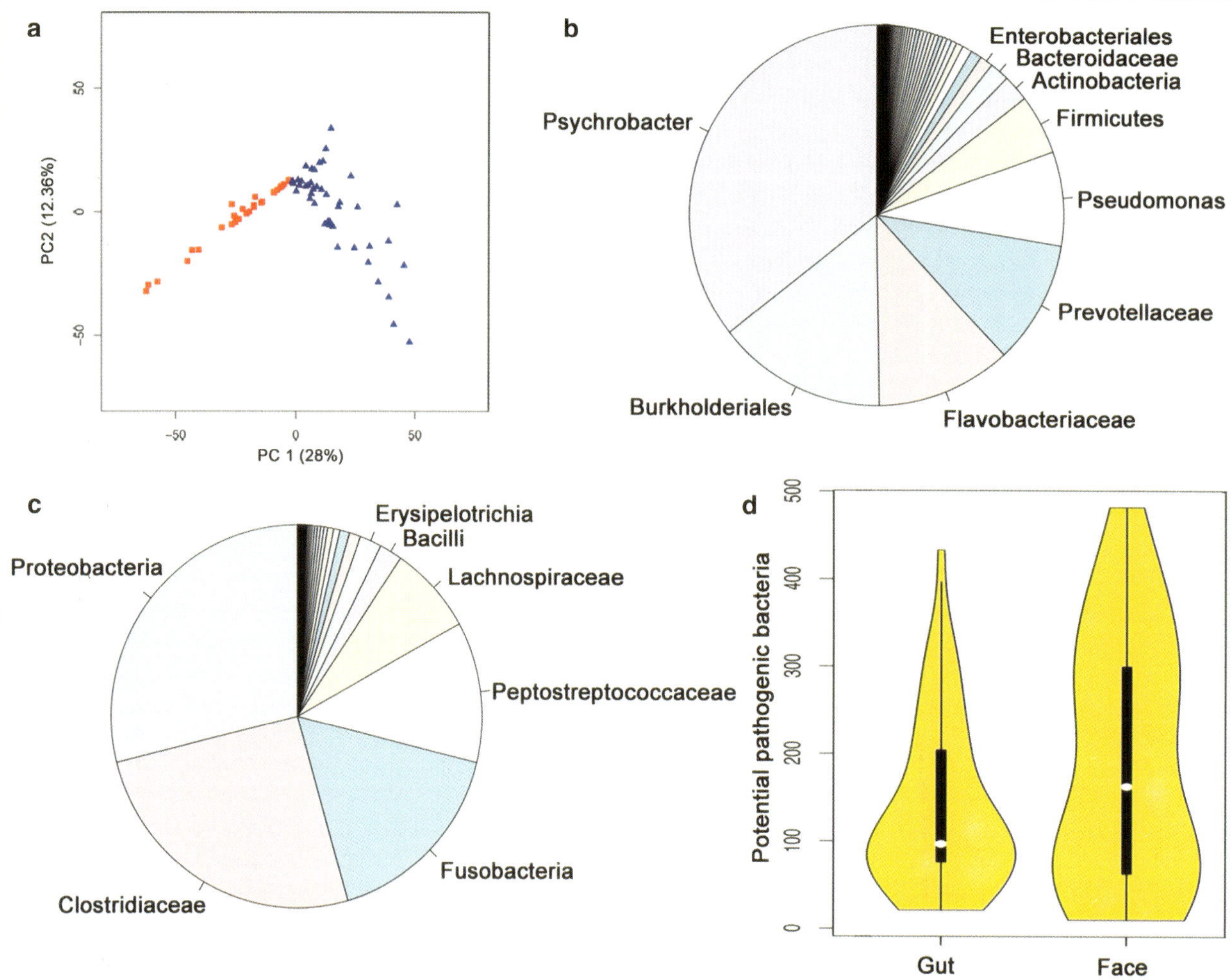

Fig. 6 Vulture facial skin and gut microbiome composition. **a** Principal component (PC) 1 (28% of the variation) and PC 2 (12.4%) of the abundance of all genes from all the KEGG metabolic classes together of the facial skin (red squares) and gut (blue triangles) samples. **b** Taxonomic profile of the facial skin and **c** gut microbiota. **d** Distribution of the number of identified potentially pathogenic bacteria in the gut and facial skin datasets

would lead to large variation in the facial skin microbiota than the more ecologically constrained gut microbiota. In general, the identified taxa from the gut and facial skin microbiomes can be hypothesized to derive from (i) host, such as *Methanobrevibacter smithii* in the gut, and (ii) environment and carcass, e.g. *Xanthomonas* and *Actinobacillus pleuropneumoniae*. Determination of the carcass microbiota would be necessary for further evaluation of this grouping; however, it was not possible to obtain samples of the carcass the sampled vultures were feeding from. Given that the most abundant facial skin microbes can be associated to a variety of microbial attributes ranging from producers of antifungals to usual intestinal bacteria and plant and soil related bacteria, it is clear that there is a large environmental and carcass microbiota input to the vulture's highly variable facial skin microbiome. On the other hand, those most abundant in the gut were related mainly to intestinal or faecal bacteria, reflecting the digestive and more specialized functions expected to occur in the gut. Our data confirms previous PCR-based results [17] that identify *Clostridia* and *Fusobacteria* as dominant taxa in the gut microbiome (Figs. 2, 6c). As expected, we identified clear traits (bacterial taxa and genes) in the gut microbiome for carrying out digestive and nutritional activities.

Reduced core host microbiome

In order to differentiate the constant host microbiome from the one derived from variable and external influences (i.e. microbes derived from the carcass and the environment), we defined two types of microbiome cores. A relaxed core containing those elements (microbial species and genes) present in at least 50% of the samples, and a strict core with those present in at least 80% of the samples. We found that the relaxed core contained ~43% and ~22.7% of the facial skin and gut taxa, respectively, and the strict core only contained ~1% of the taxa in both gut and facial skin datasets. Notably, the distinction between carcass and established constant host-derived microbiome was complicated, even after the cores were defined. For example, the foodborne pathogen *Salmonella enterica* was present in the gut core (Fig. 6b). We additionally identified genes in the facial skin and gut microbiome functional strict cores that are related to putrescine, one of the main molecules produced in a carcass (Additional files 5 and 6). We found ~26× more habitat-specialized microbes in the facial skin than in the gut microbiome (facial skin = 8373, gut = 320), most likely due to the fact that a mammalian corpse is a disturbance habitat that selects for a specialized microbial community [13]. Some of these community species likely derive from the carrion microbiota. For example, we identified phenol degrading bacteria in the vulture facial skin, such as *Acinetobacter calcoaceticus* [70] (max. mapping $\text{reads}_{\text{facial skin}} = 478$, max. mapping $\text{reads}_{\text{gut}} = 6$), for which we identified its gene coding for phenol 2-monooxygenase in the NR gene catalogue. Phenolic compounds can act against foodborne pathogens and spoilage bacteria [71], suggesting that they derive from carrion dwellers, adapted to their competitive environment, instead of being part of the core vulture facial skin microbiome. Thus, we suggest that the vulture microbiome is a result of its scavenging diet, with part of the carcass microbiome leaving a profound footprint in the vulture microbiome.

Pathogenicity challenges

Given the identification of a strong carcass microbiome signature in the vulture microbiome, we next characterized all potential pathogens dealt with by the vultures. We defined potential pathogens as taxa and functions that, while present in the vulture microbiome without conferring an apparently negative health effect, could be deadly for non-scavengers. Most of the significantly more abundant potential pathogens found in the facial skin microbiome ($P < 0.05$) are known to produce anthrax-like illnesses, periodontitis, pneumonia, and tuberculosis in mammals, while those found more abundantly in the gut are known to cause gastroenteritis, gas gangrene, food poisoning, and dysentery in humans (Figs. 6d, 7a, b). We identified several pathogenic plasmids in the gut microbiome, such as the Shiga toxin 1-converting phage BP-4795, which transmits virulence genes to the infected *E. coli* [62], as well as genes in the facial skin microbiome related to pathogenicity, such as haemolysins (Additional file 6). Our untargeted metagenomics approach also identified non-bacterial potential pathogens in the gut, such as the round worm *T. trichiura*, causing trichuriasis in humans [66], and the apicomplexan parasite *E. brunetti*, responsible for haemorrhagic intestinal coccidiosis in poultry [67]. These results highlight the

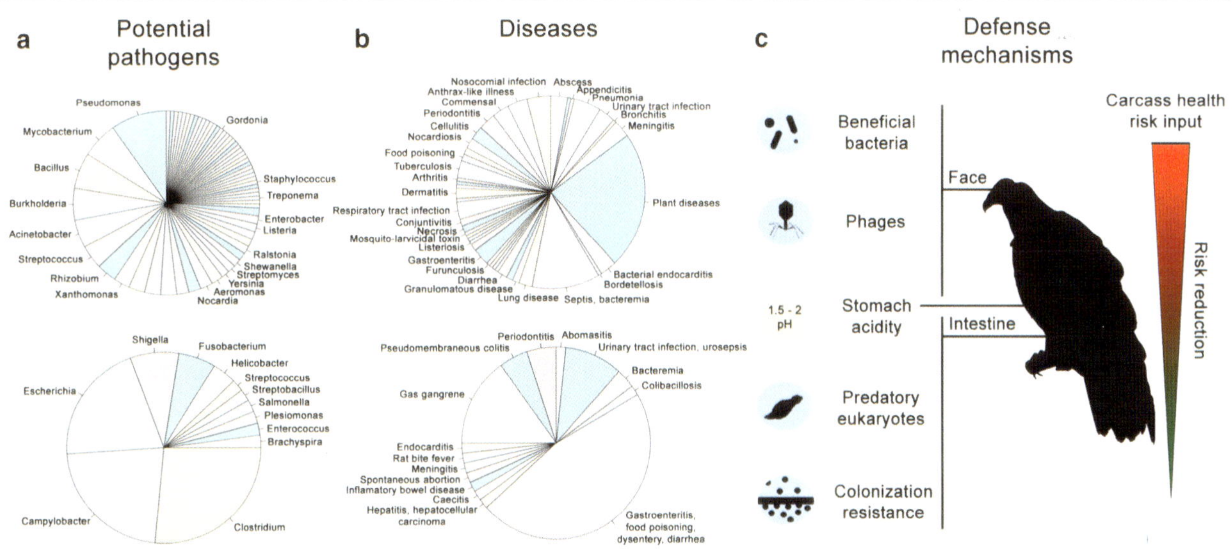

Fig. 7 Health challenges faced by the vulture. **a** Vultures are confronted with a wide variety of carcass-derived microbes (**b**) that pose serious pathogenic risks to non-scavenging species. **c** Different potential microbiome-mediated defence mechanisms account for the vulture's ability to tolerate and reduce the health-risk potential that a carcass represents as it passes through its digestive system

health-challenging environment dealt by the vulture due to its scavenging diet.

Stomach acidity protection

The vulture stomach acidity has been suggested to prevent potential pathogens from reaching the gut [14, 17]. However, postprandial pH values observed in the stomach of black and turkey vultures appear to be no more acidic than those reported for domestic fowl and non-scavenging birds that consume large animal prey [72]. Instrument readings of the pH are usually higher in a stomach with food contents, since the gastric acid is sparse and diluted by the water content in the lumpy food items. Sequential and independent probe values in the stomach can often provide different readings, even when the probe is used in the same location. This is reflected in the large standard deviations observed in the previously reported pH readings of black vultures (pH 3.8 ± 1.25) [72]. The measurements were less acidic, and neutral in some occasions in the duodenum (pH 6.1 ± 0.48) and lower intestine (pH 6.0 ± 0.3) [72]. Given that the carcass microbiome enters the vulture's body mainly along with the ingested food items, the pH measurements suggest that the gastrointestinal acidity is not an efficient filter against all the potential pathogens present in a scavenging diet, rather it plays the general role of primary selection, which is not enough for all the potential pathogens in the carcass.

Most of the potential pathogens identified were restricted to few samples, and the abundance of the pathogens was not consistent across samples after count normalization. These observations could be due to variation in the carcass microbiome, or efficient elimination of the potential pathogens by the vulture. In the comparison of the facial skin and gut microbiomes, we found that the facial skin had more species of potential pathogens than the gut ($P = 0.036$) (Fig. 6d, Table 2). However, there was no statistical difference in their abundance ($P = 0.82$), and the gut still harboured various potential pathogens. Interestingly, among the non-bacterial identifications we found the Chinese liver fluke, *Clonorchis sinensis* in 22 of the facial skin samples and 39 of the gut samples (66.6% of the facial skin and 83% of the gut samples). This liver fluke feeds on bile and causes problems in fat digestion, and it is able to reach the gut of the hosts given its acidity resistance [73].

Microbiome mediated protection

It has been shown that microbes provide protection to the host against pathogenic bacteria, thus we hypothesized that the vulture microbiome plays a protective role in terms of combating, preventing or maintaining in balance the abundance of potential pathogens. Accordingly, we identified functional and taxonomic protective elements that could be classified as related to (i) beneficial bacterial taxa and functions, (ii) phages, (iii) predatory eukaryotes, and (iv) colonization resistance (Fig. 7c, Additional file 5).

Beneficial bacterial taxa

Consistent with our microbiome-mediated protection hypothesis, we identified *Hylemonella gracilis* as part of

Table 2 Top 10 potential disease-causing bacteria identified in the facial skin and gut

Pathogen	Disease	$\bar{x}$ facial skin	Rank facial skin	$\bar{x}$ gut	Rank gut
Stenotrophomonas maltophilia K279a	Bacteraemia, bronchitis, pneumonia, urinary tract infection	75,292	1	18,298	7
Clostridium perfringens ATCC 13124	Gas gangrene	61,879	2	166,694.6	1
Plesiomonas shigelloides 302-73	Gastroenteritis	48,642	3	134,119	2
Clostridium perfringens str. 13	Gas gangrene	41,308	4	125,717.5	3
Pseudomonas fluorescens A506	Commensal (plant)	31,324.9	5	271.2	49
Clostridium perfringens SM101	Gas gangrene	30,361.2	6	109,973.2	4
Acinetobacter lwoffii SH145	Nosocomial infections	19,950.2	7	3.2	149
Aeromonas salmonicida subsp. salmonicida A449	Furunculosis	14,347.4	8	45.4	92
Acidovorax avenae subsp. avenae ATCC 19860	Bacterial leaf blight, brown stripe, red stripe	13,111.2	9	998.7	30
Propionibacterium propionicum F0230a	Commensal	11,896.8	10	73.64	80
Campylobacter lari RM2100	Gastroenteritis, diarrhoea	4791	26	53,435	5
Campylobacter jejuni subsp. doylei 269.97	Bacteraemia	477.2	108	24,733.9	6
Campylobacter jejuni RM1221	Food poisoning	327.4	120	13,136.9	9
Fusobacterium nucleatum subsp. nucleatum ATCC 25586	Periodontitis	2166	57	13,456.6	8
Clostridium perfringens E str. JGS1987	Gastroenteritis, gas gangrene	3398.2	39	12,724.7	10

the facial skin core, which has been shown to prevent long term colonization by *Yersinia pestis* [74]. Other beneficial bacteria present in both gut and facial skin microbiomes include *Lactobacillus sakei*, an antilisterial bacterium [75]. We also identified several genes for the biosynthesis of antibiotics such as carbapenem, tetracycline, macrolides, and ansamycins, as well as resistance genes towards them (Additional file 6). The identification of insecticide, fungicide, and antiparasite related taxa and genes in the facial skin microbiome suggests protective mechanisms against possible eukaryotic pathogens present in the carcass (Additional file 6). For example, *Pseudomonas entomophila,* which causes lethality in flies [76], and for which we identified a gene coding for an insecticidal toxin SepC/Tcc class in the facial skin NR gene set catalogue (Additional file 5). The production of antibiotics to outcompete for resources is known in soil microbiomes, and recently similar strategies have been reported in the human nasal microbiome from commensal bacteria against pathogens [77]. Our results suggest that the vulture's facial skin microbiome plays a similar defensive role. Regarding the gut microbiome, commensal *Clostridia* are known to play an important role in the production of butyrate that the colonocytes use [78]. Notably, *C. butyricum* was among the most abundant *Clostridia* in the gut microbiome. Future studies would be needed to go beyond the description presented here to test for competitive exclusion among bacteria in the vulture gut microbiome [79, 80].

Beneficial bacterial functions

Besides containing potential pathogenic microbes, carcasses also contain toxic and carcinogenic compounds [81], which pose health risks to the vulture, particularly to its facial skin, which is in direct contact with such compounds. Among the bacteria identified in higher abundance in the facial microbiome was *Arthrobacter phenanthrenivorans,* which is able to degrade phenanthrene, a skin-irritating polycyclic aromatic hydrocarbon (PAH). PAH are xenobiotic pollutants with negative health-effects found to be emitted from animal carcass [82], and previously reported in high concentrations in other vulture species [83]. Interestingly, the largest variation on the metabolism of xenobiotics biodegradation was in the facial skin dataset (Additional file 6), with PAHs degradation metabolism being the most abundant subclass from the xenobiotics degradation pathway in both facial skin and gut. These findings suggest a microbiome protective role for the vulture against such compounds. In regards to the gut microbiome, the second most abundant *Fusobacteria* in the gut from the NR gene set was the gut butyrate-producing *F. varium* [84], for which we also identified its gene formate C-acetyltransferase, which is involved in butanoate metabolism, as the most abundant gene in the gut dataset. Interestingly, besides the use of butyrate for the colonocytes, it has been shown that butyrate glycerides have antimicrobial activity against *C. perfringens* and *Salmonella typhimurium* [85].

Phage controlled pathogen abundance

Phages in the human gut microbiome have been shown to play a protective role and the increasing identification of antibiotic resistance genes in pathogenic bacteria has led to the proposition of using phages as alternative therapies [86]. Given the identification of potential antibiotic resistance genes in the vulture facial skin and gut microbiomes (Additional file 5), we investigated the possible role of phages in eliminating or balancing the abundance of potential pathogens. In the facial skin microbiome, *Clostridium* phages positively correlated with *C. perfringens* and *C. botulinum,* whereas in the gut we observed enterobacteria phages correlating to *Escherichia fergusonii* (Additional file 7). Furthermore, in the taxonomic annotations of the gut functional core, we identified the *Salmonella* phage SPN3US (Additional file 7), which has shown effective inhibition of *S. enterica* [87]. From the facial skin functional strict core, the most abundant virus was phage BPP-1 (Additional file 7), which infects pathogenic *Bordetella* bacteria [88]. These findings show that the phage sets in both facial skin and gut microbiomes are related to the presence of the potential pathogens most abundant in the corresponding sample type. They also suggest that phages could represent an alternative defence mechanism for the control, and possibly elimination of potential pathogens, as in phage therapy [89] (Additional file 5).

Predatory defence mechanism

In spite of being important elements in the gut microbiome, gut microbial eukaryotes remain largely unexplored. Thus, we investigated whether vulture gut microbial eukaryotes played any protective role. We identified the invertebrate *Adineta vaga,* which feeds on dead bacteria and protozoans, to be ~6.8× more abundant in the gut core than in the facial skin core. This identification suggests that a predatory mechanism may be exploited for defence in the vulture's gut.

Biofilm formation and colonization resistance

Biofilms are assemblages of microbes associated within a matrix composed of extracellular polymeric substances that facilitate their adhesion to the surface, protection against antimicrobials, and better nutrient acquisition.

The abundance of *Fusobacteria* in the gut has been suggested to play a particularly relevant role in lumen biofilm formation in the gastrointestinal tract [90]. To explore this hypothesis, we searched for proteins related to biofilm formation (Additional file 7). In the core of the gut functional potential we identified biofilm related proteins from *F. mortiferum*, such as rubrerythrin, as well as from *C. perfringens*, such as UDP-glucuronic acid epimerase. Given that bacteria form biofilms in which they can thrive under different patterns of gene expression [91], this suggests that the identified potential pathogenic *Clostridia* and *Fusobacteria* from the gut microbiome might not pose pathogenic risks and instead offer colonization resistance against other external pathogens (Additional file 5). To further explore the possible colonization resistance role of *Clostridia* and *Fusobacteria*, we examined the gut functional core for toxins with potential effects on the vulture. We identified only few potentially pathogenic toxin coding genes from *Fusobacterium* (Additional file 7). Considering that *F. varium* has been shown to affect its human host in a beneficial manner by antagonizing colonization by pathogenic agents [92], we suggest that an important role of the gut *Fusobacteria* could be the formation of biofilms and colonization resistance, without representing a serious pathogenic threat. We identified the pathogenicity genes perfringolysin O and phospholipase C in the gut microbiome from *C. perfringens*. However, we also identified genes for the biosynthesis of short chain fatty acids from *Clostridia*, which can provide protection against inflammatory responses [93]. Thus, we could classify the observed *Clostridia* into two types, (i) the potentially pathogenic, mainly represented by *C. perfringens* and (ii) the non-pathogenic, which may contribute to biofilm formation and health defence (Additional file 4).

Conclusions

Our findings strongly suggest that the turkey and black vultures have adapted to their scavenging diet with the help of their facial skin and gut microbiomes. Surprisingly, most of their microbiome consists of a large variable pool of environmental and carcass-derived microbiota, with only a small set of constant inhabitants. In particular, the presence of a wide variety of microbes reported as pathogenic to non-scavengers (mammals and other birds) without an apparent or a reported pathogenic effect on the vultures calls for deeper study. Further studies would be required to determine whether the microbes reported here are pathogenic to the wild vultures or if they serve as reservoirs, and to determine what is their zoonotic potential. A better characterization of wild-life as potential pathogenic reservoirs (with microbiological, epidemiological and surveillance data) would allow for better informed wild-life protection programs, particularly for those species in endangered status, such as some species of vultures (e.g. the white-backed vulture [94]). We highlight the identification within the vultures' facial skin and gut microbiomes of defence mechanisms that are alternative to the use of antimicrobials, such as the use of predatory microbes, and the protective nature of colonization resistance through biofilm formation by Fusobacteria and Clostridia. However, further microbiology studies would be needed to isolate the relevant microbes and validate the antimicrobial mechanisms reported here from the vultures' microbiomes.

The establishment of these suggested protective mechanisms in the vulture microbiome unveiled by metagenomics analyses highlights the important role that vultures play in their ecosystem. This role is the essential but underrated service of cleaning up carcasses that otherwise would spread microbial elements pathogenic to species without a specialized microbiome like that of the vultures. In conclusion, our results show the importance of complementing genomic analyses with metagenomics on the host microbiome in order to obtain a clearer understanding of the host-microbial alliance that aids the evolution of extreme dietary adaptations.

Additional files

Additional file 1. The number of sequencing reads at the different filtering stages and metadata information on the samples (sheet 1). It also contains the read mapping counts to the various whole genome databases with MGmapper using the facial skin (sheet 2) and gut (sheet 3) datasets, as well as the bacterial taxonomic identifications from the 16S results in the study by Roggenbuck et al. [17] not found in the metagenomic bacterial taxonomic identification (sheet 4).

Additional file 2. The identified differentially abundant bacteria of the facial skin microbiome compared to the gut microbiome using a t-test (sheet 1) and a Wilcoxon test (sheet 2). It also contains a summary of the taxonomic identifications from the whole-genomic databases (sheet 3) and a summary of the abundance of the identified differentially abundant species (sheet 4).

Additional file 3. The comparative results of the facial skin and gut microbiome taxonomic content (sheet 1) and microbial attributes (sheet 2) identified with MEGAN. It also contains stats on the facial skin and gut microbiome functional annotation (sheet 3) and the bacterial total genes from each pathway from KEGG (sheet 4).

Additional file 4. Identified potential pathogens in the vultures' facial skin and gut microbiomes (sheet 1–4). The document also contains identified Clostridia toxin/antitoxins (sheet 5), pathogenic genes (sheet 6), strains with sporulation potential (sheet 7), and short chain fatty acids (sheet 8).

Additional file 5. Extra results and discussions on the vultures' facial skin and gut microbiomes.

Additional file 6. The identified proteins related to xenobiotics metabolism from the facial skin and gut microbiomes (sheets 1 and 2), as well as the identified genes from the facial skin and gut microbiomes related to putrescine and other carcass compounds (sheets 3 and 4). It also contains the identified resistance genes (sheets 5 and 6), and information on other identified genes related to pathogenicity (e.g. haemolysins) and health protection (e.g. antiparasitics) (sheet 7).

Additional file 7. The correlation values of the microbes from the facial skin (sheet 1) and gut (sheet 2) microbiomes. It also contains supporting information on identified phages (sheet 3), biofilm formation genes (sheet 4), and *E. coli* toxin/anti-toxin genes (sheet 5), as well as the identified toxins from Fusobacteria (sheet 6) and Clostridia (sheet 7).

Authors' contributions

MLZM performed the metagenomics analyses. KMV and MLZM performed the search for the resistance genes and potentially pathogenic microbes. MLZM, LHH, MTPG, MR, SR, and TSP interpreted the results. MLZM wrote the manuscript. LHH, MTPG, MR, SR, and TSP provided significant input on the manuscript drafting. All authors read and approved the final manuscript.

Author details

[1] Centre for GeoGenetics, Natural History Museum of Denmark, University of Copenhagen, Øster Voldgade 5-7, 1350 Copenhagen K, Denmark. [2] Department for Bioinformatics and Microbe Technology, Novozymes A/S, 2880 Bagsværd, Denmark. [3] Undergraduate Program on Genomic Sciences, Center for Genomic Sciences, National Autonomous University of Mexico, Av. Universidad s/n Col. Chamilpa, 62210 Cuernavaca, Morelos, Mexico. [4] Section for Microbiology and Biotechnology, Department of Environmental Science, Aarhus University, Frederiksborgvej 399, 4000 Roskilde, Denmark. [5] Center for Biological Sequence Analysis, Department of Bio and Health Informatics, Technical University of Denmark, Anker Engelunds Vej 1 Bygning 101A, 2800 Kgs. Lyngby, Denmark. [6] Novo Nordisk Foundation Center for Protein Research, Faculty of Health and Medical Sciences, University of Copenhagen, Blegdamsvej 3, 2200 Copenhagen N, Denmark. [7] Norwegian University of Science and Technology, University Museum, 7491 Trondheim, Norway. [8] Centre of Excellence for Omics-Driven Computational Biodiscovery (COMBio), Faculty of Applied Sciences, AIMST University, 08100 Bedong, Malaysia.

Acknowledgements

We thank the Danish National High-Throughput DNA Sequencing Centre for the generation of the sequencing data. We are also grateful to George Pacheco and Lillian Anne Petersen for DNA extractions and library preparations. We also gratefully acknowledge the Danish National Supercomputer for Life Sciences—Computerome (computerome.dtu.dk) for the computational resources to perform the sequence analyses. We thank Prof. Gary Graves (Smithsonian Institution) for providing the vulture facial skin and gut samples and valuable input on the manuscript drafting. We also thank Brian Schmidt and Christina Gebhard (both Smithsonian Institution) for necropsying vultures; Blaine Hyle, Talon Redding, William Simmons and J. D. Freye (all USDA) for collecting vultures; and Keith Wehner, Blaine Hyle and Brett Dunlap (all USDA) for providing critical logistic support in Nashville. The Alexander Wetmore Fund of the Smithsonian Institution provided funding for fieldwork. Søren Brunak thanks the Novo Nordisk Foundation (Grant NNF14CC0001).

Competing interests

The authors declare that they have no competing interests.

Funding

MLZM and MTPG thank Lundbeck Foundation Grant R52-A5062 for funding their research.

References

1. Jarvis ED, Mirarab S, Aberer AJ, Li B, Houde P, Li C, et al. Whole genome analyses resolve early branches in the tree of life of modern birds. Science. 2014;346:1320–31.
2. de Lucas M, Ferrer M, Bechard MJ, Muñoz AR. Griffon vulture mortality at wind farms in southern Spain: distribution of fatalities and active mitigation measures. Biol Conserv. 2012;147:184–9.
3. Mckean S, Mander M, Diederichs N, Ntuli L, Mavundla K, Williams V, et al. The impact of traditional use on vultures in South Africa. Vulture News. 2013;65:15–36.
4. Snyder NFR, Snyder H. The California condor: a saga of natural history and conservation. Cambridge: Academic Press; 2000. p. 410.
5. Houston DC. The ecology of Serengeti vultures. Oxford: Oxford Press; 1972.
6. Houston DC. The role of griffon vultures *Gyps africanus* and *Gyps ruppellii* as scavengers. J Zool. 1974;172:35–46.
7. Grigg NP, Krilow JM, Gutierrez-Ibanez C, Wylie DR, Graves GR, Iwaniuk AN. Anatomical evidence for scent guided foraging in the turkey vulture. Sci Rep. 2017. https://doi.org/10.1038/s41598-017-17794-0.
8. Koenig R. Ornithology. Vulture research soars as the scavengers' numbers decline. Science. 2006. https://doi.org/10.1126/science.312.5780.1591.
9. Margalida A, Colomer MA. Modelling the effects of sanitary policies on European vulture conservation. Sci Rep. 2012;2:753.
10. Anzen DH. Herbivores and the number of tree species in tropical forests. Am Nat. 1970;104(940):501–28.
11. Vollaard EJ, Clasener HA. Colonization resistance. Antimicrob Agents Chemother. 1994;38:409–14.
12. Loeffler AG, Hart MN. Chapter 26—Infectious diseases. In: Introduction to human disease: pathophysiology for health professionals. 6th ed. Burlington: Jones & Bartlett Learning; 2014. p. 396–7.
13. Metcalf JL, Xu ZZ, Weiss S, Lax S, Van Treuren W, Hyde ER, et al. Microbial community assembly and metabolic function during mammalian corpse decomposition. Science. 2015;351:158–62.
14. Chung O, Jin S, Cho YS, Lim J, Kim H, Jho S, et al. The first whole genome and transcriptome of the cinereous vulture reveals adaptation in the gastric and immune defense systems and possible convergent evolution between the Old and New World vultures. Genome Biol. 2015;16:215.
15. Mateos-Hernndez L, Crespo E, Fuente JDL, de la Lastra JMP. Identification of key molecules involved in the protection of vultures against pathogens and toxins. In: Baptista GR, editor. An integrated view of the molecular recognition and toxinology—from analytical procedures to biomedical applications. Rijeka: InTech; 2013.
16. Houston DC, Cooper JE. The digestive tract of the whiteback griffon vulture and its role in disease transmission among wild ungulates. J Wildl Dis. 1975;11:306–13.
17. Roggenbuck M, Bærholm Schnell I, Blom N, Bælum J, Bertelsen MF, Pontén TS, et al. The microbiome of New World vultures. Nat Commun. 2014. https://doi.org/10.1038/ncomms6498.
18. Ley RE, Lozupone CA, Hamady M, Knight R, Gordon JI. Worlds within worlds: evolution of the vertebrate gut microbiota. Nat Rev Microbiol. 2008;6:776–88.
19. Ley RE, Hamady M, Lozupone C, Turnbaugh PJ, Ramey RR, Bircher JS, et al. Evolution of mammals and their gut microbes. Science. 2008;320:1647–51.
20. Semova I, Carten JD, Stombaugh J, Mackey LC, Knight R, Farber SA, et al. Microbiota regulate intestinal absorption and metabolism of fatty acids in the zebrafish. Cell Host Microbe. 2012;12:277–88.
21. Hooper LV, Littman DR, Macpherson AJ. Interactions between the microbiota and the immune system. Science. 2012;336:1268–73.
22. Buffie CG, Pamer EG. Microbiota-mediated colonization resistance against intestinal pathogens. Nat Rev Immunol. 2013;13:790–801.
23. Qin J, Li Y, Cai Z, Li S, Zhu J, Zhang F, et al. A metagenome-wide association study of gut microbiota in type 2 diabetes. Nature. 2012;490:55–60.
24. Ley RE, Turnbaugh PJ, Klein S, Gordon JI. Microbial ecology: human gut microbes associated with obesity. Nature. 2006;444:1022–3.
25. Sokol H, Pigneur B, Watterlot L, Lakhdari O, Bermúdez-Humarán LG, Gratadoux J-J, et al. *Faecalibacterium prausnitzii* is an anti-inflammatory commensal bacterium identified by gut microbiota analysis of Crohn disease patients. Proc Natl Acad Sci. 2008;105:16731–6.
26. Bolger AM, Lohse M, Usadel B. Trimmomatic: a flexible trimmer for Illumina sequence data. Bioinformatics. 2014;30:2114–20.
27. Zhang G, Li B, Li C, Gilbert M, Jarvis E, Consortium TAG, et al. Comparative genomic data of the avian phylogenomics project. GigaSci Database. 2014;3:26.
28. Kultima JR, Sunagawa S, Li J, Chen W, Chen H, Mende DR, et al. MOCAT: a metagenomics assembly and gene prediction toolkit. PLoS ONE. 2012;7:1–6.

29. Petersen TN, Lukjancenko O, Thomsen MCF, Maddalena Sperotto M, Lund O, Møller Aarestrup F, et al. MGmapper: reference based mapping and taxonomy annotation of metagenomics sequence reads. PLoS ONE. 2017;12:e0176469.
30. Li H, Durbin R. Fast and accurate short read alignment with Burrows–Wheeler transform. Bioinformatics. 2009;25:1754–60.
31. Nielsen HB, Almeida M, Juncker AS, Rasmussen S, Li J, Sunagawa S, et al. Identification and assembly of genomes and genetic elements in complex metagenomic samples without using reference genomes. Nat Biotechnol. 2014;32:822–8.
32. Peterson J, Garges S, Giovanni M, McInnes P, Wang L, Schloss JA, et al. The NIH human microbiome project. Genome Res. 2009;19:2317–23.
33. Zankari E, Hasman H, Cosentino S, Vestergaard M, Rasmussen S, Lund O, et al. Identification of acquired antimicrobial resistance genes. J Antimicrob Chemother. 2012;67:2640–4.
34. DeSantis TZ, Hugenholtz P, Larsen N, Rojas M, Brodie EL, Keller K, et al. Greengenes, a chimera-checked 16S rRNA gene database and workbench compatible with ARB. Appl Environ Microbiol. 2006;72:5069–72.
35. Quast C, Pruesse E, Yilmaz P, Gerken J, Schweer T, Yarza P, et al. The SILVA ribosomal RNA gene database project: improved data processing and web-based tools. Nucleic Acids Res. 2013;41:D590–6.
36. R Core Team. R: a language and environment for statistical computing. Vienna: R Foundation for Statistical Computing; 2013.
37. Huson DH, Weber N. Microbial community analysis using MEGAN. Methods Enzymol. 2013;531:465–85.
38. Edgar RC. Search and clustering orders of magnitude faster than BLAST. Bioinformatics. 2010;26:2460–1.
39. Gillespie JJ, Wattam AR, Cammer SA, Gabbard JL, Shukla MP, Dalay O, et al. PATRIC: the comprehensive bacterial bioinformatics resource with a focus on human pathogenic species. Infect Immun. 2011;79:4286–98.
40. Van Belkum A. Classification of bacterial pathogens. COGEM Res Rep CGM. 2011;2011-07:1–113.
41. Ho Sui SJ, Fedynak A, Hsiao WWL, Langille MGI, Brinkman FSL. The association of virulence factors with genomic islands. PLoS ONE. 2009;4:e8094.
42. Buchfink B, Xie C, Huson DH. Fast and sensitive protein alignment using DIAMOND. Nat Methods. 2014;12:59–60.
43. Peng Y, Leung HCM, Yiu SM, Chin FYL. IDBA-UD: a de novo assembler for single-cell and metagenomic sequencing data with highly uneven depth. Bioinformatics. 2012;28:1420–8.
44. Hyatt D, Chen G-L, Locascio PF, Land ML, Larimer FW, Hauser LJ. Prodigal: prokaryotic gene recognition and translation initiation site identification. BMC Bioinform. 2010;11:119.
45. UniProt Consortium. The universal protein resource (UniProt). Nucleic Acids Res. 2008;36:D190–5.
46. Kanehisa M, Goto S. KEGG: Kyoto encyclopedia of genes and genomes. Nucleic Acids Res. 2000;28:27–30.
47. Luo R, Liu B, Xie Y, Li Z, Huang W, Yuan J, et al. SOAPdenovo2: an empirically improved memory-efficient short-read de novo assembler. Gigascience. 2012. https://doi.org/10.1186/2047-217x-1-18.
48. Gibson MK, Forsberg KJ, Dantas G. Improved annotation of antibiotic resistance determinants reveals microbial resistomes cluster by ecology. ISME J. 2015;9:207–16.
49. Eddy SR. Accelerated profile HMM searches. PLoS Comput Biol. 2011;7:e1002195.
50. Martínez I, Lattimer JM, Hubach KL, Case JA, Yang J, Weber CG, et al. Gut microbiome composition is linked to whole grain-induced immunological improvements. ISME J. 2013;7:269–80.
51. Rey FE, Faith JJ, Bain J, Muehlbauer MJ, Stevens RD, Newgard CB, et al. Dissecting the in vivo metabolic potential of two human gut acetogens. J Biol Chem. 2010;285:22082–90.
52. Leisner JJ, Laursen BG, Prévost H, Drider D, Dalgaard P. *Carnobacterium*: positive and negative effects in the environment and in foods. FEMS Microbiol Rev. 2007;31:592–613.
53. Suzuki M, Yamamoto T, Kawai Y, Inoue N, Yamazaki K. Mode of action of piscicocin CS526 produced by *Carnobacterium piscicola* CS526. J Appl Microbiol. 2005;98:1146–51.
54. Mirray WD, Khan AW, van den Berg L. *Clostridium saccharolyticum* sp. nov., a saccharolytic species from sewage sludge. Int J Syst Bacteriol. 1982;32:132–5.
55. He YL, Ding YF, Long YQ. Two cellulolytic *Clostridium* species: *Clostridium cellulosi* sp. nov. and *Clostridium cellulofermentans* sp. nov. Int J Syst Bacteriol. 1991;41:306–9.
56. Chassard C, Delmas E, Lawson PA, Bernalier-Donadille A. *Bacteroides xylanisolvens* sp. nov., a xylan-degrading bacterium isolated from human faeces. Int J Syst Evol Microbiol. 2008;58:1008–13.
57. George HA, Johnson JL, Moore WE, Holdeman LV, Chen JS. Acetone, isopropanol, and butanol production by *Clostridium beijerinckii* (syn. *Clostridium butylicum*) and *Clostridium aurantibutyricum*. Appl Environ Microbiol. 1983;45:1160–3.
58. Madihah MS, Ariff AB, Khalil MS, Suraini AA, Karim MI. Anaerobic fermentation of gelatinized sago starch-derived sugars to acetone-1-butanol-ethanol solvent by *Clostridium acetobutylicum*. Folia Microbiol. 2001;46:197–204.
59. Frodyma ME, Downs D. The panE gene, encoding ketopantoate reductase, maps at 10 minutes and is allelic to apbA in *Salmonella typhimurium*. J Bacteriol. 1998;180:4757–9.
60. Grice EA, Kong HH, Renaud G, Young AC, Bouffard GG, Blakesley RW, et al. A diversity profile of the human skin microbiota. Genome Res. 2008;18:1043–50.
61. Chain PSG, Lang DM, Comerci DJ, Malfatti SA, Vergez LM, Shin M, et al. Genome of *Ochrobactrum anthropi* ATCC 49188T, a versatile opportunistic pathogen and symbiont of several eukaryotic hosts. J Bacteriol. 2011;193:4274–5.
62. Creuzburg K, Recktenwald J, Kuhle V, Herold S, Hensel M, Schmidt H. The Shiga toxin 1-converting bacteriophage BP-4795 encodes an NleA-like type III effector protein. J Bacteriol. 2005;187:8494–8.
63. Jakhetia R, Talukder KA, Verma NK. Isolation, characterization and comparative genomics of bacteriophage SfIV: a novel serotype converting phage from *Shigella flexneri*. BMC Genomics. 2013;14:677.
64. Harkinezhad T, Geens T, Vanrompay D. *Chlamydophila psittaci* infections in birds: a review with emphasis on zoonotic consequences. Vet Microbiol. 2009;135:68–77.
65. Klementowicz JE, Travis MA, Grencis RK. *Trichuris muris*: a model of gastro-intestinal parasite infection. Semin Immunopathol. 2012;34:815–28.
66. Jung RC, Beaver PC. Clinical observations on *Trichocephalus trichiurus* (whipworm) infestation in children. Pediatrics. 1951;8:548–57.
67. Shirley MW, Smith AL, Tomley FM. The biology of avian *Eimeria* with an emphasis on their control by vaccination. Adv Parasitol. 2005;60:285–330.
68. East IJ, Eisemann CH. Vaccination against *Lucilia cuprina*: the causative agent of sheep blowfly strike. Immunol Cell Biol. 1993;71:453–62.
69. Wertheim HFL, Nghia HDT, Taylor W, Schultsz C. *Streptococcus suis*: an emerging human pathogen. Clin Infect Dis. 2009;48:617–25.
70. Paller G, Hommel RK, Kleber HP. Phenol degradation by *Acinetobacter calcoaceticus* NCIB 8250. J Basic Microbiol. 1995;35:325–35.
71. Nazzaro F, Fratianni F, De Martino L, Coppola R, De Feo V. Effect of essential oils on pathogenic bacteria. Pharmaceuticals. 2013;6:1451–74.
72. Graves G. Field measurements of gastrointestinal pH of New World vultures in Guyana. J Raptor Res. 2017;51:465–9.
73. Hou PC. The pathology of *Clonorchis sinensis* infestation of the liver. J Pathol Bacteriol. 1955;70:53–64.
74. Pawlowski DR, Raslawsky A, Siebert G, Metzger DJ. Identification of *Hylemonella gracilis* as an antagonist of *Yersinia pestis* persistence. J Bioterror Biodef. 2011. https://doi.org/10.4172/2157-2526.s3-004.
75. Bredholt S, Nesbakken T, Holck A. Industrial application of an antilisterial strain of *Lactobacillus sakei* as a protective culture and its effect on the sensory acceptability of cooked, sliced, vacuum-packaged meats. Int J Food Microbiol. 2001;66:191–6.
76. Vodovar N, Vinals M, Liehl P, Basset A, Degrouard J, Spellman P, et al. *Drosophila* host defense after oral infection by an entomopathogenic *Pseudomonas* species. Proc Natl Acad Sci. 2005;102:11414–9.
77. Zipperer A, Konnerth MC, Laux C, Berscheid A, Janek D, Weidenmaier C, et al. Human commensals producing a novel antibiotic impair pathogen colonization. Nature. 2016;535:511–6.
78. Pryde SE, Duncan SH, Hold GL, Stewart CS, Flint HJ. The microbiology of butyrate formation in the human colon. FEMS Microbiol Lett. 2002;217:133–9.
79. Freilich S, Zarecki R, Eilam O, Segal ES, Henry CS, Kupiec M, et al. Competitive and cooperative metabolic interactions in bacterial communities. Nat Commun. 2011. https://doi.org/10.1038/ncomms1597.

80. Louca S, Doebeli M. Transient dynamics of competitive exclusion in microbial communities. Environ Microbiol. 2016;18:1863–74.
81. Phan NT, Kim KH, Jeon EC, Kim UH, Sohn JR, Pandey SK. Analysis of volatile organic compounds released during food decaying processes. Environ Monit Assess. 2012;184:1683–92.
82. Chen SJ, Hsieh LT, Chiu SC. Emission of polycyclic aromatic hydrocarbons from animal carcass incinerators. Sci Total Environ. 2003;313:61–76.
83. Dhananjayan V, Muralidharan S. Levels of polycyclic aromatic hydrocarbons, polychlorinated biphenyls, and organochlorine pesticides in various tissues of white-backed vulture in India. Biomed Res Int. 2013. https://doi.org/10.1155/2013/190353.
84. Dzink JL, Socransky SS. Amino acid utilization by *Fusobacterium nucleatum* grown in a chemically defined medium. Oral Microbiol Immunol. 1990;5:172–4.
85. Namkung H, Yu H, Gong J, Leeson S. Antimicrobial activity of butyrate glycerides toward *Salmonella typhimurium* and *Clostridium perfringens*. Poult Sci. 2011;90:2217–22.
86. Sulakvelidze A, Alavidze Z, Morris JG. Bacteriophage therapy. Antimicrob Agents Chemother. 2001;45:649–59.
87. Kagawa H, Ono N, Enomoto M, Komeda Y. Bacteriophage chi sensitivity and motility of *Escherichia coli* K-12 and *Salmonella typhimurium* Fla-mutants possessing the hook structure. J Bacteriol. 1984;157:649–54.
88. Liu M, Deora R, Doulatov SR, Gingery M, Eiserling FA, Preston A, et al. Reverse transcriptase-mediated tropism switching in *Bordetella* bacteriophage. Science. 2002;295:2091–4.
89. Focà A, Liberto MC, Quirino A, Marascio N, Zicca E, Pavia G, et al. Gut inflammation and immunity: what is the role of the human gut virome? Mediat Inflamm. 2015. https://doi.org/10.1155/2015/326032.
90. Keenan SW, Engel AS, Elsey RM. The alligator gut microbiome and implications for archosaur symbioses. Sci Rep. 2013;3:2877.
91. Prigent-Combaret C, Vidal O, Dorel C, Lejeune P. Abiotic surface sensing and biofilm-dependent regulation of gene expression in *Escherichia coli*. J Bacteriol. 1999;181:5993–6002.
92. Ushijima T, Ozaki Y. Potent antagonism of *Escherichia coli*, *Bacteroides ovatus*, *Fusobacterium varium*, and *Enterococcus faecalis*, alone or in combination, for enteropathogens in anaerobic continuous flow cultures. J Med Microbiol. 1986;22:157–63.
93. Vinolo MAR, Rodrigues HG, Nachbar RT, Curi R. Regulation of inflammation by short chain fatty acids. Nutrients. 2011;3:858–76.
94. Birdlife International. *Gyps africanus* (amended version of 2016 assessment). The IUCN Red List of Threatened Species. 2017;2017:e.T22695189A118592149.

24

Determination of the expression of three fimbrial subunit proteins in cultured *Trueperella pyogenes*

Mengcheng Liu[1,2†], Bing Wang[1,2†], Hongmin Liang[1,2], Bo Ma[1,2], Junwei Wang[1,2] and Wenlong Zhang[1,2*]

Abstract

Background: *Trueperella pyogenes* is a commensal and a significant opportunistic pathogen in animals. A variety of identified or putative virulence factors are considered to significantly contribute to the occurrence of *T. pyogenes* infection in different species. However, these virulence factors are not fully understood.

Results: In the current study, the genes encoding putative fimbrial proteins, i.e. Fim A, Fim C, and Fim E, were cloned. Recombinant Fim A (rFim A), Fim C (rFim C), and Fim E (rFim E) were prepared and used to generate rabbit anti-rFim A, anti-rFim C, and anti-rFim E serum, respectively. Using these sera, we found that only Fim E was constitutively expressed in *T. pyogenes*. The expression level of Fim E in *T. pyogenes* peaked within 6–10 h of culture period in pH 7.5. Fim E protein expression was unaffected by anaerobic condition, but was inhibited by the microaerophilic condition. Tube agglutination tests indicated that Fim E was exhibited on the surface of *T. pyogenes* cells because anti-rFim E serum caused strong agglutination. Additionally, the blots for Fim A detection showed nonspecific reactions. Furthermore, the tube agglutination tests showed that anti-Fim A serum failed to cause agglutination of *T. pyogenes* cells, which indicated that Fim A was not, or poorly, expressed in cultured *T. pyogenes*. Anti-rFim C serum caused strong agglutination. However, the blots for Fim C detection showed a strong nonspecific reaction. Thus, the expression of Fim C was difficult to be determined using the current method.

Conclusions: Fim E was expressed in cultured *T. pyogenes*. However, Fim A was either not or poorly expressed in cultured *T. pyogenes*. Moreover, Fim C expression was not determined using the current strategy.

Keywords: Expression, Fim A, Fim C and Fim E, *Trueperella pyogenes*, Virulence factors

Background

Trueperella pyogenes is a Gram-positive rod-shaped bacterium [1]. This organism is a commensal and a common opportunistic pathogen in different domestic and wild animals [2–4]. Moreover, human beings can be infected by this bacterium; however, the infections are generally related to occupational exposure [5].

The ability of the *T. pyogenes* in causing infections in different species could be, at least partially, attributed to various virulence factors that are encoded in its genome [1]. The virulence factors of this bacterium include exotoxins (pyolysin), exoenzymes (proteases and DNase), and adhesins [1]. Among these virulence factors, components that mediate the adhesion of the organism to host cells play essential roles in establishing the infection [6, 7]. For *T. pyogenes*, these host cell adhesive factors not only work in establishing the infection but also when the organism acts as a commensal on the various mucous membranes of the hosts. Thus, investigations have been conducted on adhesins to help understand the pathogenicity of *T. pyogenes* and its mechanism in terms of switching from a commensal to a pathogen. Many adhesive components, such as collagen-binding protein A, fibronectin-binding protein, and fimbriae, that might

*Correspondence: zhangwenlong@neau.edu.cn
†Mengcheng Liu and Bing Wang contributed equally to current study
[1] College of Veterinary Medicine, Northeast Agricultural University, Changjiang Road 600, Harbin 150030, Heilongjiang, People's Republic of China
Full list of author information is available at the end of the article

mediate the adhesion of this organism to the host tissue, have been reported [1]. The genes encoding these adhesive components have been extensively used as molecular markers for identifying, genotyping, or predicting the virulence of *T. pyogenes* [3, 8]. However, evidence of adhesin expression in *T. pyogenes* cells is extremely limited [9–11]. *T. pyogenes* has been reported to express fimbriae [1]; however, the properties and constitution of this structure have not been studied. Putative fimbrial subunit proteins, such as Fim A, Fim B, Fim C, Fim E, and Fim J, have been reported to be expressed in *T. pyogenes*. However, only the genes, mRNAs, or the existence of specific antibodies against these proteins in *T. pyogenes*-infected animals have been detected [1, 12, 13].

In the current study, we aimed to determine the expression of three putative fimbrial subunit proteins, namely, Fim A, Fim C, and Fim E, in cultured *T. pyogenes*. However, only the expression of Fim E was detected. These results will contribute to the work on molecular pathogenesis regarding *T. pyogenes*.

Methods

Bacterial culture

Single colonies of *T. pyogenes* strains 0912 and 1005 were obtained by inoculating the bacteria on Martin broth agar plates (AOBOX Biotechnology Co., Beijing, China) with 10% sheep blood. The isolates originated from the lung of cattle that had dies due to pneumonia in China. The agar plates with the inoculum were incubated at 37 °C for 48 h. For the enrichment culture of the bacteria, single colonies of each *T. pyogenes* strain were inoculated into liquid Martin broth medium (AOBOX Biotechnology Co., Beijing, China) with 10% fetal bovine serum (FBS) and shaken at 37 °C for 24 h. The cultures were adjusted to reach an optical density (OD) 600 nm value of 1.2 using fresh culture medium, and then inoculated into fresh culture medium at a ratio of 2%.

In some of the experiments, the pH of liquid Martin broth medium was adjusted to different end points, using HCl (1 mol/L) or NaOH (1 mol/L), as indicated in the results.

For the anaerobic culturing of the bacteria, liquid paraffin was used to seal the surface of the liquid Martin broth medium. After inoculation, a 48-h static culture was used for bacterial proliferation. Moreover, the bacteria were cultured in a microaerophilic environment. Briefly, the bacteria were inoculated into the Martin broth agar plates with 10% sheep blood. The plates were placed in a jar. AnaeroPack-MicroAero (Mitsubishi Gas Chemical Company, Tokyo, Japan) was used to generate a microaerophilic environment. After 24 h, the lawn from the culture was harvested by washing the plates with sterile phosphate buffer saline (PBS).

In most of the above experiments, bacterial growth was determined by measuring the OD 600 nm values of the cultures. The purity of the cultures was determined by using streak plate method and Gram staining.

Cloning and expression of *fimA*, *fimC*, and *fimE* genes

The genome of the bacteria was extracted using a Bacterium genome extraction kit (Tiangen Biotech, Beijing, China) according to the manufacturer's instruction. The genes encoding the Fim A, C, and E proteins were amplified and cloned using the primers listed in Table 1. The genes were inserted into a prokaryotic expression vector, pET-30a (+) (Novagen, Madison, USA) through the corresponding restriction sites. The transformants were sequenced by BGI International using a T7 promoter and a terminator primer. The recombinant plasmids were named pET-30a (+)-*fimA*, pET-30a (+)-*fimC*, and pET-30a (+)-*fimE*.

All these recombinant plasmids were transformed into *Escherichia coli* Rosetta (DE3)™ competent cells (Novagen, Madison, USA). The positively transformed *E. coli* were cultured at 37 °C until they reached an OD 600 nm value of 0.6–0.8. Recombinant Fim A (rFim A), Fim C (rFim C), and Fim E (rFim E) were expressed by inducing with 1 mmol/L isopropyl-β-D-1-thiogalactoside (IPTG) for 4 h and were then purified using nickel-charged resin (Merck, Shanghai, China). The purified proteins were dialyzed against PBS with 5% glycerol at 4 °C for 48 h. The proteins were quantified using Bradford Protein

Table 1 Primers used for gene cloning and plasmid construction

Names of the primers	Nucleotide (5′ to 3′)	Restrict sites
fimA forward	C<u>GAGCTC</u>ATGGGTGCACTGGTGACGGC	*Sac* I
fimA backward	CCC<u>AAGCTT</u>TTAGGCATTACGACGACGAGCGAC	*Hind* III
fimC forward	CGC<u>GGATCC</u>GTGTTTACGGTGGTAACC	*EcoR* I
fimC backward	CCC<u>AAGCTT</u>TTAGCTACGACGACGAGCGTG	*Hind* III
fimE forward	C<u>GAGCTC</u>ATGAAGCGAAACAAGTTACGTGC	*Sac* I
fimE backward	CCC<u>AAGCTT</u>TTAGACGTCCTTGCGTCGGTT	*Hind* III

Restriction enzyme recognition sites are underlined in each sequence and listed in the right column

Assay Kit (Beyotime, Beijing, China), according to the manufacturer's instructions and stored at − 80 °C until use. The signal peptides of these proteins were predicted using DNAMAN (LynnonBiosoft, San Ramon, USA).

Preparation of rabbit sera against *T. pyogenes*, Fim A, Fim C, and Fim E

T. pyogenes strain 1005 was cultured in 50 mL Martin broth medium with 10% FBS. The culture was harvested after being incubated at 37 °C for 20 h, and then inactivated by treating with 0.5% formaldehyde at 37 °C for 72 h. The inactivated culture was centrifuged and the precipitation was resuspended in 20 mL normal saline (0.9% NaCl w/v). Aluminum hydroxide gel suspension was prepared as described in a previous study [14]. The inactive *T. pyogenes* culture was mixed with aluminum hydroxide gel suspension at a volume ratio of 5:1.

The protocol of the animal experiment was approved by the Ethics Committee on the Use and Care of Animals, Northeast Agricultural University, China.

Rabbit anti-*T. pyogenes* strain 1005 serum was prepared through subcutaneous inoculation of a New Zealand rabbit with 1 mL mixture of inactive *T. pyogenes* (4.1×10^9 cells) and aluminum hydroxide gel twice with an interval of 15 days. Seven days after the second inoculation, the rabbit was boosted with 1 mL live *T. pyogenes* (4.1×10^9 cells). Seven days after the boosting, serum was collected from the rabbit and stored at − 20 °C.

Rabbit anti-rFim A, anti-rFim C, and anti-rFim E sera were prepared by immunizing New Zealand rabbits with the corresponding recombinants. Each recombinant protein was used to immunize one rabbit. Each rabbit received two inoculations at a 2-week interval. A mixture of 500 μg recombinant protein and Freund's complete adjuvant (Sigma-Aldrich, Shanghai, China) was used for the first inoculation, and a mixture of 500 μg recombinant protein and Freund's incomplete adjuvant (Sigma-Aldrich, Shanghai, China) was used for the second inoculation. Three days after the second immunization, serum was collected and stored at − 20 °C.

Determination of the reactivity of recombinant proteins to anti-*T. pyogenes* serum

The reactivity of the three recombinant proteins to rabbit anti-*T. pyogenes* serum were determined by using western blot assay. Purified rFim A, rFim C, and rFim E (10 μg each) were separated via sodium dodecyl sulfate polyacrylamide gel electrophoresis (SDS-PAGE) and were transferred onto nitrocellulose (NC) membranes. The NC membranes were blocked with 10% skim milk in PBST (0.05% v/v Tween 20 in PBS) for 1 h at room temperature. The membranes were then washed with PBST 5 times. The anti-*T. pyogenes* serum was diluted (1:10,000) and incubated with the NC membranes at 4 °C overnight and washed with PBST five times. Horseradish peroxidase (HRP) conjunct goat anti-rabbit IgG (ZSGB-bio, Beijing, China) was diluted (1:5000) and incubated with the NC membranes for 1 h at room temperature.

To verify the presence of the three recombinant proteins used for the analysis, a parallel immunoblot assay was performed using anti-histidine tag monoclonal antibodies (1:5000) (ZSGB-bio, Beijing, China) and anti-mouse HRP conjunct secondary antibodies (1:5000) (ZSGB-bio, Beijing, China) that were incubated with the NC membranes at 4 °C overnight and for 1 h at room temperature.

Determination of the expression of Fim A, Fim C, and Fim E in cultured *T. pyogenes*

The expression of Fim A, Fim C, and Fim E in cultured *T. pyogenes* were determined by using western blot assay. Briefly, the *T. pyogenes* strain 0912 and strain 1005 cultures were harvested, and the collected cultures were centrifuged at 4 °C. The precipitations were washed with sterile PBS twice. Moreover, the bacteria were resuspended in sterile PBS and ultrasonically broken down (500 W) for 10 min (5 s with intervals of 3 s). The products were centrifuged at 4 °C, and the supernatants were harvested for further analysis. The concentrations of the proteins in supernatants were determined using Bradford Protein Assay Kit (Beyotime, Beijing, China). Afterward, the samples were adjusted using the same concentration. A total of 40 μg of proteins in samples were separated through SDS-PAGE. The expression of Fim A, Fim C, and Fim E in the samples were determined using rabbit anti-rFim A (1:5000), rFim C (1:2000), and rFim E (1:2000) sera, respectively. The primary antibodies were incubated with the NC membranes at 4 °C overnight. HRP conjugated goat anti-rabbit IgG (ZSGB-bio, Beijing, China) was diluted (1:5000) and incubated with the NC membrane for 1 h at room temperature.

Tube agglutination test

T. pyogenes strains 0912 and 1005 cells were cultured at 37 °C until the OD 600 nm value reached 1.75. The cultures, in volumes of 50 mL, were centrifuged at 4 °C. The supernatants were discarded and the precipitates were washed twice with sterile PBS. The final precipitations were resuspended in 25 mL sterile normal saline. The bacterial suspensions were used as antigens for the tube agglutination test.

Tube agglutination test was utilized to determine the reactivity of the anti-rFim A, anti-rFim C, and anti-rFim E sera to *T. pyogenes* cells. The twofold serially diluted sera by normal saline (0.5 mL) was mixed with equal volumes of bacterial suspension. The tubes were incubated at 37 °C for 30 min. Unimmunized rabbit serum was added in every set of the test as controls.

Results

Cloning *fimA*, *fimE*, and *fimC* genes of *T. pyogenes*

The *fimA*, *fimC*, and *fimE* genes were amplified from genomes of *T. pyogenes* strains 0912 and 1005. The *fimA*, *fimC*, and *fimE* genes from *T. pyogenes* strain 0912 were 1362, 1374, and 1755 base pair (bp), respectively. The *fimA* and *fimC* genes of *T. pyogenes* strain 1005 showed the same length as the genes from strain 0912, whereas three nucleotide (382–384) deletions were observed in the *fimE* gene from *T. pyogenes* strain 1005, in comparison with *fimE* gene from strain 0912. The homologies of *fimA*, *fimC*, and *fimE* genes from the two strains were 98.83%, 99.04%, and 96.75%, respectively. The homologies of the deduced primary structures of Fim A, Fim C, and Fim E protein from the two strains were 98.01%, 99.43%, and 96.23%, respectively.

The primary structures of putative Fim A, Fim C, and Fim E proteins of *T. pyogenes* strain 0912 were analyzed using DNAMAN, which predicted signal peptides with lengths of 22, 27, and 30 amino acids (aa) at the carboxyl terminals of the three proteins, respectively. As reported previously [12], the deduced primary structures of Fim A, Fim C and Fim E proteins possess a cell wall sorting signal (CWSS), which is composed of a LPLTG motif and located approximately 30 aa away from the C terminus of these proteins (amino acid sequences of the three putative proteins of *T. pyogenes* strain 0912 are provided in Additional file 1).

Preparation and identification of rFim A, rFim C, and rFim E

As the target proteins from the two strains showed relatively high homology, only genes from *T. pyogenes* strain 0912 were expressed in *E. coli*. The rFim A and rFim C showed a molecular weight of approximately 58 kDa, whereas rFim E weighed approximately 72 kDa (Fig. 1a). Furthermore, western blot assay showed that rFim E, but not rFim A and rFim C, reacted with the anti-*T. pyogenes* serum (Fig. 1b). Results indicated that only anti-Fim E antibodies were elicited when the rabbit was immunized with *T. pyogenes*.

Determination of the expression of Fim A, Fim C, and Fim E in cultured *T. pyogenes* strain 0912

Trueperella pyogenes strain 0912 was cultured for 4 h. The western blot assay indicated that only Fim E (predicted molecular weight was 56.6 kDa, without signal peptide and amino acids behind CWSS) was detected in the bacterium (Fig. 2). The blots for Fim A (predicted molecular weight is 42.2 kDa) and Fim C (predicted molecular weight was 41.1 kDa) detection showed nonspecific reaction bands. However, at the predicted area on the blots, none of the bands showed stronger reactivity than those of the other bands with the corresponding antiserum.

Determination of the effects of different cultural conditions on the expression of Fim A, Fim C, and Fim E in *T. pyogenes* strains 0912 and 1005

We initially determined the influence of culture period on the expression of the three proteins. As shown in Fig. 3, we sampled *T. pyogenes* strains 0912 and 1005 cultures at 4, 6, 8, 10, 12, 16, 20, and 24 h post-inoculation. The expression of Fim E was observed in *T. pyogenes* strains 0912 and 1005 and was detectable in all samples collected at different time points. The expression of Fim E peaked at 6 h for strain 0912, and 10 h for strain 1005.

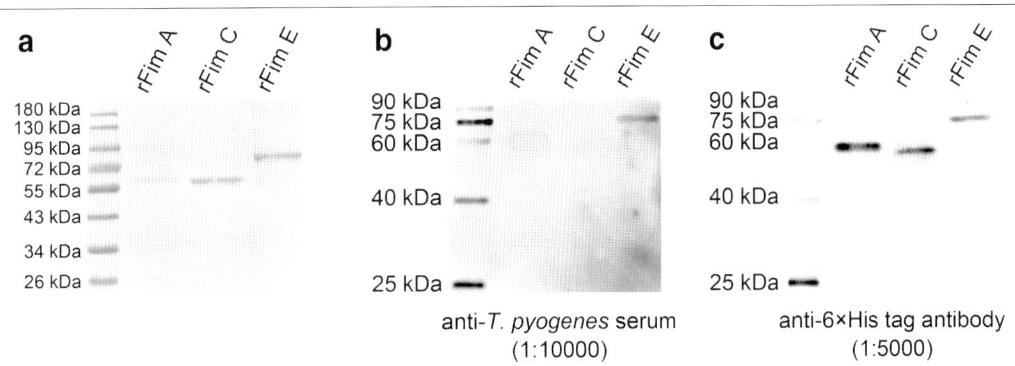

Fig. 1 Analysis of the molecular weight and immunoreactivity of the rFim A, rFim C, and rFim E proteins by SDS-PAGE and western blot assays. **a** Purified rFim A, rFim C, and rFim E were analyzed via SDS-PAGE. The predicted molecular weight of rFim A, rFim C, and rFim E was 58 kDa, 58 kDa, and 72 kDa, respectively. **b** Immunoreactivity of rFim A, rFim C, and rFim E to rabbit anti-*T. pyogenes* serum. The serum was diluted 1:10,000. **c** Determination of the existence and the amount of rFim A, rFim C, and rFim E on the NC membrane via immunoblot assay using anti-histidine tag monoclonal antibody. The antibody was diluted 1:5000

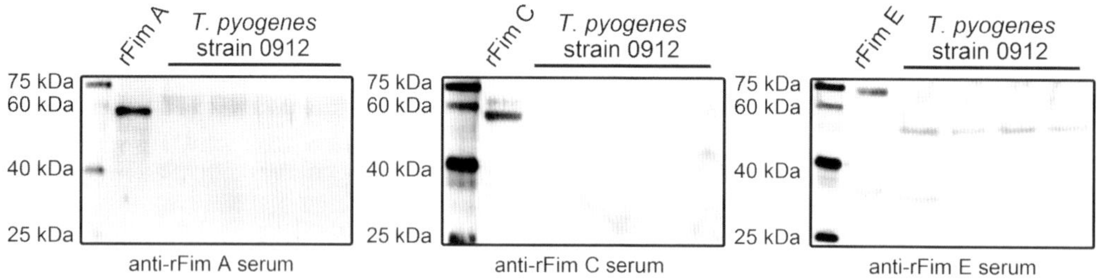

Fig. 2 Analyzing the expression of Fim A, Fim C, and Fim E in cultured *T. pyogenes* strain 0912 by western blot assays. The samples for immunoblot assay were harvested from four different batches of cultured *T. pyogenes* strain 0912, all cultured for 4 h

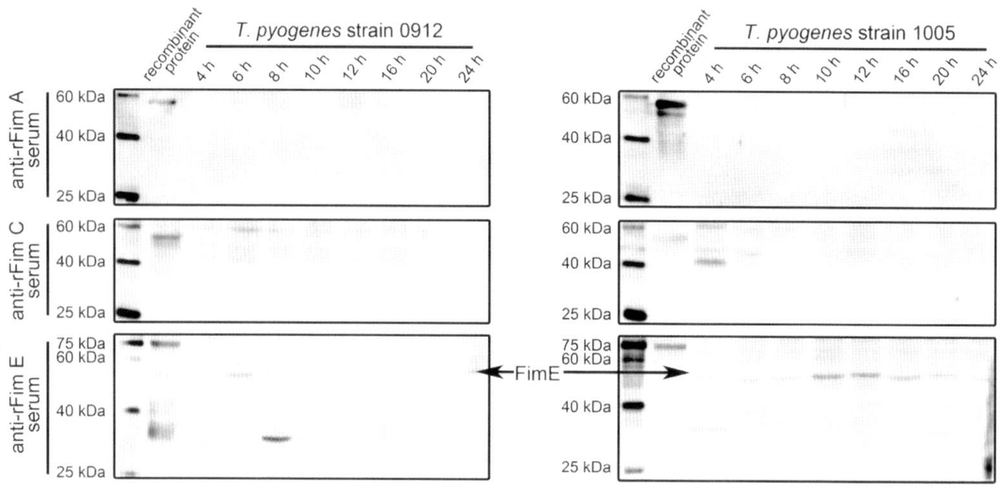

Fig. 3 Analyzing the effect of culture period on the expression of Fim A, Fim C, and Fim E in *T. pyogenes* strain 0912 and strain 1005 by western blot assays. *T. pyogenes* strain 0912 and strain 1005 cells were cultured for 24 h. Samples were collected at 4, 6, 8, 10, 12, 16, 20, and 24 h. The experiment was repeated at least three times

The blots for Fim A and Fim C detection showed many nonspecific reaction bands.

We determined the influence of pH on the expression of the three proteins in *T. pyogenes* strains 0912 and 1005. Effective proliferation of *T. pyogenes* was observed at pH 6.5, 7.5, and 8.5 within 8 h and were partially inhibited at pH 4.5, 5.5, 9.5, and 10.5. Figure 4 show that Fim E expression could be observed in organisms cultured at pH 5.5–8.5. The blots for Fim A and Fim C detection still showed many nonspecific reaction bands.

We finally tried to investigate the influence of anaerobic environment and microaerophilic environment on the expression of the three proteins in *T. pyogenes* strain 0912. Proliferation of the organism in anaerobic environments was not as efficient as proliferating in aerobic conditions. Figure 5 indicates that anaerobic environment did not affect the expression of the three recombinant proteins, and only the Fim E was detectable in the western blot assay. The microaerophilic environment improved the growth rate and promoted the production of pyolysin of the microorganisms on the plates (data not shown). However, Fim E was not detected in the microorganism by western blot assay using anti-rFim E serum, thus indicating that the microaerophilic environment could have inhibited the expression of Fim E (Fig. 5). Moreover, Fim A and Fim C were not detected in *T. pyogenes* cultured in the microaerophilic environment (Fig. 5).

Tube agglutination test

Results of tube agglutination test showed that rabbit anti-rFim C and anti-rFim E sera caused noticeable agglutination of *T. pyogenes* strains 0912 and 1005 cells at dilution ratios as high as 1:1280 and 1:640 (Fig. 6), respectively. Results indicated that the antigens targeted by the rabbit anti-rFim C and anti-rFim E sera were exposed on the surface of the organism.

In contrast, rabbit anti-rFim A serum and the serum collected from an unimmunized rabbit did not cause

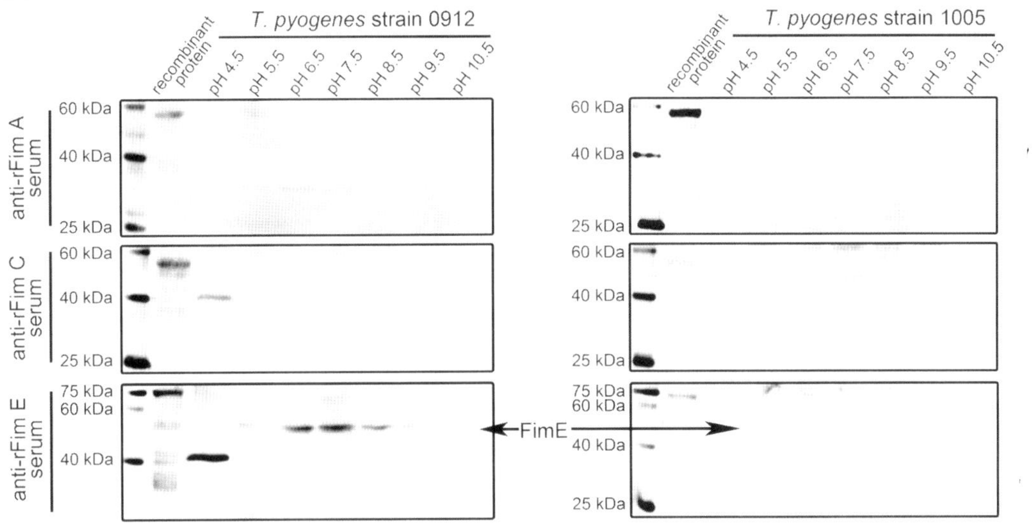

Fig. 4 Analyzing the effect of pH value on the expression of Fim A, Fim C, and Fim E in *T. pyogenes* strain 0912 and strain 1005 by western blot assays. *T. pyogenes* strain 0912 and strain 1005 cells were cultured at pH 4.5, 5.5, 6.5, 7.5, 8.5, 9.5, and 10.5 conditions for 8 h. The experiment was repeated at least three times

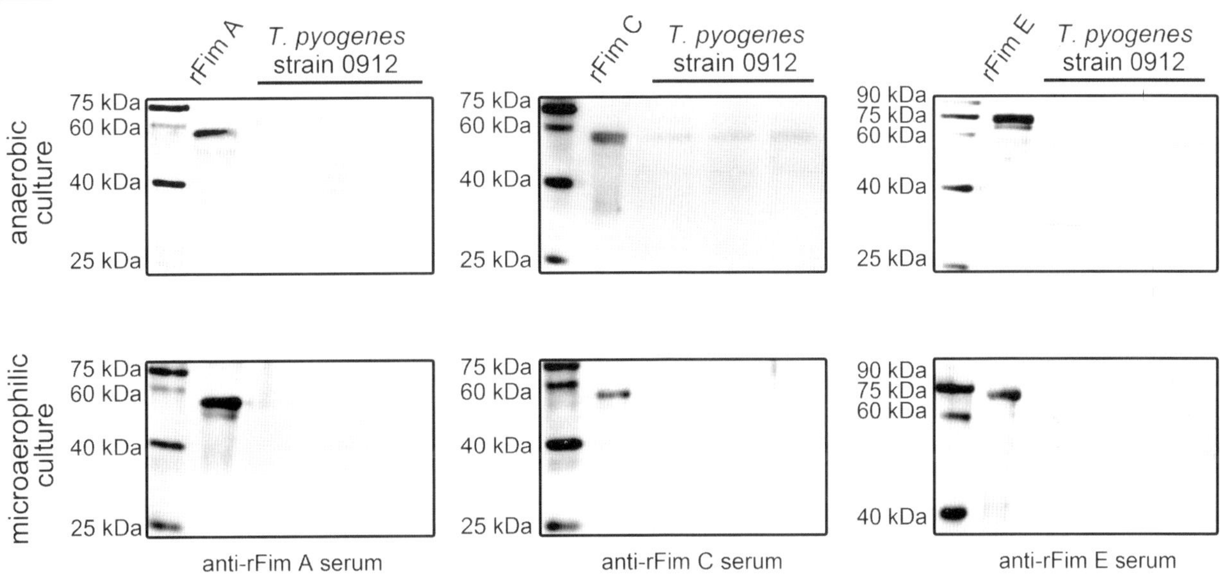

Fig. 5 Analysis of the effects of anaerobic and microaerophilic environment on the expression of Fim A, Fim C, and Fim E in *T. pyogenes* strain 0912 by western blot assays. The samples for immunoblot assay were harvested from three different batches of cultured *T. pyogenes* strain 0912, cultured for 48 h in anaerobic environment or 24 h in microaerophilic environment

noticeable agglutination of *T. pyogenes* cells within 30 min even at a dilution ratio of as low as 1:40 (Fig. 6).

Discussion

The pathogenesis of infections caused by the opportunistic pathogen *T. pyogenes* remain poorly characterized. Opportunistic pathogenic infections take place when the host immune systems are affected by adverse factors, such as shipping, wounds, extreme weather, and primary pathogenic infections, that facilitate the colonization and invasion of these pathogens [15, 16]. In addition, the changes in expression profiles of the various virulence factors of pathogens might be essential in establishing infections. Jost and Billington [1] speculated that genetically regulated differential expression levels of virulence factors are among the reasons for the transformation of

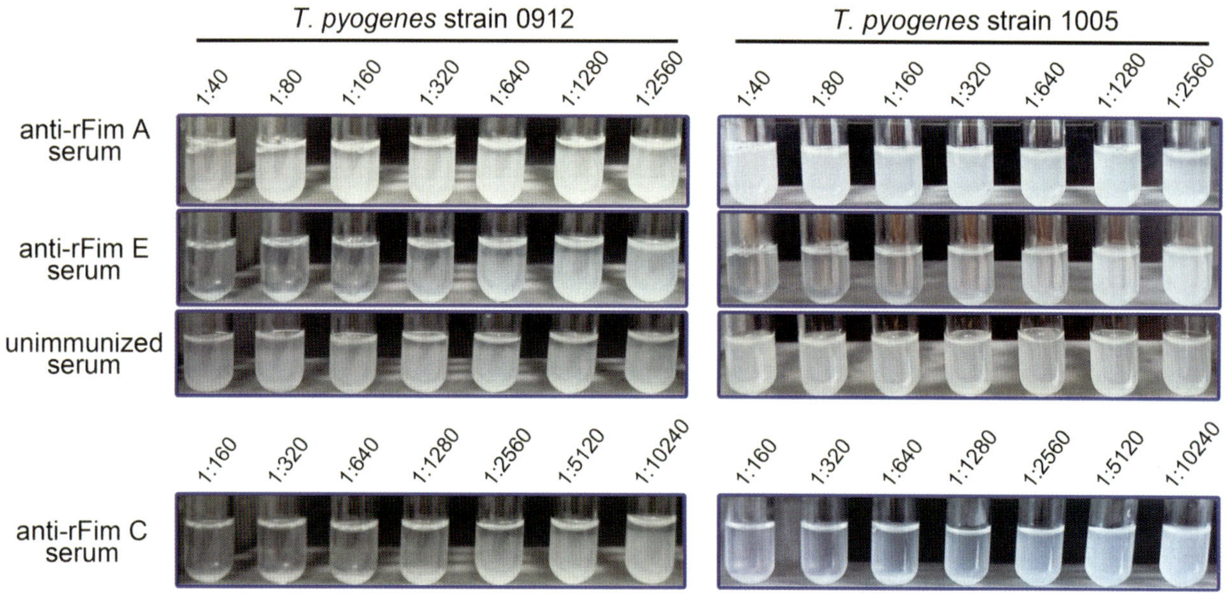

Fig. 6 Analysis the reactivity of anti-rFim A, rFim C, and rFim E serum to intact *T. pyogenes* cells via tube agglutination test. *T. pyogenes* strain 0912 and strain 1005 cells were cultured for 8 h. Anti-rFim C and anti-rFim E serum caused agglutination of *T. pyogenes* strain 0912 and strain 1005 cells. Anti-rFim A serum failed to cause agglutination of *T. pyogenes* strain 0912 and strain 1005 cells. The experiment was repeated twice

a commensal to a pathogenic organism in *T. pyogenes* infection. Thus, investigating the expression profiles of the virulence factors of *T. pyogenes* would help in comprehensively understand its pathogenesis. In the current study, the expression of three putative fimbriae proteins (Fim A, Fim C, and Fim E) in cultured *T. pyogenes* were investigated. The results showed that Fim E protein expression was evident; however, Fim A protein expression was not detected. Moreover, the expression of Fim E was inhibited by microaerophilic conditions.

We first determined the presence of Fim A-, Fim C-, and Fim E-specific antibodies in rabbit anti-*T. pyogenes* serum by immunizing rabbits with the bacterium. The results showed that only rFim E reacted to the anti-serum (Fig. 1), thereby indicating the lack of Fim A- and Fim C-specific antibodies in the serum. Formaldehyde treatment caused the overdenaturation of Fim A and Fim C, which might have caused the phenomenon. However, Fim E molecules in cultured *T. pyogenes* would also be denatured by the formaldehyde treatment and successfully elicited specific antibodies in rabbit. This implied that the molecules in the *T. pyogenes* were not overdenatured by the formaldehyde treatment. Additionally, the anti-*T. pyogenes* serum was prepared by immunizing the rabbit with formaldehyde-inactivated and live *T. pyogenes*. The protocol in the experiment proved the existence of antibodies that were specific to all the components of *T. pyogenes* cells in the serum. Hence, we assumed that the *fimA* and *fimC* genes were either not expressed or expressed in relatively low levels in cultured *T. pyogenes*, thereby leading to the failure of eliciting specific antibodies against the two proteins.

Then, we directly examined the expression of Fim A, Fim C, and Fim E in cultured *T. pyogenes*. Results in Figs. 2, 3, 4 indicate that only Fim E could be steadily detected in cultured *T. pyogenes* using western blot assay. The blots for Fim C detection showed strong nonspecific reaction bands (Figs. 2, 3, 4). Meanwhile, the anti-*T. pyogenes* serum failed to detect rFim C (Fig. 1). Thus, we could not draw a conclusion related to the expression profile of Fim C in cultured *T. pyogenes*; however, the anti-rFim C serum caused strong agglutination of *T. pyogenes*. Bisinotto [12] reported that anti-Fim C serum has been detected in cattle with *T. pyogenes* infection, and that the expression of Fim C by *T. pyogenes* is observable in vivo. To exactly determine the expression of Fim C in *T. pyogenes*, specific tools, such as monoclonal antibodies against Fim C, are needed. The expression of Fim A was not observed in *T. pyogenes* lysates using western blot assay (Figs. 2, 3, 4); meanwhile, the anti-rFim A serum did not cause agglutination in *T. pyogenes* within 30 min. Several immunoblots showed reactive components and similar molecular weights to the predicted molecular weight of Fim A in *T. pyogenes* lysates (*T. pyogenes* strain 1005 sampled at 16, 20, and 24 h in Fig. 3 and *T. pyogenes* strain 0912 cultured in pH 5.5 and 6.5 conditions in Fig. 4). Thus, we tested the reactivity of *T. pyogenes* cultured under these conditions to anti-rFim

A serum via tube agglutination assay. Results showed no or only weak reaction between *T. pyogenes* and anti-rFim A serum (data not shown). These data indicated the Fim A was not, or poorly, expressed in cultured *T. pyogenes* in this experiment. The experiment exhibited two limitations: (1) only two isolated strains of *T. pyogenes* were involved and (2) a standard ATCC strain of *T. pyogenes* was lacking. Thus, further investigation is needed to determine whether the results of these experiments are universal in *T. pyogenes* strains, using more *T. pyogenes* strains isolated from different animal species and with different types of *T. pyogenes* infections.

Based on the results of the experiments, the microaerophilic condition promoted the proliferation of *T. pyogenes,* but inhibited the expression of Fim E in vitro. *Neisseria meningitidis* has been reported to posttranslationally modify one of its pili for the detachment of individual bacterium cells from the colony and colonizing new sites after several rounds of cell division while attached to a host cell [17]. This implies that the bacteria can regulate the expression of adhesins by controlling their attachment and detachment during infections. We speculated that the rapid proliferation of *T. pyogenes* in microaerophilic condition may spread *T. pyogenes* cells, thereby leading to the downregulation of adhesin protein expression. However, in the present study, the microaerophilic culture was only achieved when the organism was cultured on the plate. This led to another speculation that the expression of Fim E in *T. pyogenes* decreased due to the changes in the culturing method, but not because of the gaseous environment. This hypothesis should be addressed in future studies.

T. pyogenes has been reported to be less efficient to produce fimbriae under standard growth conditions [1]. Yanagawa and Honda [18] reported that only a small portion of cultured *T. pyogenes* have fimbriae (10%), and that the number of fimbriae on each piliated bacterial cell is less than 10. On the basis of our results, we speculated that the poor expression of fimbriae was at least partially attributed to the poor expression of Fim A, if the putative Fim A indeed participates in the assembly of *T. pyogenes* fimbriae.

Jost and Billington [1] and Bisinotto [12] reported the existence of antibodies against Fim A in *T. pyogenes*-infected cattle, thus indicating the expression of Fim A by *T. pyogenes* in vivo. Moreover, Bicalho [19] reported that the increased transcription of *fimA* gene of *T. pyogenes* is associated with the occurrence of metritis and endometritis in postpartum dairy cows. However, the results of Bisinotto's study inferred the poor expression of Fim A by *T. pyogenes* compared with the expression levels of Fim C and Fim E, because the OD value of the ELISA for Fim A-specific antibody detection was noticeably lower than those of the ELISA for Fim C and Fim E-specific antibody detection [12].

An interesting phenomenon in Bisinotto's report is that the titers of antibodies against Fim C and Fim E were associated with the presence of *T. pyogenes* in the uterus of cattle (constantly detectable if the *T. pyogenes* was detected in the cattle and consistently higher than that of herdmates without *T. pyogenes*), but were not significantly related to the day relative to calving. In contrast, the titers of antibodies against Fim A were not associated with the presence of *T. pyogenes.* However, the increase of the concentration of Fim A-specific antibodies was significantly related to the day relative to calving in cows with *T. pyogenes* [12]. Thus, we speculated that the expression of Fim C and Fim E by *T. pyogenes* in vivo are constitutive, whereas the expression of Fim A might be regulated by several factors related to the calving of the cattle.

Another possible mechanism related to the upregulation of Fim A expression in vivo might be a quorum-sensing response. Duarte [20] reported that the genome of *T. pyogenes* involves the *lsrACDBFGE* operon, which is related to the quorum-sensing signal response AI-2. Huang [21] reported that N-acyl homoserine lactones, a type of quorum-sensing molecule, significantly decreased the expression levels of virulence genes of residual *T. pyogenes* in a mouse model. These data infer the importance of quorum sensing in regulating the expression of virulence factors in *T. pyogenes.* Wagener [22] reported that the proportion of *T. pyogenes*-positive cows increased from 0.5% at day 0–85% at 15th day postpartum, as determined via traditional bacterial isolation method, thereby indicating the proliferation of *T. pyogenes* in the uterus of the cattle. Moreover, Williams [23] reported that the growth density of *T. pyogenes* from uterine lumen swabs collected from postpartum cows peaked in samples collected at the 14th day postpartum. The proliferation of the organism in the cattle uterus might raise the concentration of quorum-sensing molecules in tissues and upregulate the Fim A expression.

Combining the results of the previous and current studies, we speculated that the poor expression of Fim A restricts the formation of additional fimbriae by *T. pyogenes* in normal circumstances, and that *T. pyogenes* shows commensal characteristics. When the environmental conditions changed, the upregulation of Fim A expression promoted fimbriae assembly. Additional fimbriae and the upregulation of other virulence factor expressions facilitated the invasion of *T. pyogenes* into deep tissues. In future studies, genetic technology-mediated overexpression of Fim A protein in *T. pyogenes,* followed by the counting of fimbriae, might be a practical strategy to further study the role of Fim A in *T. pyogenes* infection.

Conclusions

We determined the expression profile of the three putative fimbriae proteins, namely, Fim A, Fim C, and Fim E, in in vitro cultured *T. pyogenes*. Based on our results, only Fim E could be detected via western blot method. The expression of Fim E could be inhibited by microaerophilic condition. Our results would be helpful for comprehensively understanding the pathogenesis of *T. pyogenes* infections and developing *T. pyogenes* vaccines. The expression profile and role of Fim A and Fim C in *T. pyogenes* should be further studied, using more sensitive and specific tools and proper strategies.

Abbreviations

aa: amino acids; bp: base pair; CWSS: cell wall sorting signal; NC: nitrocellulose; FBS: fetal bovine serum; HRP: horse radish peroxidase; IPTG: isopropyl-β-D-1-thiogalactoside; OD: optical density; PBS: phosphate buffer saline; rFim A: recombinant Fim A; rFim C: recombinant Fim C; rFim E: recombinant Fim E; SDS-PAGE: sodium dodecyl sulfate polyacrylamide gel electrophoresis; *T. pyogenes*: *Trueperella pyogenes*.

Authors' contributions

WZ designed the experiments, analyzed the results, supervised the work, and drafted the manuscript. ML prepared the recombinant proteins and antisera and performed the western blot assays and tube agglutination tests. BW cloned the genes and HL provided help to purify the recombinant proteins. BM and JW supervised the work. All authors read and approved the final manuscript.

Author details

[1] College of Veterinary Medicine, Northeast Agricultural University, Changjiang Road 600, Harbin 150030, Heilongjiang, People's Republic of China. [2] Key Laboratory of Animal Pathogen Biology of Ministry of Agriculture and Rural Affairs of the People's Republic of China, Northeastern Science Inspection Station, Harbin 150030, Heilongjiang, People's Republic of China.

Competing interests

The authors declare that they have no competing interests.

Funding

This work was supported by National Natural Science Foundation of China (Grant Nos. 31672529 and 31402177), the University Nursing Program for Young Scholars with Creative Talents in Heilongjiang Province (Grant No. UNPYSCT-2017019), the "Academic Backbone" Project of Northeast Agricultural University (Grant No. 17XG09).

References

1. Jost BH, Billington SJ. *Arcanobacterium pyogenes*: molecular pathogenesis of an animal opportunist. Antonie Van Leeuwenhoek. 2005;88:87–102.
2. Nagib S, Glaeser SP, Eisenberg T, Sammra O, Lammler C, Kampfer P, et al. Fatal infection in three Grey Slender Lorises (*Loris lydekkerianus nordicus*) caused by clonally related *Trueperella pyogenes*. BMC Vet Res. 2017;13:273.
3. Risseti RM, Zastempowska E, Twaruzek M, Lassa H, Pantoja JCF, de Vargas APC, et al. Virulence markers associated with *Trueperella pyogenes* infections in livestock and companion animals. Lett Appl Microbiol. 2017;65:125–32.
4. Wickhorst JP, Hassan AA, Sheet OH, Eisenberg T, Sammra O, Alssahen M, et al. *Trueperella pyogenes* isolated from a brain abscess of an adult roebuck (*Capreolus capreolus*). Folia Microbiol. 2018;63:17–22.
5. Kavitha K, Latha R, Udayashankar C, Jayanthi K, Oudeacoumar P. Three cases of *Arcanobacterium pyogenes*-associated soft tissue infection. J Med Microbiol. 2010;59:736–9.
6. Patel S, Mathivanan N, Goyal A. Bacterial adhesins, the pathogenic weapons to trick host defense arsenal. Biomed Pharmacother. 2017;93:763–71.
7. Solanki V, Tiwari M, Tiwari V. Host-bacteria interaction and adhesin study for development of therapeutics. Int J Biol Macromol. 2018;112:54–64.
8. Rogovskyy AS, Lawhon S, Kuczmanski K, Gillis DC, Wu J, Hurley H, et al. Phenotypic and genotypic characteristics of *Trueperella pyogenes* isolated from ruminants. J Vet Diagn Invest. 2018;30:348–53.
9. Esmay PA, Billington SJ, Link MA, Songer JG, Jost BH. The *Arcanobacterium pyogenes* collagen-binding protein, CbpA, promotes adhesion to host cells. Infect Immun. 2003;71:4368–74.
10. Jost BH, Songer JG, Billington SJ. Cloning, expression, and characterization of a neuraminidase gene from *Arcanobacterium pyogenes*. Infect Immun. 2001;69:4430–7.
11. Jost BH, Songer JG, Billington SJ. Identification of a second *Arcanobacterium pyogenes* neuraminidase and involvement of neuraminidase activity in host cell adhesion. Infect Immun. 2002;70:1106–12.
12. Bisinotto RS, Filho JCO, Narbus C, Machado VS, Murray E, Bicalho RC. Identification of fimbrial subunits in the genome of *Trueperella pyogenes* and association between serum antibodies against fimbrial proteins and uterine conditions in dairy cows. J Dairy Sci. 2016;99:3765–76.
13. Zhao K, Liu M, Zhang X, Wang H, Yue B. In vitro and in vivo expression of virulence genes in *Trueperella pyogenes* based on a mouse model. Vet Microbiol. 2013;163:344–50.
14. Zhang W, Wang P, Wang B, Ma B, Wang J. A combined *Clostridium perfringens*/*Trueperella pyogenes* inactivated vaccine induces complete immunoprotection in a mouse model. Biologicals. 2017;47:1–10.
15. Confer AW. Update on bacterial pathogenesis in BRD. Anim Health Res Rev. 2009;10:145–8.
16. Zhang W, Liu X, Liu M, Ma B, Xu L, Wang J. Development of a multiplex PCR for simultaneous detection of *Pasteurella multocida*, *Mannheimia haemolytica* and *Trueperella pyogenes*. Acta Vet Hung. 2017;65:327–39.
17. Moorthy S, Keklak J, Klein EA. Perspective: adhesion mediated signal transduction in bacterial pathogens. Pathogens. 2016;5:23. https://doi.org/10.3390/pathogens5010023.
18. Yanagawa R, Honda E. Presence of pili in species of human and animal parasites and pathogens of the genus *Corynebacterium*. Infect Immun. 1976;13:1293–5.
19. Bicalho ML, Machado VS, Oikonomou G, Gilbert RO, Bicalho RC. Association between virulence factors of *Escherichia coli*, *Fusobacterium necrophorum*, and *Arcanobacterium pyogenes* and uterine diseases of dairy cows. Vet Microbiol. 2012;157:125–31.
20. Duarte VDS, Treu L, Campanaro S, Dias RS, Silva CCD, Giacomini A, et al. The complete genome sequence of *Trueperella pyogenes* UFV1 reveals a processing system involved in the quorum-sensing signal response. Genome Announc. 2017;5:e00639–717. https://doi.org/10.1128/genomea.00639-17.
21. Huang T, Song X, Zhao K, Jing J, Shen Y, Zhang X, et al. Quorum-sensing molecules *N*-acyl homoserine lactones inhibit *Trueperella pyogenes* infection in mouse model. Vet Microbiol. 2018;213:89–94.
22. Wagener K, Grunert T, Prunner I, Ehling-Schulz M, Drillich M. Dynamics of uterine infections with *Escherichia coli*, *Streptococcus uberis* and *Trueperella pyogenes* in post-partum dairy cows and their association with clinical endometritis. Vet J. 2014;202:527–32.
23. Williams EJ. Drivers of post-partum uterine disease in dairy cattle. Reprod Domest Anim. 2013;48:53–8.

Salmonella enterica subspecies *enterica* serovar Choleraesuis in a German wild boar population: occurrence and characterisation

Ulrich Methner[1*], Sabine Merbach[2] and Martin Peters[2]

Abstract

Background: The swine-adapted serovar Choleraesuis of *Salmonella enterica* subspecies *enterica* is found rarely in domestic pigs in Germany. However, a considerable and increasing number of S. Choleraesuis organisms have been isolated from wild boars in Germany in recent years. To investigate a possible epidemiological context, S. Choleraesuis strains from a regional German wild boar population and other hosts were characterised by genotyping methods.

Results: Macrorestriction analysis, biochemical differentiation and antimicrobial susceptibility typing enabled the identification of several clusters of S. Choleraesuis. Some clusters occurred almost permanently in a certain district, whereas other groups circulated among different wild boar herds in larger regions. Non-porcine hosts were infected with the same cluster as the wild boars.

Conclusions: The emergence of S. Choleraesuis in wild boars might be caused by a higher prevalence in the wild boar population, but also the higher awareness to infections with African swine fever may have resulted in a higher number of examined animals. Separation of wild boar populations and, as a result, also the diverse S. Choleraesuis organisms might be due to natural barriers and artificial barriers like arterial roads. The findings of S. Choleraesuis in domestic pigs emphasize the importance of strict biosecurity measures to prevent transmission from wild boars of this but also other pathogens. To avoid risks for humans by zoonotic pathogens regular inspections of meat from wildlife need to be conducted.

Keywords: Epidemiology, Germany, *Salmonella* Choleraesuis, Typing, Wild boar

Background

Pigs might be infected with different non-host adapted *Salmonella* serovars, which rarely produce systemic infections but are able to colonise the alimentary tract and gut-associated lymphoid tissue [1]. *S.* Typhimurium and *S.* Derby are the worldwide most commonly detected non-typhoid serovars in pigs, however, all *Salmonella* organisms isolated from pigs are considered a hazard for public health [2]. *Salmonella enterica* subspecies *enterica* serovar Choleraesuis is defined as host-adapted but not host-restricted on the basis that 99% of incidents are associated with pigs [3] and causes paratyphoid in swine with clinical manifestations of enterocolitis and septicaemia [4, 5]. However, it does naturally infect also other host species, including man, in which the disease can be severe. Although *S.* Choleraesuis is not often detected from human sources in the United States [6] and the European Union [2], it is an important serovar in several Asian countries. In Thailand [7] and Taiwan [8] *S.* Choleraesuis is not only frequently isolated from humans but identified as the main cause of salmonellosis. During 1950s and 1960s, *S.* Choleraesuis was the predominant serovar isolated from pigs worldwide [1]. Subsequently its prevalence has declined in numerous countries to a point where it was infrequently reported [9, 10]. At present time, this serovar is still prevalent in North America and Asia [11], but is rarely detected in Australia and

*Correspondence: ulrich.methner@fli.de
[1] Institute of Bacterial Infections and Zoonoses at the Friedrich-Loeffler-Institute, Federal Research Institute for Animal Health, Naumburger Str. 96a, 07743 Jena, Germany
Full list of author information is available at the end of the article

Western European countries [12]. A baseline survey on the prevalence of *Salmonella* in slaughter pigs in the EU from 2006 to 2007 revealed that *S.* Choleraesuis was detected in 4 out of the 25 participating Member States in altogether only 10 out of 2600 lymph nodes examined [12]. In Germany, the National Reference Laboratory for *Salmonella* received from 2001 to 2008 not a single strain of *S.* Choleraesuis isolated from domestic pigs for further typing [personal communication, Szabo] indicating that the swine adapted serovar was not resident in the pig population in Germany. In contrast, *S.* Choleraesuis was isolated in regional laboratories in some federal states from wild boars. Reports on the occurrence of *S.* Choleraesuis in wild boars in Germany are infrequent and concern mainly single cases [13–16] or one epidemiological study [17]. Since 2013, the number of *S.* Choleraesuis organisms isolated from wild boars in Germany and sent to the National Reference Laboratory for *Salmonella* for further typing increased considerably from 17 in 2013 to 180 in 2017 [personal communication, Szabo], indicating a marked rise in prevalence in the German wild boar population. In a regional diagnostic laboratory in the federal state North Rhine-Westphalia a strong increase of septic salmonellosis in wild boars due to *S.* Choleraesuis was also observed during the last years. The swine adapted serovar was isolated in this region in a few cases even from domestic pigs, two foxes (*Vulpes vulpes*), a badger (*Meles meles*) and a red deer (*Cervus elaphus*). The aim of the present study was to characterise the *S.* Choleraesuis strains from the different hosts by phenotyping and genotyping methods in order to investigate a possible epidemiological connection.

Methods

Bacterial strains

A total of 31 strains of *S.* Choleraesuis isolated [18] from 31 wild boars of different age, i.e. shoats, piglets under 12 months, yearlings between 12 and 24 months, and adults over 24 months were included in the study. This selection of strains represents the entire spectrum of isolates found in the administrative district of Arnsberg in the German federal state North Rhine-Westphalia in 2017. Altogether 46 wild boars were examined from the same district in this period. *S.* Choleraesuis was detected in 39 animals, but strains from eight wild boars were excluded from the study as they were isolated at the same place of origin on the same day. The age of the animals was estimated based on tooth eruption as well as wear and tear of teeth of the lower jaw [19]. Additionally, five isolates of *S.* Choleraesuis from domestic pigs, two strains from foxes and one strain each from a badger and a red deer detected in 2017 or 2018 in this region were also included. Depending on the presence of gross lesions, tissue samples from affected organs (e.g. liver, spleen, lung, bone lesions, segments of the intestine, and intestinal content) were collected and examined according to the standard method [18]. All *Salmonella* isolates were serotyped using poly- and monovalent anti-O as well as anti-H sera (SIFIN) according to the Kauffmann-White scheme [20], the biochemical profile of the strains was determined to differentiate between biovars *S.* Choleraesuis sensu stricto and *S.* Choleraesuis variatio Kunzendorf [21], using the identification system API 20E (Analytical Profile Index 20 tubes test for Enterobacteriaceae, bioMerieux, Nürtingen, Germany).

Antimicrobial susceptibility testing

Antimicrobial susceptibility of the *S.* Choleraesuis strains was assessed by determining the minimum inhibitory concentration (MIC) using the broth microdilution method with Sensititre™ EUVSEC plates (Trek Diagnostic Systems Ltd, East Grinstead, United Kingdom). Epidemiological cut-off values according to the European Committee on Antimicrobial Susceptibility Testing (EUCAST) were used [22]. Antimicrobial susceptibilities to sulfamethoxazole (SMX), trimethoprim (TMP), ciprofloxacin (CIP), tetracycline (TET), meropenem (MERO), azithromycin (AZI), nalidixic acid (NAL), cefotaxime (FOT), chloramphenicol (CHL), tigecycline (TGC), ceftazidime (TAZ), colistin (COL), ampicillin (AMP) and gentamicin (GEN) were examined.

Genotyping using pulsed-field gel electrophoresis (PFGE)

Macrorestriction analysis was carried out as described previously [17].

Pathomorphological and histological examination of the animals

A complete post-mortem examination was carried out by veterinarians on all wild boar carcasses submitted to the regional diagnostic laboratory in the federal state North Rhine-Westphalia by hunters or local veterinary authorities. African and Classical swine fever were ruled out by means of PCR, *Brucella* infection and Aujeszky's disease have been excluded by serological methods. Wild boars examined were found dead or were shot by hunters because of overt clinical disease (abnormal behaviour, lost escape behaviour). Road killed animals were not submitted. Animals weighed between 1.5 and 53 kg. Depending on the state of decomposition samples of brain, lung, heart, liver, spleen, kidney, and intestine were fixed in 10% neutral buffered formalin. From animals with swollen feet, metaphyses of long bones were included. Bones were decalcified using hydrochloric acid (Osteomoll, Merck, Darmstadt, Germany). The formalin fixed tissue was further processed for histology using routine techniques. Sections were cut at 5 µm and stained with hematoxylin and eosin for microscopic examination. Domestic pigs and non-porcine game animals with *S.* Choleraesuis findings were necropsied in order to determine the cause of illness and death. Processing of samples from these animals for histology was identical as described above.

Results

Serological and biochemical characterisation of *S.* Choleraesuis

All isolates were typed according to the Kauffmann-White scheme and revealed the complete antigenic formula (6, 7: c: 1, 5) for *S.* Choleraesuis. All 40 *S.* Choleraesuis strains from different hosts were H_2S positive and, therefore, could be referred to as biovar Kunzendorf (Table 1). The isolates revealed also identical fermentation patterns for sorbitol (SOR), melibiose (MEL) and arabinose (ARA). Therefore, only one "Analytical Profile Index" of the *S.* Choleraesuis isolates was identified (6 504 510: H_2S+, SOR+, MEL−, ARA−).

Antimicrobial susceptibilities

All 40 *S.* Choleraesuis strains tested were sensitive to 12 out of 14 antimicrobial compounds. The organisms were all resistant to ciprofloxacin (MIC = 0.12 µg/mL). Twenty five out of the 40 strains revealed a MIC of 256 µg/mL for sulfamethoxazole and were, therefore, sensitive to this antimicrobial substance. The other 15 *S.* Choleraesuis isolates were resistant to sulfamethoxazole (MIC > 1024 µg/mL) (Table 1). This distinctive feature was also used to differentiate the *S.* Choleraesuis strains beyond the macrorestriction cluster. MIC values of 256 µg/mL were designated as 1 and MIC values of > 1024 µg/mL were termed as 2 and added to the single macrorestriction cluster to further distinguish between the *S.* Choleraesuis organisms (Table 1). Levels of susceptibility against the other antimicrobial substances did not reveal differences between the strains, the resistance pattern of the *S.* Choleraesuis strains was nearly identical. MIC values (µg/mL) of the strains were: TMP (0.5), TET (8), MERO (0.06), AZI (16), NAL (8), FOT (< 0.25), CHL (16), TGC (1–2), TAZ (1), COL (< 1), AMP (4) and GEN (2).

Table 1 Characteristics of *Salmonella* Choleraesuis strains

Animal origin (number of strains)	MIC[a] (µg/mL) to SMX	Macrorestriction pattern		Macrorestriction cluster[d]
		Xba I X[b]	*Spe* I S[c]	
Wild boars (n = 18)	256	1	1	A1
Domestic pigs (n = 2)	256	1	1	A1
Badger (n = 1)	256	1	1	A1
Deer (n = 1)	256	1	1	A1
Wild boars (n = 2)	> 1024	1	1	A2
Domestic pigs (n = 2)	> 1024	1	1	A2
Wild boars (n = 7)	> 1024	2	2	B2
Foxes (n = 2)	> 1024	2	2	B2
Wild boars (n = 2)	256	1	3	C1
Wild boars (n = 2)	> 1024	1	3	C2
Domestic pigs (n = 1)	256	1	4	D1

Analytical profile index: 6 504 510 (identical in all strains)

[a] MIC to sulfamethoxazole (SMX):1 = 256; 2 = > 1024 (addition to macrorestriction cluster[d])

[b] Pattern numbers correspond to lane numbers in Fig. 1

[c] Pattern numbers correspond to lane numbers in Fig. 1

[d] Macrorestriction cluster as combination of macrorestriction patterns[b, c] and MIC[a]

Macrorestriction analysis

Two different restriction endonucleases, *Xba*I and *Spe*I (Fig. 1) were used to cleave whole-cell DNA of 40 *S.* Choleraesuis isolates originating from different regions in the district of Arnsberg in the federal state North Rhine-Westphalia (Table 1). *Xba*I digestion yielded two (X1 to X2) different patterns, *Spe*I digestion resulted in four (S1 to S4) patterns. Results of macrorestriction analysis allowed the assignment of the 40 *S.* Choleraesuis strains examined in this study to macrorestriction clusters A, B, C and D (Table 1).

Combining of phenotyping and genotyping results

The different susceptibility patterns of the *S.* Choleraesuis organisms to sulfamethoxazole enabled a further distinction of the macrorestriction clusters A, B, C and D in A1, A2, B2, C1, C2 and D1 (Table 1). The distribution of the strains according to both their affiliation to the different macrorestriction clusters and their place of origin in the district of Arnsberg in the federal state North Rhine-Westphalia are presented in Fig. 2. It could be shown that the discriminative groups are predominant in different regions. *S.* Choleraesuis strains isolated from both wild boars and foxes belonging to cluster B2 were found only in the west whereas strains of group C (C1 and C2) originated only from the east of this region. Clusters A1 and A2 were detected in the centre of the district Arnsberg, however, nearly completely separated from cluster B2. Also in this region the strains isolated from a badger, a red deer and a domestic pig did belong to the same group (A1) as the strains from wild boars. The few strains from cluster A2 were rather widely distributed in the Arnsberg district and two of them were isolated from domestic pigs. One strain isolated from a domestic pig revealed a unique macrorestriction pattern (D1), which was not

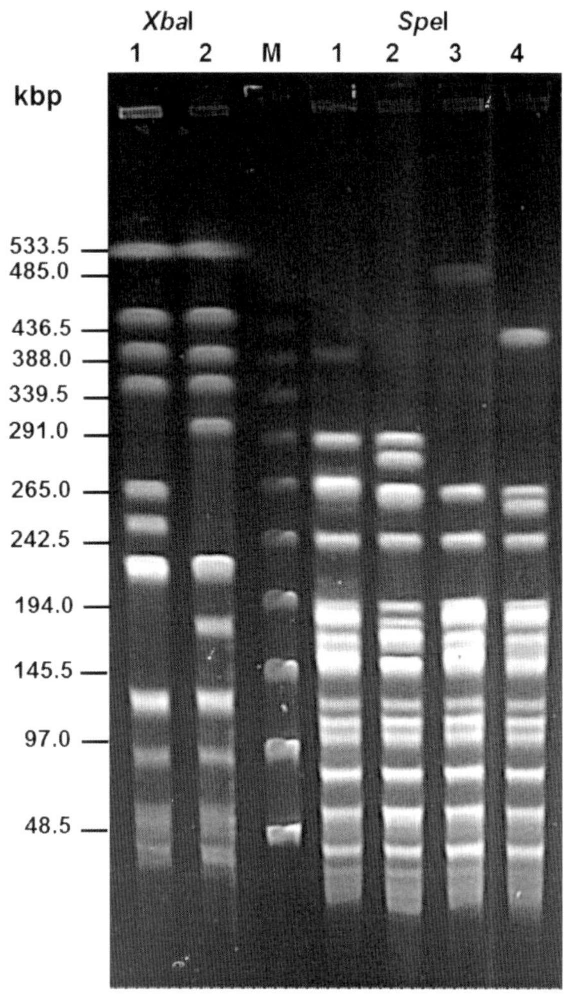

Fig. 1 *Xba*I (X1, X2) and *Spe*I (S1, S2, S3, S4) macrorestriction patterns of 40 *Salmonella*. Choleraesuis strains from 31 wild boars, 5 domestic pigs, 2 badgers, 1 fox and 1 red deer

detected from any other host. In total, macrorestriction cluster A1 was the most widespread type in this district, reaching even regions in the south of the Arnsberg area and still further towards the federal state of Hessen.

Pathological findings in wild boars and other hosts

Nearly all boars (especially shoats and juveniles) examined showed signs of septicaemia. Pneumonia, congested liver with miliary necroses, enlarged spleen and hyperaemic lymph nodes were observed regularly. The animals revealed haemorrhages associated with endothelial damage and microvascular thrombosis in multiple organs like lungs, kidneys and in a few cases also in the epiglottis. Enterocolitis was not detected in any of the wild boars. Five animals were suffering from severe osteomyelitis and physitis with swollen feet. Histologically, necrotising hepatitis and splenitis as well as fibrinopurulent necrotising bronchopneumonia were the hallmarks of *S.* Choleraesuis infection in wild boars. In most cases, it was possible to cultivate pure colonies of the agent from different organs directly without pre-enrichment in buffered peptone water. The pathological findings in domestic pigs were less pronounced. One pig showed signs of septic salmonellosis with necrotising hepatosplenitis. The other domestic pigs suffered from bronchopneumonia and polyarthritis, in these animals the agent was isolated only from the intestine. From the two foxes, *S.* Choleraesuis was detected from a splenic abscess and the liver, respectively. The swine adapted *Salmonella* serovar was also isolated from liver, spleen and intestine of a badger suffering from focal cerebellar encephalomalacia, bronchopneumonia and necrotising hepatitis as well as from the intestine of a red deer. This animal originating from a game animal enclosure with public access was in poor nutritional condition, had a severe lung worm infestation, multiple abscesses in lung, lung lymph nodes and spleen, and a chronic peritonitis.

Discussion

The occurrence of the swine-adapted serovar *S.* Choleraesuis in domestic pigs is considered as major problem for the pig industry in Asia and North America [11]. Only occasional findings are reported from Australia and Europe [12]. The recent report on zoonoses in the European Union provided no evidence on the occurrence of *S.* Choleraesuis, neither in pigs nor in humans [2]. In Germany, *S.* Choleraesuis was isolated from pigs or pork in 2014 in only two cases [23] indicating that the swine adapted serovar is not resident in the domestic pig population in this country. Reports on clinical cases or outbreaks of *S.* Choleraesuis in domestic pigs [16, 24] are also seldom. In contrast, the number of *S.* Choleraesuis isolates from wild boars sent to the German National Reference Laboratory for *Salmonella* increased from 17 in 2013 to 180 in 2017 [personal communication, Szabo], suggesting a rising prevalence in the German wild boar population. Strains of other serovars of *Salmonella* from wild boars in Germany were submitted only in a few cases for further typing. Several reasons may be responsible for this development: (i) a real increase of *S.* Choleraesuis in wild boars as result of the increased number of animals in the wild boar population [25], (ii) the higher awareness to possible African swine fever infections [26] as similarities in gross lesions with *S.* Choleraesuis infections [16] might have resulted in a higher number of animals sent to regional diagnostic laboratories, and (iii) an increase in virulence due to a possibly newly emerged clone of *S.* Choleraesuis. The diagnostic laboratory of the administrative district Arnsberg notified also an increase of septic salmonellosis due to *S.* Choleraesuis in wild boar

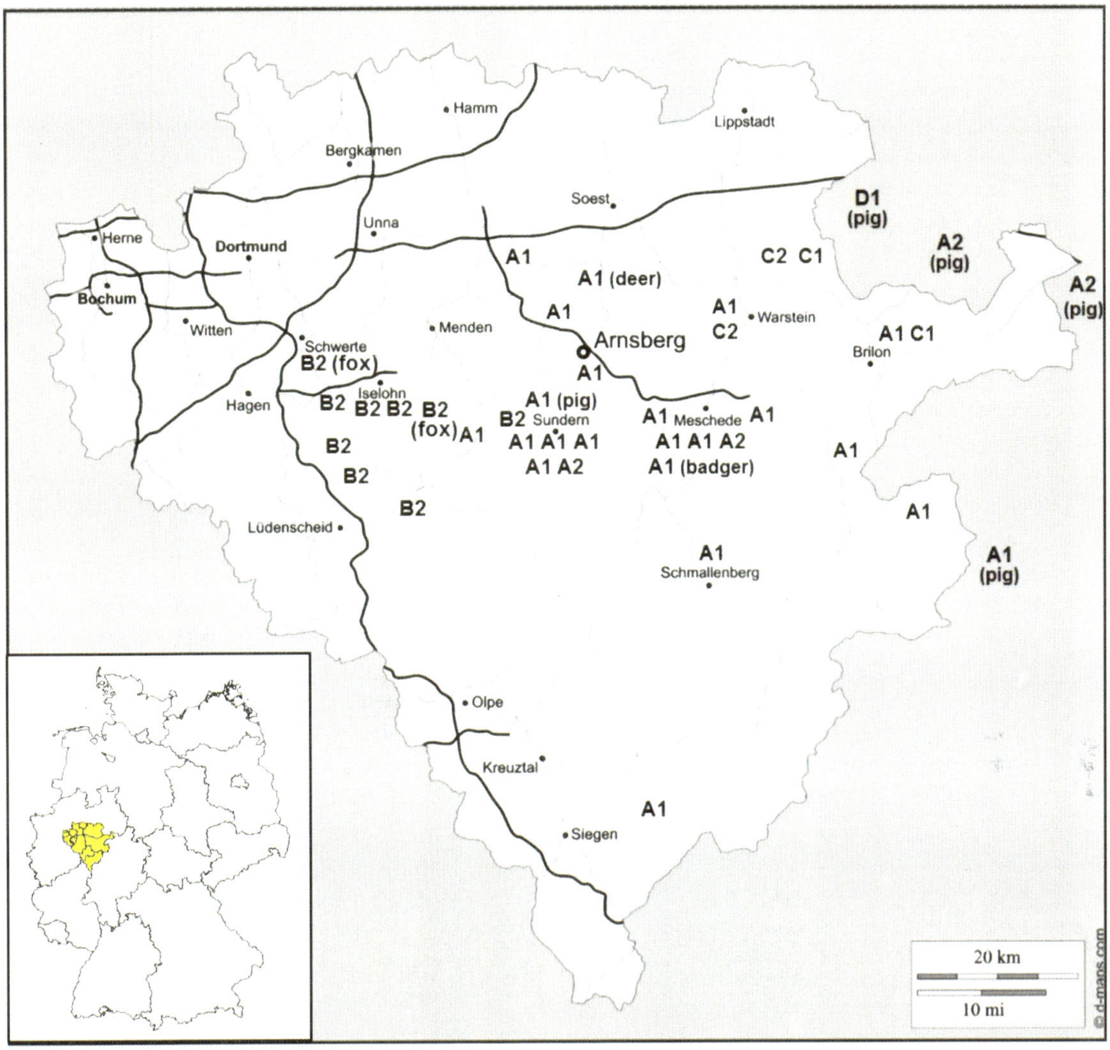

Fig. 2 Distribution of macrorestriction clusters (A1, A2, B2, C1, C2, D1) of *Salmonella* Choleraesuis isolates from wild boars, domestic pigs, foxes, badger and red deer according to their place of origin in the administrative district of Arnsberg in the federal state North Rhine-Westphalia in Germany

submissions from 2006 (0 of 10) to 2017 (36 of 46). The generalised lesions in wild boars but also in other hosts in this study confirmed earlier observations and indicated the highly invasive character of this pig-adapted serovar [15–17, 24, 27]. The strong similarities in gross lesions after infection with *S.* Choleraesuis and African swine fever demand a high awareness of hunters, farmers, veterinarians and competent authorities in the control of these diseases. However, despite the actual threat by African swine fever, other diseases (classical swine fever, other septicaemic bacterial infections e.g. with *Streptococcus suis* and *Mycoplasma suis* or *Brucella suis* biovar 2) in pigs must also be considered in the differential diagnosis [28].

To detect a possible epidemiological connection between the *S.* Choleraesuis strains originating from both, different regions and hosts, PFGE as well as biochemical differentiation and antimicrobial susceptibility typing were applied to discriminate among the isolates [29, 30]. Several PFGE analyses of *S.* Choleraesuis isolates have provided reliable information on the discrimination among field isolates, between wild-type and vaccine strains, but also on the association between isolates of human and porcine origin [8, 17, 24, 29, 31]. In this study the macrorestriction analysis with two different enzymes subdivided 40 *S.* Choleraesuis isolates into 4 macrorestriction clusters A, B, C and D. The different sulfamethoxazole susceptibility patterns of the strains enabled at least partly a further differentiation of these clusters in A1/A2, B2, C1/C2 and D1. Although the biochemical characterisation of serovar *S.* Choleraesuis might be a valuable tool for the further phenotypical discrimination [17, 20, 21, 24], all strains examined in this study did belong to biovar Kunzendorf (H_2S positive) and revealed only one "Analytical Profile Index" so that an additional distinction of the macrorestriction groups was not possible. The finding that single macrorestriction cluster occur almost permanently in only certain regions of the district Arnsberg indicates (i) that wild boars live and move only in special parts of the region or (ii) that there are barriers between regions which do not allow an exchange of the *Salmonella* organisms between different hordes of wild boars and (iii) that the *S.* Choleraesuis strains belonging to the different clusters persist and circulate in the wild boar populations in the corresponding regions. The distribution of the single cluster in this study is in great accordance with earlier results gained in another region in Germany located in a distance of about 300 kilometres [17]. Interestingly, the macrorestriction cluster of *S.* Choleraesuis strains identified in both regions did not reveal any accordance, indicating that an exchange of the organism over these long distances did not occur. The incidence of a special macrorestriction cluster in only a particular area might also be due to the amount of feed available. If there is plenty of feed the boars will stay in a territory of ca. 15 square kilometres, however, this territory may be considerably enlarged if there is a lack of feed [25]. Under these circumstances different wild boar hordes or single animals may share the same region and possibly exchange not only *S.* Choleraesuis organisms but also other pathogens. Whether this is the case in parts of the Arnsberg district is open. Also in areas with more than one macrorestriction cluster it is unknown whether these clusters occur each in one horde or in different hordes. Another factor contributing to the separation of single *S.* Choleraesuis cluster or rather the wild boar packs are with high probability barriers like motorways or other traffic routes used in high frequency. This holds true for the Arnsberg district but also other regions [17]. Therefore, it might be assumed that both natural barriers like mountains, mountain ranges or wide rivers as well as artificial barriers like arterial roads which are difficult to cross cause the separation of wild boars and, as well as their pathogens. The fact that in different non-porcine hosts like a deer, two foxes, a badger and a domestic pig the identical macrorestriction cluster was detected as in the wild boars from the corresponding region indicates, that the wild boars are the source of the infection with the swine adapted serovar *S.* Choleraesuis. Of special importance, also in view of the possible transfer of pathogens from wild boars to domestic pigs is the type of *S.* Choleraesuis cluster in domestic pigs. As wild boars or carrier wild boars might be considered as natural reservoir of *S.* Choleraesuis [11, 17], the route of transmission of this agent to the domestic pig population might be an indicator of infection routes also for other pathogens like African swine fever-virus, Classical swine fever-virus, *Brucella suis* or *Trichinella spiralis* [32, 33] and, therefore, give valuable information for the prevention of this transfer. Although the domestic pigs in this study revealed clusters of *S.* Choleraesuis identified in wild boars, it can only be suspected that wild boars are the source for the infection. Even a questionnaire in the pig farms did not yield sufficient information to finally confirm this route (data not shown). The pigs were not in free-range production and in the farms only single pigs were affected. The difficulties in analysing these routes of infection were also reported for both single cases of *S.* Choleraesuis infections [16] and large pig herds [24]. Therefore, hygiene and biosecurity measures are extremely important to prevent transmission of *Salmonella* and other pathogens from the wild boar population to domestic pigs.

The fact that *S.* Choleraesuis is the dominating serovar in the German wild boar population and that other *Salmonella* serovars are detected far less frequently [34] might indicate that wild boars are not an important host or source for foodborne salmonellosis in humans. On the contrary, studies from other countries [35–37] report on the occurrence of a wide range of *Salmonella* serovars belonging to different subspecies in wild boars. Nevertheless, because of the risk to transfer *Salmonella* and other zoonotic pathogens to humans there is a permanent need to reinforce attention on game meat inspection in order to improve the safety of pork from wild boars. Therefore, both regular inspection of meat from wildlife by official veterinarians and advice of hunters and persons who prepare and consume wild boar meat are essential measures for reducing risks to human and domestic pig health.

Conclusions

Because of the increased emergence of *S.* Choleraesuis in the German wild boar population, the study aimed to investigate an epidemiological connection of this host-adapted serovar in wild boars and other hosts. Phenotyping and genotyping methods enabled the identification of several clusters of *S.* Choleraesuis. These groups persist either in a certain regional wild boar population or circulate in different hordes in larger areas. The separation of the wild boar hordes or the *S.* Choleraesuis strains, respectively, might be due to natural and artificial barriers like arterial roads. The detection of *S.* Choleraesuis in single cases of domestic pigs indicates the possible transmission of pathogens from wild boars and requires the establishment of an effective biosecurity system at animal farms. The inspection of meat from wildlife needs to be conducted to avoid zoonotic infections.

Authors' contributions

UM coordinated the study, performed serotyping, macrorestriction analysis, MIC determination, data evaluation and wrote the manuscript. MP and SM carried out pathomorphological examinations, performed bacteriological analysis and coordinated topographical data. All authors read and approved the final manuscript.

Author details

[1] Institute of Bacterial Infections and Zoonoses at the Friedrich-Loeffler-Institute, Federal Research Institute for Animal Health, Naumburger Str. 96a, 07743 Jena, Germany. [2] Chemisches und Veterinäruntersuchungsamt Westfalen, Zur Taubeneiche 10-12, 59821 Arnsberg, Germany.

Acknowledgements

The skilled technical assistance of Lisa Rüter, Silke Keiling and Sigrid Trautmann (FLI Jena) as well as Daniela David, Jutta Juchmann and Felix Wiedemann (CVUA Westfalen) is gratefully acknowledged. We particularly thank Prof. Dr. Konrad Sachse for critical reading of the manuscript and language editing.

Competing interests

The authors declare that they have no competing interests.

Funding

This research did not receive any specific grant from funding agencies in the public, commercial, or not-for-profit sectors.

References

1. Stevens MP, Gray JT. *Salmonella* infections in pigs. In: Barrow PA, Methner U, editors. *Salmonella* in domestic animals. 2nd ed. Wallingford: CABI International; 2013. p. 263–94.
2. European Food Safety Authority (EFSA). The European Union summary report on trends and sources of zoonoses, zoonotic agents and food-borne outbreaks in 2016. EFSA J. 2017;15:5077.
3. Uzzau S, Brown DJ, Wallis T, Rubino S, Leori G, Bernhard S, et al. Host adapted serotypes of *Salmonella enterica*. Epidemiol Infect. 2000;125:229–55.
4. Reed WM, Olander HJ, Thaker HL. Studies of the pathogenesis of *Salmonella* Typhimurium and *Salmonella* Choleraesuis var. kunzendorf infection in weaning pigs. Am J Vet Res. 1986;47:75–83.
5. Gray JT, Fedorka-Cray PJ. Survival and infectivity of *Salmonella* Choleraesuis in swine feces. J Food Prot. 2001;64:945–9.
6. Centers for Disease Control and Prevention (CDC). National *Salmonella* surveillance Annual Report, 2015. Atlanta, Georgia: US Department of Health and Human Services, CDC; 2017.
7. Bangtrakulnonth A, Pornreonwong S, Pulsrikarn C, Sawanpanyalert P, Hendriksen RS, Lo Fo Wong DM. Salmonella serovars from humans and other sources in Thailand, 1993–2002. Emerg Infect Dis. 2004;10:131–6.
8. Chang CC, Lin YH, Chang CF, Yeh KS, Chiu CH, Chu C, et al. Epidemiologic relationship between fluoroquinolone-resistant *Salmonella enterica* serovar Choleraesuis strains isolated from humans and pigs in Taiwan (1997 to 2002). J Clin Microbiol. 2005;43:2798–804.
9. Laval A, Morvan H, Despez G, Corbion B. Salmonellosis in swine. In: Reports and communications, *Salmonella* and Salmonellosis, Ploufragan/St Brieuc, France, 15–17 September 1993, p. 164–74.
10. Helmuth R, Kasbohrer A, Geue L, Rabsch W, Protz W. Pilot study on the prevalence of *Salmonella* in slaughter pigs in Germany. In: Proceedings of the 2nd International Symposium on epidemiology and control of *Salmonella* in pork, Copenhagen, Denmark, 20–22 August 1997. p. 103–6.
11. Fedorka-Cray PJ, Gray JT, Wray C. *Salmonella* infections in pigs. In: Wray C, Wray A, editors. *Salmonella* in domestic animals. CAB International: Wallingford; 2000. p. 1191–207.
12. European Food Safety Authority (EFSA). Report of the task force on zoonoses data collection on the analysis of the baseline survey on the prevalence of *Salmonella* in slaughter pigs, Part A. EFSA J. 2008;135:1–111.
13. Plötner J, Bussemer J, Otta J, Schmidt O, Winkler H. Zu einer *Salmonella*-choleraesuis-Infektion im Schwarzwildbestand zweier benachbarter Jagdgebiete. Mh Vet-Med. 1979;34:860–1.
14. Weber A, Broos H, Wachowitz R, Heil G, Schultze-Rhonhof J. Nachweis von *Salmonella* choleraesuis beim einheimischen Schwarzwild (Sus scrofa). Tierärztl Umschau. 1990;45:411–4.
15. Müller M, Weber A, Tucher R, Naumann L. Osteomyelitis bei einem Wildschwein (Sus scrofa) durch *Salmonella* Choleraesuis. Tierärztl Umschau. 2004;59:700–2.
16. Eddicks M, Hausleitner R, Eddicks L, Blutke A, Straubinger RK, Wolf G, et al. Nachweis von *Salmonella* Choleraesuis var. Kunzendorf bei einem Mastschwein mit septikämischer Salmonellose. Ein Fallbericht. Tierärztliche Praxis Großtiere. 2016;44:381–7.
17. Methner U, Heller M, Bocklisch H. *Salmonella enterica* subspecies *enterica* serovar Choleraesuis in a wild boar population in Germany. Eur J Wildl Res. 2010;56:493–502.
18. International Organization for Standardization (ISO): ISO 6579-1:2017 (E). Microbiology of the food chain-horizontal method for the detection, enumeration and serotyping of *Salmonella*—Part 1: detection of *Salmonella* spp., 2017. http://www.iso.org.
19. Briedermann L. Schwarzwild. Stuttgart: Franckh-Kosmos Verlags-GmbH & Co. KG; 2009.
20. Grimont PAD, Weill FX. Antigenic formulae of the *Salmonella* serovars. In: WHO collaborating centre for reference and research on *Salmonella*, 9th edition. Paris: Institut Pasteur; 2007. http://www.pasteur.fr/sante/clre/cadrecnr/salmomsindex.html.
21. Le Minor L, Beaud R, Laurent B, Monteil V. Etude des *Salmonella* possedant les facteurs antigeniques 6,7:c:1,5. Ann Inst Pasteur/Microbiol. 1985;138B:225–34.
22. European Committee on Antimicrobial Susceptibility Testing (EUCAST). Breakpoints tables for interpretation of MICs and zone diameters. Version 3.1. Geneva, Switzerland; 2013. http://www.eucast.org.
23. Bundesinstitut für Riskobewertung (BfR): Agents of zoonoses in Germany in 2014. BfR Wissensch. 2016;06/2016:275. http://www.bfr.bund.de.
24. Pedersen K, Sørensen G, Löfström C, Leekitcharoenphon P, Nielsen B, Wingstrand A, et al. Reappearance of *Salmonella* serovar Choleraesuis var. Kunzendorf in Danish pig herds. Vet Microbiol. 2015;176:282–91.
25. Deutscher Jagdverband. https://www.jagdverband.de/sites/default/files/2018-%20Jahresstrecke%20Schwarzwild.jpg.
26. Verordnung zur Durchführung eines Monitorings auf das Virus der Klassischen und der Afrikanischen Schweinepest bei Wild- und Hausschweinen (Schweinepest-Monitoring-Verordnung - SchwPestMonV). 9. November 2016, BGBl. I, p. 2518.
27. Kingsley RA, Bäumler AJ. Host adaptation and the emergence of infectious disease: the *Salmonella* paradigm. Mol Microbiol. 2000;36:1006–14.
28. Zimmermann JJ, Karriker LA, Ramirez A, Schwartz KJ, Stevenson GW, editors. Diseases of swine. 10th ed. New York: Wiley Blackwell; 2012.
29. Weide-Botjes M, Liebisch B, Schwarz S, Watts JL. Molecular characterization of *Salmonella enterica* subsp. *enterica* serovar Choleraesuis field isolates and differentiation from homologous live vaccine strains Suisaloral and SC-54. J Clin Microbiol. 1996;34:2460–3.
30. Chiu CH, Su LH, Chu C, Chia JH, Wu TL, Lin TY. Isolation of *Salmonella* enterica serotype Choleraesuis resistant to ceftriaxone and ciprofloxacin. Lancet. 2004;363:1285–6.
31. Asai T, Namimatsu T, Osumi T, Kojima A, Harada K, Aoki H, et al. Molecular typing and antimicrobial resistance of *Salmonella* enterica subspecies enterica serovar Choleraesuis isolates from diseased pigs in Japan. Comp Immunol Microbiol Infect Dis. 2008. https://doi.org/10.1016/j.simid.2008.08.004.
32. Kruse H, Kirkemo AM, Handeland K. Wildlife as source of zoonotic infections. Emerg Infect Dis. 2004;10:2067–72.
33. Gottstein B, Pozio E, Nöckler K. Epidemiology, diagnosis, treatment, and control of trichinellosis. Clin Microbiol Rev. 2009;22:127–45.
34. Bundesamt für Verbraucherschutz und Lebensmittelsicherheit (BVL): Reports of Food Safety—Zoonoses Monitoring 2016; BVL Report 12.2; 2017. p. 18.

Descriptive study for culling and mortality in five high-producing Spanish dairy cattle farms (2006–2016)

Ramon Armengol[1,3*] and Lorenzo Fraile[1,2]

Abstract

Background: High turnover rate in dairy farms due to culling and mortality is associated with poor animal welfare, an increase in production costs and lower economic benefits for the dairy farm. Understanding cow elimination better would help to formulate specific prevention measures and improve the efficiency of milk production in dairy farms. Culling and mortality data from five standard high-producing dairy farms in Spain were analysed over a period of 11 years (2006–2016). Data were collected by the same veterinary team and using the same software system.

Results: Significant between-herd differences in eliminated cows were observed for type of elimination (slaughter or death on the farm), age at elimination, cause of elimination, number of lactations and production parameters, such as total days in milk, life milk yield, litres per day of productive life and litres per day of life. Culling and mortality were higher during the hot season and for cows of second and third parities. Between-herd differences were observed. Reproductive disorders (30.2%) were the most frequent reason for elimination, with low production (23.4%) being the second most frequent reason. Accidents on the farm (7.7%) were a more frequent cause of elimination than metabolic diseases (7.2%), locomotor disorders (2.4%) and obstetrics (2.4%).

Conclusions: Veterinary teams or farmers' associations can use culling and mortality information for benchmarking cow farms if data collection and analysis is standardised for comparability. The analysis of culling and mortality information should help farmers to improve efficiency.

Keywords: Benchmarking, Dairy cow, Culling, Mortality

Background

Culling (removal of a live cow from the farm for slaughter), mortality (death of an animal on the farm, whether euthanized or unassisted) and sale (selling cows to other farms) are normal events in intensive dairy production systems. In any livestock production system, net farm revenue is affected by income and costs. The sale of milk is the most important factor for income in dairy farms and the rearing and purchase of replacements are important costs for the farm [1].

A high turnover rate negatively affects the farm´s average milk production due to the fact that replacements produce less milk than the substituted animals in the short term [2, 3]. Moreover, a high turnover rate directly increases the cost of replacement at the farm level. Thus, a thorough analysis of the causes of elimination and death of these cows is imperative to improving productive efficiency. It is also increasingly a concern for dairy product consumers and animal welfare, because a high and sustained turnover rate is an indicator of poor welfare status [4]. Ideally, farmers should voluntarily decide which cows go to slaughter based on production and should be able to replace these cows with first lactation cows with a higher potential of production.

Spain and the southern part of Europe have a long heat stress risk season (May–October) that can affect the reproductive performance and immunologic status of cows [5]. Moreover, the prevalence of metabolic

*Correspondence: rarmengol@ca.udl.cat
[3] Present Address: Department of Animal Science, University of Lleida, ETSEA, Av. Alcalde Rovira Roure, 191, E25198 Lleida, Spain
Full list of author information is available at the end of the article

disorders, mastitis and infectious diseases and/or their severity can also be significantly affected by climate [6]. Thus, weather conditions could affect culling and mortality parameters throughout the year.

The causes of culling and mortality in dairy cows are associated with reproductive status and disorders [7–9], milk production [10], metabolic and post-partum disorders, mammary gland disorders and lameness [11–13]. A portion of culling and mortality events on dairy farms can be attributed to undesirable factors in the production system. These causes vary depending on age, parity and stage of lactation of the dairy cow [12, 14]. In some areas of the world, the proportion of dairy cows eliminated by a particular cause may vary throughout the year according to extrinsic factors on the farm, such as climate [15]. Moreover, each farm has its own elimination policy for dairy cows and the percentage of animals involuntarily culled or dying on the farm is specific to each farm. Studying the causes and percentages of elimination and mortality at different times of the year can help identify seasonal problems in the production system. This type of analysis can also inform future investment decisions to improve animal welfare and production. Using the same criteria and analysis system is necessary to advice farmers and benchmark different farms. The main aim of the study was to describe the causes of culling and mortality on selected high-producing dairy farms and establish benchmarking indicators.

Methods

Study population

Five standard high-production commercial dairy herds from North-eastern Spain (Huesca in Aragon and Lleida in Catalonia), of the Holstein Fresian breed, were selected from the database of a veterinary practice. Selection criteria for including a farm were: use of the same farm software, same codification for culling and mortality reasons, similar management systems and the same veterinary team carrying out clinical and/or anatomo-pathological examination for diagnosing the causes of culling and mortality. A high-producing dairy farm with Holstein cows produces at least 10,000 l of milk by cow in 305 days of lactation [16]. The study was carried out on five high-production commercial dairy farms over a period of 11 years (1st January 2006 to 31st December 2016). Farms housed between 140 and 600 lactating Holstein cows (bovine females that had calved at least once) with a production of 10,300–12,300 kg of milk by cow (3.6% fat and 3.3% protein) in 305 days. Cows were housed in sawdust-bedded free-stall barns or sawdust-bedded free-stall cubicles, and were fed a total mixed ration consisting of corn silage, grass silage, and concentrates and cows were never grazed. Cows were milked twice (at 6 a.m. and 6 p.m.) or three times a day (at 4 a.m., 12 p.m., and 8 p.m.) and individual milk yield was recorded daily. Each lactating cow was sampled and analysed by the Official Milk Recording Centre for milk quality (fat, protein and lactose concentration) and somatic cell count per ml once a month. Because of data ownership issues, official milk quality parameters were not available for this study. Herd size of the farms under study was stable throughout the period (±3%). Breeding management was carried out by artificial insemination with Holstein semen. Cows were bred on observed oestrus or diagnosed by a computerised pedometry system (Afimilk, Kibbutz Afikim, 1514800, Israel). It was decided not to inseminate first lactation and multiparous cows before 90 and 70 days postpartum, respectively.

For the purpose of this study, the year was divided into four periods as detailed in Table 1. Finally, farms 1, 3 and 4 had cooling systems based on the use of fans and showers, farm 2 used showers and farm 5 had no cooling system.

Destiny and cause of elimination

The destiny of eliminated cows was classified into two groups: slaughtered or dead on the farm. The average annual herd turnover rate was defined as the mean number of eliminated cows per year over the 11-year period divided by the mean number of cows present during the 11-year period [17]. In the included farms, the sale of animals for further productive purposes did never

Table 1 Description of the characteristics of the different periods of the year

Period	1	2	3	4
Months	1st January–31st March	1st April–30th June	1st July–30th September	1st October–31st December
Avg maximum temp (°C)	12.7	25.1	31.1	15.6
Avg minimum temp (°C)	0.8	14.3	17.4	5.2
Avg relative humidity (%)	71	55	57	79

Avg average, *Temp* temperature

occur. The cause of elimination was established based on the classification proposed by the USDA in the National Animal Health Monitoring Scheme [1, 18]. The cause of elimination was established consensually between the veterinarian and the farmer, taking into account the veterinary diagnosis and the productive, genetic improvement and milk quality criteria of the farmer. Although the software is able to capture different possible causes of elimination, the database only retains the primary cause of elimination in the cow's individual history. The causes of elimination are detailed below.

Reproductive causes

Cows with reproductive pathology such as abortion, ovarian cysts, anovulatory cows, non-pregnant first lactation and multiparous cows up to 350 and 250 days in milk (DIM), respectively. Non-pregnant cows remained on the farm until their average daily milk production was under 22 l/day.

Mammary gland causes

Mastitis (clinical, subclinical or chronic) of any of the quarters, cistern or teat morphological defects.

Production causes

Cows that are not producing enough milk within 40–200 DIM according to the prediction of milk yield provided by the farm software (approximately 22 l/day over 7 consecutive days) without an overt clinical problem and without taking into account their pregnancy status.

Locomotor causes

Limping cows and morphological leg defects.

Metabolic/digestive causes

Abomasal torsion, dilation or displacement, diarrhoea, ketosis, fatty liver, hypocalcaemia, hypomagnesaemia, hypokalaemia, acidosis and downer cow syndrome.

Respiratory causes

Bovine respiratory syndrome confirmed by clinical or necropsy examination.

Dystocia/obstetrics causes

Clinical problems related to calving such as dystocia, uterine torsion, prolapsed uterus or vagina. Uterine, vaginal or vulvar trauma as a consequence of parturition were also included. Nervous and musculoskeletal system lesions as a consequence of dystocia were included if they occurred within the first 7 days after parturition.

Accidental causes

Trauma with equipment, tools or buildings on the farm. Errors in drug administration, intoxication with chemicals and traumatic reticulitis were included in this section.

Infectious causes

Cows positive for infectious diseases included in an eradication program such as neosporosis, bovine viral diarrhoea and paratuberculosis.

Unknown causes

Unknown cause of death and lack of data on the cow elimination report.

Collection of data

Clinical, reproduction, production and management data were recorded using specific software (Afifarm, Afimilk, Kibbutz Afikim, 1514800, Israel). The following individual data of the eliminated cows were recorded from the herd database: identification of farm, identification of the cow, date of birth, date of artificial insemination, bull, pregnancy diagnosis, disease diagnosed (date), clinical signs, analytical data, treatment (date and drug), change of pen, preventive hoof trimming, vaccination (date and product), date of calving, date of dry-off, date of death, destiny (slaughtered or dead at farm), cause of elimination, age at death (DL) and number of lactations at elimination (NL). Moreover, individual production data for each cow under study were life milk yield (LMY) (milk produced throughout the cow's life), total days in milk (tDIM), litres per day of productive life (LPL) (LPL was calculated as LMY/tDIM) and litres per day of life (LDL) (LDL was calculated as LMY/DL).

Statistical analysis

All statistical analyses were carried out using SAS V.9.1.3 (SAS institute Inc, Cary, NC, USA). For all analyses, the individual cow was used as the study unit. The significance level was set at 0.05. The variables included in the statistical analyses were classified as nominal (farm, destiny and cause of elimination), ordinal (NL and period of the year) or continuous: DL, LMY, tDIM, LPL and LDL. All the cows with five or more lactations were grouped to carry out the statistical analysis. Shapiro–Wilk's and Levene tests were used to evaluate the normality of the distribution of the continuous variables and the homogeneity of variances, respectively.

Descriptive statistics were performed for all the variables by farm and as an average of the five farms. For clarity in the figures, the causes of elimination have been grouped into "major causes" (causes of elimination with a percentage higher than 15%), "intermediate cause" (causes of elimination with values between 8 and 15%) and "minor causes" (elimination causes with values lower than 8%). Contingency tables (Chi square or Fisher exact tests) were used when the association between nominal and ordinal variables was assessed. To study the association between nominal or ordinal variables with the continuous non-normally distributed variables, the Wilcoxon test (with the Mann–Whitney U test to compare each pair of values) was used. To analyse the association between continuous normally distributed variables and nominal or ordinal variables, an ANOVA test (with Student's t-test to compare each pair of values) was used.

Results

Productive data of cows eliminated

A total of 4811 cows from five dairy farms were either sent to slaughter or died on the farm from 2006 to 2016. On average, eliminated cows had a DL of 1939 ± 11 days, the NL was 3 ± 0.1, the LMY was 31,120 ± 303 l, the tDIM was 984 ± 9 days, the LPL was 29.9 ± 0.2 l and the LDL was 14.4 ± 0.1 l. Significant differences ($P < 0.05$) were observed between farms for most of the studied parameters with the exception of farms 1 and 5 (Table 2, Additional file 1: Table S1 and Additional file 2: Table S2). Annual herd turnover rate ranged from 25 to 35% on the five farms and the overall percentage of eliminated cows during the first, second, third, fourth and after the fourth parity was 20.4, 22.9, 21.7, 16.2 and 18.8%, respectively. These percentages in eliminated cows considering number of parity were significantly different ($P < 0.05$) between farms (Fig. 1). Finally, production parameters in slaughtered compared to dead cows were significantly different ($P < 0.05$): NL (3 ± 0.1 vs 3.2 ± 0.1), DL (1958 ± 12 vs 1861 ± 23 days), tDIM (1003 ± 10 vs 902 ± 19 days), LMY (31,426 ± 338 vs 29,852 ± 685 l) and LPL (29.8 ± 0.1 vs 30.8 ± 03 l) (Table 2).

Destiny and cause of elimination

During the period under study, 80.6% of the eliminated cows were slaughtered and 19.4% died on the farm. Cows were sent to slaughter every 20 days on average

Table 2 Average (± SEM) and confidence intervals (95%) for production parameters of eliminated cows (slaughtered and dead) over 11 years (2006–2016) in five farms

Farm	1	2	3	4	5	Average		
						Eliminated cows	Slaughtered cows	Dead cows
Number of milking cows (n)	140 ± 4	340 ± 9	600 ± 15	420 ± 8	181 ± 6	NA	NA	NA
Number of daily milkings	2	3	3	3	2	NA	NA	NA
NL	3.4 ± 0.1^{a}	3.6 ± 0.1^{b}	2.9 ± 0.1^{c}	2.7 ± 0.1^{d}	3.2 ± 0.1^{a}	3 ± 0.1	3 ± 0.1^{A}	3.2 ± 0.1^{B}
	(3.1–3.6)	(3.5–3.7)	(2.8–3.0)	(2.6–2.8)	(3.1–3.3)	(3.0–3.1)	(2.9–3.1)	(3.1–3.3)
DL (days)	2092 ± 45^{a}	2171 ± 26^{b}	1943 ± 23^{c}	1775 ± 15^{d}	$1935 \pm 26^{c,e}$	1939 ± 11	1958 ± 12^{A}	1861 ± 23^{B}
	(2004.3–2181.1)	(2120.9–2221.3)	(1897.7–1989.1)	(1745.0–1804.1)	(1884.9–1985.3)	(1913.3–1960.7)	(1935–1981)	(1815–1906)
tDIM (days)	1127 ± 38^{a}	1203 ± 21^{b}	948 ± 18^{c}	842 ± 12^{d}	1002 ± 22^{e}	984 ± 9	1003 ± 10^{A}	902 ± 19^{B}
	(1054.6–1202.3)	(1160.8–1245.3)	(912.7–982.6)	(819.5–867.9)	(980.1–1031.5)	(967.8–1001.9)	(984–1022)	(865–939)
LMY (litres)	$38{,}607 \pm 1353^{a,d}$	$39{,}001 \pm 765^{a}$	$31{,}183 \pm 629^{b}$	$23{,}897 \pm 374^{c}$	$34{,}134 \pm 787^{d}$	31,120 ± 303	$31{,}426 \pm 338^{A}$	$29{,}852 \pm 685^{B}$
	(35,467.3–40,782.6)	(37,499.9–40,503.8)	(29,949.6–32,417.3)	(23,156.3–24,623.5)	(32,589.8–35,678.3)	(30,527.4–31,716.2)	(30,763–32,089)	(28,507–31,196)
LPL (litres)	32.4 ± 0.4^{a}	30.8 ± 0.2^{b}	31.5 ± 0.2^{c}	27.0 ± 0.2^{d}	32.7 ± 0.2^{a}	29.9 ± 0.2	29.8 ± 0.1^{A}	30.8 ± 03^{B}
	(31.7–33.1)	(30.3–31.2)	(31.2–31.9)	(26.7–27.3)	(32.1–33.1)	(29.8–30.2)	(29.6–30)	(30.3–31.3)
LDL (litres)	16.6 ± 0.4^{a}	16.2 ± 0.2^{a}	14.6 ± 0.2^{b}	12.2 ± 0.1^{c}	15.9 ± 0.2^{a}	14.4 ± 0.1	14.4 ± 0.1^{A}	14.2 ± 0.2^{A}
	(16.0–17.5)	(15.8–16.5)	(14.3–15.0)	(11.9–12.4)	(15.6–16.4)	(14.2–14.6)	(14.3–14.6)	(13.7–14.6)

NL, DL, LMY, tDIM, LPL and LDL is number of lactations, days of life, life milk yield, total days in milk, litres per day of productive life and litres per day of life, respectively

NA non-applicable

$^{a-e}$ Means within a row with different superscripts differ between farms ($P < 0.05$)

^{A,B} Means within a row with different capital superscripts differ between slaughtered and dead cows ($P < 0.05$)

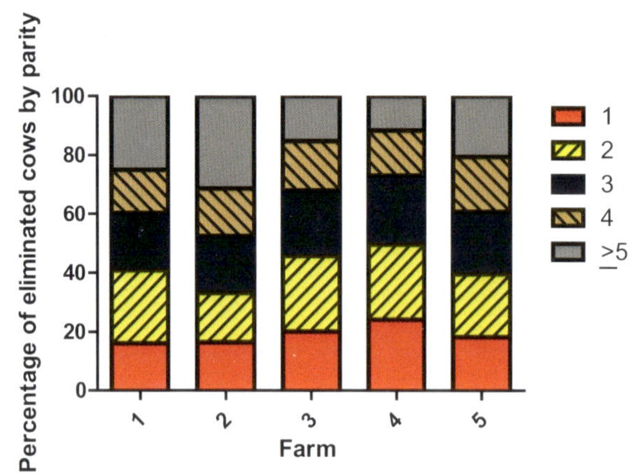

Fig. 1 Percentage of eliminated cows by parity and farm

and carcasses of dead cows were removed within a mandatory period of 48 h. Significant differences ($P < 0.05$) were observed between farms such that the highest percentage of dead cows was observed on farms 2 and 5 (20.9 and 25.4%, respectively), whereas the lowest percentage was observed on farm 1 (12.5%). Reproductive disorders (30.2%), production (23.4%) and mammary gland disorders (13.5%) were the three main causes of cow elimination representing 67% of all the events. Secondly, accidents (7.7%), metabolic or digestive disorders (7.2%) and infectious diseases (6.5%) represented 21.4% of the cow eliminations. Thirdly, locomotor disorders (3.6%), dystocia or obstetrics (2.4%) and respiratory causes (0.7%) were a minor group representing 6.7% of all the events. Finally, the cause of elimination was unknown in 4.7% of the cases. The percentage for each cause of elimination and for slaughtered and dead cows by farm is shown in Table 3. Reproductive disorders were the major cause for elimination on farms 1, 2, 3 and 5, whereas the major cause for elimination on farm 4 was productive reasons. Significant differences ($P < 0.05$) were observed between farms regarding the reason for cow elimination. The causes of elimination were significantly different ($P < 0.05$) between slaughtered and dead cows. In particular, reproductive disorders, production causes

Table 3 Description of the cause of elimination for cows in the eliminated, slaughtered and dead cows in five farms over 11 years (2006–2016)

Farm	1	2	3	4	5	Average		
						Eliminated cows	Slaughtered cows	Dead cows
Herd turnover (%)	26	25	27	30	35	28.1 (27.0–29.2)	NA	NA
Slaughter (%)	87.5	79.1	81.1	82.2	74.6	80.6 (80.3–82.5)	NA	NA
Dead on the farm (%)	12.5	20.9	18.9	17.8	25.4	19.4 (17.5–19.7)	NA	NA
Reason for elimination								
Reproduction (%)	32.8	27.4	40.4	23.7	34.3	30.2 (28.9–31.5)	37.3 (35.8–38.8)	0.7 (0.3–1.5)
Mammary gland (%)	17.7	22.2	10.6	5.7	22.4	13.5 (12.6–14.5)	13.9 (12.9–15.1)	11.6 (9.7–13.8)
Production (%)	14.5	22.3	16.5	31.8	18.0	23.4 (22.2–24.6)	28.9 (27.6.30.4)	0 NA
Locomotor (%)	5.2	4.2	4.3	2.5	3.7	3.6 (3.1–4.2)	3.6 (3–4.2)	3.5 (2.5–4.9)
Metabolic/digestive (%)	13.4	7.8	11.6	2.5	8.6	7.2 (6.5–7.9)	4.1 (3.5–4.7)	20.1 (17.7–22.8)
Respiratory (%)	2.6	0.8	0.7	0.0	1.1	0.7 (0.6–0.8)	0.3 (0.1–0.5)	2.1 (1.3–3.3)
Dystocia/obstetrics (%)	2.0	3.5	2.9	1.5	2.7	2.4 (2.0–2.9)	0.4 (0.2–0.7)	10.7 (8.9–12.8)
Accident (%)	9.3	2.2	6.6	11.2	8.1	7.7 (7.0–8.6)	1.6 (1.3–2)	33.3 (30.3–36.3)
Infectious disease (%)	1.2	3.2	2.4	14.4	0.3	6.5 (5.8–7.3)	6.9 (6.2–7.8)	4.7 (3.5–6.3)
Unknown (%)	1.2	6.2	4.1	6.6	0.7	4.7 (4.2–5.4)	2.7 (2.2–3.3)	13.2 (11.2–15.6)

Confidence intervals (95%) between brackets at the average column and infectious causes were significantly more frequent ($P < 0.05$) in slaughtered than in dead cows whereas metabolic/digestive, dystocia/obstetrics, accident, respiratory and unknown causes, were significantly less frequent ($P < 0.05$) in slaughtered than in dead cows.

The cause for elimination differed significantly ($P < 0.05$) depending on the parity of the cow (Fig. 2a–c) but the pattern varied depending on the cause. Reproductive and production causes were the most frequent causes of elimination in cows of all parities. Reproductive cause progressively and significantly ($P < 0.05$) decreased in importance, especially after more than three lactations. Productive cause also decreased significantly ($P < 0.05$) in importance between the first and fourth parities, but increased in cows with five or more parities at the same level of first lactation cows. Accidents were the third main cause of elimination for cows of first and second lactation, but progressively and significantly ($P < 0.05$) decreased in importance. The percentage of eliminated cows due to mammary gland disease, metabolic diseases and unknown causes increased significantly ($P < 0.05$) as the cows got older. Dystocia showed a significant increase ($P < 0.05$) in importance between the second and third lactations. Infectious diseases were more important in third lactation cows compared to younger cows and showed a decreasing trend in cows eliminated with four or more lactations. Finally, the percentage of elimination due to locomotor and respiratory causes did not show any statistically significant changes ($P > 0.05$) during the cows' lifespan.

For all farms, the percentage of cows that died on the farm was significantly ($P < 0.05$) affected by period. Proportion of dead cows was significantly higher during period 2 (22.4%) and 3 (22.4%) when compared to period 1 (17.9%) and 4 (16.4%). The causes of elimination were also significantly affected by the time of year but the pattern was different taking into account the different causes (Fig. 3a–c). Reproductive and metabolic/digestive causes showed the highest values during periods 1 and 4 that were significantly higher ($P < 0.05$) than for period 2 and 3, whereas accidents and infectious diseases showed the highest values during periods 2 and 3 that were significantly higher ($P < 0.05$) than for periods 1 and 4. On the other hand, elimination due to unknown and locomotor causes peaked at periods 3 and 4, respectively without showing significant differences ($P > 0.05$) with the other periods. The remaining causes of elimination did not show significant variation throughout the year.

Discussion

This study used data from five dairy herds in Spain from 2006 to 2016 that are typical of the intensive milk production sector in southern Europe, but also in other countries and areas of the world. Defining culling criteria and a cause of mortality can be biased depending on how data are collected, who is responsible for the data collection and on the data analysis system [1]. All data analysed in the study were collected using the same software system and the same team of veterinarians. Use of the same criteria and analysis system is necessary to advice farmers and benchmark different farms. This point is critical because the reason for culling can be biased depending on how data are collected, who is responsible for this data collection and the data analysis system [17]. Despite similarities in management, nutrition, collection and data analysis, veterinarian diagnosis and treatment of diseases, key points of herd performance such as age at death, mortality and culling reasons, tDIM and LMY differed significantly between herds. In this study, these differences could be more related to intrinsic factors of each farm such as care of animals by workers, differences between farmer's criteria when deciding to treat a sick cow or euthanize it, hygiene and design of facilities than number of milking cows or milk yield. Climate conditions may also have an effect on mortality and cause of death. We suggest that analysing between-herd differences and benchmarking farms is useful to improve the day-by-day management and animal care on the farms.

The DL and LMY of eliminated cows in our study was similar to the value reported in a study from the Netherlands [19]. On the other hand, tDIM was lower than values described by others [20, 21]. Finally NL (3.0 ± 0.1) was lower than the value described by Africor (3.3 ± 0.1) [22] but higher than a Swedish study with multiple dairy breeds (2.3 ± 1.4) [9]. Thus, there is great variability in the productive parameters of eliminated cows published in the literature and comparison to other studies is difficult given the different methods of collection of production data. Some of these studies analyse data based on information provided by official control agencies that estimate production. This makes it imperative to obtain data for a particular geographical area and for particular production characteristics in order to define benchmarking strategies.

In this study, annual average herd turnover rate on the farms ranged between 25 and 35%. The terms used in the literature to define the causes for the elimination of cows, due to either culling or mortality, and whether this elimination is voluntary and planned or involuntary and unplanned, can be confusing. In any case, the percentage of turnover rates ranges from 21.3% in Ireland [23] and up to 40% in Australia [24], 25.4% in the Netherlands [19], 26% in northwest Spain [7], 22.6 and 30% in the UK [25, 26], between 28.2 and 33.5% in Canada [27] and 36% in the USA [28]). In contrast, between-herd differences for herd turnover rates are 10% in this research study,

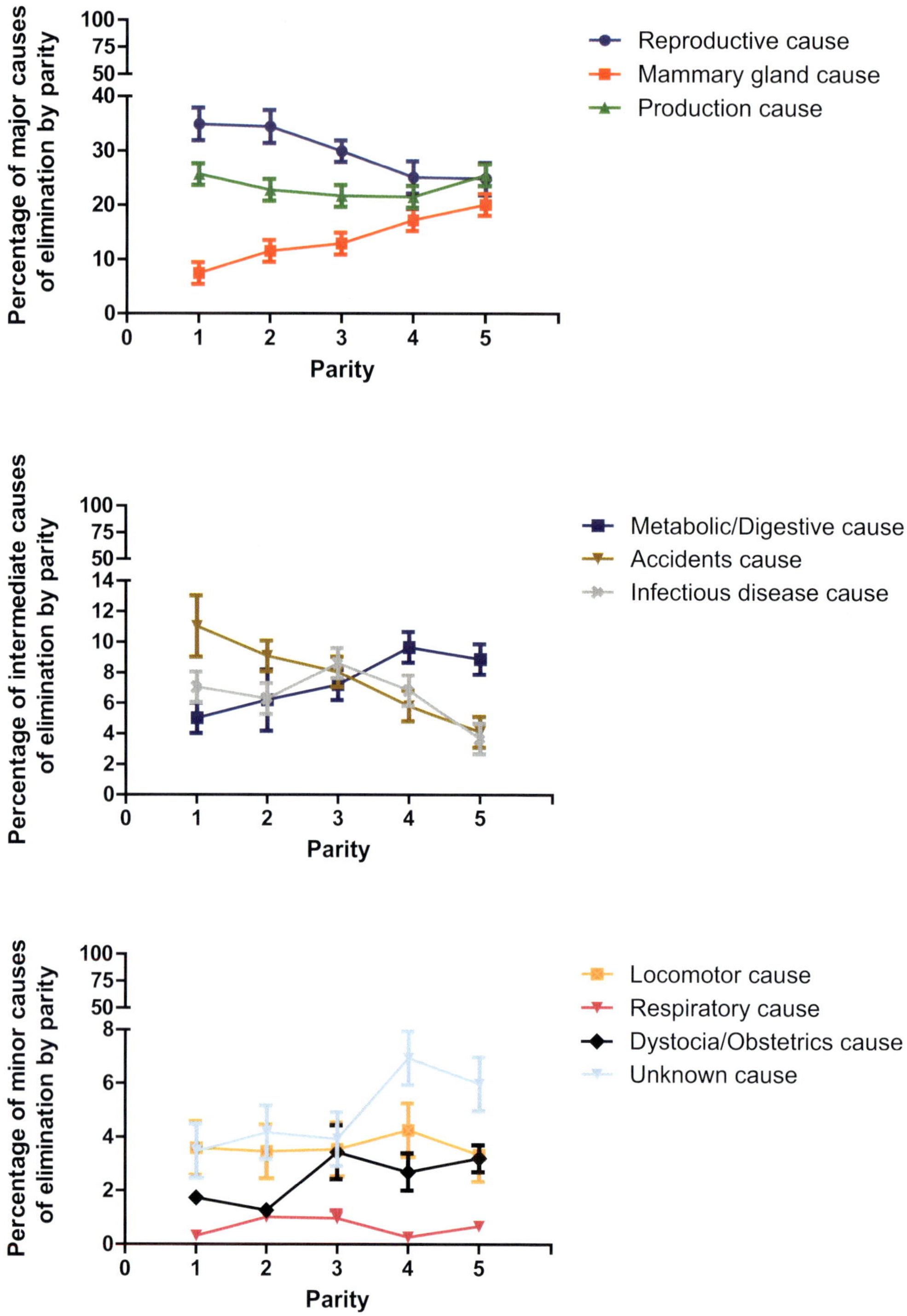

Fig. 2 Percentage (with 95% confidence interval) of major, intermediate and minor causes of elimination by cow parity. In the figure, parity equal to or higher than five is represented by five. The causes of elimination have been grouped into "major causes" (causes of elimination with a percentage higher than 15%), "intermediate cause" (causes of elimination with values between 8 and 15%) and "minor causes" (elimination causes with values lower than 8%)

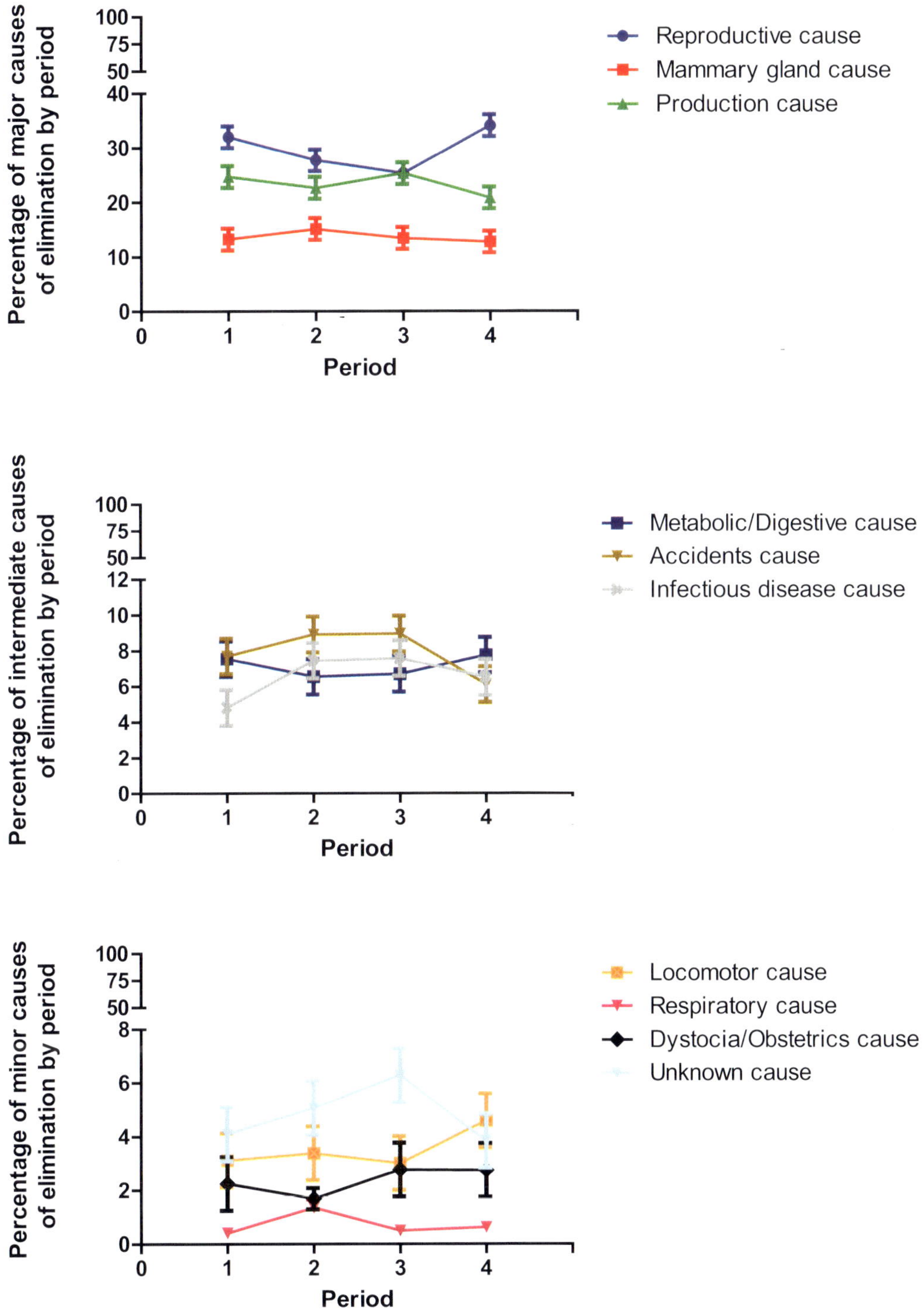

Fig. 3 Percentage (with 95% confidence interval) of major, intermediate and minor causes of elimination by period of year. The year was divided into four periods: 1 (1st January–31st March), 2 (1st April–30th June), 3 (1st July–30th September) and 4 (1st October–31st December). The causes of elimination have been grouped into "major causes" (causes of elimination with a percentage higher than 15%), "intermediate cause" (causes of elimination with values between 8 and 15%) and "minor causes" (elimination causes with values lower than 8%)

whereas, in other studies in Europe between-herd differences where 50.3% in the Netherlands (herd turnover range 6.2–56.5%) and 24% in the UK (range 11.5–35.5%). These two studies included a greater number of farms, which may have had different production and management systems [29], which could explain these differences. On the other hand, results from the current report agree with those from a study conducted in Poland, with a culling rate between 20 and 35% [30] and rates of 28.1–35.2% reported in another study carried out in the USA with farms whose size was similar to those included in our study [4]. In our study, turnover rates for second and third parity cows (22.9 and 21.7% respectively) were significantly higher than first, fourth and after fourth parity cows (20.4, 16.2 and 18.8%, respectively). Farmers and technicians of the included farms are aware that a cow needs more than one parity to achieve economic amortization. This reference value on economic amortization is based on economic data from the farms under study and is supported by recent research [31]. It could be a reasonable explanation why farmers increase the culling rate during the second and third parity. After the fourth parity, turnover rate decreases probably because cows have demonstrated good production and reproductive performance [14].

In our study, 19.4% of the eliminated cows died on the farm. This result is similar to that reported by other studies with the proportion of dead cows between 17.2 and 20.6% in northwestern Spain and USA [7, 10] but higher than 10.6 and 14.8% reported previously for USA [28, 32]. The proportion of dead cows may be a consequence of socio-psychological differences between countries and regions in terms of practices around euthanasia and death [33]. We suggest that farmers in our study area were more likely to treat sick animals and keep them on the farm than they are in other countries, which would explain the differences in proportion of cows dying on the farms compared to other studies. Another factor that may affect the proportion of dead cows could be the intensity of the heat stress season. It has been shown that this period is a risk factor in significantly increasing mortality on farms and the proportion of dead cows could be extremely high on farms without optimal anti-heat stress systems [14, 15, 34]. Other factors to explain the higher levels of dead cows in this study compared to others [28, 32], could be injured animals due to accidents, mainly related to slippery floors. Additionally, the transport of sick or injured cows to slaughter is strictly regulated and farmers can be penalized with large fines. Thus, they may prefer to have a problematic animal die on the farm instead of sending it to the slaughterhouse. Overall, between-herd differences were observed in this parameter. The percentage of dead cows could be a good parameter for benchmarking farms, since many factors are at play including building design, management, disease prevention and elimination policy.

Regarding the overall data analysis, the most important cause of elimination was reproductive issues followed by low milk production and mammary gland disease. The order of the causes of elimination agreed with other studies, but the proportions for each reason were different between studies. Thus, the percentage of elimination due to reproductive causes was higher (30.2%) than the value described in the USA (17%) [10], Canada (18%) [27], Sweden (24.8%) [35] and north-west Spain (24.7%) [7]. Low milk production was the second most important cause of elimination (23.4%) in our study and it was higher than the value found for USA (12.1%) [10], Canada (6–7%) [27] and Sweden (6.2%) [35]. Mammary gland disease was the third main cause of removal (13.5%), and this percentage was lower than the value reported in Sweden (22.5%) [35] and Spain (15.6%) [7] but similar to the values reported in the USA (12.1%) [14], and Canada (11.3–12.5%) [27]. The next most important causes of elimination were accidents and metabolic and digestive disorders, which also showed a high variability between studies. The percentage of eliminated cows due to accidents on the farm in the current study (7.7%) was higher than the value found for Canada (3.8%) [27], but it was lower than the values reported in Denmark (5–19%) [18]. Finally, the percentage of eliminated cows due to metabolic and digestive diseases (7.2%) was higher than the values reported in Sweden (2.2%) [35].

Elimination of animals positive for infectious diseases was responsible for 6.5% of eliminated cows. Other studies report information on infectious diseases as a cause for elimination, including bovine leucosis or paratuberculosis, but comparisons cannot be carried out due to different ways of collecting information. The percentage of eliminated cows due to foot and leg problems (3.6%) was lower than the value described in USA (8.1%) [10], Spain (8.0%) [7], Canada (7.2–7.8%) [27] and Sweden (6.6%) [35]. Problems at calving were responsible for 2.4% of eliminations. This percentage was higher than the report (0.6%) from Canada [27] but lower than a study that reviewed mortality data worldwide (2.0–46.0%) [18]. A lack of information regarding the reasons for elimination was found in 4.7% of dead animals. This cause of elimination defined as "unknown" is also observed in other studies at similar proportions (4–5%) [10, 36]. Some studies and data centres show a higher proportion (17–20%) of unknown causes of elimination [27, 37]. When a comparison of causes of elimination was carried out between herds, differences were observed suggesting that the analysis of the cause of elimination can also be a proper indicator for benchmarking and improving production systems of farms [29, 38]. Causes of elimination also differed significantly in relation to parity and in a logical pattern. For instance, the importance of mammary gland and metabolic diseases as causes of elimination increased with age in our study. As previously reported by others, the risk of mastitis increases significantly as the number of lactations increases compared to first lactation cows (for second, third and fourth or more lactation cows respectively: RR = 1.57/2.41/3.40) [39]. In the case of metabolic diseases, cows with 3 or more parities have an increased relative risk of subclinical hypocalcaemia (RR = 1.7; 95% CI 1.2–2.3) [40] and ketosis (RR = 1.64; 95% CI 1.59–1.69) when compared to second lactation cows [41]. A comparison of the cause of cow elimination should be carried out carefully among different countries but should also be detailed between farms with very similar characteristics to compare them and identify problems of animal welfare and management, with the objective of providing specific and personalised solutions.

The season of the year significantly affected mortality, increasing during the hottest seasons as reported in other studies. A one unit increase in Heat Stress Index results in a 3% increase in the on-farm mortality rate (RR = 1.03; 95% CI 1.03–1.04) [15] whereas one study reported an increase of 4.7% in mortality associated with a 1 °C increase in Heat Stress Index in Italy [42]. Another study carried out in Belgium showed significant heat-related increases in dairy cattle mortality, (RR = 1.09; 95% CI 1.02–1.17, for moderate heat and RR = 1.26; 95% CI 1.08–1.48, for extreme heat) [34]. These results agree with a Swedish study where the risk of mortality increased during the hot season versus autumn and winter [38]. Differences were also observed between herds, since farms without anti-heat stress systems had higher mortality rates during the warm season. This is of particular interest when proposing investments to mitigate heat stress on farms located in areas or countries where climate change may have an impact. These farms should adapt their production system to the changing climate conditions. Season also significantly affects the cause for removing a cow. As an example, reproductive disorders and metabolic/digestive diseases as causes of elimination increased during period 4 (Sep–Dec). A reasonable explanation could be that these cows suffer from heat stress during the dry off period and suffered from a negative energy balance before parturition [6, 43].

Conclusions

This study shows that the causes of elimination can be significantly different between dairy farms even though they have similar productive systems, similar health status, close veterinary diagnosis and herd software data compilation. These differences could be due mainly to the farmer's personality, differences in the cow management and facility design. Applying benchmarking strategies based on data from eliminated cows can be very useful to demonstrate that the elimination plan is not suitable, the management of the animals may be improved or that poorly designed farm facilities may have a negative impact on the efficiency of the farm. In summary, the analysis of the causes of cow elimination can be of great technical interest for the farmer but the same classification of causes and veterinary diagnosis must be used in dairy farms to draw comparable conclusions.

Additional files

Additional file 1: Table S1. Distribution of the number of milking cows, number of lactations (NL) and days of life (DL) of eliminated cows by farm over 11 years (2006–2016).

Additional file 2: Table S2. Distribution of the total days in milk (tDIM), life milk yield (LMY), litres per day of productive life (LPL) and litres per day of life (LDL) of eliminated cows by farm over 11 years (2006–2016).

Abbreviations

DF: dead on the farm; DIM: days in milk; DL: age at death; DS: dead due to slaughter; LDL: litres per day of life; LMY: life milk yield; LPL: litres per day of productive life; NL: number of lactations at elimination; tDIM: total days in milk.

Authors' contributions

RA was project coordinator, selected farms and collected the data. RA and LF conceived the study and wrote the manuscript. LF performed the data analysis. Both authors read and approved the final manuscript.

Author details

[1] Departament de Ciència Animal, ETSEA, University of Lleida, Av. Alcalde Rovira Roure 191, E25198 Lleida, Spain. [2] Agrotecnio Center, Av. Alcalde Rovira Roure, 80, E25198 Lleida, Spain. [3] Present Address: Department of Animal Science, University of Lleida, ETSEA, Av. Alcalde Rovira Roure, 191, E25198 Lleida, Spain.

Acknowledgements

The authors are grateful to Dr. Carolina Naranjo Freixa for helping in the review of the manuscript and farm owners for their time and interest.

Competing interests

The authors declare that they have no competing interests.

Funding

This research did not receive any specific grant from funding agencies in the public, commercial, or not-for-profit sectors.

References

1. Compton CWR, Heuer C, Thomsen PT, Carpenter TE, Phyn CVC, McDougall S. A systematic literature review and meta-analysis of mortality and culling in dairy cattle. J Dairy Sci. 2017;100:1–16.
2. Renkema JA, Stelwagen J. Economic evaluation of replacement rates in dairy herds I. Reduction of replacement rates through improved health. Livest Prod Sci. 1979;6:15–27.
3. Rogers GW, Van Arendonk JAM, McDaniel BT. Influence of production and prices on optimum culling rates and annualized net revenue. J Dairy Sci. 1988;71:3453–62.
4. De Vries A, Olson JD, Pinedo PJ. Reproductive risk factors for culling and productive life in large dairy herds in the eastern United States between 2001 and 2006. J Dairy Sci. 2010;93:613–23.
5. García-Ispierto I, López-Gatius F, Santolaria P, Yániz JL, Nogareda C, López-Béjar M, De Rensis F. Relationship between heat stress during the peri-implantation period and early fetal loss in dairy cattle. Theriogenology. 2006;65:799–807.
6. De Rensis F, Scaramuzzi RJ. Heat stress and seasonal effects on reproduction in the dairy cow—a review. Theriogenology. 2003;60:1139–51.
7. Fouz R, Yus E, Sanjuán ML, Diéguez FJ. Causas de eliminación en rebaños bovinos lecheros de raza frisona en Control Lechero Oficial. ITEA. 2014;110:171–86.
8. Stevenson MA, Lean IJ. Descriptive epidemiological study on culling and deaths in eight dairy herds. Aust Vet J. 1998;76:482–8.
9. Schneider MP, Strandberg E, Emanuelson U, Grandinson K, Roth A. The effect of veterinary-treated clinical mastitis and pregnancy status on culling in Swedish dairy cows. Prev Vet Med. 2007;80:179–92.
10. Pinedo PJ, De Vries A, Webb DW. Dynamics of culling risk with disposal codes reported by Dairy Herd Improvement dairy herds. J Dairy Sci. 2010;93:2250–61.
11. Gröhn YT, Eicher SW, Ducrocq V, Hertl JA. Effect of diseases on the culling of Holstein dairy cows in New York State. J Dairy Sci. 1998;81:966–78.
12. Rajala-Schultz PJ, Grohn YT. Culling of dairy cows. Part I. Effects of diseases on culling in Finnish Ayrshire cows. Prev Vet Med. 1999;41:195–208.
13. Chiumia D, Chagunda MGG, Mac Rae AI, Roberts DJ. Predisposing factors for involuntary culling in Holstein–Friesian dairy cows. J Dairy Res. 2013;80:45–50.
14. Seegers H, Beaudeau F, Fourichon C, Bareille N. Reasons for culling in French Holstein cows. Prev Vet Med. 1998;36:257–71.
15. Williams KEB, Berke O, Pearl DL, Hand K, Kelton DF. Heat stress related dairy cow mortality during heat waves and control periods in rural Southern Ontario from 2010–2012. BMC Vet Res. 2015;11:291.
16. Dobson H, Smith RF, Royal MD, Knight CH, Sheldon IM. The high producing dairy cow and its reproductive performance. Reprod Domest Anim. 2007;42:17–23. https://doi.org/10.1111/j.1439-0531.2007.00906.x.
17. Fetrow J, Nordlund KV, Norman HD. Culling: nomenclature, definitions, and recommendations. J Dairy Sci. 2006;89:1896–905.
18. Thomsen PT, Houe H. Dairy cow mortality: a review. Vet Q. 2006;28:122–9.
19. Mohd N, Steeneveld W, Hogeveen H. The average culling rate of Dutch dairy herds over the years 2007–2010 and its association with herd reproduction, performance and health. J Dairy Res. 2014;81:1–8.
20. de Lopez Maturana E, Ugarte E, Gonzalez-Recio O. Impact of calving ease on functional longevity and herd amortization costs in Basque Holsteins using survival analysis. J Dairy Sci. 2007;90:4451–7.
21. Hultgren J, Svensson C. Heifer rearing conditions affect length of productive life in Swedish dairy cows. Prev Vet Med. 2009;89:255–64.
22. Official Holstein Friesian association in north-west Spain (Galicia): Africor. 2016. https://issuu.com/transmediacomunicacion/docs/africor_lugo_memoria_2016_93515defa5e95a. Accessed Sep 2017.
23. Maher P, Good M, More SJ. Trends in cow numbers and culling rate in the Irish cattle population, 2003–2006. Ir Vet J. 2008;61:455–63.
24. National service body for the Australian dairy industry. DairyAustralia. 2017. http://www.dairyaustralia.com.au/~/media/Documents/Stats%20and%20markets/S%20and%20O/20176/Situation%20And%20Outlook%20June%202017.pdf. Accessed June 2017.
25. Bell MJ, Wall E, Russell G, Roberts DJ, Simm G. Risk factors for culling in Holstein–Friesian dairy cows. Vet Rec. 2010;167:238–40.
26. Whitaker DA, Macrae AI, Burrough E. Disposal and disease rates in British dairy herds between April 1998 and March 2002. Vet Rec. 2004;155:43–7.
27. The Canadian Dairy Information Centre (CDIC). 2017. http://dairyinfo.gc.ca. Accessed Sep 2017.
28. Smith JW, Ely LO, Chapa AM. Effect of region, herd size, and milk production on reasons cows leave the herd. J Dairy Sci. 2000;83:2980–7.
29. Raboisson D, Cahuzac E, Sans P, Allaire G. Herd-level and contextual factors influencing dairy cow mortality in France in 2005 and 2006. J Dairy Sci. 2011;94:1790–803.
30. Olechnowicz J, Jaskowski JM. Reasons for culling, culling due to lameness, and economic losses in dairy cows. Med Weter. 2011;67:618–21.
31. Boulton AC, Rushton J, Wathes DC. An empirical analysis of the cost of rearing heifers from birth to first calving and the time taken to repay these costs. Animal. 2017;11:1372–80.
32. Hadley GL, Wolf CA, Harsh SB. Dairy cattle culling patterns, explanations, and implications. J Dairy Sci. 2006;89:2286–96.
33. Beaudeau F, Van der Ploeg JD, Boileau B, Seegers H, Noordhuizen JPTM. Relationships between culling criteria in dairy herds and farmers' management styles. Prev Vet Med. 1996;25:327–42.
34. Cox B, Gasparrini A, Boudewijn C, Delcloo A, Bijnens E, Vangronsveld J, Nawrot T. Mortality related to cold and heat. What do we learn from dairy cattle? Environ Res. 2016;149:231–8.
35. Ahlman T, Berglund B, Rydhmer L, Strandberg E. Culling reasons in organic and conventional dairy herds and genotype by environment interaction for longevity. J Dairy Sci. 2011;94:1568–75.
36. Thomsen PT, Kjeldsen AM, Sorensen JT, Houe H. Mortality (including euthanasia) among Danish dairy cows (1990–2001). Prev Vet Med. 2004;62:19–33.
37. Fusi F, Angelucci A, Lorenzi V, Luca Bolzoni L, Bertocchi L. Assessing circumstances and causes of dairy cow death in Italian dairy farms through a veterinary practice survey (2013–2014). Prev Vet Med. 2017;137(Pt A):105–8.
38. Alvåsen K, Mörk MK, Sandgren CH, Thomsen PT, Emanuelson U. Herd-level risk factors associated with cow mortality in Swedish dairy herds. J Dairy Sci. 2012;95:4352–62.
39. Ramirez NF, Keefe G, Dohoo I, Sánchez J, Arroyave O, Cerón J, Jaramillo M, Palacio LG. Herd- and cow-level risk factors associated with subclinical mastitis in dairy farms from the High Plains of the northern Antioquia, Colombia. J Dairy Sci. 2014;97:1–10.
40. Neves RC, Leno BM, Stokol T, Overton TR, McArt JAA. Risk factors associated with postpartum subclinical hypocalcemia in dairy cows. J Dairy Sci. 2017;100:3796–804.
41. Tatone EH, Duffield TF, LeBlanc SJ, DeVries TJ, Gordon JL. Investigating the within-herd prevalence and risk factors for ketosis in dairy cattle in Ontario as diagnosed by the test-day concentration of β-hydroxybutyrate in milk. J Dairy Sci. 2017;100:1308–18.
42. Crescio MI, Forastiere F, Maurella C, Ingravalle F, Rua G. Heat-related mortality in dairy cattle: a case crossover study. Prev Vet Med. 2010;97:191–7.
43. Raboisson D, Mounié M, Maigné E. Diseases, reproductive performance, and changes in milk production associated with subclinical ketosis in dairy cows: a meta-analysis and review. J Dairy Sci. 2014;97:7547–63.

Canine angiostrongylosis in Sweden: a nationwide seroepidemiological survey by enzyme-linked immunosorbent assays and a summary of five-year diagnostic activity (2011–2015)

Giulio Grandi[1,2*], Eva Osterman Lind[1], Roland Schaper[3], Erik Ågren[4] and Manuela Schnyder[5]

Abstract

Background: For the first time in Sweden, *Angiostrongylus vasorum* was detected on the island of Sydkoster in foxes and dogs in 2003. After sporadic detection of the parasite in foxes in southern Sweden, the first positive canine faecal sample on the mainland was found in 2011. Since then a total of 2882 faecal samples have been analysed with the Baermann test at the National Veterinary Institute (SVA) during the years 2011–2015; 20 of them being positive. Contemporaneously, of over 525 fox necropsies, only three were found to be infected. To gather a more accurate knowledge of *A. vasorum* occurrence in Sweden, a large scale seroepidemiological survey was performed and totally 3885 serum samples from dogs were tested for both the presence of circulating antigens and of specific antibodies to *A. vasorum*.

Results: In total, 0.10% (n = 4, 95% Confidence Intervals, CI 0.03–0.26%) of the dogs were positive for both antigen and antibodies, whereas 0.51% (n = 20, CI 0.31–0.79%) of the tested dogs were only antigen positive and 0.88% (n = 34, CI 0.61–1.22%) only positive for specific antibodies. Seropositive animals, as well as the majority of *A. vasorum*-positive faecal samples tested during the same period, were spread over central and southern Sweden. Annual prevalence of positive faecal dog samples and of necropsied *A. vasorum* positive foxes (coming from southern Sweden) varied from 0.3 to 0.9% (overall: 0.7%, CI 0.4–1.1%) and 0.0 to 1.4% (overall: 0.3%, CI 0.1–0.9%), respectively.

Conclusions: The findings confirmed that *A. vasorum* has become established in various geographical areas of central and southern Sweden. Veterinarians and dog owners should be aware of the potential risks of infection in large areas of the country, since canine angiostrongylosis may be a fatal disease if left untreated.

Keywords: *Angiostrongylus vasorum*, Antigen, Antibodies, Serology, Dog

Background

Angiostrongylus vasorum, the French heartworm, is a nematode parasite of dogs. The worm resides in the right side of the heart and in the pulmonary arteries. The red fox (*Vulpes vulpes*) and other wild canids act as definitive hosts as do dogs, while intermediate hosts, terrestrial gastropod molluscs, are needed to complete the life cycle. Frogs and birds may be involved as paratenic hosts [1–4]. Although *A. vasorum* was reported from France in the 19th century [5], a more detailed characterization of the clinical features related to the infection as well as improvement of diagnostic methods mainly took place during the last 20 years.

Clinical signs may vary greatly but coagulopathy and lung lesions have been identified as the two main reasons

*Correspondence: giulio.grandi@slu.se
[2] Department of Biomedical Sciences and Veterinary Public Health (BVF), Swedish University of Agricultural Sciences, PO Box 7028, Ulls väg 26, SE-757 56 Uppsala, Sweden
Full list of author information is available at the end of the article

for a potentially fatal outcome of the disease in dogs. Clinical manifestations of coagulopathy can range from subcutaneous haematomas, epistaxis to neurological signs depending on the site of bleeding. The lung damage is related to microinjuries and inflammatory processes taking place both when eggs of *A. vasorum* are caught in the lung capillaries and when the hatched larvae migrate to the air passages. Tissue injuries intensify and may lead to the classical textbook clinical presentation of the disease characterized by dyspnoea, exercise intolerance, coughing, followed by lethargy and weakness [6].

A more accurate description of the geographical distribution of *A. vasorum* can be obtained using detection methods characterized by high sensitivity and specificity; such a description can be useful to promote better prevention measures and to increase disease awareness in areas where the risk of infection is present [7]. Traditionally the diagnosis relies on the detection of first stage larvae (L1) from faeces, but the excretion of L1 only takes place when lung lesions have already developed and furthermore, the Baermann technique has limitations in sensitivity and specificity [7]. For these reasons, other techniques such as Polymerase Chain Reaction (PCR) and serology have been developed and tested on individuals and—in the case of serology—in large scale studies. *A. vasorum* PCR protocols using specific primers targeting the ITS-2 region are usually able to detect a single L1 of *A. vasorum* [8–10]. Enzyme-Linked Immunosorbent Assays (ELISAs) have also developed to detect circulating parasite antigens [11] or antibodies against the parasite in serum samples [12, 13]. The diagnostic approach usually follows or completes a clinical assessment of individual patients, while large scale surveys are conducted on large numbers of randomly collected samples from individuals, distinguishing between infected and non-infected animals and therefore giving information on the occurrence and prevalence of *A. vasorum* in a given population.

During the past decades, the endemic foci of infection have expanded and new ones have been reported. The relative importance of different factors related to this apparent spread is still unclear. Increased urbanization of the red fox acting as wildlife reservoir [14] and increased movement of domestic dogs both within and between countries [15] are certainly involved. Climatic changes influencing the distribution of intermediate hosts may also play a role [16]. Beside historically endemic areas, like southern France, part of the British Isles and Denmark, there is a list of countries in South, Central and East Europe where the presence of the parasite has consistently been recorded. Recently an increased prevalence of the parasite in foxes [17, 18] and dogs [19, 20] has been reported in e.g. the United Kingdom (UK) and in Italy. Moreover, new autochthonous cases have been described in other countries such as Belgium [21], Slovakia [22] and Serbia [23]. During the past years, it has been possible to obtain a more complete picture of parasite prevalence in dog populations through large scale serological studies carried out in some countries, for example in Germany and UK [24], Italy [25], Switzerland [26], Poland [27], Hungary [7], Slovakia [28], Bulgaria [29], Belgium [30] and Portugal [31].

In Scandinavia, *A. vasorum* was initially detected in 1983 in Denmark in a dog that had travelled several times to southern France [32]. In Danish foxes, *A. vasorum* was first reported in 1992 [33], and the prevalence in foxes in the same area (northern Zealand) rose from 48.7% in 1993 [34] to 90% in 2002 [35]. Despite a prevalence of 9.7% of *A. vasorum* infections was found in Danish dogs in 2004 [36], an overall prevalence of 2.2% was reported in hunting dogs in 2013 [37]. In Norway the parasite was identified for the first time in a red fox in March 2016 [38]. In Sweden, *A. vasorum* infection was first diagnosed in 2003, both in a dog and in a red fox (*Vulpes vulpes*) from the island of Sydkoster (Västra Götaland county) [39], and since then further individual cases of *A. vasorum* infections have been identified in dogs and red foxes on the mainland as well.

The aim of the present study was to determine the prevalence and geographical distribution of *A. vasorum* in Swedish dogs by using serological analyses and data from routine diagnostic activity performed at the National Veterinary Institute (SVA).

Methods

Prevalence study using ELISAs

Sera of 3885 dogs were collected from the Clinical Chemistry Laboratory (CCL) of the University Animal Hospital (UDS-SLU, Uppsala) and from the SVA. Sera from CCL (n = 1212) were collected from February to April 2014, either from dogs attending the University Animal Hospital (n = 495) or were sent to CCL from other veterinary clinics of the country (n = 717). Sera collected from the SVA (n = 2674) were submitted from veterinary clinics during 2013 for the analysis of tick-borne bacterial pathogens such as *Anaplasma phagocytophilum* and *Borrelia* spp. For each sample the postal code of the residence of the dog owner was recorded. No other data could be retained due to confidentiality issues.

An aliquot of the samples was sent to the Institute of Parasitology, Vetsuisse Faculty, University of Zurich, Switzerland, for analysis for the presence of circulating *A. vasorum* antigens using monoclonal (mAb Av 56/1/2) and polyclonal antibodies in a sandwich ELISA with a sensitivity of 95.7% and a specificity of 94.0%, as previously described [11]. In brief, tests were performed in 96-well microtiter plates (Maxisorp, Nunc Roskilde,

Denmark) coated overnight at 4 °C with 2.5 μg/mL of mAb Av 56/1/2 that had been obtained by the fusion of spleen cells of mice immunised against adult *A. vasorum* excretory/secretory (E/S) antigen with myeloma cells, based on the protocol of de StGroth and Scheidegger [40]. Plates were then washed and saturated for 30 min at 37 °C with PBS-Tween-20 (PBS-T). Serum dilutions (100 μL/well, 1:2 in PBS–T) were incubated for 1 h at 37 °C. After further washing steps, hyperimmune polyclonal rabbit serum (100 μL/well) from rabbits also immunised with adult *A. vasorum* E/S antigen was added in a concentration of 1:500, incubated for 1 h at 37 °C and plates again washed before adding 100 μL/well goat anti-rabbit IgG conjugated to alkaline phosphatase and diluted in PBS–T (1:2500). After the repetition of the incubation and washing steps, 100 μL/well of substrate (*p*-nitrophenyl phosphate) were added. Absorbance values were read at 405 nm (OD405) with a Multiscan RC ELISA reader (Thermo Labsystems, Helsinki, Finland). The ELISA has been shown to detect circulating antigens starting at 5 weeks post infection (wpi) and at 10 wpi virtually all dogs are persistently positive. After anthelmintic treatment, antigens can be detectable until 9 weeks post treatment [11]. Additionally, a sandwich ELISA (sensitivity 81.0%, specificity 98.8%) using *A. vasorum* adult somatic antigen purified by monoclonal antibodies (mAb Av 5/5) was used for specific antibody detection [14]. Briefly, plates were coated overnight at 4 °C with *A. vasorum* adult somatic antigen (5 μg/mL), washed and saturated. Sera were used in a standard dilution of 1:200 in PBS-T with 10% foetal calf serum; 100 μL diluted sera/well were incubated at 37 °C in a humid chamber for 1 h. After washing steps, specific affinity-purified, alkaline phosphatase conjugated goat anti-dog IgG (γ) antibodies were used at a dilution of 1:250 in PBS-T (100 μL/well). Substrate was added after the washing steps and absorbance values obtained as described above. The ELISA has been shown to detect antibodies from 3 to 6 wpi and to remain positive as long as the animal is infected. After anthelmintic treatment, antibodies may remain detectable until 9 weeks post treatment [13].

All test runs included a background control, a conjugate control, three positive control sera from three experimentally infected dogs and two negative control sera from uninfected dogs, as previously described [11, 13]. Test thresholds were regionally determined with 300 randomly selected samples based on the mean value of optical density (A_{405} nm) plus 3 standard deviations.

The collected data were embedded into a geographical information system (GIS) using the program RegioGraph 10 (GfK GeoMarketing, Bruchsal, Germany) to visualize the regional distribution of *A. vasorum* antigen- and/or antibody-positive samples. The locations of positive samples were displayed on maps with administrative and postcode boundaries based on the three-digit postcodes of Sweden as points of reference.

Excel 2007 for Windows (Microsoft Corporation, Redmond, USA) was used to calculate the prevalence values and the 95% confidence interval (CI) of prevalence values.

Data from routine diagnostic activity, 2011–2015

Dogs

Faecal samples (Table 2) submitted to the SVA by veterinary clinics or private dog owners were tested with a modified larval recovery method [41]. The SVA requires at least three samples from three different droppings collected over 3 days from each dog in order to perform the analysis. All samples originated from dogs showing clinical signs, either respiratory or other clinical signs compatible with *A. vasorum* infection, and therefore cannot be considered representative of the general canine population.

Red foxes

Red foxes (Table 2) received at the SVA for diagnostic necropsies or submitted by hunters for pathogen screening were examined specifically for *A. vasorum* and lungworms by visual inspection of the cardiovascular and respiratory systems. During 2011, 3000 hunted red foxes were submitted for the national *Echinococcus multilocularis* surveillance program. Over 500 heart and lung sets were examined for parasites that year. A joint database was created in order to produce Table 2.

Results

A total of 0.10% (n = 4, 95%, CI 0.03–0.26%) of the dogs were positive in both ELISAs, while 0.51% (n = 20, CI 0.31–0.79%) were antigen positive only and 0.88% (n = 34, CI 0. 1–1.22%) were positive for specific antibodies only (Table 1). The geographical distribution of positive samples is shown in Fig. 1. Samples positive in both tests were found only in the counties of Gävleborg, Uppsala and Kronoberg (Fig. 1).

Endemic canine cases of *A. vasorum* were diagnosed once in 2011 and 2012, respectively. Subsequently, the parasite was sporadically found (4–9 times per year). A progressively increasing number of faecal samples was submitted to the SVA throughout this period.

Detailed figures on the number of examined faecal samples as well as the number of foxes necropsied at the SVA between 2011 and 2015 are provided in Table 2.

Table 1 Serological results of 3885 dog serum samples from Sweden tested for the presence of circulating antigens of *Angiostrongylus vasorum* and of specific antibodies to *A. vasorum*

	Positive samples (n)	%	95% confidence intervals
Antibody-positive	38	0.98	0.69–1.34
Antibody-positive only	34	0.88	0.61–1.22
Antigen positive	24	0.62	0.40–0.92
Antigen positive only	20	0.51	0.31–0.79
Antibody and antigen positive	4	0.10	0.03–0.26

Discussion

The first Swedish fox being positive for *A. vasorum* was identified in 2003 on the island of Sydkoster, in the county of Västra Götaland (see Fig. 1). Six years later, in the beginning of 2009, the parasite was found in the lungs of four out of 269 foxes examined within an *E. multilocularis* surveillance program; again, the positive animals originated from Sydkoster. After this finding, a targeted survey aimed at finding other foci of *A. vasorum* was performed in 2009 on 137 foxes from south-western Sweden. Eight foxes were found to be infected, of which seven were from Sydkoster (64% of the foxes collected on this island within the survey) and one from the municipality of Osby (county of Skåne), which was the first *A. vasorum* case described on mainland Sweden [42]. Even though many red foxes have been necropsied thereafter, the parasite has been identified only three additional times, in 2011, 2013 and 2014 (Table 2). The fox that tested positive in 2011 is particularly interesting because it originated from the municipality of Kalvsvik (county of Kronoberg), in the same area where one of the four dogs being both positive for antibodies and antigen was found. No double positive samples were identified in the county where the majority of positive foxes were previously found (Västra Götaland).

The implications of positive results and the performance of the two assays used in the present study have been evaluated independently by determining sensitivities and specificities [11, 13]. In the present study, the number of sera positive for antibody or antigen detection only could indicate an apparently low correlation between the two ELISAs used. However, when combined, these test parameters change: using the OR rule (the combined results are considered positive if either individual test is positive), sensitivity increases by loss of specificity, while using the AND rule (the combined results are considered positive only if both individual tests are positive), specificity reaches 99.9%, while sensitivity decreases to 82.0% [24]. Importantly, these values are influenced by the prevalence of *A. vasorum* within a determined population: the positive predictive values of the serological tests, represented by the proportion of positive test results that indicate a truly positive sample, is highest with the AND rule and this may of particular value in study areas where little is known on the occurrence of the parasite: reliability of a positive sample is high. However, at low prevalence, such high positive predictive values are reached at the expense of low sensitivity [24].

Therefore, a combined positive result indicate a dog that harbours an active *A. vasorum* infection inducing the production of antibodies; it has higher specificity than that of a single positive test (for antigen or antibody detection), although sensitivity is lower. However, as such a test combination is reflected by high positive predictive values, its use is of particular interest in areas of expected low endemicity, as it may occur in countries with relatively new introduction of the parasite like in Sweden.

This is supported by large scale studies from Germany [24] and Poland [27]: applying similar methodologies, seroprevalences of *A. vasorum* were higher than the ones detected in Swedish dogs. Intermediate prevalence figures have been recorded in Italy [25] and in the UK [24], whereas the highest prevalence so far was recorded in Hungary [7]. The seroprevalence of antibody-positive dogs in Sweden was the lowest recorded so far. Dogs positive for antibodies only may have acquired the infection recently, i.e. 3 weeks before (while antigen is detected earliest 5 wpi), but they also could be parasite-free, i.e. after anthelmintic treatment or spontaneous clearance of infection. The data confirmed that the level of exposure to the parasite in Sweden is still quite low. This is in accordance with the extremely low number of infected foxes detected so far, which are considered as a reservoir contributing to the establishment of the parasite [26, 33], as supported by constantly higher prevalences in foxes is than in dogs in corresponding areas [43]. In this context it needs to be added that the difficulty to identify positive foxes with low worm burdens combined with low disease awareness in an early phase of investigations may have contributed missing positive foxes, and that dissection may not be considered as a gold standard [44].

Another indirect demonstration of the low endemic presence of the parasite in Sweden is given by the results of faecal examinations performed at the SVA,

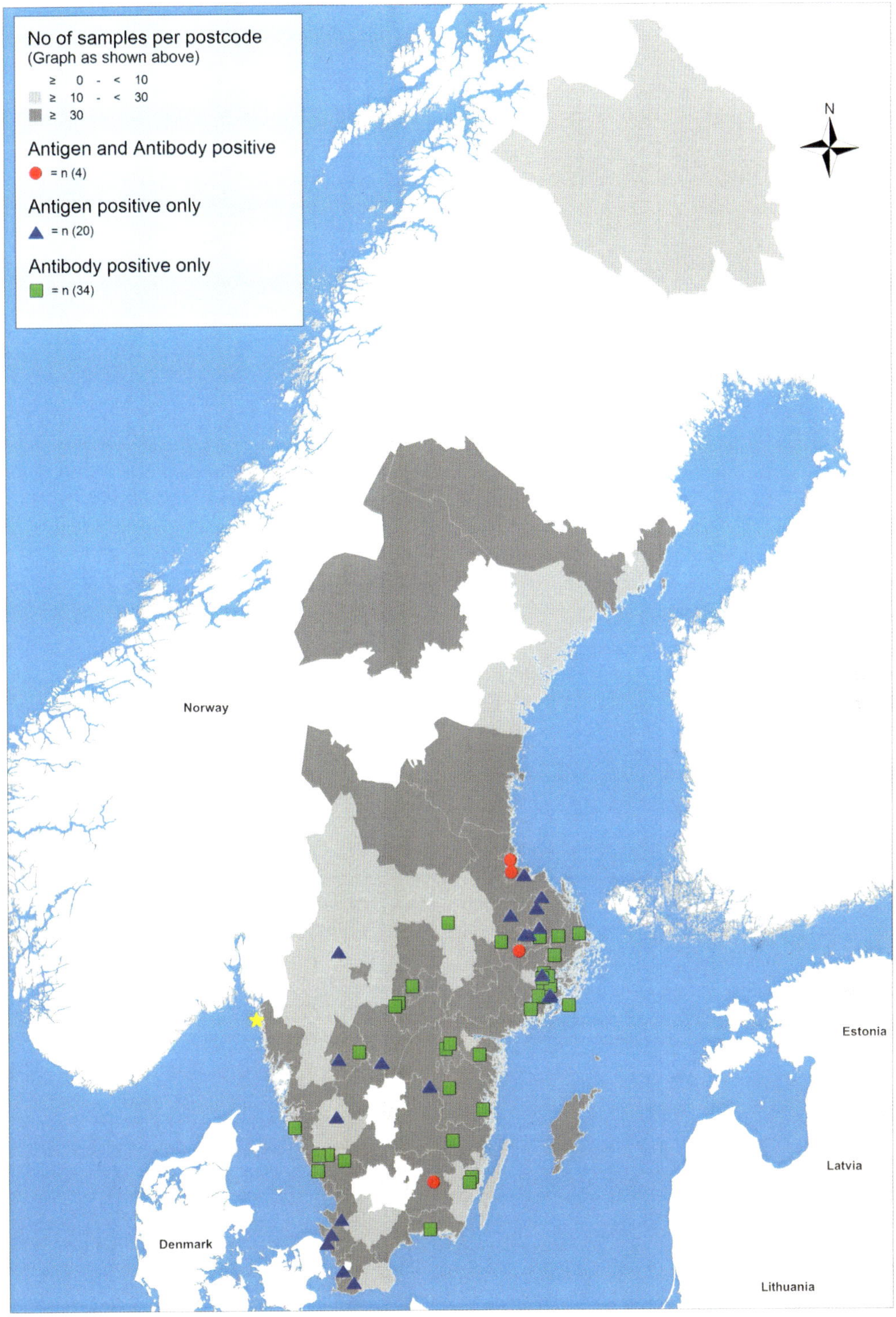

Fig. 1 Detection of *Angiostrongylus vasorum* circulating antigens and specific antibodies in serum samples from 3885 dogs from Sweden. Dark grey areas represent the origin of the tested dog sera. The first place of finding of *A. vasorum* in Sweden (island of Sydkoster) is marked with a yellow star

Table 2 Results from the diagnostic activity concerning *A. vasorum* related methodologies carried out at the SVA between 2011 and 2015

	Year					Total
	2011	2012	2013	2014	2015	
Groups	Numbers					
Dogs, Baermann tested samples	298	355	504	693	1032	2882
A. vasorum positive canine faecal samples (%)	1 (0.3; 0.0–1.9)	1 (0.3; 0.0–1.6)	4 (0.8; 0.2–2)	5 (0.7; 0.2–1.7)	9 (0.9; 0.4–106)	20 (0.7; 0.4–1.1)
County of origin*	M	O	M, S, K, Y	AB, C, D, H, M	AB, BD, E, O, M, Y, Z	–
Red foxes necropsied	525	88	164	70	100	947
A. vasorum positive foxes (%)	1 (0.2; 0–1.1)	0 (0.0; 0.3.3)	1 (0.6; 0.0–3.4)	1 (1.4; 0.0–7.7)	0 (0; 0.0–3.0)	3 (0.3; 0.1–0.9)
County of origin*	G	–	O	O	–	

Codes for Swedish counties: AB: Stockholm, BD: Norrbotten; C: Uppsala, D: Södermanland, E: Östergötland, G: Kronoberg; H: Kalmar, K: Blekinge, M: Skåne; O: Västra Götaland; S: Värmland; Y: Västernorrland; Z: Jämtland

presupposing that samples obtained from clinically ill dogs do not represent the general canine population. After the first description of an autochthonous case in a dog in 2003, the first dog was not diagnosed until 2011 by a Baermann analysis. Because of the relatively common (8–9%) occurrence of *Crenosoma vulpis*, the fox lungworm, Baermann examinations are being regularly performed at the SVA. After the first report of *A. vasorum* in Sweden the number of examinations have steadily increased, however, despite this increase, the number of *A. vasorum* positive findings has remained low (Table 2).

Detection of the parasite both in foxes and dogs in Denmark and Sweden, but only one recent finding in a red fox in Norway and still no occurrence of the parasite in Finland suggest that *A. vasorum* may have been introduced from Denmark and/or Germany. Southern Sweden is often visited by tourists from these countries, especially during the summer, and they are often accompanied by their dogs. Another interesting aspect is the partial overlapping of geographical distribution of samples positive by serology with samples positive at coprological examination (data not shown). In fact, all the positive samples (faecal or serum samples) originated from geographic areas that in a prediction model have been shown to be suitable for the establishment of the parasite [16], although it cannot be excluded that some of the positive dog cases found in the present study are not endemic but may have been imported from other endemic foci instead. The presence of an abundant fox population especially in agricultural regions, coinciding with the well-established circulation of lungworms (*C. vulpis*) that use molluscan intermediate like *A. vasorum*, is a situation with high risk for spreading of the parasite in Scandinavia. This is for instance supported by data from neighbouring Denmark, where the occurrence of the parasite in foxes has increased rapidly during the last 20 years.

Conclusions

The results confirmed that *A. vasorum* is endemically present in Sweden: not limited to restricted areas such as the Island of Sydkoster and the municipality of Osby in Scania, but also in foci in widespread areas of the country. Since suitable conditions for the establishment of *A. vasorum* apparently exist in southern Sweden and potentially also in other areas of Sweden, disease awareness among practitioners, dog owners and hunters, and an according strategical deworming management is recommended, despite the currently low prevalence. This may be particularly important in the case of dogs living or visiting highly endemic areas, in order to avoid further introduction of the parasite into new areas (with the potential to create new foci), and to prevent clinical disease due to angiostrongylosis. Regular deworming should be considered in dogs which belong to "high risk categories", such as young dogs and/or dogs having free roaming activity that show risk behaviour like indiscriminate ingestion of items from their environment.

Authors' contributions

GG, EOL and MS planned the study, GG collected the samples, MS analysed the samples and interpreted the results. RS provided graphical materials, GG and MS wrote the manuscript. EÅ provided data and wrote sections regarding wildlife surveillance programs and occurrence of *A. vasorum* in foxes. EOL, EÅ and RS commented on the manuscript. All authors read and approved the final manuscript.

Author details

[1] Department of Microbiology, National Veterinary Institute, Ulls väg 2B, SE-756 51 Uppsala, Sweden. [2] Department of Biomedical Sciences and Veterinary Public Health (BVF), Swedish University of Agricultural Sciences, PO Box 7028, Ulls väg 26, SE-757 56 Uppsala, Sweden. [3] Bayer Animal Health GmbH, 51368 Leverkusen, Germany. [4] Department of Pathology and Wildlife Diseases, National Veterinary Institute, Ulls väg 2B, SE-756 51 Uppsala, Sweden. [5] Institute of Parasitology Vetsuisse Faculty, University of Zurich, Winterthurerstrasse 266a, 8057 Zurich, Switzerland.

Acknowledgements

Henrik Uhlhorn, SVA, is thanked for the assistance in gathering data from red foxes and for comments on the manuscript. Inger Lilliehöök, Clinical Chemistry Laboratory of the University Animal Hospital is thanked for the permission and help given to collect part of serum samples; Susanne André and Therese Råsbäck are thanked for the assistance in collecting serum samples from the SVA. Charlotta Thornberg, SVA, is thanked for helping in recording sample data. Nina Gillis-Germitsch and Stefan Müller from the Institute of Parasitology in Zurich are acknowledged for their great support for laboratory analyses. Eva Wattrang (SVA) is acknowledged for language revision of the manuscript.

Competing interests

The authors declare that they have no competing interests. Roland Schaper is employee at Bayer Animal Health, Leverkusen, Germany.

Funding

This study was funded in part by "Jan Skogsborg" Foundation aimed at the improvement of research and education regarding canine diseases and in part by Bayer AB, Solna, Sweden. Both funding bodies contributed to cover the costs of the serological analyses. Bayer AB contributed also to the creation of the Figures of the present article.

References

1. Guilhon J. Research on the life cycle of the canine vascular strongyle [in French]. Bull Acad Vét. 1963;36:431–42.
2. Guilhon J, Bressou C. Role of limacidae in the life cycle of *Angiostrongylus vasorum* (Baillet, 1866) [in French]. C R Acad Sc. 1960;251:2252–3.
3. Bolt G, Monrad J, Frandsen F, Henriksen P, Dietz HH. The common frog (*Rana temporaria*) as a potential paratenic and intermediate host for *Angiostrongylus vasorum*. Parasitol Res. 1993;79:428–30.
4. Mozzer LR, Lima WS. *Gallus gallus domesticus*: paratenic host of *Angiostrongylus vasorum*. Vet Parasitol. 2015;207:81–4. https://doi.org/10.1016/j.vetpar.2014.11.003.
5. Serres E. Entozoa found in the right ear, the corresponding ventricle and the pulmonary artery of a dog [in French]. J Vétérinaires du Midi. 1854;7:70.
6. Chapman PS, Boag AK, Guitian J, Boswood A. *Angiostrongylus vasorum* infection in 23 dogs (1999–2002). J Small Anim Pract. 2004;45:435–40.
7. Schnyder M, Schaper R, Lukacs Z, Hornok S, Farkas R. Combined serological detection of circulating *Angiostrongylus vasorum* antigen and parasite-specific antibodies in dogs from Hungary. Parasitol Res. 2015;114(Suppl 1):S145–54. https://doi.org/10.1007/s00436-015-4520-1.
8. Helm J, Gilleard JS, Jackson M, Redman E, Bell R. A case of canine *Angiostrongylus vasorum* in Scotland confirmed by PCR and sequence analysis. J Small Anim Pract. 2009;50:255–9. https://doi.org/10.1111/j.1748-5827.2009.00741.x.
9. Jefferies R, Morgan ER, Shaw SE. A SYBR green real-time PCR assay for the detection of the nematode *Angiostrongylus vasorum* in definitive and intermediate hosts. Vet Parasitol. 2009;166:112–8. https://doi.org/10.1016/j.vetpar.2009.07.042.
10. Al-Sabi MN, Deplazes P, Webster P, Willesen JL, Davidson RK, Kapel CM. PCR detection of *Angiostrongylus vasorum* in faecal samples of dogs and foxes. Parasitol Res. 2010;107:135–40. https://doi.org/10.1007/s00436-010-1847-5.
11. Schnyder M, Tanner I, Webster P, Barutzki D, Deplazes P. An ELISA for sensitive and specific detection of circulating antigen of *Angiostrongylus vasorum* in serum samples of naturally and experimentally infected dogs. Vet Parasitol. 2011;179:152–8. https://doi.org/10.1016/j.vetpar.2011.01.054.
12. Verzberger-Epshtein I, Markham RJ, Sheppard JA, Stryhn H, Whitney H, Conboy GA. Serologic detection of *Angiostrongylus vasorum* infection in dogs. Vet Parasitol. 2008;151:53–60.
13. Schucan A, Schnyder M, Tanner I, Barutzki D, Traversa D, Deplazes P. Detection of specific antibodies in dogs infected with *Angiostrongylus vasorum*. Vet Parasitol. 2012;185:216–24. https://doi.org/10.1016/j.vetpar.2011.09.040.
14. Deplazes P, Hegglin D, Gloor S, Romig T. Wilderness in the city: the urbanization of *Echinococcus multilocularis*. Trends Parasitol. 2004;20:77–84.
15. Bourne DE. Pet travel: should vets do more? Companion Anim. 2015;20:212–21.
16. Morgan ER, Jefferies R, Krajewski M, Ward P, Shaw SE. Canine pulmonary angiostrongylosis: the influence of climate on parasite distribution. Parasitol Int. 2009;58:406–10. https://doi.org/10.1016/j.parint.2009.08.003.
17. Taylor CS, Garcia Gato R, Learmount J, Aziz NA, Montgomery C, Rose H, et al. Increased prevalence and geographic spread of the cardiopulmonary nematode *Angiostrongylus vasorum* in fox populations in Great Britain. Parasitology. 2015;142:1190–5. https://doi.org/10.1017/s0031182015000463.
18. Santoro M, D'Alessio N, Di Prisco F, Neola B, Restucci B, Pagano TB, et al. *Angiostrongylus vasorum* infection in red foxes (*Vulpes vulpes*) in southern Italy. Acta Parasitol. 2015;60:356–9. https://doi.org/10.1515/ap-2015-0050.
19. Aziz NA, Daly E, Allen S, Rowson B, Greig C, Forman D, et al. Distribution of *Angiostrongylus vasorum* and its gastropod intermediate hosts along the rural-urban gradient in two cities in the United Kingdom, using real time PCR. Parasit Vectors. 2016;9:56. https://doi.org/10.1186/s13071-016-1338-3.
20. Traversa D, Di Cesare A, Meloni S, Frangipane di Regalbono A, Milillo P, Pampurini F, et al. Canine angiostrongylosis in Italy: occurrence of *Angiostrongylus vasorum* in dogs with compatible clinical pictures. Parasitol Res. 2013;112:2473–80. https://doi.org/10.1007/s00436-013-3412-5.
21. Jolly S, Poncelet L, Lempereur L, Caron Y, Bayrou C, Cassart D, et al. First report of a fatal autochthonous canine *Angiostrongylus vasorum* infection in Belgium. Parasitol Int. 2015;64:97–9. https://doi.org/10.1016/j.parint.2014.10.008.
22. Miterpakova M, Hurnikova Z, Zalewski AP. The first clinically manifested case of angiostrongylosis in a dog in Slovakia. Acta Parasitol. 2014;59:661–5. https://doi.org/10.2478/s11686-014-0289-0.
23. Simin S, Spasojevic Kosic L, Kuruca L, Pavlovic I, Savovic M, Lalosevic V. Moving the boundaries to the South-East: first record of autochthonous *Angiostrongylus vasorum* infection in a dog in Vojvodina province, northern Serbia. Parasit Vectors. 2014;7:396. https://doi.org/10.1186/1756-3305-7-396.
24. Schnyder M, Schaper R, Bilbrough G, Morgan ER, Deplazes P. Seroepidemiological survey for canine angiostrongylosis in dogs from Germany and the UK using combined detection of *Angiostrongylus vasorum* antigen and specific antibodies. Parasitology. 2013;140:1442–50. https://doi.org/10.1017/s0031182013001091.
25. Guardone L, Schnyder M, Macchioni F, Deplazes P, Magi M. Serological detection of circulating *Angiostrongylus vasorum* antigen and specific antibodies in dogs from central and northern Italy. Vet Parasitol. 2013;192:192–8. https://doi.org/10.1016/j.vetpar.2012.10.016.
26. Lurati L, Deplazes P, Hegglin D, Schnyder M. Seroepidemiological survey and spatial analysis of the occurrence of *Angiostrongylus vasorum* in Swiss dogs in relation to biogeographic aspects. Vet Parasitol. 2015;212:219–26. https://doi.org/10.1016/j.vetpar.2015.08.017.
27. Schnyder M, Schaper R, Pantchev N, Kowalska D, Szwedko A, Deplazes P. Serological detection of circulating *Angiostrongylus vasorum* antigen- and parasite-specific antibodies in dogs from Poland. Parasitol Res. 2013;112(Suppl 1):109–17. https://doi.org/10.1007/s00436-013-3285-7.
28. Miterpáková M, Schnyder M, Schaper R, Hurníková Z, Čabanová V. Serological survey for canine angiostrongylosis in Slovakia. Helminthologia. 2015;52:205–10. https://doi.org/10.1515/helmin-2015-0034.
29. Pantchev N, Schnyder M, Vrhovec MG, Schaper R, Tsachev I. Current Surveys of the Seroprevalence of *Borrelia burgdorferi*, *Ehrlichia canis*, *Anaplasma phagocytophilum*, *Leishmania infantum*, *Babesia canis*, *Angiostrongylus vasorum* and *Dirofilaria immitis* in Dogs in Bulgaria. Parasitol Res. 2015;114(Suppl 1):S117–30. https://doi.org/10.1007/s00436-015-4518-8.
30. Lempereur L, Martinelle L, Marechal F, Bayrou C, Dalemans AC, Schnyder M, et al. Prevalence of *Angiostrongylus vasorum* in southern Belgium, a coprological and serological survey. Parasit Vectors. 2016;9:533. https://doi.org/10.1186/s13071-016-1820-y.
31. Alho AM, Schnyder M, Schaper R, Meireles J, Belo S, Deplazes P, et al. Seroprevalence of circulating *Angiostrongylus vasorum* antigen and parasite-specific antibodies in dogs from Portugal. Parasitol Res. 2016;115:2567–72. https://doi.org/10.1007/s00436-016-5001-x.
32. Finnerup E. *Angiostrongylus vasorum* in dogs [in Danish]. Dansk VetTidsskr. 1983;66(8):338–40.

33. Bolt G, Monrad J, Henriksen P, Dietz HH, Koch J, Bindseil E, et al. The fox (*Vulpes vulpes*) as a reservoir for canine angiostrongylosis in Denmark. Field survey and experimental infections. Acta Vet Scand. 1992;33:357–62.
34. Willingham AL, Ockens NW, Kapel CM, Monrad J. A helminthological survey of wild red foxes (*Vulpes vulpes*) from the metropolitan area of Copenhagen. J Helminthol. 1996;70:259–63.
35. Saeed I, Maddox-Hyttel C, Monrad J, Kapel CM. Helminths of red foxes (*Vulpes vulpes*) in Denmark. Vet Parasitol. 2006;139:168–79. https://doi.org/10.1016/j.vetpar.2006.02.015.
36. Tønsberg H, Saeed I, Koch J. Parasitological study of hunting dogs and foxes in Odsherred—an epidemiological study of the prevalence [in Danish]. Dansk VetTidsskr. 2004;87:14–8.
37. Al-Sabi MN, Kapel CM, Johansson A, Espersen MC, Koch J, Willesen JL. A coprological investigation of gastrointestinal and cardiopulmonary parasites in hunting dogs in Denmark. Vet Parasitol. 2013;196:366–72. https://doi.org/10.1016/j.vetpar.2013.03.027.
38. French heartworm [in Norwegian]. 2017. http://www.vetinst.no/sykdom-og-agens/fransk-hjerteorm. Accessed 21 Sept 2017.
39. Åblad B, Christensson D, Osterman Lind E, Ågren E, Mörner T. *Angiostrongylus vasorum* established in Sweden [in Swedish]. Svensk VetTidn. 2003;55:11–5.
40. de StGroth SF, Scheidegger D. Production of monoclonal antibodies: strategy and tactics. J Immunol Methods. 1980;35:1–21.
41. Deplazes P, Eckert J, Mathis A, von Samson-Himmelstjerna G, Zahner H. Parasitology in veterinary medicine. Wageningen Academic Publishers: Wageningen; 2016.
42. Malmsten J, Ågren E. Disease situation in wildlife animals in Sweden in 2009—Annual report from the Wildlife Monitoring Program at the National Veterinary Institute. SVA:s rapportserie 19. 2009. p. 19.
43. Koch J, Willesen JL. Canine pulmonary angiostrongylosis: an update [in Swedish]. Vet J. 2009;179:348–59. https://doi.org/10.1016/j.tvjl.2007.11.014.
44. Gillis-Germitsch N, Kapel CMO, Thamsborg SM, Deplazes P, Schnyder M. Host-specific serological response to *Angiostrongylus vasorum* infection in red foxes (*Vulpes vulpes*): implications for parasite epidemiology. Parasitology. 2017;144:1144–53. https://doi.org/10.1017/S0031182017000427.

Permissions

All chapters in this book were first published in AVS, by BioMed Central; hereby published with permission under the Creative Commons Attribution License or equivalent. Every chapter published in this book has been scrutinized by our experts. Their significance has been extensively debated. The topics covered herein carry significant findings which will fuel the growth of the discipline. They may even be implemented as practical applications or may be referred to as a beginning point for another development.

The contributors of this book come from diverse backgrounds, making this book a truly international effort. This book will bring forth new frontiers with its revolutionizing research information and detailed analysis of the nascent developments around the world.

We would like to thank all the contributing authors for lending their expertise to make the book truly unique. They have played a crucial role in the development of this book. Without their invaluable contributions this book wouldn't have been possible. They have made vital efforts to compile up to date information on the varied aspects of this subject to make this book a valuable addition to the collection of many professionals and students.

This book was conceptualized with the vision of imparting up-to-date information and advanced data in this field. To ensure the same, a matchless editorial board was set up. Every individual on the board went through rigorous rounds of assessment to prove their worth. After which they invested a large part of their time researching and compiling the most relevant data for our readers.

The editorial board has been involved in producing this book since its inception. They have spent rigorous hours researching and exploring the diverse topics which have resulted in the successful publishing of this book. They have passed on their knowledge of decades through this book. To expedite this challenging task, the publisher supported the team at every step. A small team of assistant editors was also appointed to further simplify the editing procedure and attain best results for the readers.

Apart from the editorial board, the designing team has also invested a significant amount of their time in understanding the subject and creating the most relevant covers. They scrutinized every image to scout for the most suitable representation of the subject and create an appropriate cover for the book.

The publishing team has been an ardent support to the editorial, designing and production team. Their endless efforts to recruit the best for this project, has resulted in the accomplishment of this book. They are a veteran in the field of academics and their pool of knowledge is as vast as their experience in printing. Their expertise and guidance has proved useful at every step. Their uncompromising quality standards have made this book an exceptional effort. Their encouragement from time to time has been an inspiration for everyone.

The publisher and the editorial board hope that this book will prove to be a valuable piece of knowledge for researchers, students, practitioners and scholars across the globe.

List of Contributors

Sina Reinartz and Ottmar Distl
University of Veterinary Medicine Hannover, Foundation, Institute for Animal Breeding and Genetics, Bünteweg 17p, 30559 Hannover, Germany

Maren Hellige and Karsten Feige
University of Veterinary Medicine Hannover, Foundation, Clinic for Horses, Bünteweg 9, 30559 Hannover, Germany

Peter Wenning
University of Veterinary Medicine Hannover, Foundation, Clinic for Cattle, Bischofsholer Damm 15, 30173 Hannover, Germany

Anna Malmsten and Anne-Marie Dalin
Division of Reproduction, Department of Clinical Sciences, Swedish University of Agricultural Sciences, Uppsala, Sweden

Gunnar Jansson
Grimsö Wildlife Research Station, Department of Ecology, Swedish University of Agricultural Sciences, 730 91 Riddarhyttan, Sweden

Nils Lundeheim
Department of Animal Breeding and Genetics, Swedish University of Agricultural Sciences, Uppsala, Sweden

Jenny Larsson, Nils Fall and Magdalena Jacobson
Department of Clinical Sciences, Swedish University of Agricultural Sciences, Uppsala, Sweden

Maria Lindberg
Farm and Animal Health, Kungsängens Gård hus 6 B, SE-753 23 Uppsala, Sweden

Pia Gustås and Anne-Sofie Lagerstedt
Department of Clinical Sciences, Faculty of Veterinary Medicine and Animal Husbandry, Swedish University of Agricultural Sciences, Uppsala, Sweden

Sofia Honkavaara
Department of Clinical Sciences, Faculty of Veterinary Medicine and Animal Husbandry, Swedish University of Agricultural Sciences, Uppsala, Sweden
Evidensia Specialistdjursjukhuset Helsingborg, Bergavägen 3, 250 23 Helsingborg, Sweden

Kjerstin Pettersson
University Animal Hospital, Swedish University of Agricultural Sciences, Uppsala, Sweden

Anna Byström
Department of Anatomy, Physiology and Biochemistry, Faculty of Veterinary Medicine and Animal Husbandry, Swedish University of Agricultural Sciences, Uppsala, Sweden

Agata Rybicka and Magdalena Król
Department of Physiological Sciences, Faculty of Veterinary Medicine, Warsaw University of Life Sciences, Warsaw, Poland

Severiano R. Silva, Rita Payan-Carreira, Cristina M. Guedes and Simão Coelho
Zootecnia Department, Centro de Ciência Animal E Veterinária, Universidade de Trás-os-Montes e Alto Douro, 5000-801 Vila Real, Portugal

Ana Sofia Santos
EUVG-Escola Universitária Vasco da Gama, Campus Universitário, Bloco B, Lordemão, 3020-210 Coimbra, Portugal
CITAB, Universidade de Trás-os-Montes e Alto Douro, Quinta de Prados, 5000-801 Vila Real, Portugal

Désirée Müllhaupt, Patrick Kircher, Nadja Pfammatter and Stefanie Ohlerth
Clinic for Diagnostic Imaging, Vetsuisse Faculty, University of Zurich, Winterthurerstrasse 258c, 8057 Zurich, Switzerland

Sandra Wenger and Jean-Michel Hatt
Clinic for Zoo Animals, Exotic Pets and Wildlife, Vetsuisse Faculty, University of Zurich, Winterthurerstrasse 260, 8057 Zurich, Switzerland

Torun Wallgren, Rebecka Westin and Stefan Gunnarsson
Department of Animal Environment and Health, Swedish University of Agricultural Sciences, Skara, Sweden

Muhammad Majeed, Gokhlesh Kumar, Mansour El-Matbouli and Mona Saleh
Clinical Division of Fish Medicine, University of Veterinary Medicine, Veterinärplatz 1, 1210 Vienna, Austria

Sarah Schlosser
VetCore Facility for Research, University of Veterinary Medicine, Vienna, Austria

Odd Viking Höglund
Department of Clinical Sciences, Uppsala, Sweden

Johanna Lövebrant
Alingsås Veterinärstuga AB, Björkekärrsvägen 26, 441 91 Alingsås, Sweden

Ulf Olsson
Unit of Applied Statistics and Mathematics, Swedish University of Agricultural Sciences, Uppsala, Sweden

Katja Höglund
Department of Anatomy, Physiology and Biochemistry, Swedish University of Agricultural Sciences, Uppsala, Sweden

Jonas Johansson Wensman
Department of Clinical Sciences, Swedish University of Agricultural Sciences, Uppsala, Sweden

Ayman Samman and Margaret J.Hosie
MRC-University of Glasgow Centre for Virus Research, Glasgow, UK

Anna Lindhe and Louise Treiberg Berndtsson
Department of Virology, Immune Biology and Parasitology, National Veterinary Institute, Uppsala, Sweden

Jean-Christophe Thibault
Global Technical Services,Merial, Lyon, France

Azzurra Santoro
Department of Veterinary Medicine, University of Perugia, Via San Costanzo 4, 06126 Perugia, Italy

Maarja Tagel, Kärt Must and Miia Laine
Institute of Veterinary Medicine and Animal Sciences, Estonian University of Life Sciences, Kreutzwaldi 62, 51014 Tartu, Estonia

Brian Lassen
Institute of Veterinary Medicine and Animal Sciences, Estonian University of Life Sciences, Kreutzwaldi 62, 51014 Tartu, Estonia
Department of Veterinary Disease Biology, Faculty of Health and Medical Sciences, University of Copenhagen, Grønnegårdsvej 15, 1870 Frederiksberg C, Denmark

Pikka Jokelainen
Institute of Veterinary Medicine and Animal Sciences, Estonian University of Life Sciences, Kreutzwaldi 62, 51014 Tartu, Estonia
Faculty of Veterinary Medicine, University of Helsinki, Helsinki, Finland
Statens Serum Institut, Artillerivej 5, 2300 Copenhagen S, Denmark

Silvia Bellini
Istituto Zooprofilattico Sperimentale della Lombardia ed Emilia Romagna (IZSLER), Brescia, Italy

Domenico Rutili
Private Consultant, Perugia, Italy

Vittorio Guberti
Istituto Superiore per la Protezione e la Ricerca Ambientale (ISPRA), Ozzano Emilia, Bologna, Italy

Christine Brøkner
Department of Veterinary Clinical and Animal Sciences, Faculty of Health and Medical Sciences, University of Copenhagen, Grønnegaardsvej 3, 1870 Frederiksberg, Denmark

Anne-Helene Tauson
Department of Veterinary Clinical and Animal Sciences, Faculty of Health and Medical Sciences, University of Copenhagen, Grønnegaardsvej 3, 1870 Frederiksberg, Denmark
Department of Animal and Aquacultural Sciences, Norwegian University of Life Sciences, Ås, Norway

Dag Austbø and Jon A. Næsset
Department of Animal and Aquacultural Sciences, Norwegian University of Life Sciences, Ås, Norway

Dominique Blache
School of Animal Biology, Faculty of Natural and Agricultural Sciences, University of Western Australia, 35 Stirling Highway, Crawley, Perth, WA 6009, Australia

Knud Erik B. Knudsen
Department of Animal Science, Aarhus University, Blichers Allé 20, 8830 Tjele, Denmark

Hanne H. Hansen
Department of Large Animal Sciences, Faculty of Health and Medical Sciences, University of Copenhagen, Grønnegaardsvej 2, 1870 Frederiksberg, Denmark

Heidi Hiitiö, Johanna Vakkamäki, Heli Simojoki and Satu Pyörälä
Department of Production Animal Medicine, Faculty of Veterinary Medicine, University of Helsinki, Paroninkuja 20, 04920 Saarentaus, Finland

Tiina Autio and Sinikka Pelkonen
Veterinary Bacteriology Research Unit, Finnish Food Safety Authority Evira, Neulaniementie 4, 70210 Kuopio, Finland

Jouni Junnila
Oy 4Pharma Ltd., Mannerheimintie 44 A,00260 Helsinki, Finland

Beata Dolka, Artur Żbikowski, Izabella Dolka and Piotr Szeleszczuk
Department of Pathology and Veterinary Diagnostics, Faculty of Veterinary Medicine, Warsaw University of Life Sciences-SGGW, Nowoursynowska 159c St., 02-776 Warsaw, Poland

Lisbeth Rem Jessen, Tina Møller Sørensen, Zenia Littau Lilja and Maja Kristensen
Department of Veterinary Clinical Sciences, University of Copenhagen, Dyrlægevej 16, 1870 Frederiksberg C, Denmark

Tine Hald
National Food Institute, Technical University of Denmark, Kemitorvet, Building 204, 2800 Kgs. Lyngby, Denmark

Peter Damborg
Department of Veterinary and Animal Sciences, University of Copenhagen, Stigbøjlen 4, 1870 Frederiksberg C, Denmark

Christina Nathues
Veterinary Public Health Institute, Department of Clinical Research & Veterinary Public Health, Vetsuisse Faculty, University of Bern, Schwarzenburgstrasse 155, 3097 Liebefeld, Switzerland
Federal Food Safety and Veterinary Office, Schwarzenburgstrasse 155, 3003 Bern, Switzerland

Eltje Janssen, Andrea Duengelhoef and Elisabeth grosse Beilage
Field Station for Epidemiology, University of Veterinary Medicine Hannover, Buescheler Strasse 9, 49456 Bakum, Germany

Heiko Nathues
Clinic for Swine, Department of Clinical Veterinary Medicine, Vetsuisse Faculty, University of Bern, Bremgartenstrasse 109a, 3012 Bern, Switzerland

Maria Torsein
Farm & Animal Health, Uddetorp Röda huset, 532 96 Skara, Sweden
Department of Animal Environment and Health, Swedish University of Agricultural Sciences, Skara, Sweden

Charlotte Berg
Department of Animal Environment and Health, Swedish University of Agricultural Sciences, Skara, Sweden

Ann Lindberg
Department of Disease Control and Epidemiology, National Veterinary Institute, 751 89 Uppsala, Sweden

Catarina Svensson
Department of Clinical Sciences, Swedish University of Agricultural Sciences, Uppsala, Sweden

Karin Persson Waller
Department of Clinical Sciences, Swedish University of Agricultural Sciences, Uppsala, Sweden
Department of Animal Health and Antimicrobial Strategies, National Veterinary Institute, 751 89 Uppsala, Sweden

Sören Krogh Jensen
Department of Animal Science,Aarhus University, Research Centre Foulum, Tjele, Denmark

Hirotaka Tokushige, Asuka Kushiro, Atsushi Okano, Tatsuya Maeda and Hideki Ito
Racehorse Clinic, Miho Training Center, Japan Racing Association (JRA), 2500-2 Mikoma, Miho-mura, Inashiki-gun, Ibaraki 300-0493, Japan

Ai Wakuno
Racehorse Clinic, Ritto Training Center, JRA, 1028 Misono, Ritto-shi, Shiga 520-3085, Japan

Shun-ichi Nagata
Analytical Chemistry Section, Laboratory of Racing Chemistry, 1731-2 Tokami-cyo, Utsunomiya-shi, Tochigi 320-0851, Japan

Minoru Ohta
Equine Research Institute, JRA, 1400-4 Shiba, Shimotsuke-shi, Tochigi 329-0412, Japan

Anna Fredrika Boström, Heli Katariina Hyytiäinen, and Anna Katrina Hielm-Björkman
Department of Equine and Small Animal Medicine, Faculty of Veterinary Medicine, University of Helsinki, Helsinki, Finland

Petteri Koho
Rehabilitation Orton, Tenholantie 10, 00280 Helsinki, Finland

Sigitas Cizinauskas
Small Animal Hospital Aisti, Virtatie 9, 01600 Vantaa, Finland

Christian Sonne, Jean-Pierre Desforges, Igor Eulaers, Emilie Andersen-Ranberg, Kim Gustavson and Rune Dietz
Department of Bioscience, Arctic Research Centre (ARC), Aarhus University, Faculty of Science and Technology, Frederiksborgvej 399, Roskilde, Denmark

Bjørn Munro Jenssen
Department of Bioscience, Arctic Research Centre (ARC), Aarhus University, Faculty of Science and Technology, Frederiksborgvej 399, Roskilde, Denmark
Department of Biology, Norwegian University of Science and Technology, 7491 Trondheim, Norway
Department of Arctic Technology, The University Centre in Svalbard, Longyearbyen, Norway

Robert James Letcher
Ecotoxicology and Wildlife Health Division, Environment and Climate Change Canada, National Wildlife Research Centre, Carleton University, Ottawa, ON K1A 0H3, Canada

Bjarne Styrishave
Toxicology Laboratory, Department of Pharmacy, Faculty of Health and Medical Sciences, University of Copenhagen, Universitetsparken 2, 2100 Copenhagen, Denmark

Marie Lisandra Zepeda Mendoza
Centre for GeoGenetics, Natural History Museum of Denmark, University of Copenhagen, Øster Voldgade 5-7, 1350 Copenhagen K, Denmark

Karla Manzano Vargas
Centre for GeoGenetics, Natural History Museum of Denmark, University of Copenhagen, Øster Voldgade 5-7, 1350 Copenhagen K, Denmark
Undergraduate Program on Genomic Sciences, Center for Genomic Sciences, National Autonomous University of Mexico, Av. Universidad s/n Col. Chamilpa, 62210 Cuernavaca, Morelos, Mexico

Thomas Sicheritz-Pontén
Centre for GeoGenetics, Natural History Museum of Denmark, University of Copenhagen, Øster Voldgade 5-7, 1350 Copenhagen K, Denmark
Center for Biological Sequence Analysis, Department of Bio and Health Informatics, Technical University of Denmark, Anker Engelunds Vej 1 Bygning 101A, 2800 Kgs. Lyngby, Denmark
Centre of Excellence for Omics-Driven Computational Biodiscovery (COMBio), Faculty of Applied Sciences, AIMST University, 08100 Bedong, Malaysia

M. Thomas P. Gilbert
Centre for GeoGenetics, Natural History Museum of Denmark, University of Copenhagen, Øster Voldgade 5-7, 1350 Copenhagen K, Denmark
Norwegian University of Science and Technology, University Museum, 7491 Trondheim, Norway

Michael Roggenbuck
Department for Bioinformatics and Microbe Technology, Novozymes A/S, 2880 Bagsværd, Denmark

Lars Hestbjerg Hansen
Section for Microbiology and Biotechnology, Department of Environmental Science, Aarhus University, Frederiksborgvej 399, 4000 Roskilde, Denmark

Søren Brunak
Center for Biological Sequence Analysis, Department of Bio and Health Informatics, Technical University of Denmark, Anker Engelunds Vej 1 Bygning 101A, 2800 Kgs. Lyngby, Denmark
Novo Nordisk Foundation Center for Protein Research, Faculty of Health and Medical Sciences, University of Copenhagen, Blegdamsvej 3, 2200 Copenhagen N, Denmark

Mengcheng Liu, Bing Wang, Hongmin Liang, Bo Ma, Junwei Wang and Wenlong Zhang
College of Veterinary Medicine, Northeast Agricultural University, Changjiang Road 600, Harbin 150030, Heilongjiang, People's Republic of China
Key Laboratory of Animal Pathogen Biology of Ministry of Agriculture and Rural Affairs of the People's Republic of China, Northeastern Science Inspection Station, Harbin 150030, Heilongjiang, People's Republic of China

Ulrich Methner
Institute of Bacterial Infections and Zoonoses at the Friedrich-Loeffler-Institute, Federal Research Institute for Animal Health, Naumburger Str. 96a, 07743 Jena, Germany

Sabine Merbach and Martin Peters
Chemisches und Veterinäruntersuchungsamt Westfalen, Zur Taubeneiche 10-12, 59821 Arnsberg, Germany

Lorenzo Fraile
Departament de Ciència Animal, ETSEA, University of Lleida, Av. Alcalde Rovira Roure 191, E25198 Lleida, Spain
Agrotecnio Center, Av. Alcalde Rovira Roure, 80, E25198 Lleida, Spain

Ramon Armengol
Departament de Ciència Animal, ETSEA, University of Lleida, Av. Alcalde Rovira Roure 191, E25198 Lleida, Spain
Department of Animal Science, University of Lleida, ETSEA, Av. Alcalde Rovira Roure, 191, E25198 Lleida, Spain

Eva Osterman Lind
Department of Microbiology, National Veterinary Institute, Ulls väg 2B, SE-756 51 Uppsala, Sweden

Giulio Grandi
Department of Microbiology, National Veterinary Institute, Ulls väg 2B, SE-756 51 Uppsala, Sweden
Department of Biomedical Sciences and Veterinary Public Health (BVF), Swedish University of Agricultural Sciences, Ulls väg 26, SE-757 56 Uppsala, Sweden

Roland Schaper
Bayer Animal Health GmbH,51368 Leverkusen, Germany

Erik Ågren
Department of Pathology and Wildlife Diseases, National Veterinary Institute, Ulls väg 2B, SE-756 51 Uppsala, Sweden

Manuela Schnyder
Institute of Parasitology Vetsuisse Faculty, University of Zurich, Winterthurerstrasse 266a, 8057 Zurich, Switzerland

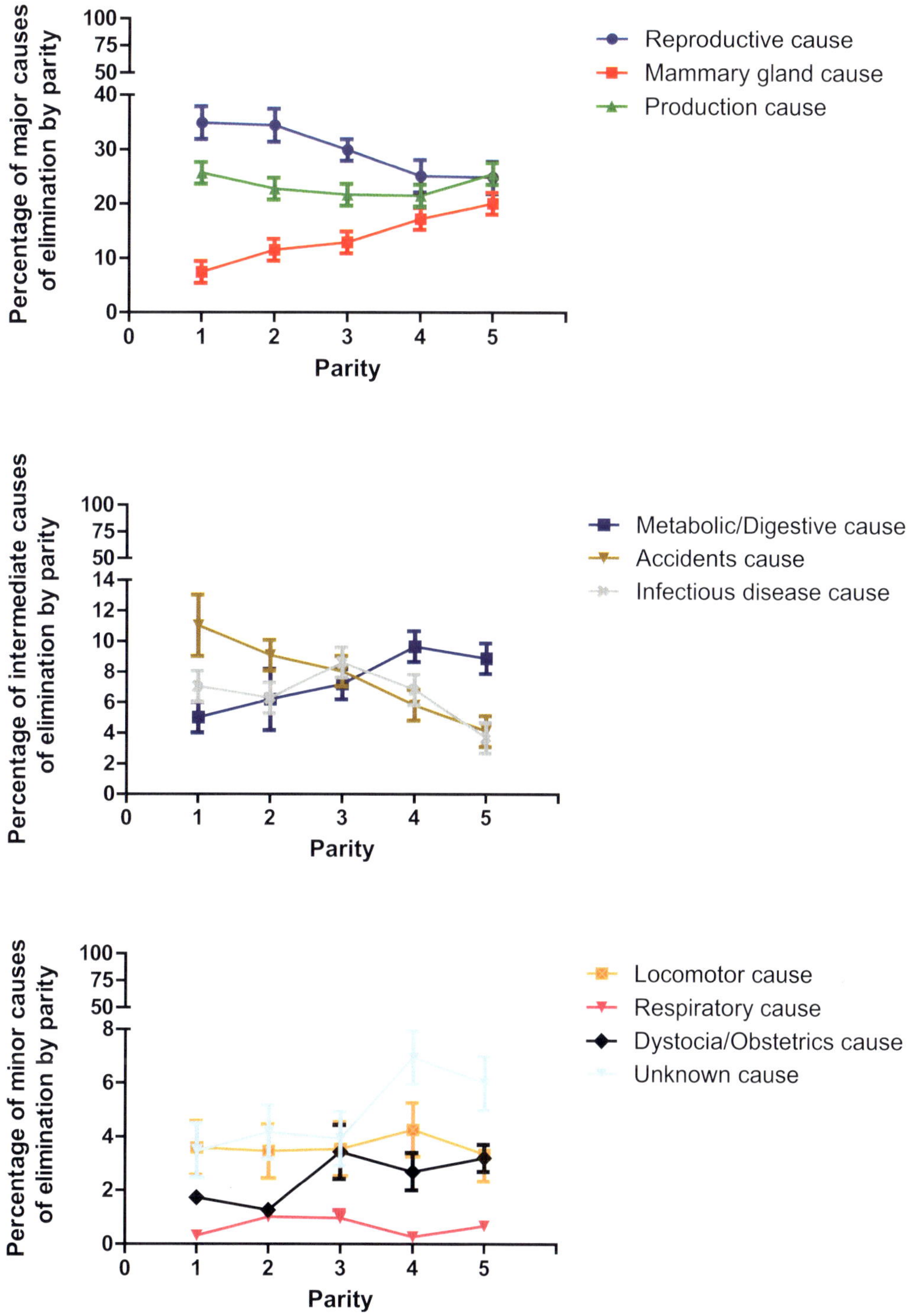

Fig. 2 Percentage (with 95% confidence interval) of major, intermediate and minor causes of elimination by cow parity. In the figure, parity equal to or higher than five is represented by five. The causes of elimination have been grouped into "major causes" (causes of elimination with a percentage higher than 15%), "intermediate cause" (causes of elimination with values between 8 and 15%) and "minor causes" (elimination causes with values lower than 8%)

and infectious causes were significantly more frequent ($P < 0.05$) in slaughtered than in dead cows whereas metabolic/digestive, dystocia/obstetrics, accident, respiratory and unknown causes, were significantly less frequent ($P < 0.05$) in slaughtered than in dead cows.

The cause for elimination differed significantly ($P < 0.05$) depending on the parity of the cow (Fig. 2a–c) but the pattern varied depending on the cause. Reproductive and production causes were the most frequent causes of elimination in cows of all parities. Reproductive cause progressively and significantly ($P < 0.05$) decreased in importance, especially after more than three lactations. Productive cause also decreased significantly ($P < 0.05$) in importance between the first and fourth parities, but increased in cows with five or more parities at the same level of first lactation cows. Accidents were the third main cause of elimination for cows of first and second lactation, but progressively and significantly ($P < 0.05$) decreased in importance. The percentage of eliminated cows due to mammary gland disease, metabolic diseases and unknown causes increased significantly ($P < 0.05$) as the cows got older. Dystocia showed a significant increase ($P < 0.05$) in importance between the second and third lactations. Infectious diseases were more important in third lactation cows compared to younger cows and showed a decreasing trend in cows eliminated with four or more lactations. Finally, the percentage of elimination due to locomotor and respiratory causes did not show any statistically significant changes ($P > 0.05$) during the cows' lifespan.

For all farms, the percentage of cows that died on the farm was significantly ($P < 0.05$) affected by period. Proportion of dead cows was significantly higher during period 2 (22.4%) and 3 (22.4%) when compared to period 1 (17.9%) and 4 (16.4%). The causes of elimination were also significantly affected by the time of year but the pattern was different taking into account the different causes (Fig. 3a–c). Reproductive and metabolic/digestive causes showed the highest values during periods 1 and 4 that were significantly higher ($P < 0.05$) than for period 2 and 3, whereas accidents and infectious diseases showed the highest values during periods 2 and 3 that were significantly higher ($P < 0.05$) than for periods 1 and 4. On the other hand, elimination due to unknown and locomotor causes peaked at periods 3 and 4, respectively without showing significant differences ($P > 0.05$) with the other periods. The remaining causes of elimination did not show significant variation throughout the year.

Discussion

This study used data from five dairy herds in Spain from 2006 to 2016 that are typical of the intensive milk production sector in southern Europe, but also in other countries and areas of the world. Defining culling criteria and a cause of mortality can be biased depending on how data are collected, who is responsible for the data collection and on the data analysis system [1]. All data analysed in the study were collected using the same software system and the same team of veterinarians. Use of the same criteria and analysis system is necessary to advice farmers and benchmark different farms. This point is critical because the reason for culling can be biased depending on how data are collected, who is responsible for this data collection and the data analysis system [17]. Despite similarities in management, nutrition, collection and data analysis, veterinarian diagnosis and treatment of diseases, key points of herd performance such as age at death, mortality and culling reasons, tDIM and LMY differed significantly between herds. In this study, these differences could be more related to intrinsic factors of each farm such as care of animals by workers, differences between farmer's criteria when deciding to treat a sick cow or euthanize it, hygiene and design of facilities than number of milking cows or milk yield. Climate conditions may also have an effect on mortality and cause of death. We suggest that analysing between-herd differences and benchmarking farms is useful to improve the day-by-day management and animal care on the farms.

The DL and LMY of eliminated cows in our study was similar to the value reported in a study from the Netherlands [19]. On the other hand, tDIM was lower than values described by others [20, 21]. Finally NL (3.0 ± 0.1) was lower than the value described by Africor (3.3 ± 0.1) [22] but higher than a Swedish study with multiple dairy breeds (2.3 ± 1.4) [9]. Thus, there is great variability in the productive parameters of eliminated cows published in the literature and comparison to other studies is difficult given the different methods of collection of production data. Some of these studies analyse data based on information provided by official control agencies that estimate production. This makes it imperative to obtain data for a particular geographical area and for particular production characteristics in order to define benchmarking strategies.

In this study, annual average herd turnover rate on the farms ranged between 25 and 35%. The terms used in the literature to define the causes for the elimination of cows, due to either culling or mortality, and whether this elimination is voluntary and planned or involuntary and unplanned, can be confusing. In any case, the percentage of turnover rates ranges from 21.3% in Ireland [23] and up to 40% in Australia [24], 25.4% in the Netherlands [19], 26% in northwest Spain [7], 22.6 and 30% in the UK [25, 26], between 28.2 and 33.5% in Canada [27] and 36% in the USA [28]). In contrast, between-herd differences for herd turnover rates are 10% in this research study,

Index

A

Acepromazine, 73-74, 76-79

African Swine Fever, 91-92, 94-95, 98-99, 213, 216-218

Alfaxalone-medetomidine, 159-160, 162-164

Angiostrongylus Vasorum, 231, 234-235, 237-238

Antibiotic Treatments, 116, 135

Antibodies, 34-35, 67, 70-72, 80-88, 90, 99, 121, 123-125, 142, 148, 151, 158, 181, 205-207, 210-212, 231-235, 237-238

Antigen, 34-35, 37, 71, 86, 88, 121-124, 127, 183, 231, 233-234, 237

Aphanomyces Invadans, 65-66, 68-70, 72

Avian Influenza, 119-120, 125-127

B

Benchmarking, 220-221, 225, 228-229

Blood Pressure, 73-79, 159-162, 164

C

Cancer Stem Cell, 38

Canine Mammary Tumor, 32-33, 37-38

Cleft Lip And Jaw, 1, 3-6

Colonization Resistance, 185, 198-201

Colostrum, 14, 17, 21-22, 145-158

Computed Tomography, 3-5, 45-46, 53

Constant Rate Infusion, 159, 164-165

Cresty Neck Score, 39, 43-44

D

Dietary Fibre, 100-102

E

Epizootic Ulcerative Syndrome, 65, 72

Equine Anesthesia, 159-160

Escherichia Coli, 14, 22, 118, 195, 203, 205, 212

F

Feline Calicivirus, 80, 82-83

Fimbrial Subunit Proteins, 204-205

G

Glycaemic, 100-104

H

H5n1, 119-120, 122, 125-127

I

Image Analysis, 39-41, 44

Inactivated Vaccine, 119-120, 125-127, 212

Insulinemic, 100-104

Inter-rater Reliability, 166-169, 171-172

L

Lactations, 220, 222-223, 225, 229

Lc-ms/ms, 65, 68

Locomotion, 24, 28, 30-31, 70, 167, 171-173

M

Macrorestriction Analysis, 213-215, 217, 219

Microbiome, 185-203

Mycoplasma Hyopneumoniae, 142, 144

N

Neoplasms, 32-33, 37-38

O

Oestrus, 7-11, 221

Oomycetes, 65-66, 69-70

Ornithodoros Genus, 91-92

Ornithodoros Spp., 96

Orofacial Malformation, 1

Orthopaedics, 24

Ovulation Rate, 7-8, 11

P

Persistent Organic Pollutants, 174, 181-183

Physiotherapy, 166-168, 170, 172-173

Polymerase Chain Reaction, 127, 137-138, 232

Porcine Reproductive And Respiratory Syndrome Virus (prrsv), 137

Post-mortem Nape Fat Measurements, 39

Pregnancy Rate, 7, 9-11

Pyoderma, 128-132, 134-135

R

Rational Antimicrobial Use, 128, 134

Rugae Palatinae, 1-2, 5

S

Salmonella Choleraesuis, 213, 215, 217, 219

Salmonella Enterica, 197, 213, 219

Scavenging, 93, 185-186, 195, 197-198, 200
Sevoflurane, 159-165
Somatic Cell Count, 105, 113-114, 117-118, 221
Subclinical Mastitis, 105-112, 114
Surgical Stress, 73-78
Sus Scrofa Domesticus, 84

T
T. Pyogenes, 204-212
Tail Biting, 54-59, 61-64
Tail Docking, 54-55, 63-64
Thorax, 45-47, 51, 53
Thymus, 45-46, 48-49, 52
Toxoplasma Gondii, 84, 86-88, 90
Toxoplasmosis, 84-85, 90
Transition Milk, 145, 150-154, 157
Treadmill Walking, 24-25, 27-31

U
Urinary Tract Infections, 128, 132-133

V
Vaccine Strain, 80-83, 120, 124
Virulence Factors, 22, 65-66, 69, 72, 202, 204, 210-212
Virus Neutralization, 80-83